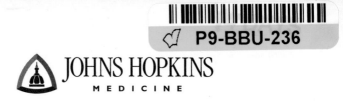
JOHNS HOPKINS
M E D I C I N E

JOHNS HOPKINS

HIV Guide

Management of HIV Infection and Its Complications

2012 EDITION

Edited by

Joel E. Gallant, MD, MPH

Paul A. Pham, PharmD

The Johns Hopkins University School of Medicine

JONES & BARTLETT
L E A R N I N G

World Headquarters
Jones & Bartlett Learning
5 Wall Street
Burlington, MA 01803
978-443-5000
info@jblearning.com
www.jblearning.com

Jones & Bartlett Learning books and products are available through most bookstores and online book-sellers. To contact Jones & Bartlett Learning directly, call 800-832-0034, fax 978-443-8000, or visit our website, www.jblearning.com.

Substantial discounts on bulk quantities of Jones & Bartlett Learning publications are available to corporations, professional associations, and other qualified organizations. For details and specific discount information, contact the special sales department at Jones & Bartlett Learning via the above contact information or send an email to specialsales@jblearning.com.

The *Johns Hopkins HIV Guide* is an independent publication and has not been authorized, sponsored, or otherwise approved by the owners of the trademarks or service marks referenced in this product.

The authors, editor, and publisher have made every effort to provide accurate information. However, they are not responsible for errors, omissions, or for any outcomes related to the use of the contents of this book and take no responsibility for the use of the products and procedures described. Treatments and side effects described in this book may not be applicable to all people; likewise, some people may require a dose or experience a side effect that is not described herein. Drugs and medical devices are discussed that may have limited availability con-trolled by the Food and Drug Administration (FDA) for use only in a research study or clinical trial. Research, clinical practice, and government regulations often change the accepted standard in this field. When consider-ation is being given to use of any drug in the clinical setting, the healthcare provider or reader is responsible for determining FDA status of the drug, reading the package insert, and reviewing prescribing information for the most up-to-date recommendations on dose, precautions, and contraindications, and determining the appropriate usage for the product. This is especially important in the case of drugs that are new or seldom used.

Our goal is to provide health professionals focused, core prescribing information in a convenient, organized, and concise fashion. The information provided in the *Johns Hopkins HIV Guide* is designed to support, not replace, the relationship that exists between a patient/site visitor and his/her physician. The guide is intended as a quick and convenient reminder of information you have already learned elsewhere; it is not meant to be a replacement for training, experience, continuing medical education, or studying the latest drug prescribing literature.

Production Credits
Executive Publisher: Christopher Davis
Senior Acquisitions Editor: Nancy Anastasi Duffy
Special Projects Editor: Kathy Richardson
Senior Production Editor: Daniel Stone
Marketing Manager: Rebecca Rockel
Manufacturing and Inventory Control
    Supervisor: Amy Bacus
Print Buyer: Jessica O'Donnell

Composition: diacriTech
Cover Design: Scott Moden
Cover Image: Top image © Tischenko
Irina/ShutterStock, Inc.; Bottom image
© Sybille Yates/ShutterStock, Inc.
Printing and Binding: Edward Brothers Malloy
Cover Printing: Edward Brothers Malloy

ISBN: 978-0-7637-8548-2

6048

Printed in the United States of America
16 15 14 13 12   10 9 8 7 6 5 4 3 2 1

Contributors

Editors

Joel E. Gallant, MD, MPH, FACP, FIDSA
Professor of Medicine &
Epidemiology
Division of Infectious Diseases
Johns Hopkins University
School of Medicine

Paul A. Pham, PharmD
Research Associate
Division of Infectious
Diseases
Johns Hopkins University
School of Medicine

Authors

Paul G. Auwaerter, MD, FACP, FIDSA
Associate Professor of
Medicine
Divisions of Infectious
Diseases and
General Internal Medicine
Johns Hopkins University
School of Medicine

Andrew F. Angelino, MD
Associate Professor of
Psychiatry
Department of Psychiatry
and Behavioral Sciences
Johns Hopkins University
School of Medicine

John G. Bartlett, MD
Professor of Medicine
Division of Infectious Diseases
Johns Hopkins University
School of Medicine

Gail V. Berkenblit, MD, PhD
Assistant Professor of
Medicine
Division of General Internal
Medicine
Johns Hopkins University
School of Medicine

Joel N. Blankson, MD, PhD
Associate Professor of
Medicine
Director, Inpatient HIV Unit
Division of Infectious
Diseases
Johns Hopkins University
School of Medicine

Todd T. Brown, MD, PhD
Assistant Professor of
Medicine
Division of Endocrinology
and Metabolism
Johns Hopkins University
School of Medicine

Joseph Cofrancesco Jr., MD, MPH, FACP
Associate Professor of
Medicine
Divisions of General Internal
Medicine and Infectious
Diseases
Director, Institute for
Excellence in Education
Johns Hopkins University
School of Medicine

Andrea L. Cox, MD, PhD
Associate Professor of
Medicine
Division of Infectious
Diseases
Johns Hopkins University
School of Medicine

James P. Dunn, MD
Associate Professor of
Ophthalmology
Division of Ocular
Immunology
The Wilmer Eye Institute
Johns Hopkins University
School of Medicine

Christopher P. Eckstein, MD
Division of Neurology
University of South Alabama
Health System

Maureen M. Forrestel, PharmD
Pharmacist
Columbia, MD

Khalil G. Ghanem, MD, PhD
Associate Professor of
Medicine
Johns Hopkins University
School of Medicine
Director, STD/HIV/TB
Clinical Services
Baltimore City Health
Department

Amita Gupta, MD, MHS
Associate Professor
of Medicine and
International Health
Deputy Director, Center for
Clinical Global Health
Education
Johns Hopkins University
School of Medicine

Daniel Harrison, MD
Assistant Professor of
Neurology
Department of Neurology
Johns Hopkins University
School of Medicine

Christopher J. Hoffmann, MD, MPH
Assistant Professor of
Medicine
Division of Infectious
Diseases
Johns Hopkins University
School of Medicine

Jeffrey Hsu, MD
Assistant Professor of
Psychiatry
Department of Psychiatry
and Behavioral Sciences
Johns Hopkins University
School of Medicine

Noreen A. Hynes, MD, MPH
Associate Professor
Director, Geographic
Medicine Center
Division of Infectious
Diseases
Johns Hopkins University
School of Medicine

David J. Kouba, MD, PhD, FAACS
Associate Clinical Professor
of Dermatology
The Toledo Clinic
Wayne State University

Noah Lechtzin, MD, MHS
Assistant Professor of
Medicine
Division of Pulmonary and
Critical Care Medicine
Johns Hopkins University
School of Medicine

Mark Levis, MD, PhD
Associate Professor
Division of Hematologic
Malignancies
Johns Hopkins University
School of Medicine

Michael Levy, MD, PhD
Assistant Professor of
Neurology
Department of Neurology
Johns Hopkins University
School of Medicine

Spyridon S. Marinopoulos, MD
Assistant Professor of Medicine
Division of General Internal
Medicine
Johns Hopkins University
School of Medicine

Robin McKenzie, MD
Associate Professor of
Medicine
Division of Infectious
Diseases
Johns Hopkins University
School of Medicine

Michael Melia, MD
Assistant Professor of
Medicine
Division of Infectious
Diseases
Johns Hopkins University
School of Medicine

Richard D. Moore, MD, MHS
Professor of Medicine
Division of General Internal
Medicine
Johns Hopkins University
School of Medicine

Dionissis Neofytos, MD, MPH
Assistant Professor of
Medicine
Transplant and Oncology
Infectious Disease Program
Division of Infectious Diseases
Johns Hopkins University
School of Medicine

Scott Newsome, DO
Assistant Professor of
Neurology
Division of Neuroimmunology
and Neuroinfectious
Diseases
Johns Hopkins University
School of Medicine

Eric Nuermberger, MD
Associate Professor
of Medicine and
International Health
Division of Infectious Diseases
Johns Hopkins University
School of Medicine

Kathleen R. Page, MD
Assistant Professor of
Medicine
Division of Infectious Diseases
Johns Hopkins University
School of Medicine

John N. Ratchford, MD
Assistant Professor of
Neurology
Department of Neurology
Johns Hopkins University
School of Medicine

Jeffrey Rumbaugh, MD, PhD
Assistant Professor of
Neurology
Department of Neurology
Emory University

Raj Sindwani, MD, FACS
Section Head
Rhinology, Sinus and Skull
Base Surgery
Cleveland Clinic

Patrick R. Sosnay, MD
Assistant Professor of
Medicine
Division of Pulmonary and
Critical Care Medicine
Affiliate Faculty - Institute
of Genetic Medicine
Johns Hopkins University
School of Medicine

Lisa A. Spacek, MD, PhD
Adjunct Assistant
Professor of Medicine
Division of Infectious
Diseases
Johns Hopkins University
School of Medicine

Timothy R. Sterling, MD
Professor of Medicine
Division of Infectious
Diseases
Vanderbilt University School
of Medicine

Chloe Lynne Thio, MD
Associate Professor of
Medicine
Division of Infectious
Diseases
Johns Hopkins University
School of Medicine

Glenn J. Treisman, MD, PhD
Professor of Psychiatry and
Behavioral Sciences
Professor of Medicine
Department of Psychiatry
and Behavioral Sciences
Johns Hopkins University
School of Medicine

Nina Wagner-Johnston, MD
Assistant Professor of Medicine
Division of Medical Oncology
Washington University School of Medicine

Barbara E. Wilgus, MSN, CRNP
Nurse Practitioner
Division of Infectious Diseases
Johns Hopkins University School of Medicine

Joseph M. Vinetz, MD
Professor of Medicine
Division of Infectious Diseases
School of Medicine
University of California, San Diego

The POC-IT Center

Paul G. Auwaerter, MD, FACP, FIDSA
Executive Director
Chief Medical Officer

Steven A. Libowitz
Senior Director

Nicole Sokol
Guides Manager

Danielle Meinsler
Guides Administrator

Contents

Diagnosis

Drugs

Management

Pathogens

Foreword

The *Johns Hopkins POC-IT HIV Guide* was initially a project and product of the Division of Infectious Diseases at Johns Hopkins University School of Medicine. It was launched in 2000 as a website and was then adapted for use with handheld devices in April 2001. The idea was then, and remains, to present timely and accurate recommendations for the management of HIV in a format concise enough to fit the small screen of a handheld device. This approach forced extraordinary discipline in economy of language, restricting the authors to include only the most practical and important issues of clinical practice. The result is that clinicians can usually locate, access, and apply information at the point of care in under a minute. The adaptation of this material for this new print publication—the *Johns Hopkins HIV Guide: Management of HIV Infection and Its Complications* captures these important features.

Preface

Clinicians need accurate, concise, and easy-to-use information at point-of-care. The *Johns Hopkins HIV Guide: Management of HIV Infection and Its Complications* has been designed to meet the ever more urgent needs of time-strapped clinicians by distilling complex material into need-to-know information that is easily accessible, rapidly viewable, and up to date, helping health care professionals raise the standards of care and improve patient safety.

DRUG ADMINISTRATION AND GENERAL ABBREVIATIONS

μL	microliter
μmol	micromole
Abnl	abnormal
Ab	antibodies
Abx	antibiotic(s)
ac	before meal
admin	administered
ADR	adverse drug reaction
ART	antiretroviral therapy
AUC	area under the concentration time curve
c	copies
ca	cancer
caps	capsule
CCR5	chemokine receptor 5
cg	centigram
CFU	colony forming units
cm	centimeter
cm^2	centimeters squared
CNS	central nervous system
Cx	culture
CXR	chest X-ray
CVVH	continuous veno-venous hemofiltration
CVVHD	continuous veno-venous hemodialysis
d/c	discontinue, discharge
DDx	differential diagnosis
dL	deciliter
DS	double strength
Dx	diagnosis
g	gram
GNB	gram-negative bacilli
H$_2$O	water
HAART	highly active antiretroviral therapy
HD	hemodialysis
Hg	mercury
HPF	high powered field
hr, hrs	hour, hours
hs	at bedtime (hours of sleep)
HSV	herpes simplex virus
Hx	history
IM	intramuscular
IU	international unit
IV	intravenous
kg	kilogram
L	liter
m	meter
m^2	meters squared
mcg or μg	microgram
mEq	milliequivalent
mg	milligram
MIC	minimum inhibitory concentration
min	minutes
mL	milliliter
mm	millimeter
mm^3	cubic millimeters

mmol	millimole
mo, mos	month, months
mU	milliunits
N	normal (solution) or total sample size
ng	nanogram
nl	normal
nm	nanometer
OI	opportunistic infection
OTC	over-the-counter
oz	ounce
PCR	polymerase chain reaction
PE	physical exam
plt	platelet
PMN	polymorpho-nuclear leukocytes
PO	by mouth
PRN or prn	as needed
PSI	pounds per square inch
pt	patient
qmo	every month
qwk	every week
RBC	red blood cell
ROM	range of motion
r/o	rule out
Rx	treatment
rxn	reaction
s	second
sol'n	solution
s/p	status post
SQ	subcutaneously
SS	single strength
Sx	symptoms
TAMs	thymidine analog mutations
Txp	transplant
U	unit
US	ultrasound
vol	volume
w/	with
w/i	within
w/o	without
WBC	white blood cell
wk, wks	week, weeks
wnl	within normal limits
×	times/for
yr, yrs	year, years

COMMONLY USED DRUG NAME ABBREVIATIONS

3TC	lamivudine
ABC	abacavir
APAP	acetaminophen
ATV	atazanavir
ATV/r	atazanavir/ritonavir
AZT	zidovudine
d4T	stavudine
ddI	didanosine
DLV	delavirdine
DRV	darunavir
DRV/r	darunavir/ritonavir
EFV	efavirenz
ENF	enfuvirtide
ETR	etravirine
FPV	fosamprenavir
FPV/r	fosamprenavir/ritonavir
FTC	emtricitabine
G-CSF	filgastrim
IDV	indinavir
IDV/r	indinavir/ritonavir
LPV/r	lopinavir/ritonavir
MVC	maraviroc
NFV	nelfinavir
NVP	nevirapine
PCP	phencyclidine
RAL	raltegravir
RFB	rifabutin
RPV	rilpivirine
RTV	ritonavir
SQV	saquinavir
SQV/r	saquinavir/ritonavir
T-20	enfuvirtide
TDF	tenofovir DF
TPV	tipranavir
TPV/r	tipranavir/ritonavir

SECTION 1
DIAGNOSIS

Complications of Therapy

HEPATOTOXICITY

Joel E. Gallant, MD, MPH and Christopher J. Hoffmann, MD, MPH

PATHOGENESIS

- Distinct mechanisms of ART-related hepatotoxicity: Idiosyncratic reactions and dose dependent cytotoxicity: most common cause; most ART agents, NRTI, NNRTI, PI (may be dose dependent). Order of risk: ddI>d4T>AZT>ABC>3TC, FTC, TDF; NVP>>EFV; TPV, full dose RTV >> other PIs.
- Hypersensitivity reaction: early NVP and ABC (ABC hepatotoxicity can occur in absence of ABC hypersensitivity reaction and among HLAB*5701 -negative pts).
- Mitochondrial toxicity: NRTIs; esp. d4T, ddI, AZT.
- Immune reconstitution inflammatory syndrome (IRIS): all agents during CD4 increase.
- General risk factors: HBV and/or HCV co-infection (esp. genotype 3), older age, previous hepatotoxicity, alcoholism, cirrhosis, obesity, substance abuse, baseline abnormal transaminases, other hepatotoxic medications (eg: anti-tuberculosis therapy). Note: sustained virologic response on HCV therapy decreases HCV-associated risk.
- NVP hypersensitivity risk factors: female sex and higher CD4 (>250 for women, >400 for men) at time of ART initiation.
- ABC hypersensitivity risk factor: HLA B*5701 haplotype.
- Lactic acidosis risk factors: female, higher BMI.

CLINICAL

- Definition of hepatotoxicity: drug-related elevation in ALT/AST in absence of another etiology.
- Hepatotoxicity predominately hepatocellular (increase in ALT, AST with minimal initial change in bilirubin or alk phos). Consider other Dx if high bilirubin without high ALT or for high alk phos. Indirect hyperbilirubinemia may due to ATV or IDV therapy and not associated with hepatotoxicity.
- Presentation related to etiology.
- Idiosyncratic reactions: most common: onset <6 mos after ART initiation, often asymptomatic and lasting <3 wks. Dose-dependent reactions: generally result of cumulative drug exposure and occur >6 mos on drug. Both often asymptomatic with spontaneous resolution but can progress to severe livery injury.
- Hypersensitivity: onset 4–6 wks after ART initiation, presents with fever, rash, constitutional Sx. (Note: can be confused with acute viral infection such as influenza).
- Mitochondrial toxicity: onset usually >6 mos after initiation of d4T, ddI, or AZT; presents with lactic acidosis, nausea, anorexia, dyspnea, hepatomegaly, steatosis, and weight loss.
- IRIS: usually presents after <6 mos of ART and after robust CD4 rise. Associated with reconstituted immune response to antigens (e.g., HBV, MAC).

DIAGNOSIS

Differential Diagnosis

- **Viral hepatitis:** acute infection or flare with HAV, HBV, HCV, HDV. HBV can lead to flare spontaneously, with reactivation during waning immunity, and with loss of suppression of HBV DNA by 3TC or other anti-HBV agents due to discontinuation or resistance.
- **Acute viral infection:** CMV, EBV.
- **Bacterial infections:** TB, MAC, and *Bartonella henselae*.
- **Malignancy:** lymphoma.
- **Toxins:** acetaminophen, alcohol, antiretroviral agents, other medications (including naturopathic products).
- **Influenza:** rash, fever, constitutional Sx; no significant elevation in ALT.

Diagnosis

- Measure transaminases before starting ART. If normal, may be checked monthly for 1st 3 mos. If stable, can be increased to 3-mo intervals. Most hepatotoxicity diagnosed by routine ALT testing.
- Suspect hepatotoxicity if patients present with malaise, anorexia, nausea, fevers, rash (especially with NVP or ABC hypersensitivity hepatitis), or weight loss.

TREATMENT
Art
- Stop or modify ART if: (1) symptomatic hepatitis, (2) lactic acidosis, (3) jaundice, (4) evidence of ABC or NVP hypersensitivity, or (5) ALT >10×.
- Presence of constitutional Sx, elevated lactate, or evidence of hepatic dysfunction (coagulopathy or elevated ammonia) suggest severe toxicity and is medical emergency; discontinue ART and provide close monitoring, usually as inpatient.
- Provide supportive care. (1) Mitochondrial toxicity sometimes treated with riboflavin or thiamine therapy, but no data. Full resolution of hyperlactemia may take months. (2) Hypersensitivity sometimes treated with prednisone, but no data. Do not restart causative medication (NVP or ABC). Attempt to identify cause, usually continue ART and underlying OI; may treat with nonsteroidal anti-inflammatory drugs (NSAIDs) or prednisone to control Sx. Evaluate carefully to avoid missing other causes and stopping ART unnecessarily.
- Asymptomatic elevations <10× ULN can be managed with close clinical monitoring (repeat ALT/AST until elevation resolves).
- If ALT elevated >5× ULN or persistently elevated, evaluate for other causes (see previous Differential Diagnosis section); consider flare of HBV or reactivation even if negative serologies recently obtained.
- Asymptomatic elevations 5–10× ULN must be managed on case-by-case basis. Patients without liver disease may do well without discontinuation of therapy but with close monitoring until ALT elevation is resolved.
- Elevations >10× ULN require close monitoring and generally discontinuation of ART until ALT elevation has resolved.
- If drugs stopped or switch needed, switch to drugs with less hepatotoxicity: NRTIs: 3TC, FTC, TDF, ABC; NNRTIs: EFV; PI: no conclusive data, except that TPV/r more hepatotoxic than others. No drug absolutely contraindicated in patients with chronic hepatitis, though ABC contraindicated in patients with severe hepatic disease (because of hepatic metabolism), and dose reduction of some PIs recommended. Dual PIs more hepatotoxic than single PIs. Boosting with low-dose RTV (100–200 mg/day) doesn't increase hepatotoxicity, but greater hepatotoxicity with TPV/r 500/200 mg twice daily.

Anti-TB Therapy
- Clinical assessment monthly when receiving treatment for TB. Warn patients of Sx of hepatitis (dark urine, fever >3 days, malaise).
- Obtain transaminases with any Sx consistent with hepatitis and routinely at 1 and 3 mos.
- If ALT/AST >5× ULN: discontinue INH, RIF, PZA; consider use of EMB, SM, and FQ.
- When transaminases have normalized, reintroduce primary drugs one at a time.

SELECTED REFERENCES
Soriano V, Puoti M, Garcia-Gascó P, et al. Antiretroviral drugs and liver injury. *AIDS*, 2008; 22: 1–13.
Comments: Clear and concise review of hepatotoxicity causes and management.

Núñez M, Clinical syndromes and consequences of antiretroviral-related hepatotoxicity. *Hepatology*, 2010; 52: 1143–55.
Comments: Clear, updated review of ART-associated hepatotoxicity.

Ouyang DW, Shapiro DE, Lu M, et al. Increased risk of hepatotoxicity in HIV-infected pregnant women receiving antiretroviral therapy independent of nevirapine exposure. *AIDS*, 2009; 23: 2425–30.
Comments: Analysis of hepatotoxicity during pregnancy in United States cohort of women receiving ART.

Joshi D, O'Grady J, Dieterich D, Gazzard B, Agarwal K. Increasing burden of liver disease in patients with HIV infection. *Lancet*, 2011; 377: 1198–209.
Comments: Comprehensive review of issues of liver disease among people living with HIV. Includes overview of hepatotoxicity.

HYPERLIPIDEMIA

Lisa A. Spacek, MD, PhD, Gail V. Berkenblit, MD, PhD, and Joseph Cofrancesco, Jr., MD, MPH

DEFINITION
- Lipid profile estimate of LDL based on Friedewald equation: HDL = TC – LDL – 0.2 × TG; assumes TG ≤400 mg/dL.

- Hypercholesterolemia = TC >240 mg/dL.
- Severe hypertriglyceridemia >500 mg/dL.

CLINICAL

- Advanced HIV disease in patients not on ART associated with increased TG and decreased TC.
- Dyslipidemia, often hypercholesterolemia, seen with ART.
- Lipid abnormalities may be less responsive to Rx, and drug interactions preclude the use of some statins, (i.e., lovastatin, simvastatin, pitavastatin).
- NRTIs: increase LDL and TG, d4T>AZT>ABC; ABC and ddI associated with increased MI risk in some studies, esp in patients with multiple cardiac risk factors. Causal relationship and mechanism still unclear.
- PIs: RTV-boosted PIs increase LDL, HDL, TG; DRV/r and ATV/r have less effect on lipid profile than LPV/r. TG increased with LPV/r and FPV/r, less for DRV/r and ATV/r. TC increases an average of 30 mg/dL on PIs. Usually seen within 2–3 mos of starting PI.
- NNRTIs increase LDL, HDL, TG; EFV > NVP.
- INSTI: RAL has favorable lipid profile.
- CCR5 Antagonist: Post hoc analysis of MERIT study found MVC to improve lipid profile. Inactivation of CCR5 is protective against atherosclerosis in mouse model.

DIAGNOSIS

- Obtain lipid profile after 8–12 hr fast: check at baseline, before initiating or changing ART, 3–6 mos afterwards; and annually if at target cholesterol.
- Hx: evaluate for atherosclerotic disease (CHD, PVD), diabetes, and CHD risk factors: smoking; age (men >45, women >55); HTN; HDL <40 (subtract 1 risk factor if HDL >60); family history of premature CHD (male 1st degree relative <55, female 1st degree relative <65).
- PE: often unrevealing, though may detect vascular disease, xanthomas, xanthelasma, and, in severe hypertriglyceridemia, lipemia retinalis.
- Count number of risk factors and determine risk of coronary heart disease (CHD). If >2 risk factors, calculate 10-yr risk of CHD.
- Rx of hypercholesterolemia focuses on LDL reduction (based on NCEP guidelines; see Table 1-1).
- LDL goal: (1) high risk (CHD, non-coronary atherosclerotic disease, diabetes): LDL <100. (Optional goal <70 for very high risk) (2) >2 risk factors: LDL <130. (Optional goal <100 for moderately high risk.) (3) 0–1 risk factor: LDL <160.
- TG goal: normal <150, borderline 150–199, high 200–499, very high >500. Medical therapy indicated for fasting TG levels >500. TG >1000–2000: risk of pancreatitis.
- If cannot obtain fasting profile, use non-HDL cholesterol (TC – HDL = non-HDL). Targets for non-HDL = LDL target + 30.

TREATMENT

General Principles

- Counsel on risk factor modification: smoking, cocaine, diet, exercise.
- Refer to nutritionist for diet and weight management. Exercise program for elevated TG.
- If diet, exercise and lipid-lowering therapy insufficient, change to NNRTI or to PI with more favorable lipid profile if possible.
- 10-year risk calculator available at *http://www.nhlbi.nih.gov/guidelines/cholesterol*.

Pharmacologic Therapy

- HMG-CoA reductase inhibitors (statins) most potent agents for lowering LDL. Statin levels may be altered by PIs; start at low doses and cautiously increase. Atorvastatin and rosuvastatin shown to have greater effect on TC, LDL and non-HDL than pravastatin. Avoid lovastatin and simvastatin. See HMG-CoA reductase inhibitor p. 342 for detailed drug interactions with ART.
- Coadministration of pravastatin and DRV/r increases levels of statin, use lowest possible initial dose of pravastatin and monitor.
- Begin atorvastatin 10–20 mg (max 80 mg, but most do not exceed 40 mg with PIs) once-daily or rosuvastatin 5 mg PO at bedtime (max 40 mg).
- Fibric acids preferred for high TG. Start with gemfibrozil 600 mg PO twice daily or fenofibrate 48–200 mg PO once daily.
- Avoid bile acid sequestrants (interfere with ART absorption).
- Niacin an option, but may worsen insulin resistance. Can cause flushing; patients may take ASA 81 mg (if no contraindication) 1/2 hr before dose and gradually escalate dose.

TABLE 1-1. NATIONAL CHOLESTEROL EDUCATION PROGRAM GUIDELINES

Risk Category	Goal LDL (mg/dL)	Initiate Lifestyle Modification (LDL mg/dL)	Initiate Drug Therapy (LDL mg/dL)
High risk: Known CHD or CHD-equivalent (10-year risk >20%)	<100 (optional, 70)	Any LDL	>100 (<100 consider)
Moderately high risk: 2+ risk factors (10%–20% 10-yr risk*)	<130 (optional,100)	Any LDL	>130 (100–129 consider)
Moderate risk: 2+ risk factors (10-yr risk <10%*)	<130	>130	>160
Lower risk: 0–1 risk factor	<160	>160	>190 (160–189 consider)

*10 year risk calculator available at www.nhlbi.nih.gov/guidelines/cholesterol

DIAGNOSIS

FOLLOW-UP
Monitoring
- Repeat fasting lipid profile 6–12 wks after starting or changing lipid lowering therapy, then every 6 mos once stable.
- Check LFTs at baseline then 6–12 wks after initiation of therapy, then every 3–6 mos depending on patient's clinical situation.
- Both statins and fibric acid can cause myopathy; combination with fenofibrate may have less risk than gemfibrozil. Routine CK monitoring not recommended in asymptomatic patients, but patients should report myalgias. Discontinue Rx temporarily if myositis occurs, then consider restarting at lower dose.

SELECTED REFERENCES
Panel on Antiretroviral Guidelines for Adults and Adolescents. Guidelines for the use of antiretroviral agents in HIV-1-infected adults and adolescents. Department of Health and Human Services; January 10, 2011; 1–166. http://aidsinfo.nih.gov/contentfiles/AdultandAdolescentGL.pdf. Accessed March 30, 2011.
Comments: Table 15a lists drug interactions between PIs and statins. With the exception of SQV/r and pravastatin, all other PI/statin combinations result in increased statin AUC.

Aberg JA, Kaplan JE, Libman H, et al. Primary care guidelines for the management of persons infected with human immunodeficiency virus: 2009 update by the HIV medicine Association of the Infectious Diseases Society of America. *Clin Infect Dis*, 2009; 49: 651–81.
Comments: IDSA guidelines include comments on hyperlipidemia, reference HIVMA/IDSA/ACTG recommendations (2003), and endorse National Cholesterol Education Program Guidelines, which determine LDL goal based on risk for coronary artery disease.

Thompson MA, Aberg JA, Cahn P, et al. Antiretroviral treatment of adult HIV infection: 2010 recommendations of the International AIDS Society-USA panel. *JAMA*, 2010; 304: 321–33.
Comments: IAS-USA guidelines endorse Framingham risk algorithm with caveat that CVD risk in setting of HIV infection may be underestimated.

European AIDS Clinical Society. Prevention and management of non-infectious co-morbidities in HIV. November 1, 2009. http://www.europeanaidsclinicalsociety.org/Guidelines/G2.htm. Accessed July 17, 2011.
Comments: European guidelines endorse use of rosuvastatin.

Reinsch N, Neuhaus K, Esser S, et al. Are HIV patients undertreated? Cardiovascular risk factors in HIV: results of the HIV-HEART study. *Eur J Cardiovasc Prev Rehabil*, 2011; Feb 28. [Epub ahead of print]
Comments: Cross-sectional study of 803 patients determined prevalence of cardiovascular risk factors for CHD and 10-year risk for CHD. The most common were smoking (51.2%), high TG (39.0%), high LDL (27.5 %), and HTN (21.4%). In total, 60.3%, 21.6%, and 18.1% of patients categorized as being at low (<10%), moderate (10%–20%), and high (>20%) were at a 10-year risk for CHD, respectively.

Singh S, Willig JH, Mugavero MJ, et al. Comparative effectiveness and toxicity of statins among HIV-infected patients. *Clin Infect Dis*, 2011; 52: 387–95. Epub 2010 Dec 28.

Comments: Retrospective cohort study of 700 patients initiated on ART found greater likelihood of reaching NCEP goals for LDL with atorvastatin (OR, 2.1; P = .001) and rosuvastatin (OR 2.1; P = .03) than pravastatin with similar toxicity rates.

MacInnes A, Lazzarin A, Di Perri G, et al. MVC can improve lipid profiles in dyslipidemic patients with HIV: results from the MERIT trial. *HIV Clin Trials*, 2011; 12: 24–36.
Comments: Post hoc analysis of MERIT study data compared 360 patients on MVC vs 361 patients on EFV. MVC not associated with elevations in TC, LDL, or TG, and showed beneficial effects on lipid profiles of dyslipidemic patients.

Crane HM, Grunfeld C, Willig JH, et al. Impact of NRTIs on lipid levels among a large HIV-infected cohort initiating antiretroviral therapy in clinical care. *AIDS*, 2011; 25: 185–95.
Comments: Observational cohort study of 2267 ART-naïve HIV+ patients started on TDF/FTC or 3TC vs other NRTI backbones found highest LDL with ddI/3TC and highest TG with d4T/3TC. TDF/FTC or 3TC associated with lipid levels lower than other combinations.

Mills AM, Nelson M, Jayaweera D, et al. Once-daily darunavir/ritonavir vs. lopinavir/ritonavir in treatment-naive, HIV-1-infected patients: 96-week analysis. *AIDS*, 2009; 23: 1679–88.
Comments: ARTEMIS 96-wk data: 698 patients on DRV/r 800/100 once-daily OR LPV/r 800/200 twice-daily with TDF/FTC found DRV/r associated with smaller increases in TG and TC than LPV/r.

IMMUNE RECONSTITUTION INFLAMMATORY SYNDROME (IRIS)

Kathleen R. Page, MD

CLINICAL

- Paradoxical deterioration in clinical status after ART initiation despite improved immune function due to inflammatory response against infectious antigen, which may or may not have been Dx'd at initiation of ART.
- Typically occurs in patients with low initial CD4 (usually <50) and rapid decline in VL; onset usually within 6 wks of ART initiation, but sometimes several mos later.
- Inciting pathogens: *M. avium* complex, *M. tuberculosis* (30% of cases), and other mycobacteria, CMV, *Cryptococcus*, phencyclidine (PCP), *Leishmania*, HSV, VZV, HBV, HCV, JC virus, HHV-8 (Kaposi and Castleman), JC virus (PML), and others.
- Common Sx (varies according to causative pathogen): fever, localized lymphadenophathy/lymphadenitis, abscesses, pneumonia, vitritis, CNS disease, hepatitis, and dermatologic manifestations.
- Presentations of OIs may be atypical (e.g., MAC: localized granulomatous lymphadenopathy without mycobacteremia; CMV: vitritis; PML: enhancing CNS lesions; *Cryptococcus*: marked CSF leukocytosis).
- Autoimmune diseases (e.g., sarcoidosis, Grave's disease) may be exacerbated.
- Despite high risk (>25%) of paradoxical worsening in patients with active TB after initiation of ART, overall mortality improved in coinfected patients with CD4 <100 treated with ART.

DIAGNOSIS

- Compatible presentation after initiation of ART (usually within 6 wks, with rising CD4 and decrease in VL).
- DDx includes new OI, malignancy (e.g., lymphoma), treatment failure for OI, and drug toxicity (especially with hepatitis).

TREATMENT

General Principles

- Treat underlying active infection (refer to specific pathogen module).
- Continue ART, unless inflammatory response is life threatening.
- Anti-inflammatory therapy (NSAIDs and/or corticosteroids).
- Response to corticosteroids typically rapid. Slow taper may be required.
- Most studies support early initiation of ART during the treatment of an active OI.
- Prolonged delays in ART initiation should be avoided to prevent additional morbidity and mortality from untreated HIV.

PATHOGEN-SPECIFIC CONSIDERATIONS

- **MAC (lymphadenitis):** NSAIDs; if Sx persist, 20–40 mg/day prednisone with slow taper, titrating to recurrence of symptoms. Abscesses may be surgically drained.

DIAGNOSIS

- **Tuberculosis:** prednisone 20–40 mg/day for 2 wks with slow taper. In patients with active TB not on ART, ART should be initiated during continuation phase of TB therapy. However, immediate or very early initiation of ART (within 4 wks of initiation of TB therapy) indicated in patients with CD4 <50.
- **CMV vitritis:** systemic or periocular steroid; 50% respond.
- **Hepatitis:** consider using TDF + either 3TC or FTC in patients infected with HBV coinfection. Consider discontinuing ART if serious drug toxicity suspected. Risk of reversible drug-related hepatotoxicity highest with full-dose RTV (rarely used), but tends to occur >6 wks into therapy. NVP hepatotoxicity occurs early (within 6 wks); may be associated with rash and can be fatal, but rarely observed with pretreatment CD4 <250.
- **Cryptococcal meningitis:** usually Cx negative, but higher CSF opening pressure. Steroids, serial LPs to manage elevated CSF pressure. IDSA guidelines recommend initiating ART within 2–10 wks of Dx. Consider screening for asymptomatic antigenemia prior to ART initiation in patients with CD4 <100 living in high incidence areas, such as sub-Saharan Africa or Southeast Asia.

SELECTED REFERENCES

Ratnam I, Chiu C, Kandala NB, Easterbrook PJ. Incidence and risk factors for immune reconstitution inflammatory syndrome in an ethnically diverse HIV type 1-infected cohort. *Clin Infect Dis*, 2006; 42: 418–27.
Comments: Retrospective study of 199 patients initiating ART in a clinic in London. 44 of 199 (23%) developed IRIS, with dermatologic manifestations accounting for majority of cases. 50% of IRIS events related to genital herpes. Independent risk factors for IRIS were young age at initiation of ART, baseline CD4 percent <10%, and CD4:CD8 cell ratio <0.15.

Zolopa A, Andersen J, Powderly W, et al. Early antiretroviral therapy reduces AIDS progression/death in individuals with acute opportunistic infections: a multicenter randomized strategy trial. *PLoS One*, 2009; 4: e5575.
Comments: A5164 randomized 282 subjects with AIDS-related OIs (TB excluded), to early or deferred ART. Early ART (within 14 days of starting OI treatment) improved survival/AIDS progression compared to delayed ART (after completion of acute OI therapy).

Grant PM, Komarow L, Andersen J, et al. Risk factor analyses for immune reconstitution inflammatory syndrome in a randomized study of early vs. deferred ART during an opportunistic infection. *PLoS One*, 2010; 5: e11416.
Comments: Analysis of A5164 randomized trial identified the following risk factors associated with IRIS: the presence of a fungal infection, lower CD4 counts and higher baseline VL, and higher CD4 counts and lower VL on treatment. However, early initiation of ART or timing of ART was not associated with IRIS.

Havlir D, Ive P, Kendall M, et al. International randomized trial of immediate vs early ART in HIV+ patients treated for TB: ACTG 5221 STRIDE Study. Paper presented at: Conference on Retroviruses and Opportunistic Infections; February 28, 2011; Boston, MA.
Comments: Open-label, randomized, strategy study comparing immediate ART (2 wks after TB treatment start) to early ART (8 to 12 wks) among HIV+ subjects with CD4+ cells <250 treated for confirmed or suspected TB. Except for patients with CD4 ≤50, immediate ART did not reduce AIDS and death compared to early ART. Among patients with CD4 ≤50, immediate ART resulted in lower rates of AIDS and death.

F.X. Blanc, T. Sok, D. Laureillard, et al. A Significant enhancement in survival with (two weeks) vs. late (eight weeks) initiation of highly active antiretroviral treatment (HAART) in severely immunosupressed HIV-infected adults with newly diagnosed tuberculosis. International AIDS Conference, July 2010, Vienna Abstract THLBB106.
Comments: CAMELIA was a randomized study of 661 pts. co-infected with TB and HIV and CD4 <200. One arm received HAART 2 weeks after initiation of TB treatment and the second arm received HAART 8 weeks after initiation of treatment. Mortality was reduced 34% in the early HAART group. Immune reconstitution syndrome was more common in the early treatment group, but easy to manage clinically.

Karim SA, Naidoo K, Padayatchi N, et al. Optimal timing of ART during TB therapy: findings of the SAPiT trial. Paper presented at: Conference on Retroviruses and Opportunistic Infections; February 28, 2011; Boston, MA
Comments: Open-label randomized controlled trial in South Africa in sputum AFB smear-positive patients (n = 642) with HIV and CD4 counts <500 comparing early therapy (ART initiated within 4 wks of TB treatment initiation, n = 214) and late therapy (ART initiated within the first 4 wks of the continuation phase of TB treatment, n = 215). In patients with CD4 counts <50, early ART initiation was associated with better AIDS-free survival, albeit with increased risk of IRIS. However, in patients with CD4 ≤50, delaying initiation of ART to the first 4 wks of continuation phase of TB reduced the risk of IRIS and drug switches without compromising AIDS-free survival.

Abdool Karim SS, Naidoo K, Grobler A, et al. Timing of initiation of antiretroviral drugs during tuberculosis therapy. *N Engl J Med*, 2010; 362: 697–706.

Comments: Open-label, randomized, controlled trial with 642 patients with TB/HIV coinfection to start ART either during tuberculosis therapy or after the completion of TB treatment. Mortality was lower in patients initiating ART during TB therapy in all CD4 strata.

Müller M, Wandel S, Colebunders R, et al. Immune reconstitution inflammatory syndrome in patients starting antiretroviral therapy for HIV infection: a systematic review and meta-analysis. *Lancet Infect Dis*, 2010; 10: 251–61.

Comments: Systematic review of 54 cohort studies of 13,103 patients starting ART, of whom 1699 developed IRIS. The risk of IRIS was associated with CD4 cell count at the start of ART, with a high risk in patients with CD4 <50.

DIABETES MELLITUS AND INSULIN RESISTANCE

Todd T. Brown, MD, PhD and Joseph Cofrancesco, Jr., MD, MPH

CLINICAL

- IR common in HIV+ patients on ART.
- DM less common, but still 2–4× higher than in general population.
- IR also caused by fat accumulation (lipodystrophy). In general population (and presumably in HIV+ patients), IR increases risk for coronary artery disease.
- Risk factors for IR/DM: abdominal fat accumulation, peripheral lipoatrophy, family Hx of DM, obesity, age, HCV, low CD4 nadir, black/Hispanic race.
- Consider role of other medications: corticosteroids, GH, megestrol acetate, immunosuppressants, atypical antipsychotics.
- Older PIs (IDV, full dose RTV) have marked effects on IR. Of the current PIs, LPV/r > DRV/r and ATV/r. Independent effect of low dose RTV on IR controversial.

DIAGNOSIS

- DM = fasting glucose >126 mg/dL confirmed with a repeat test, or Sx of DM and a random plasma glucose >200 mg/dL.
- HgbA1c underestimates glycemia in HIV+ patients on ART (~HgbA1c 0.8% less than expected). Caution should be used for using HgbA1c for Dx in HIV+ patients given potential for false negatives with current American Diabetes Association (ADA) criteria (DM= HgbA1c ≥6.5%).
- Impaired fasting glucose (IFG) = 100–125 mg/dL, at risk for developing DM per ADA definition.
- If unclear, consider 2-hr 75-g oral glucose tolerance test (OGTT), more sensitive than fasting glucose: 140–199 = impaired glucose tolerance (IGT), >200 = DM.
- IGT or IFG is considered pre-DM. HgbA1c 5.7–6.4 considered pre-DM in general population.
- Check fasting glucose at baseline, prior to and 3 and 6 mos after ART initiation, then yearly if normal.
- No accepted role for clinical use of insulin levels to assess IR.

TREATMENT

Diet, Exercise, Risk Factor Modification

- Balanced diet and regular exercise crucial. ADA diet consisting of 50% carbohydrates (higher-fiber, unrefined preferred), 30% fat (unsaturated preferred), and 20% protein recommended.
- Nutrition consultation recommended.
- Modest weight loss (10%) in those with BMI >25 reduces glucose intolerance and can prevent onset of DM in non-HIV infected population at risk. Lifestyle modification shown to improve metabolic parameters in HIV-infected patients.
- Aggressive risk factor modification for coronary disease: lipid control, HTN control (generally with angiotensin-converting enzyme inhibitors [ACE-I] or angiotensin II receptor blocker [ARB]), smoking cessation, cocaine avoidance, ASA therapy.

Medications (Oral)

- First-line treatment for DM: metformin, pioglitazone.
- **Metformin:** reduces hepatic IR. Associated with reduced visceral fat, BP, TG (10%–20%) in HIV+ patients. Some studies have shown decreased limb fat with metformin; use with caution in patients with lipoatrophy. Serum creatinine >1.5 mg/dL an absolute contraindication due to lactic acidosis

risk. Also enhanced theoretical risk with NRTIs, liver disease, and CHF. GI upset most common. Start at 500 mg once daily, titrate 500 mg weekly to 2 g twice daily (max dose 850 3 ×/day).

- **Pioglitazone:** reduces peripheral IR as peroxisome proliferator-activated receptor (PPAR) gamma agonists. Modest effect on lipoatrophy. Some decrease in TG with pioglitazone. Pioglitazone: start at 15 mg, titrate up to 45 mg/day. Max effect seen after several wks. Fluid retention common. Avoid with CHF, liver disease. Reduced bone density and fractures associated with pioglitazone use.
- Combination of metformin and thiazolidinediones (TZDs) not established in HIV+ patients, but synergy expected.
- Use sulfonylureas, meglitinides, exenatide, sitagliptin, or acarbose as second-line therapies.
- Metformin can be considered along with lifestyle changes in those with pre-diabetes.

Insulin
- Consider low dose (10–15 units) bedtime glargine, detimer, or NPH insulin in combination with oral antidiabetic agents if failing oral agents. Insulin effective for glucose control with individualized regimen.
- Consider referral to diabetes expert.

Modification of ART
- Consider switching off older PIs provided viral control not jeopardized (data limited).
- Although data limited, some PIs (e.g. ATV, DRV), may cause less insulin resistance.

FOLLOW-UP
Monitoring
- **Lifestyle changes only:** self-monitored blood glucose weekly.
- **Oral agents:** monitor fasting glucose every morning.
- **Insulin:** monitor glucose 2–4 ×/day.
- **Screening:** patients with pre-DM should be screened at 3–6 mo intervals. After Dx of DM, monitor HgbA1c q3–6 mos, depending on control. Goal <7%, with caveat regarding accuracy of A1c in HIV-infected persons.
- Monitoring for complications: dilated fundoscopic exam by ophthalmology, spot urine for microalbumin and foot exam with inspection, monofilament, and vibration testing at baseline and q6–12 mos.

SELECTED REFERENCES
The International Expert Committee. International Expert Committee report on the role of the A1C assay in the diagnosis of diabetes. *Diabetes Care*, 2009; 32: 1327–34.
Comments: Excellent discussion regarding Dx of DM and rationale for using A1c.

Kim PS, Woods C, Georgoff P, et al. A1c underestimates glycemia in HIV infection. *Diabetes Care*, 2009; 32: 1591–3.
Comments: Important prospective study showing underestimation of glycemia in HIV+ patients by ~30 mg/dL.

Brown TT, Tassiopoulos K, Bosch RJ, Shikuma C, McComsey GA. Association between systemic inflammation and incident diabetes in HIV-infected patients after initiation of antiretroviral therapy. *Diabetes Care*, 2010; 33: 2244–9. Epub 2010 Jul 27.
Comments: Systemic inflammation after ART initiation associated with incident DM, suggesting role for inflammation in pathogenesis of DM in HIV+ patients.

American Diabetes Association. Diagnosis and classification of diabetes mellitus. *Diabetes Care*, 2011; 34(Suppl 1): S62–S69.
Comments: Latest recommendations from ADA in general population.

Wohl DA, McComsey G, Tebas P, et al. Current concepts in the diagnosis and management of metabolic complications of HIV infection and its therapy. *Clin Infect Dis*, 2006; 43: 645–53.
Comments: A review of Dx and treatment of metabolic complications in HIV, including insulin resistance and diabetes, written by members of ACTG Complications Sub-Committee.

Mehta SH, Moore RD, Thomas DL, Chaisson RE, Sulkowski MS. The effect of HAART and HCV infection on the development of hyperglycemia among HIV-infected persons. *J Acquir Immune Defic Syndr*, 2003; 33: 577–84.
Comments: With an adjusted relative hazard of 2.28 (95% CI, 1.23–4.22), this study established HCV as an independent risk factor for hyperglycemia.

LACTIC ACIDOSIS

Richard D. Moore, MD, MHS

CLINICAL

- **Incidence:** mild, asymptomatic hyperlactatemia: 8%–15%; symptomatic hyperlactatemia: 0.5%–12%.
- **Symptoms:** fatigue; weakness; myalgias; and GI distress, including abdominal pain, abdominal distention, nausea/vomiting, diarrhea. Later can advance to dyspnea, orthostasis, organ failure (hepatic, renal), cardiovascular collapse, and death.
- **Mortality:** 7% with lactate 5–10 mM, 20%–30% with lactate 10–15 mM, 50%–60% with lactate >15 mM.
- **Caused by NRTI use:** d4T > ddI, AZT. May not occur with 3TC, FTC, ABC, TDF, though listed in package insert as a class effect.
- Associated with mitochondrial DNA gamma polymerase inhibition and decrease in mitochondrial DNA.
- **May be accompanied** by hepatic steatosis (fatty liver), pancreatitis. Fatal liver failure can occur (earliest reports in AZT-treated patients).
- **Increased risk** with lower CD4, older age, female sex. Do not use ddI + d4T in pregnancy (FDA warning).

DIAGNOSIS

- Lactate >2 mM. Venous blood drawn without tourniquet into chilled fluoride-oxalate tube. Blood must be put on ice after phlebotomy, processed in lab within 4 hrs. Should not exercise 24 hrs before level drawn.
- Low bicarb, anion gap >16 ($Na - [Cl + CO2)]$), elevated CPK, LDH, amylase, lipase, AST, ALT. These tests not sensitive or specific. Can have hyperlactatemia with normal bicarbonate and anion gap.
- Ultrasound or CT of liver may show steatosis.
- Asymptomatic elevation of lactate to 2–5 mM range does not reliably predict higher elevations and symptoms. Most with mild elevation do not progress.
- Mild Sx may not correlate well with lactate levels.

TREATMENT
Treatment of Hyperlactatemia and Lactic Acidosis

- Lactate >5 mM may not require treatment in absence of Sx (routine lactate monitoring not recommended).
- Symptomatic patients (lactate typically >5 mM) should discontinue NRTIs.
- Consider switch to ABC or TDF if on d4T, ddI, or AZT with mild lactate elevation and minimal Sx. Combination of TDF and full-dose ddI has been associated with severe lactic acidosis.
- Lactate >10–15 mM may require urgent supportive management. Seriously ill persons may require IV hydration, mechanical ventilation, pressors, dialysis.
- Anecdotal reports of benefit from L-carnitine (50–100 mg/kg/day IV in divided doses q4hrs by slow infusion), thiamine (100 mg IV), riboflavin (100 mg PO once daily), vitamin C (500 mg PO or IV once daily), coenzyme Q (1.5 mg/kg IV once daily) but no clinical trials of efficacy.

FOLLOW-UP
Relapse

- Monitor lactate initially if alternative NRTIs restarted.

SELECTED REFERENCES

Lactic Acidosis International Study Group. Risk factors for lactic acidosis and severe hyperlactataemia in HIV-1-infected adults exposed to antiretroviral therapy. *AIDS*, 2007; 21: 2455–64.
Comments: International Study Group findings. Risk factors for hyperlactatemia include dideoxynucleosides, female sex, low CD4.

Tan D, Walmsley S, Shen S, Paboud J. Mild to moderate symptoms do not correlate with lactate levels in HIV-positive patients on nucleoside reverse transcriptase inhibitors. *HIV Clin Trials*, 2006; 7: 107–15.
Comments: Mild Sx did not correlate with lactate levels (up to 4.5 mmol/L) in this cross-sectional observational study.

Lonergan JT, McComsey GA, Fisher RL, et al. Lack of recurrence of hyperlactatemia in HIV-infected patients switched from stavudine to abacavir or zidovudine. *J Acquir Immune Defic Syndr*, 2004; 36: 935–42.

Comments: Lack of recurrence of hyperlactatemia after stopping d4T, letting lactate return to normal, then starting AZT or ABC.

Carr A. Lactic acidemia in infection with human immunodeficiency virus. *Clin Infect Dis*, 2003; 36: S96–S100.
Comments: Greatest risk in pregnancy. Mild hyperlactatemia common, but uncommonly leads to severe illness. Asymptomatic hyperlactatemia should not be treated.

Ogedegbe AE, Thomas DL, Diehl AM. Hyperlactataemia syndromes associated with HIV therapy. *Lancet Infect Dis*, 2003; 3: 329–37.
Comments: Review of etiology, signs and Sx, and management of hyperlactatemia and lactic acidosis syndromes associated with HIV and HIV treatment.

Côté HC, Brumme ZL, Craib KJ, et al. Changes in mitochondrial DNA as a marker of nucleoside toxicity in HIV-infected patients. *NEJM*, 2002; 346: 811–20.
Comments: Study showing effect of NRTIs on mitochondria and mitochondrial function.

LIPODYSTROPHY

Lisa A. Spacek, MD, PhD and Joseph Cofrancesco, Jr., MD, MPH

CLINICAL

- **Lipoatrophy (LA):** fat loss in face, proximal extremities (LE > UE), buttocks, and SQ tissue throughout body, including SQ abdominal fat. Must be differentiated from wasting, a consequence of HIV-disease progression and/or OIs involving loss of muscle and fat. Lipoatrophy associated with use of ART, especially thymidine analog NRTIs. Associated with hyperlipidemia, insulin resistance, and mitochondrial toxicity due to thymidine analog use (d4T>AZT), generally occurring after 2–4 yrs of use. May be more likely when combined with EFV vs boosted PI.
- **Fat accumulation (FA):** neck/dorsocervical fat pad, visceral abdomen, lipomas, breasts. Must be differentiated from normal increase in weight often seen with control of HIV. Risk factors include: (a) host factors: age >40, gender, baseline body composition, race/ethnicity, and genetics; (b) disease factors: CD4 nadir, more severe/longer duration of disease, degree of immune reconstitution; and (c) medication factors: duration of ART. More common with PI use, associated with hyperlipidemia and insulin resistance.

DIAGNOSIS

- In clinical practice, patient history and PE most commonly used.
- **LA:** close examination of extremities, buttock, and SQ tissue of abdomen. Old photographs may be helpful. DEXA scans used for research purposes.
- **FA:** may be difficult to differentiate from "usual" obesity. Waist measurement or waist/hip ratio may be helpful. Examine dorsocervical area and abdominal area, with close attention to distension/visceral fat accumulation (as opposed to SQ fat accumulation). CT scan at L4/5 used to assess visceral fat, used as research tool.

TREATMENT

General

- Suppression of HIV replication is primary objective; best to notice changes early and treat associated metabolic alterations.
- Prevention and early detection yield better results.
- Studies focus on patients with established and often severe changes.

Fat Accumulation

- **Address insulin resistance if present:** consider metformin (500 mg once daily–1000 mg twice daily); effect on FA variable. May lead to worsening of LA. Metformin not approved for HIV-associated FA.
- **Exercise:** At least1 hr resistance training and aerobic exercise 3 times weekly; general weight reduction can sometimes help, but watch for further LA.
- Studies changing ART, including eliminating PIs, have failed to demonstrate significant impact on FA. There may be less FA with ATV, especially if insulin resistant, although data not conclusive.
- **Recombinant human growth hormone (rhGH):** optimal dose/dosing schedule unclear: max: 0.1 mg/kg/day or 6 mg/day; range 3–6 mg once daily or every other day if no insulin resistance

and no lipoatrophy. Multiple side effects including insulin resistance and fluid retention, and very costly. Not approved for use in HIV-associated FA. Changes reverse after cessation of rhGH.

- **Growth hormone releasing factor (tesamorelin):** FDA approved for treatment of excess abdominal fat accumulation. Modest (14%–18%) abdominal fat reduction after 26 wks, but reversal of benefits seen with discontinuation of drug. Well tolerated with ~3% higher rates of discontinuation compared to placebo. Arthralgia, myalgia, edema, and injection site reaction reported in >5% of treated patients.
- **Liposuction (U/S-guided):** for dorsocervical fat accumulation. Fat recurs in some studies.
- For gynecomastia, ensure breast tissue is not tumor; consider work up for hypogonadism.

Lipoatrophy

- Prevention is critical. Avoid thymidine analogs and possibly ddI, with preferential use of TDF or ABC.
- **Early detection and change of ARTs** (eliminate d4T and AZT, possibly ddI) to avoid further progression and to allow restoration of SQ fat. TDF, ABC, 3TC, FTC alternatives. See Toxicity and Side Effects: Switching Therapy, p. 406.
- Some studies suggest that switching from thymide analogs (especially AZT) less effective after 3 years of exposure.
- **Uridine:** preliminary results promising for those remaining on thymidine analog.
- **Dermatologic/plastic surgery:** "face fillers" classified as temporary or permanent. Many are used "off label." Undesirable side effects, including granulomas, migration, and lumpiness, can depend on purity of compound and skill of provider. Require multiple visits with high cost, generally not covered by insurance. Best results often seen with combination of techniques. Better results with milder LA. Polylactic acid and calcium hydroxylapatite approved in US for HIV-associated facial LA. Permanent fillers can sag if LA progresses.

SELECTED REFERENCES

Panel on Antiretroviral Guidelines for Adults and Adolescents. Guidelines for the use of antiretroviral agents in HIV-1-infected adults and adolescents. Department of Health and Human Services; January 10, 2011; 1–166. http://aidsinfo.nih.gov/contentfiles/AdultandAdolescentGL.pdf. Accessed March 30, 2011.
Comments: LA: d4T> ZDV, may be more likely when combined with EFV vs boosted PI. FA: trunk fat increase seen with EFV, PIs, and RAL-containing regimens, not known to be causal.

European AIDS Clinical Society. Prevention and management of non-infectious co-morbidities in HIV. November 1, 2009. http://www.europeanaidsclinicalsociety.org/Guidelines/G2.htm. Accessed April 13, 2011.
Comments: Clinically oriented document includes section on prevention and management of lipodystrophy.

Thompson, MA, Aberg JA, Cahn P, et al. Antiretroviral treatment of adult HIV infection: 2010 recommendations of the International AIDS Society-USA panel. *JAMA*, 2010; 304: 321–33.
Comments: AZT use limited by risk of lipoatrophy.

Falutz J, Potvin D, Mamputu JC, et al. Effects of tesamorelin, a growth hormone-releasing factor, in HIV-infected patients with abdominal fat accumulation: a randomized placebo-controlled trial with a safety extension. *J Acquir Immune Defic Syndr*, 2010; 53: 311–22.
Comments: Placebo-controlled switch study of 404 HIV+ patients taking tesamorelin for visceral adipose tissue (VAT). VAT reduced by approximately 18% (P< 0.001) in patients continuing tesamorelin for 12 mos. The initial improvements over 6 mos in VAT were rapidly lost in those switching from tesamorelin to placebo.

Sheth SH, Larson RJ. The efficacy and safety of insulin-sensitizing drugs in HIV-associated lipodystrophy syndrome: a meta-analysis of randomized trials. *BMC Infect Dis*, 2010; 10: 183.
Comments: Meta-analysis of 16 trials included 920 patients treated with insulin-sensitizing agents for lipodystrophy syndrome (insulin resistance, abnormal lipid metabolism, and redistribution of body fat). Metformin improved all three components. Rosiglitazone improved insulin but worsened lipids. Pioglitazone did not change insulin, TG, or LDL, but improved LDL. Neither rosiglitazone nor pioglitazone improved fat redistribution.

Domingo P, Torres-Torronteras J, Pomar V, et al. Uridine metabolism in HIV-1-infected patients: effect of infection, of antiretroviral therapy and of HIV-1/ART-associated lipodystrophy syndrome. PLoS One. 2010; 5: e13896.
Comments: Plasma uridine levels lower in HIV+ patients with isolated lipoatrophy.

Malignancies

CASTLEMAN DISEASE

Mark Levis, MD, PhD and Nina Wagner-Johnston, MD

PATHOGENS

- HIV-associated Castleman disease (CD) always associated with HHV-8, or Kaposi sarcoma-associated herpesvirus (KSHV). HHV-8 present in 40% of non-HIV cases.
- CD is likely the result of active lytic infection with HHV-8 as opposed to latent infection with HHV-8-associated primary effusion lymphoma.

CLINICAL

- Polyclonal lymphoproliferative disease characterized by angiofollicular lymph node hyperplasia: an "overreaction" of lymph node to an (unknown) antigen stimulus.
- Lab abnormalities include cytopenias, hypoalbuminemia, elevated CRP, and polyclonal hypergammaglobulinemia.
- Two categories: localized and multicentric. In HIV, CD always multicentric (typically plasmablastic). Presents with generalized lymphadenopathy, splenomegaly, fever/night sweats, and fatigue. Dyspnea and lymphoid lung infiltrates common.
- IL-6, both of viral and host origin, appears to contribute to pathogenesis of Sx and adenopathy.
- Most common with CD4 <100, but can present at any CD4 count.
- Patients often have KS as well.
- May "progress" to non-Hodgkin lymphoma.

DIAGNOSIS

- In appropriate clinical setting (low CD4, diffuse lymphadenopathy, constitutional Sx), Bx of a "reactive" lymph node with prominent follicles, sheets of plasma cells in the interfollicular regions, vascular proliferation with endothelial hyperplasia, and positive for HHV-8 DNA.
- HHV-8 DNA can be found in plasma of any patient with advanced/long-standing HIV disease, but titers higher in patients with CD.

TREATMENT
Prognosis

- Often very aggressive, rapidly fatal course in absence of treatment, but occasionally can be indolent.
- HIV-associated CD has higher mortality rate than CD in immunocompetent individuals.

General Considerations

- No established standard of care treatment.
- Successful treatment usually associated with decreased HHV-8 titers in blood.
- First-line treatment is monoclonal antibody or chemotherapy; antiviral agents second-line.
- Case reports of successful treatment of CD with ART, although anecdotal reports of "triggering" disease.
- HHV-8 DNA VL levels are comparable in plasma and in PBMCs.

Treatment Categories

- **Nonspecific:** chemotherapy w/ lymphoma regimens, such as CHOP (**c**yclophosphamide 750 mg/m^2, **h**ydroxydoxorubicin/doxorubicin 50 mg/m^2, **O**ncovin/vincristine 1.4 mg/m^2, prednisone 100 mg) every 21 days × 4–6 cycles; radiation therapy; or steroids.
- **Targeted antiproliferative:** anti-CD20 (rituximab, dose of 375 mg/m^2 weekly × 4 wks) or anti-IL6 (tocilizumab 8 mg/kg every 2 wks; not currently available in US).
- **Antiviral therapy:** valganciclovir 900 mg PO twice daily × 21 days, ganciclovir (GCV) 5 mg/kg IV × 21 days.
- Thalidomide 200 mg daily with rituximab 375 mg/m^2 given 4 times at 3-wk intervals, followed by rituximab maintenance every 3 mos for 1 year.

SELECTED REFERENCES

Mylona EE, Baraboutis IG, Lekakis LJ, Georgiou O, Papastamopoulos V, Skoutelis A. Multicentric Castleman's disease in HIV infection: a systematic review of the literature. *AIDS Rev*, 2008; 10: 25–35.
Comments: Provides a comprehensive review of CD studies and case reports in HIV+ patients.

Stary G, Kohrgruber N, Herneth AM, Gaiger A, Stingl G, Rieger A. Complete regression of HIV-associated multicentric Castleman disease treated with rituximab and thalidomide. *AIDS*, 2008; 22: 1232–4.
Comments: Experimental approach with rituximab and thalidomide effective in a case report.

Du MQ, Bacon CM, Isaacson PG. Kaposi sarcoma-associated herpesvirus/human herpesvirus 8 and lymphoproliferative disorders. *J Clin Pathol*, 2007; 60: 1350–7.
Comments: Review of the associated gene expression patterns of HHV-8 in lymphoproliferative disorders.

Sprinz E, Jeffman M, Liedke P, Putten A, Schwartsmann G. Successful treatment of AIDS-related Castleman's disease following the administration of highly active antiretroviral therapy (HAART). *Ann Oncol*, 2004; 15: 356–8.
Comments: Case report of ART as treatment for CD.

KAPOSI SARCOMA

David J. Kouba, MD, PhD and Christopher J. Hoffmann, MD, MPH

Pathogens
- HHV-8, a gamma herpes virus, also known as Kaposi sarcoma-associated herpesvirus (KSHV) is etiologic agent of all clinical variants of KS.

Clinical
- KS was once the AIDS-defining illness in ~10%–20% of cases in US; it has become rare in era of ART.
- In US and Europe, AIDS-related KS occurs overwhelmingly in MSM; evidence suggests sexual transmission of HHV-8 in that population. Incidence in HIV+ children low (4%) vs 50% of HIV+ MSM (prior to HAART), with higher prevalence with more lifetime sexual partners and history of anal sex. Prevalence of HHV-8 much higher in in general population of many African countries (>50%) and may be transmitted vertically.
- AIDS-related KS is most aggressive form of KS (others are classic/sporadic, endemic/African, iatrogenic/posttransplant).
- Clinical features variable, from single lesions to disseminated disease. Skin lesions commonly painless, oval, red-purplish or rust-colored macules, papules or plaques to deep violaceous or purple-black nodules. May appear as SQ nodules less commonly. With extensive disease may develop B symptoms (fevers, night sweats, malaise, weight loss).
- Coalescing plaques may obstruct lymphatic flow, causing significant lymphedema.
- Any skin surface may be affected, although commonly on trunk and face or oral mucosa.
- Visceral disease includes GI involvement, lymphatic and pulmonary disease. Poor prognosis with pulmonary KS, with median survival of 3–10 mos prior to the use of ART. Visceral disease may occur without identifiable skill lesions.
- Patients with history of KS are at higher risk for other HHV-8-associated malignancies (primary effusion body lymphoma and Castleman disease).

Diagnosis
- Definitive Dx by Bx for H and E. Immunostains for vascular differentiation (CD31 and CD34) will aid Dx, if pathology equivocal.
- Histopathology shows dermal infiltrate of atypical spindle cells, which splay apart collagen bundles while attempting to form rudimentary vascular slits. Diffuse erythrocyte extravasation and hemosiderin deposition into the dermis is characteristic. Plasma cell infiltrate frequently observed.
- DDx includes bacillary angiomatosis, pyogenic granuloma, cutaneous metastases of lymphoma, angiosarcoma.
- PCR can be used to detect KSHV viral DNA or serologic assays for KSHV antibodies. Several commercially available ELISA tests for various KSHV antigens exist. There is no "gold standard" test for identifying infected patients.
- HHV-8 DNA strongly predictive for the development of KS when detected in serum of HIV+ males.

Treatment
General Treatment Considerations
- ART sometimes results in resolution of cutaneous or systemic disease, though cases of KS exacerbation due to immune reconstitution have also been reported.

- Treatment required for: (1) systemic visceral involvement; (2) rapid progression; (3) interference with a vital function; (4) negative affect on quality of life.

Solitary or Few Skin Lesions (for Cosmetic Reasons)
- **Limited disease:** can monitor lesions after starting ART, small lesions will resolve.
- **Intralesional injection of vinblastine:** good option for solitary/few lesions when cosmesis is important, since cosmetic results can be excellent.
- **Aggressive cryotherapy:** multiple lesions in areas not cosmetically important, as healing times and cosmesis are inferior to excision or vinblastine injection.
- **Surgical excision:** solitary or few lesions in cosmetically sensitive locations.
- **Laser ablation:** poor healing, similar to cryotherapy; therefore should be used for debulking in cosmetically unimportant areas.
- **Radiation therapy:** larger and/or multiple lesions in one specific site not amenable to destructive modalities or excision. May cause or exacerbate lymphatic obstruction and lymphedema, especially in lower extremities.
- **Aliretinoin gel:** apply to KS lesions twice daily initially, then titrate to 3–4 x/day as tolerated. Response rate 35% at 12 wks in alitretinoin-treated patients vs 18% in placebo-treated patients.

Generalized Cutaneous/Aggressive/Systemic Visceral Involvement
- **For generalized cutaneous disease:** systemic chemotherapy (see below) or radiation therapy, either to an extended field or as total body electron-beam therapy.
- **For visceral disease:** systemic chemotherapy with liposomal anthracyclines such as doxorubicin to reduce side effects, or combinations of vincristine, doxorubicin, and bleomycin. Paclitaxel is effective chemotherapeutic option; however, usually recommended as second-line agent due to toxicity.
- **Systemic treatment includes:** interferon-alfa and chemotherapy with a single agent such as pegylated-liposomal anthracyclines (pegylated liposomal doxorubicin 20 mg/m^2 every 2–3 wks), paclitaxel (120–125 mg/m^2 every 2–3 wks), or etoposide (50–60 mg daily × 7 days every 2–3 wks).
- **Investigational treatment options:** angiogenesis inhibitors, IL-12, and HIV-tat inhibitors.
- **Steroids** may help prevent inflammatory response from severe visceral disease causing airway impingement or bowel obstruction.

FOLLOW-UP
- While limited cutaneous disease is primarily cosmetic issue, regular (3–6 mos) follow-up required to monitor for disseminated disease.
- Disseminated cutaneous disease requires regular follow-up, as lymphatic obstruction is common complication.
- Visceral disease requires regular follow-up with oncology and/or radiation oncology, depending on regimen selected.

SELECTED REFERENCES

Sullivan RJ, Pantanowitz L, Casper C, Stebbing J, Dezube BJ. HIV/AIDS: epidemiology, pathophysiology, and treatment of Kaposi sarcoma-associated herpesvirus disease: Kaposi sarcoma, primary effusion lymphoma, and multicentric Castleman disease. *Clin Infect Dis*, 2008; 47: 1209–15.
Comments: Review of epidemiology and presentation of KS in HIV.

Stebbing J, Sanitt A, Nelson M, Powles T, Gazzard B, Bower M. A prognostic index for AIDS-associated Kaposi's sarcoma in the era of highly active antiretroviral therapy. *Lancet*, 2006; 367: 1495–502.
Comments: Clinic-based analysis of KS mortality by disease involvement.

Vanni T, Sprinz E, Machado MW, Santana Rde C, Fonseca BA, Schwartsmann G. Systemic treatment of AIDS-related Kaposi sarcoma: current status and perspectives. *Cancer Treat Rev*, 2006; 32: 445–55.
Comments: Review of systemic treatment for KS.

LYMPHOMA, HODGKIN

Mark Levis, MD, PhD and Nina Wagner-Johnston, MD

PATHOGENS
- Almost always EBV-associated, unlike in HIV-negative patients.

CLINICAL

- Risk of developing Hodgkin's lymphoma (HL) approximately 10× higher in HIV+ persons vs general population. Incidence has unexpectedly increased in HAART era.
- Associated with higher CD4 counts (~200) vs NHL.
- Patients often have diffuse lymphadenopathy but with uninvolved nodes. Lymphadenopathy can make Dx and accurate staging difficult.
- Tends to present with advanced stage and in unusual locations, especially bone marrow.
- Frequently presents with "B Sx," e.g., night sweats and weight loss, which are commonly associated with other AIDS-related illnesses.
- Histologic subtypes in HIV+ population are less favorable mixed cellularity and lymphocyte-depleted variants.
- Tumor cells show strong expression of EBV latent membrane protein-1 (LMP-1).

DIAGNOSIS

- Bx of node, mass, or affected organ essential. Fine needle aspiration (FNA) is NOT preferred mode of Dx, as usually nondiagnostic in HL.
- Immunophenotyping of paraffin block or flow cytometric analysis of cell surface markers (CD3, CD5, CD10, CD15, CD20, CD30, CD45, Ki-67) in combination with molecular studies (EBV or HHV-8, cytogenetics, FISH).
- Staging work up should include chest/abdomen/pelvic CT, and/or PET/CT, bone marrow Bx and aspirate, CBC, ESR, and complete chemistries.

TREATMENT

Prognosis

- International Prognostic Scores (IPS) useful in predicting outcome. Poor risk features in this index: albumin <4 g/dL, Hgb <10.5 g/dL, male sex, age ≥45, stage IV disease, WBC >15,000, and lymphocytopenia (lymphocyte count <600 and/or less than 8% of the WBC).

General Considerations

- ART (either during or immediately following chemotherapy) essential for prolonged survival.
- AZT should be avoided as it can prolong or exacerbate chemotherapy-induced neutropenia.
- ddI and/or d4T can increase incidence of neuropathy.
- Survival rates approaching that of HIV-negative patients, with 90% surviving 1 yr.
- Fligrastim (G-CSF) routinely used during chemotherapy to shorten duration of neutropenia.

Regimens

- While Stanford V and BEACOPP regimens have been used, ABVD (doxorubicin, bleomycin, vinblastine, and dacarbazine) remains gold standard.
- A cooperative group study evaluating high dose chemotherapy and autologous stem cell rescue for patients with relapsed/refractory HIV-associated HL is underway.

SELECTED REFERENCES

Bohlius J, Schmidlin K, Boué F, et al. HIV-1-related Hodgkin lymphoma in the era of combination antiretroviral therapy: incidence and evoluation of CD4+ T-cell lymphocytes. *Blood*, 2011; 117: 6100–8. Epub 2011 Mar 2.
Comments: Case control study demonstrating that incidence of HL not reduced by ART.

Xicoy B, Ribera JM, Miralles P, et al. Results of treatment with doxorubicin, bleomycin, vinblastine and dacarbazine and highly active antiretroviral therapy in advanced stage, human immunodeficiency virus-related Hodgkin's lymphoma. *Haematologica*, 2007; 92: 191–8.
Comments: Phase II study demonstrating efficacy of ABVD regimen.

Berenguer J, Miralles P, Ribera J, et al. Characteristics and outcome of AIDS-related Hodgkin lymphoma before and after the introduction of highly active antiretroviral therapy. *J Acquir Immune Defic Syndr*, 2008; 47: 422–428.
Comments: Study demonstrating complete response rates of 70% vs 91% median OS of 39 mos and not reached for treated patients with HL prior to and after the introduction of ART, respectively.

LYMPHOMA, NON-HODGKIN

Mark Levis, MD, PhD and Nina Wagner-Johnston, MD

PATHOGENS

- Often associated with EBV, especially primary CNS lymphoma (PCNSL).

- HHV-8 (KSHV) causally associated with primary effusion/body cavity lymphoma.

CLINICAL

- Late manifestation of disease, most often associated with CD4 <100, though can occur at any CD4 count.
- No obvious environmental factors, but possible genetic predisposition: more common in men.
- Incidence of all AIDS-related lymphomas (ARL) has declined since ART, but decline less dramatic for lymphoma than for OIs, making it a common AIDS-defining illness.
- Several different variants of ARL: diffuse large B-cell lymphoma (DLBCL), immunoblastic/plasmablastic lymphoma, PCNSL, Burkitt or Burkitt-like lymphoma, and primary effusion lymphoma (PEL, body cavity lymphoma).
- Two subtypes almost uniquely associated with HIV are PEL and plasmablastic lymphoma of the oropharynx.
- EBV infection of the tumor (and EBV DNA in CSF) predictive of CNS metastasis.
- ARL typically present at advanced stage, often with extranodal and CNS involvement.

DIAGNOSIS

- When possible, obtain Bx of node or affected organ. FNA is NOT preferred mode of Dx, although it can often be used when Bx is not feasible.
- Immunophenotyping of paraffin block or flow cytometric analysis of cell surface markers (CD3, CD5, CD10, CD15, CD20, CD30, Ki-67) in combination with molecular studies (EBV or HHV-8, cytogenetics, FISH).
- Staging work up should include chest/abdomen/pelvic CT, bone marrow biopsy and aspirate, LP, CBC, LDH, and complete chemistries. Brain MRI with gadolinium should be considered in most cases.
- Role of PET in AIDS-related lymphoma remains unclear, though frequently obtained.

TREATMENT

Prognosis

- International Prognostic Index (IPI) scores useful in predicting outcome. Poor risk features: age >60, reduced performance status, elevated LDH, advanced stage (common in ARL), and more than one site of extranodal involvement.

General Considerations

- Continuation or initiation of ART advised in most situations. Most chemotherapy regimens safe to give with ART, but overlapping toxicity is a problem for some agents.
- AZT contraindicated secondary to prolongation/exacerbation of chemotherapy-induced neutropenia. ddI and/or d4T can increase risk of neuropathy.
- G-CSF routinely used during chemotherapy to shorten duration of neutropenia.
- Gastric or intestinal DLBCL is well-described presentation of ARL associated with an increased risk GI bleeding or perforation during chemotherapy (compared with GI DLBCL in non-AIDS population). Early diagnosis of perforation and prompt exploration are key. Unclear role for treating as inpatient during 1st cycle and keeping patients NPO.
- Rituximab (anti-CD20 monoclonal antibody) routinely used in ARL. Patients with CD4 < 50 are at increased risk of fatal infectious complications.
- In post-HAART era, survival following treatment for ARL approaching that for lymphoma in the non-AIDS population.

Regimens

- Effective regimens include R-CHOP (rituximab, decadron, cyclophosphamide, infusional etoposide, vincristine, doxorubicin). Reported complete remission rates are 80% or more, with 2-year survival of >50%.
- Intrathecal chemotherapy with methotrexate or cytarabine recommended if BM involvement, Burkitt histology, or EBV+.
- Burkitt lymphoma generally requires more intensive regimens, such as R-hyper-CVAD (rituximab, cyclophosphamide, doxorubicin, vincristine, alternating with methotrexate and cytarabine), or R-CODOX-M/IVAC (rituximab, cyclophosphamide, vincristine, doxorubicin, methotrexate, alternating with ifosfamide, etoposide, cytarabine).
- High-dose therapy with autologous stem cell transplantation is increasingly being used for relapsed or refractory disease.

DIAGNOSIS

SELECTED REFERENCES

Miralles P, Berenguer J, Ribera JM, et al. Prognosis of AIDS-related systemic non-Hodgkin lymphoma treated with chemotherapy and highly active antiretroviral therapy depends exclusively on tumor-related factors. *J Acquir Immune Defic Syndr*, 2007; 44: 167–73.
Comments: Describes prognostic factors associated with improved outcome.

Boué F, Gabarre J, Gisselbrecht C, et al. Phase II trial of CHOP plus rituximab in patients with HIV-associated non-Hodgkin's lymphoma. *J Clin Oncol*, 2006; 24: 4123–8.
Comments: Phase II study demonstrating feasibility of R-CHOP regimen in HIV+ patients.

Engels EA, Pfeiffer RM, Landgren O, Moore RD. Immunologic and virologic predictors of AIDS-related non-Hodgkin lymphoma in the highly active antiretroviral therapy era. *J Acquir Immune Defic Syndr*; 2010; 54: 78–84.
Comments: Risk of NHL highest in patients with low CD4 and extended periods of uncontrolled HIV viremia.

Collaboration of Observational HIV Epidemiological Research Europe (COHERE) Study Group, Bohlius J, Schmidlin K, Costagliola D, et al. Prognosis of HIV-associated non-Hodgkin lymphoma in patients starting combination antiretroviral therapy. *AIDS*, 2009; 23: 2029–37.
Comments: Gap in survival between NHL patients with and without HIV is closing. Survival remains greatly affected by CD4.

Martí-Carvajal AJ, Cardona AF, Lawrence A. Interventions for previously untreated patients with AIDS-associated non-Hodgkin's lymphoma. *Cochrane Database System Rev*, 2009; 8: 1–86.
Comments: Only 4 randomized-controlled trials available, and unable to make evidence-based treatment recommendations.

Dunleavy K, Little RF, Pittaluga S, et al. The role of tumor histogenesis, FDG-PET, and short-course EPOCH with dose-dense rituximab (SC-EPOCH-RR) in HIV-associated diffuse large B-cell lymphoma. *Blood*, 2010; 115: 3017–24.
Comments: Demonstrates effectiveness of R-EPOCH regimen and highlights poor positive predictive value of early-interim PET/CT.

Re A, Michieli M, Casari S, et al. High-dose therapy and autologous peripheral blood stem cell transplantation as salvage treatment for AIDS-related lymphoma: long-term results of the Italian Cooperative Group on AIDS and Tumors (GICAT) study with analysis of prognostic factors. *Blood*, 2009; 114: 1306–13.
Comments: Stem cell transplant is highly effective salvage regimen.

Sparano JA, Lee JY, Kaplan LD, et al. Rituximab plus concurrent infusional EPOCH chemotherapy is highly effective in HIV-associated B-cell non-Hodgkin lymphoma. *Blood*, 2010; 115: 3008–16.
Comments: Most recent results of AMC (AIDS Malignancies Consortium) group demonstrating efficacy of R-EPOCH.

LYMPHOMA, PRIMARY CNS

Mark Levis, MD, PhD and Nina Wagner-Johnston, MD

PATHOGENS
- EBV infection present in virtually 100% of HIV-associated primary CNS lymphoma (PCNSL).
- Absence of EBV-specific CD4+ T-cell function may provide an immunological basis for HIV-associated PCNSL.

CLINICAL
- Late manifestation of disease, associated with CD4 <50 (therefore, rarely an AIDS-defining illness).
- Incidence declining precipitously since advent of ART.
- Presents with variety of focal and nonfocal neurological signs and Sx. In contrast to PCNSL in non-AIDS population, is often associated with B Sx.
- Histology is immunoblastic, high-grade beta cell.
- CT chest/abdomen/pelvis often obtained to rule out systemic lymphoma with CNS metastasis. Bone marrow Bx unnecessary.

DIAGNOSIS
- Bx remains gold standard, but not always necessary for Dx. PCR for EBV DNA in CSF helpful in establishing Dx (see below).
- Enhancing lesions on CT or MRI (higher yield) generally have DDx of PCNSL vs CNS toxoplasmosis. Radiographic features characteristic of PCNSL include: (1) larger lesions, (2) multifocal lesions, (3) lesions involving corpus callosum, (4) inhomogenous enhancement (reflecting rapid growth rate with necrosis), (5) rarely involve posterior fossa.

- PET scans often used to demonstrate metabolically hyperactive lesion.
- CSF cytology for neoplastic cells occasionally positive.
- In appropriate clinical setting of low CD4, *Toxoplasma* seronegativity (IgG), large or multifocal hyperenhancing radiographic CNS lesions, and no response to 10–14 days of toxoplasmosis treatment, PCR for EBV DNA in the CSF has high sensitivity and specificity for Dx of PCNSL, often precluding need for Bx.

TREATMENT
Prognosis
- Outcome data limited in pre-HAART era since incidence of HIV-related PCNSL has dropped dramatically.
- In absence of ART, median survival 1–3 mos, and usually not improved with chemotherapy or radiation therapy (XRT).
- With ART (and chemotherapy/XRT), overall prognosis still poor (12–18 mos), but long-term survival more common than in past.

General Considerations
- Optimal treatment not yet defined.
- Initiation of ART essential for any chance of long-term survival.
- High-dose methotrexate is current treatment of choice.
- Whole brain radiation with concomitant corticosteroids also effective.

SELECTED REFERENCES
Corcoran C, Rebe K, can der Plas H, Myer L, Hardie DR. The predictive value of cerebrospinal fluid Epstein-Barr viral load as a marker of primary central nervous system lymphoma in HIV-infected persons. *J Clin Virol*, 2008; 42: 433–6.
Comments: Small series demonstrating the low positive predictive value of EBV viral load for diagnosing PCNSL.

Schroeder PC, Post MJ, Oschatz E, Stadler A, Bruce-Gregorios J, Thurnher MM. Analysis of the utility of diffusion-weighted MRI and apparent diffusion coefficient values in distinguishing central nervous system toxoplasmosis from lymphoma. *Neuroradiology*, 2006; 48: 715–20.
Comments: Discusses role of MRI in distinguishing toxoplasmosis from PCNSL.

Bayraktar S, Bayraktar UD, Ramos JC, Stefanovic A, Lossos IS. Primary CNS lymphoma in HIV positive and negative patients: comparison of clinical characteristics, outcome, and prognostic factors. *J Neurooncol*, 2011; 101: 257–65.
Comments: Retrospective review of 86 patients that highlights worse performance status, higher incidence of hemiparesis at presentation, and continued worse outcome for patients with HIV.

PRIMARY HIV INFECTION

Christopher J. Hoffmann, MD, MPH

PATHOGENS

- HIV-1 and HIV-2 (HIV-2 predominantly found in West Africa).
- HIV-1 divided into 3 groups: M (Main) group (worldwide distribution); O (Outlier) group (primarily West Africa); and N (Non-O, Non-M) group (Cameroon).
- M group further divided into subtypes or clades designated A–K.
- HIV-1 group M subtype B is predominant cause of HIV-1 infection in US.
- Majority of HIV sexually transmitted with MSM the major mode in US. Heterosexual sex is the major mode globally. Injection drug use and mother-to-child transmission are also important modes of infection.
- A "primary HIV-like syndrome" can occur after discontinuation of ART in 5% of individuals.

CLINICAL

- Sx occur in up to 50%–90% of patients within 1–4 wks of infection. Typically "flu-like" illness similar to other viral syndromes (e.g., influenza, mononucleosis) with low-grade fever, malaise, and headache. Additional symptoms may include lymphadenopathy, anorexia, and weight loss. Duration is usually 1–4 wks (median 2 wks).
- Hx: fever ± myalgias, arthralgias, rash, headache, pharyngitis, lymphadenopathy, oral or genital ulcers, thrush.
- Severity of presentation (and number of Sx) associated with peak HIV RNA level (VL).
- Exam: maculopapular rash that may extend to palms and soles (20%–67%), pharyngeal erythema, oral ulcerations, oropharyngeal candidiasis, lymphadenopathy, and splenomegally (each 10%–60%).
- Most common lab abnormalities: thrombocytopenia, leukopenia, elevated liver enzymes, atypical lymphocytes. CD4 may be acutely suppressed, usually rises to near normal after acute illness.
- Rate of CD4 decline to AIDS (<200) from 2 to >20 yrs (without ART). Rate related to VL, multiple other factors are likely important.
- All individuals with acute HIV infection progress to chronic disease.
- Risk of transmission highest during acute/early period because of high VL. In some studies, up to 50% of transmission estimated to be from individuals in acute infection period.

DIAGNOSIS

- ELISA negative or positive with previous negative test and VL>10,000 or p24 antigen positive. Seroconversion occurs 2–8 wks (mean 25 days) after acute infection = test "window period." 97% seropositive by 3 mos.
- VL: sensitivity 100%, specificity 97%. False positive rates as high as 1%, but usually associated with low levels (<1000). Viral RNA can be detected as early as 9 days after infection. VL <100,000 unlikely during acute phase; suggests that patient approaching viral set point. VL<1000 rules out ARS but not HIV infection; retest in several wks with serology + VL.
- VL reaches peak of 100,000–10,000,000. Levels decrease spontaneously without treatment by 2–3 logs approximately 2 wks after onset of Sx.
- p24 antigen: sensitivity 89%, specificity 100%, may be negative 1–2 mos following infection due to formation of Ag-Ab complexes. Can be detected as early as 2 wks after infection.
- Dx of HIV using VL or p24 antigen must be confirmed with WB, which may not be fully positive for several weeks.
- CD4 may be acutely decreased in primary HIV infection (rarely <200).
- Coinfection with STDs common (30%). Test for gonorrhea (p. 414), chlamydia (p. 424), syphilis (p. 30), and HSV (p. 71).

TREATMENT

General Considerations

- Data currently insufficient to guide optimal routine approach. 12+ mos of ART in acute infection followed by interruption may lead to a lower VL set point, though enthusiasm for discontinuation of ART has waned.

- Situations in which starting ART during acute infection is clearly indicated: highly symptomatic acute infection with significant neurological disease.
- Potential risks of early treatment: (1) toxicity, (2) resistance, especially if treatment fails to suppress high viral replication seen in PHI.
- Consider referral to clinical trial if available.

Transmitted Drug Resistance

- In Europe 3%–11% and North America 14%–24% of transmitted HIV has 1 or more resistance mutations.
- Obtain resistance test (genotype) to determine if drug-resistant virus was transmitted for future use when ART is needed.
- Routine testing for transmitted integrase resistance not currently recommended, but may be considered if integrase resistance suspected in source.

FOLLOW-UP

- Obtain CD4 count at time of DX to stage infection and level of immune suppression. Repeat every 3–6 mos. CD4 drawn during PHI may be lower than CD4 setpoint following resolution of acute syndrome.
- Obtain VL at time of DX, and follow regularly (e.g., monthly until setpoint established, then every 3–4 mos).
- If ART initiated, obtain VL at initiation and repeat after 2–8 wks. Decrease of 1 log by 2–8 wks expected if regimen efficacious. Complete suppression (<50) expected by 16–20 wks. Once undetectable, repeat VL every 3–4 mos to evaluate effectiveness and durability of therapy.

SELECTED REFERENCES

Volberding P et al: Antiretroviral therapy in acute and recent HIV infection: a prospective multicenter stratified trial of intentionally interrupted treatment. *AIDS* 23:1987, 2009 Sep. 24 [PMID:19696651].
Comment: Prospective cohort study of two strategies for brief ART use starting at Dx of acute or early HIV. 24% maintained VL <5000 for 24 wks following treatment interruption. This suggests viral set-point benefit of early ART in some pts.

Wawer MJ et al: Rates of HIV-1 transmission per coital act, by stage of HIV-1 infection, in Rakai, Uganda. *J Infect Dis* 191:1403, 2005 May 1 [PMID:15809897].
Comment: Risk of sexual transmission by time after infection.

Opportunistic Infections: Bacterial

BACILLARY ANGIOMATOSIS

Lisa A. Spacek, MD, PhD and David J. Kouba, MD, PhD

PATHOGENS
- *Bartonella henselae* and *quintana* are fastidious gram-negative bacilli, members of the class Alphaproteobacteria.
- *B. henselae*, endemic worldwide, commonly infects feral and domestic cats; vector for cat-to-cat transmission is the cat flea. Transmitted by exposure to cat flea feces, cat scratches. High organism burden in kitten saliva.
- *B. quintana*, etiologic agent of trench fever, spread by body louse.

CLINICAL
- Bacillary angiomatosis (BA), a multifocal angioproliferative disease due to hematogenously disseminated infection, occurs in advanced HIV (CD4 <100). Involves skin and regional lymph nodes. Can cause SQ and osseous lesions, hepatosplenic lesions as well as brain, lung, bowel and uterine cervical lesions.
- Bacteremia presents with fever, malaise, body aches, night sweats, and weight loss. May present as single bout of 5 days fever, recurrent fevers of 5 days duration, or uninterrupted fever.
- *Bartonella* spp. cause cat scratch disease, culture-negative endocarditis, trench fever. *B bacilliformis* infection known as Carrion's disease, includes Oroyo fever (acute hemolytic anemia) and verruga peruana (Peruvian warts).
- Cutaneous lesions: erythematous to violaceous, friable papules or nodules with or without ulceration, usually <1cm diameter.
- SQ lesions: large, skin-colored nodules, several cm in diameter that may ulcerate through epidermis.
- Bacillary peliosis (BP): involves liver, spleen, lymph nodes, presents with fever, nausea, vomiting, diarrhea, abdominal pain, elevated transaminases and/or alk phos.

DIAGNOSIS
- Dx: skin Bx with Warthin-Starry silver stain; Cx on blood or chocolate agar; best results with fresh media, requires >7 days for detection; PCR or RFLP analysis to distinguish *B. henselae* and *B. quintana*.
- Serology available at CDC; however, in patients with low CD4, 25% of *Bartonella* Cx+ patients may not develop Ab.
- DDx: KS, pyogenic granuloma, cherry hemangioma, angiokeratoma.

TREATMENT
- Preferred for BA, bacillary peliosis, bacteremia, and osteomyelitis: erythromycin 500 mg PO or IV 4 ×/day or doxycycline 100 mg PO or IV q12h, treat at least 3 mos.
- Preferred for CNS and severe infections: doxycycline 100 mg PO or IV q12h +/− rifampin (RIF) 300 mg PO or IV q12h, treat × 4 mos.
- Long-term suppression: macrolide or doxycycline as long as CD4 <200. Can be stopped after 3–4 mos and when CD4 >200 for ≥6 mos. Some recommend D/C Rx only if titers decline by fourfold.
- Alternative Rx for BA, bacillary peliosis, bacteremia and osteomyelitis: azithromycin (azithro) 500 mg PO once-daily, clarithromycin 500 mg PO twice-daily.
- Severe Jarisch-Herxheimer-like reaction can occur in 1st 48 hrs of Rx.

FOLLOW-UP
- Follow every 2–3 wks, as treatment responses can vary and length of treatment required is substantial.
- Infections persistent and often relapse due to intraerythrocyte phase of infection.

OTHER INFORMATION
- High-risk patients (CD4 <100) should be counseled regarding the risk of transmission from cats.

SELECTED REFERENCES

Kaplan JE, Benson C, Holmes KH, et al. Guidelines for prevention and treatment of opportunistic infections in HIV-infected adults and adolescents: recommendations from CDC, the National Institutes of Health, and the HIV Medicine Association of the Infectious Diseases Society of America. *MMWR Recomm Rep*; 2009; 58: 1–207.
Comments: No drug trials have evaluated treatment of bartonellosis in HIV+ patients. Erythromycin and doxycycline are first-line Rx. Doxycycline +/− rifampin Rx of choice for CNS, ophthalmic, and severe bartonellosis.

Biswas S, Rolain JM. *Bartonella* infection: treatment and drug resistance. *Future Microbiol*, 2010; 5: 1719–31.
Comments: Recent review of Rx co-authored by JM Rolain, lead author of 2004 treatment guidelines.

Angelakis E, Raoult D, Rolain JM. Molecular characterization of resistance to fluoroquinolones in *Bartonella henselae* and *Bartonella quintana*. *J Antimicrob Chemother*, 2009; 63: 1288–9. Epub 2009 Apr 15.
Comments: In vitro evidence NOT to use FQ to treat *B. henselae* and *B. quintana*.

Maguiña C, Guerra H, Ventosilla P. Bartonellosis. *Clin Derm*, 2009; 27: 271–80.
Comments: Review of infections caused by *Bartonella* spp. authored by members of Instituto de Medicina Tropical Alexander von Humboldt in Lima, Peru. Includes section on BA.

Rolain JM, Brouqui P, Koehler JE, Maguiña C, Dolan MJ, Raoult D. Recommendations for treatment of human infections caused by *Bartonella* species. *Antimicrob Agents Chemother*, 2004; 48: 1921–33.
Comments: The 2004 guidelines, authored by leaders in the field, are cited by CDC OI treatment 2009 recommendations. Detailed account of therapy for *Bartonella* spp. and associated protean diseases.

Koehler J, Sanchez M, Tye S, et al. Prevalence of *Bartonella* infection among human immunodeficiency virus-infected patients with fever. *Clin Infect Dis*, 2003; 37: 559–66.
Comments: A nested, matched case-control study of unexplained febrile illness included 33 HIV+ patients infected with *Bartonella* (median CD4, 35), found BA and elevated alkaline phosphatase associated with *Bartonella* infection (p≤0.03 for both). Noted that BA lesions may be difficult to recognize or diagnose.

MYCOBACTERIUM AVIUM COMPLEX (MAC), DISSEMINATED

Timothy R. Sterling, MD

PATHOGENS

- *M. avium, M. intracellulare.*
- Mode of transmission, acquisition unclear. May be inhaled and/or ingested.
- May be less common in Africa than in developed world.

CLINICAL

- *M. avium*, *M. intracellulare* ubiquitous in environment: water, soil.
- Colonization of GI tract, lungs often precedes disseminated disease.
- Seen almost exclusively in HIV+ patients with CD4 <50; also seen in HIV-negative patients with IFN-gamma receptor deficiency, IL-12, or IL-12 receptor deficiency.
- Signs/Sx: fevers, night sweats, weight loss, abdominal pain, diarrhea.
- Lab findings: anemia, elevated alkaline phosphatase.
- Lung disease uncommon, but can occur.
- Immune reconstitution inflammatory syndrome (IRIS) can occur in patients on ART: focal disease (e.g., lymphadenitis, spinal osteomyelitis) + constitutional Sx.

DIAGNOSIS

- Single blood Cx 90% sensitive; second Cx increases sensitivity slightly.
- Requires 10–21 days for growth in Cx (e.g., BACTEC); DNA probe identifies species.
- Cx from other sterile body sites useful (e.g., bone, lymph node). Positive Cx from sputum or stool often represent colonization rather than infection. Cx of lung Bx specimen generally felt to represent infection.

TREATMENT

Active Disease

- Clarithromycin 500 mg twice daily + EMB 15 mg/kg once daily. Addition of rifabutin (RFB) 300 mg once daily may improve survival (conflicting data—see refs) and decrease risk of macrolide resistance. Consider adding if CD4 <50, high mycobacterial load, or absence of effective ART.
- Azithromycin 500–600 mg once daily + EMB 15 mg/kg once daily.
- Clarithromycin levels increased by IDV, RTV, SQV and other PIs (see page 185).

- Clarithromycin levels decreased by RFB; RFB levels increased by clarithromycin.
- Caution with clarithromycin + EFV—high rates of rash.
- Treatment may be stopped in asymptomatic patients with >12 mos of therapy if CD4 >100 for >6 mos. Restart when CD4 <100.
- Do not use clofazamine; associated with increased mortality risk.
- Consider an FQ (moxifloxacin, levofloxacin, or ciprofloxacin) and/or aminoglycoside (amikacin or SM) when CD4 <50, high mycobacterial load, or drug-resistant disease.
- Drug susceptibility testing useful only for macrolides in persons with prior macrolide exposure.
- Caution with RFB: drug interactions with PIs, NNRTI, itraconazole, etc.

Primary Prophylaxis
- Indicated when CD4 <50; rule out disseminated MAC before initiating prophylaxis.
- **Preferred:** azithromycin 1200 mg weekly (or 600 mg twice weekly) or clarithromycin 500 mg twice daily or azithromycin 600 mg twice weekly.
- **Alternative:** RFB 300 mg once daily. First, rule out active TB.
- Combination of azithro + RFB effective, but greater toxicity.
- Prophylaxis can be stopped when CD4 >100 for >3 mos in response to ART; restart when CD4 <100.
- Combination of clarithromycin + RFB no more effective than clarithromycin alone, but higher rates of adverse effects; do not use this combination.

SELECTED REFERENCES

Kaplan JE, Benson CA, Holmes KH, et al. Guidelines for prevention and treatment of opportunistic infections in HIV-infected adults and adolescents: recommendations from CDC, the National Institutes of Health, and the HIV Medicine Association of the Infectious Diseases Society of America. *MMWR Recomm Rep*, 2009; 58: 1–206.

Comments: Most recent recommendations of CDC, NIH, and HIV Medicine Association of IDSA for treatment and prevention of OIs, including MAC.

NOCARDIOSIS

Michael Melia, MD and Paul G. Auwaerter, MD

PATHOGENS
- Member of aerobic Actinomycetes group. Grows slowly on media. Appear as branching, beaded filamentous gram-positive rods.
- Variably acid fast due to presence of intermediate mycolic acids in cell wall, distinguishes from *Actinomyces*. May produce sulfur granules, especially in mycetomas.
- Ubiquitous in environment. Most infections acquired by inhalation or direct inoculation.
- Many (possibly all) isolates previously identified as "*N. asteroides*" now known to have been misidentified based on current lab standards; type strain of *N. asteroides* does not appear to have been recovered from recent clinical isolates.
- Human pathogens include *N. abscessus* (former *N. asteroides* Type I drug susceptibility pattern), *N. brevicatena/paucivorans* complex (Type II), *N. nova* complex (III), *N. transvalensis* (IV), *N. farcinica* (V; more virulent), and *N. cyriacigeorgica* (VI), as well as *N. brasiliensis* (more common in tropics and actinomycetoma) and *N. pseudobrasiliensis*.
- Each species/complex generally has stereotyped antimicrobial susceptibility patterns.

CLINICAL
- Uncommon pathogen mainly affecting immunocompromised persons with T-cell dysfunction. Suspect in immunocompromised, especially if evaluating fevers with or without pulmonary, CNS, or cutaneous disease. Extracutaneous disease rare in the immunocompetent.
- Subacute presentation common. Most cases occur with CD4 <200. History of corticosteroid use (especially recent, high-dose) and recent CMV disease may be additional risk factors.
- Uncommon in HIV (less than 2% in several case series; up to 5% in autopsy studies). Cases have occurred despite trimethoprim-sulfamethoxazole (TMP-SMX) prophylaxis (for PCP).
- **Pulmonary:** primary site of infection in >2/3 of cases; may mimic TB. Sx nonspecific. Protean radiographic manifestations; can present with nodules, infiltrates (diffuse or

reticulonodular), cavities, or lung abscess. Pulmonary infiltrates (as opposed to nodules) more common in setting of HIV. Granulomata only occasionally seen on Bx.

- **Cutaneous:** cellulitis, ulcers, nodules, ulcers, or lymphocutaneous (sporotrichoid) presentations. Sinus tracts or soft tissue swelling should heighten suspicion. Mycetoma seen in tropics, especially Sout and Central America, mostly *N. brasiliensis*.
- **CNS:** brain abscess or mass lesions, occasionally with granulomas. CNS lesions common, up to 44% in disseminated infection; can be asymptomatic. Spinal cord lesions or meningitis rare.
- **Other sites:** disseminated infection, keratitis, sinusitis, endophthalmitis, bone and joint infection, renal, cardiac, peritonitis, bacteremia.
- Half of cases present with disseminated disease. 20% present with extrapulmonary disease only.

DIAGNOSIS

- Dx: generally made from smear or Cx of respiratory secretions, skin Bx, or aspirate of deep tissue. Bacteremia uncommon. May not grow in Cx, so Dx may require stains of secretions or tissue.
- Gram stain most sensitive method (51%–64%) to visualize *Nocardia* in clinical specimens. Modified acid-fast stain used only to confirm acid fastness of organisms detected by Gram stain. Cx yields range 70%–95% based on reported literature.
- Dx often difficult, may miss on routine specimens. Warn micro lab, especially for respiratory specimens, as selective Thayer-Martin media may increase yield. Multiple specimens also improve yield. Specimens should ideally be held for 2–3 wks before discarding.
- If present, granules should be washed, crushed, and examined for organisms.
- Obtain brain MRI in patients with pulmonary or disseminated disease even without localizing signs or Sx. Firm Dx generally obviates need for brain Bx.
- Consider *Nocardia* in TB suspects not responding to antituberculous therapy.
- Do not dismiss isolate as contaminant or colonizer, though cases described rarely.

TREATMENT

Pulmonary, Disseminated, CNS Infection

- Sulfonamides usually considered part of optimal therapy based on historical case series of successful treatment (primarily HIV-negative patients). Given high rates of intolerance with HIV, consider desensitization in patients with sulfa allergy.
- Sulfonamide-based therapy preferred often because of primarily non-HIV case series suggesting reduced mortality.
- Little data correlating antimicrobial susceptibility testing with clinical outcomes, but appropriate to use susceptibility testing to guide therapy.
- **Preferred (severe disease):** TMP-SMX (10 mg/kg/day TMP + 75 mg/kg/day SMX) IV in 3–4 divided doses PLUS amikacin 7.5 mg/kg IV q12h PLUS imipenem/cilastin 500 mg IV q6h OR ceftriaxone 2 g IV q12–24h. Streamline regimen after 3–6 wks or with clinical improvement.
- **Preferred (mild-moderate disease):** TMP-SMX (15 mg/kg/day TMP + 75 mg/kg/day SMX) IV or PO in 4 divided doses. May consider decreasing TMP/SMX dose (to TMP component 10 mg/kg/day) after clinical improvement.
- **Alternative:** imipenem/cilastatin 500 mg IV q6h + amikacin 7.5 mg/kg q12h × 2–4 wks or clinical improvement followed by oral regimen.
- **Alternative:** 3rd-generation cephalosporins, e.g., ceftriaxone 2 g IV q12–24h IV, offer good CNS penetration; often used in combination with amikacin 7.5 mg/kg q12h × 2–4 wks or clinical improvement followed by PO regimen.
- Monitoring: if on PO sulfonamide-based regimen, obtain 2-hr post-peak sulfonamide level (goal 100–150 mg/L) to guide dosing.
- Surgery or aspiration may be considered for large brain abscesses or extraneural abscesses not responding to medical therapy, although many such abscesses respond to medical therapy alone.
- Rx duration: in immune competent, generally 6 mos; 12 mos for CNS disease. Switch to oral regimen with clinical improvement. Longer parenteral therapy may be needed for slow responses.
- Use indefinite low dose oral suppression in patients with advanced HIV or significant immunosuppression to prevent relapse. **Note:** TMP-SMX DS twice daily likely sufficient, but SS once daily or DS 3 ×/wk insufficient.

Oral Alternatives

- **Caveat:** While sulfonamides and linezolid are nearly always active *in vitro*, antimicrobial susceptibility testing should guide selection of all other oral agents given variable susceptibilities between species.
- Older sulfonamides have good clinical efficacy, but maintain hydration to avoid oliguria, crystalluria.
- Sulfadiazine: 6–12 g/day in 4–6 divided doses, to obtain 2-hr postserum level 100–150 mg/L.
- Sulfisoxazole: 6–12 g/day in 4–6 divided doses, to obtain 2-hr postserum level 100–150 mg/L.
- Minocycline: 100–200 mg PO twice daily.
- Amoxicillin + clavulanate: 500 mg PO 3 times daily.
- Linezolid: 600 mg PO twice daily. Appears to have outstanding activity *in vitro* against *Nocardia* spp., but little clinical data to judge use. Those that have been published support its effectiveness, however.
- Moxifloxacin: 400 mg PO once daily. Some case reports arguing for, others against. Likely the most effective FQ.
- Clarithromycin: 500 mg PO twice daily; successful in one case report.

Species-Specific Treatment Resistance

- *N. abscessus:* often resistant to imipenem.
- *N. nova:* sensitive to ampicillin but not amoxicillin/clavulanate. Very low MICs to imipenem and amikacin. Typically clarithromycin susceptible.
- *N. transvalensis:* generally not sensitive to amikacin, ~10% strains resistant to imipenem. Often susceptible to ciprofloxacin.
- *N. farcinica:* ~10%–20% strains resistant to imipenem, high rates of resistance to amoxicillin, cephalosporins. Fluoroquinolones, particularly moxifloxacin, may be active.
- *N. cyriacigeorgica:* almost always resistant to FQs and clarithromycin; often resistant to ampicillin and amoxicillin-clavulanate.
- *N. brasiliensis:* often resistant to ciprofloxacin and clarithromycin but susceptible to minocycline and amoxicillin-clavulanate.
- *N. pseudobrasiliensis:* usually resistant to minocycline and amoxicillin-clavulanate but susceptible to ciprofloxacin and clarithromycin.
- *N. otitidiscaviarum:* often resistant to sulfonamides. *Nocardia* culture and sensitivity testing best performed in reference labs. Contact local/state health department; CDC Special Pathogens Branch at (404) 639–1510 or email dvd1spath@cdc.gov; or infectious disease specialist Richard Wallace, MD at (903) 877–7680.

Local, Lymphocutaneous Disease

- TMP-SMX (5 mg/kg TMP component) divided in 2–4 doses/day PO.
- Minocycline 100 mg PO twice daily.
- Duration of treatment usually 2–4 mos. Prolonged therapy usually required for mycetoma cure.

FOLLOW-UP

- Expect to see clinical improvement within 7–10 days. Switch to PO a judgment call, but use or parenteral ABx for 3–6 wks common before switch.
- Consider drug resistance as most likely cause of lack of response ± need for drainage or lack of drug penetration.
- Cure rates: 100% soft tissue, 90% pulmonary, as high as 80% for disseminated disease, 13%–60% for CNS disease (despite adequate therapy). Not clear that HIV-related immune suppression makes difference compared to historical series.
- Monitor for relapse for 1 yr post therapy.

SELECTED REFERENCES

Hansen G, Swanzy S, Gupta R, Cookson B, Limaye AP. In vitro activity of fluoroquinolones against clinical isolates of *Nocardia* identified by partial 16S rRNA sequencing. *Eur J Clin Microbiol Infect Dis*, 2008; 27: 115–20.

Comments: Review of *in vitro* activity of FQ against 33 *Nocardia* isolates suggesting <50% of all isolates susceptible, although 88% of *N. farcinica* isolates were susceptible to moxifloxacin (which appears to be most active FQ). CLSI breakpoints for pneumococcus were used given lack of defined *Nocardia* breakpoints for FQ other than ciprofloxacin.

Brown-Elliott BA, Brown JM, Conville PS, Wallace RJ Jr. Clinical and laboratory features of the *Nocardia* spp. based on current molecular taxonomy. *Clin Microbiol Rev*, 2006; 19: 259–82.

Comments: Lengthy review of *Nocardia*, especially focusing on new spp. identified through 16s RNA sequencing. Over 30 spp. now described as causing human disease.

Filice GA. Nocardiosis in persons with human immunodeficiency virus infection, transplant recipients, and large, geographically defined populations. *J Lab Clin Med*, 2005; 145: 156–62.

Comments: Author estimates that risk of *Nocardia* infection in AIDS patients was 140× that of general population, but less than what is seen in the BMT or organ transplant populations.

Lederman ER, Crum NF. A case series and focused review of nocardiosis: clinical and microbiologic aspects. *Medicine (Baltimore)*, 2004; 83: 300–13.

Comments: Sulfonamide-containing regimens remain standard of care, especially for *Nocardia* pulmonary infections.

Wallace RJ Jr, Septimus EJ, Williams TW Jr, et al. Use of trimethoprim-sulfamethoxazole for treatment of infections due to *Nocardia*. *Rev Infect Dis*, 1982; 4: 315–25.

Comments: An older paper from pre-HIV era that helped establish TMP-SMX as standard of care for treating *Nocardia* infections. All patients with cutaneous disease who were adherent to therapy had good clinical response. 92% (23/25) of patients with pulmonary disease were either cured, improving, or were ultimately cured after restarting therapy following initial relapse.

PELIOSIS HEPATIS

Andrea L. Cox, MD, PhD and Christopher J. Hoffmann MD, MPH

PATHOGENS

- **Definition:** blood filled venous pools (lakes) in liver that develop through neo-angiogenesis. Often accompanied by peliosis in the spleen.
- **Causes:** in HIV+ patients usually caused be infection by *Bartonella* spp. In HIV-negative (and some HIV+) patients, caused by anabolic steroids, Castleman disease, Hodgkin lymphoma, leukemia, other malignancies including hepatic tumors.
- **Pathogens:** *Bartonella henselae* and *B. quintana* (formerly known as *Rochalimea henselae* and *R. quintana*).
- *B. henselae*: linked to cat and flea exposure (major cause).
- *B. quintana*: linked to lice exposure (more associated with SQ and bone lesions), homelessness, low-income.
- Small, fastidious, gram-negative aerobic bacilli.

CLINICAL

- Occurs at low CD4 counts; usually <100.
- May be associated with IRIS and higher CD4 count during reconstitution.
- Characterized by multiple, small, dilated blood-filled cavities in hepatic and splenic parenchyma seen on imaging.
- Sx: indolent course of fevers, nausea, abdominal pain, and malaise.
- PE: hepatosplenomegaly, 10%–30% may also have bacillary angiomatosis.
- Lab: alk phos 5–10 × ULN, ALT and AST may be 2 × ULN; thrombocytopenia and pancytopenia have been reported.
- Rarely may cause hypovolemic shock in HIV+ patients due to hepatic hemorrhage.

DIAGNOSIS

- Blood Cx rarely positive for *Bartonella*, Cx sensitivity increases with use of isolator tubes or tubes containing EDTA; specific lab conditions required to enhance yield, so notify lab of suspicion for *Bartonella* infection.
- Definitive Dx by isolating organism from Cx of blood or tissue. Warthin-Starry silver staining shows masses of small, dark staining bacteria. PCR of material from a lesion more sensitive than Cx.
- Abdominal CT: hepatomegaly ± splenomegaly with hypodense lesions scattered throughout liver parenchyma. Other conditions producing similar radiographic findings: lymphoma, disseminated MAC, hepatic KS, and extrapulmonary pneumocystosis.
- Serologic methods (based on studies of cat scratch disease [CSD]): IFA and EIA. IFA IgG titer <1:64 suggests no infection; 1:64–1:256 suggests possible infection; >1:256 suggests active or recent infection. Repeat testing in 10–14 days for titers suggesting possible infection. HIV and low CD4 associated with decreased probability of seropositivity. Anti-*B. henselae* IgM recently shown to be useful in Dx of CSD.

- Given presence of Ab titers to *B. henselae* of >1:256 in 4.8% of healthy controls and lower likelihood of detectable Abs with low CD4, PCR may be more useful in patients with AIDS. Can distinguish between *Bartonella* spp.

TREATMENT
Antibiotic

- Erythromycin 500 mg PO 4 ×/day or doxycycline 100 mg PO twice daily >4 mos (some experts recommend combined erythromycin and doxycycline for severe disease).
- RIF 300 mg IV or PO twice daily may be added to erythromycin and/or doxycycline for severe disease.
- Many drug interactions with RIF and erythromycin.
- Anecdotal evidence of success with other macrolides, including azithromycin.
- Anecdotal evidence of success with FQ.

SELECTED REFERENCES
Maguiña C, Guerra H, Ventosilla P. Bartonellosis. *Clin Derm*, 2009; 27: 271–80.
Comments: Up-to-date review on *Bartonella* infections, including peliosis hepatis.

PNEUMONIA, BACTERIAL

Eric Nuermberger, MD

PATHOGENS

- CD4 >200: *Streptococcus pneumoniae, Haemophilus influenzae, Legionella* spp., *M. tuberculosis, S. aureus*, influenza.
- CD4 50–200: as above + *Pneumocystis jiroveci, Cryptococcus neoformans, Histoplasma capsulatum, Nocardia* spp., *Coccidioides immitis, Mycobacterium kansasii*, Kaposi sarcoma.
- CD4 <50: as above + *Pseudomonas aeruginosa, Aspergillus* spp., *M. avium* complex, cytomegalovirus (though MAC and CMV infrequent causes of pneumonia, even with positive Cx).
- *S. pneumoniae* most common bacterial pathogen.

CLINICAL

- Invasive pneumococcal, *H. influenzae* infections 100 × more common in HIV+ patients vs HIV-negative, and may mimic PCP.
- Risk of legionellosis may be 40 × higher in patients with AIDS vs general population.
- Suspect *P. aeruginosa* when CD4 <50, especially if bronchiectasis, neutropenia, or steroid therapy. Radiographic findings may include consolidation, patchy interstitial infiltrates, and cavitary disease.
- Suspect *S. aureus* (including MRSA) if IDU, cavitary pneumonia, hemoptysis, concomitant influenza, prior history of MRSA colonization, or infection in patient or close contact.
- Suspect TB with Sx >2 wks duration, past + PPD, Hx of TB exposure or residence in endemic country, hemoptysis, apical cavitary disease, hilar adenopathy, miliary or reticulonodular infiltrates. Empiric FQ therapy for community acquired pneumonia (CAP) may delay appropriate Dx of TB and select for resistance to this important second-line drug class.
- Increased mortality in HIV+ patients, especially in setting of CD4 <100, radiographic disease progression, and shock.

DIAGNOSIS

- **Hx:** cough, fever ± sputum production, dyspnea, pleuritic chest pain.
- **PE:** fever, tachycardia, tachypnea, rales, or signs of consolidation.
- **CXR:** showing infiltrate, although CXR pattern not always predictive of etiology.
- Good quality **sputum gram stain** obtained before ABx may establish probable etiology. Any isolation of *Pneumocystis, M. tuberculosis, Legionella, Cryptococcus*, or *Histoplasma* should be considered definitive Dx, but a copathogen could also be present.
- **Blood Cx:** have higher yield in HIV+ patients with bacterial pneumonia (obtain for inpatients). Other rapid tests include *Legionella* and pneumococcal urinary antigens, cryptococcal serum antigen.

TREATMENT

Outpatient (Empiric)

- PORT prediction rule, used to support hospitalization decision in immunocompetent patients (*Arch Intern Med* 161:441, 2001), is not validated for HIV+ patients and should not be used.
- Consider PCP if CD4 <250, no prophylaxis, indolent course, dry cough, diffuse interstitial infiltrates, hypoxemia/desaturation with exercise out of proportion to CXR findings, thrush. Empiric PCP treatment not recommended; pursue diagnosis with induced sputum ± BAL and treat accordingly.
- Recommendations for empiric treatment of bacterial pneumonia listed in no particular order.
- Azithromycin 500 mg PO × 1, then 250–500 mg PO once daily × 5 days or clarithromycin 500 mg PO twice daily or 1g (XL formulation) PO once daily × 7–10 days.
- Cephalosporin (cefuroxime 500 mg, cefpodoxime 400 mg, cefprozil 500 mg, cefditoren 400 mg, cefdinir 300 mg) PO twice daily × 7–10 days.
- Doxycycline 100 mg PO twice daily × 7–10 days.
- FQ (moxifloxacin 400 mg, or levofloxacin 500–750 mg) PO once daily × 5–7 days.
- Avoid macrolide if patient receiving macrolide prophylaxis for MAC.
- When alternatives exist, consider avoiding gemifloxacin in all patients (risk of rash unclear in HIV+ patients) and telithromycin in patients on PIs (adverse interactions).

Inpatient (Empiric)

- Give ABx within 4 hrs.
- **Preferred:** (ceftriaxone 1–2 g IV q day or cefotaxime 1–2 g IV q8h) PLUS (azithromycin 500 mg IV/PO once daily or erythromycin 500–1000 mg IV q6h or clarithromycin 500 mg PO twice daily or 1 g [XL formulation] PO once daily).
- **Preferred:** FQ (moxifloxacin 400 mg or levofloxacin 750 mg) IV/PO once-daily.
- Aspiration: clindamycin 600 mg IV q8h, FQ as above.
- Add PCP coverage (preferably TMP-SMX 5 mg/kg IV/PO q8h ± corticosteroids) if CD4 <250, no PCP prophylaxis, indolent course, dry cough, diffuse interstitial infiltrates, hypoxemia/ desaturation with exercise out of proportion to CXR findings.
- If *Pseudomonas* suspected (CD4 <50 with bronchiectasis, neutropenia, or steroid therapy): [ceftazidime 2 g IV q8h, cefepime 2 g IV q12h, or piperacillin/tazobactam 4.45 g IV q6h or 3.375 g IV q4h] PLUS ciprofloxacin 400 mg IV q12h or [gentamicin/tobramycin 5 mg/kg IV once daily + azith 500 mg IV once daily].
- Duration of therapy determined by etiology or suspected etiology and/or by clinical response. *S. pneumoniae, H. influenzae*: 7–10 days; Enterobacteriaceae, *Legionella*: 14 days; *S. aureus, P. aeruginosa*: 21 days.

FOLLOW-UP

- IV to PO switch when clinically improved, T <100, RR <24, PO >90, tolerating PO.
- For patients not responding to empiric therapy targeting routine bacterial pathogens, consider MRSA, *P. aeruginosa*, PCP, TB, and other mycobacterial infections, cryptococcosis and other fungal infections, KS, lymphoid inter stitial pneumonitis.
- Counsel re: smoking cessation.
- Vaccinate for influenze (all patients) and Pneumococcus (if CD4 >200). No perceived benefit to vaccination against *H. influenzae*.

OTHER INFORMATION

- Recommendations are those of the author and editorial staff, largely compiled from the available literature.

SELECTED REFERENCES

Malinis M, Myers J, Bordon J, et al. Clinical outcomes of HIV-infected patients hospitalized with bacterial community-acquired pneumonia. *Int J Infect Dis,* 2010; 14: e22–7.
Comments: Prospective study of 118 HIV+ patients and 2790 HIV-negative patients hospitalized for bacterial CAP found no difference in length of stay or time to clinical stability. More liver disease and alcohol/drug use seen in HIV+ patients. Majority of HIV+ patients had CD4 >200.

Kaplan JE, Benson CA, Holmes KH, et al. Guidelines for prevention and treatment of opportunistic infections in HIV-infected adults and adolescents: recommendations from CDC, the National Institutes of Health, and the HIV Medicine Association of the Infectious Diseases Society of America. *MMWR Recomm Rep*, 2009; 58: 1–206.

Comments: 2009 guidelines include comment on prevention and treatment of bacterial pneumonia. Recommends pneumococcal vaccination in light of increasing invasive infections with drug-resistant *S. pneumoniae*.

Gordin FM, Roediger MP, Girard PM, et al. Pneumonia in HIV-infected persons: increased risk with cigarette smoking and treatment interruption. *Am J Respir Crit Care Med*, 2008; 178: 630–6.

Comments: Analysis of data from Strategies for Management of Antiretroviral Therapy (SMART), which included 5472 participants at 318 sites in 33 countries. Study patients CD4 >350 at baseline. At 16 mos, 2.2% developed bacterial pneumonia. More pneumonia seen with episodic ART (HR, 1.6; 95% CI, 1.1–2.3) and cigarette smoking (HR, 1.8; 95% CI, 1.1–3.0).

Mandell LA, Wunderink RG, Anzueto A, et al. Infectious Diseases Society of America/American Thoracic Society consensus guidelines on the management of community-acquired pneumonia in adults. *Clin Infect Dis*, 2007; 44 Suppl 2: S27–72.

Comments: Recommendations for management of immunocompetent patients, but document still has wealth of information on laboratory testing, ABx selection and the role of specific pathogens.

Feldman C, Klugman KP, Yu VL, et al. Bacteraemic pneumococcal pneumonia: impact of HIV on clinical presentation and outcome. *J Infect*, 2007; 55: 125–35.

Comments: Large prospective study comparing HIV+ and HIV-negative patients. HIV+ had less severe illness overall and fewer comorbidities, but higher 14-day mortality after adjusting for age and severity of illness. Mortality increased with decreasing CD4 count.

SYPHILIS

Lisa A. Spacek MD, PhD and Khalil G. Ghanem, MD, PhD

PATHOGENS
- *Treponema pallidum:* a spirochete.

CLINICAL
- Occurs at any CD4 count. HIV+ patients may have abnormal serologic results (unusually high titers, false negatives, delayed seroreactivity, higher rates of serologic failure after Rx), but serology can be interpreted in usual manner.
- HIV+ patients at risk for accelerated pace of syphilis and worsening of HIV disease (decreased CD4 and increased VL) with early-stage syphilis. Annual serologic screening recommended.
- **Primary:** Single, painless nodule progresses to indurated ulcer at site of inoculation (chancre); usually evident 14–21 days after exposure; most commonly anogenital or oral.
- **Secondary:** usually 4–10 wks after chancre; maculopapular or papulosquamous eruption, often involves palms/soles (60%); fever, alopecia, mucous patches, condyloma lata; rarely arthritis, glomerulonephritis, hepatitis.
- **Tertiary:** 1/3 of those left untreated develop late sequelae, including cardiovascular syphilis, gummas, paresis, tabes dorsalis.
- **Latent:** no clinical findings but reactive serology; early latent <1 yr duration; late latent >1 yr duration.
- **Neurosyphilis:** Consider in HIV+ patients with neurologic signs or Sx; cranial nerve dysfunction, meningitis, stroke, ΔMS, loss of vibration sense; ocular syphilis should be considered in DDx of visual loss. Can occur at any stage of syphilis.
- Early neurosyphilis (i.e., occurring within the 1st year after infection) is frequent in HIV+ patients.

DIAGNOSIS
- **Definitive:** visualization of motile *T. pallidum* (darkfield examination) or positive DFA test in fluid from lesion or on histopathology (silver stain). Not grown in Cx.
- **Serologic testing:** nontreponemal serology (RPR, VDRL) followed by reflex treponemal testing (FTA-Abs or MHA-TP) establishes presumptive Dx; EIA testing (followed by nontreponemal test titer) becoming more common.
- **Neurosyphilis:** Positive CSF VDRL (30%–70% sensitive) or positive CSF FTA-Abs (in absence of blood contamination); elevated WBC (>10 on ART OR >20 not on ART); or protein (>) 50 mg/dL. A negative CSF FTA-Abs rules out Dx.
- LP recommended in patients with neurologic Sx. Some studies have demonstrated that clinical and CSF abnormalities consistent with neurosyphilis most likely in HIV+ pts with

syphilis and CD4 ≤350 and/or RPR titer of ≥1:32. However, without neurologic Sx, CSF examination in this setting not associated with improved clinical outcomes, and no longer recommended in CDC guidelines.

TREATMENT
- Staging at time of Dx determines Rx; clinical stages may overlap and manifestations are protean; neurologic manifestations can occur with any stage.
- Immune reconstitution using ART may help decrease risk of serological failure and neurosyphilis.
- Parenteral penicillin (PCN) is drug of choice in ALL stages of syphilis; no resistance observed despite decades of PCN use.

Primary or Secondary Syphilis
- **Preferred:** benzathine PCN G 2.4 million units IM ×1.
- **Alternative (PCN allergic):** doxycycline 100 mg twice daily × 14 days.

Latent and Tertiary Syphilis Excluding Neurosyphilis
- Early latent syphilis (<1 yr duration): benzathine PCN G 2.4 million units IM × 1.
- Late latent (>1 yr duration), latent of unknown duration, or tertiary syphilis, excluding neurosyphilis: benzathine PCN G 2.4 million units IM every week × 3 doses.
- **Alternative:** doxycycline 100 mg twice daily × 28 days.

Neurosyphilis
- **Preferred:** aqueous crystalline PCN G 18–24 million units daily as 3–4 million units q4 hrs (or continuously) × 10–14 days.
- **Alternative:** procaine PCN 2.4 million units IM once daily × 10–14 days (along with probenecid 500 mg 4 ×/day). Avoid probenecid in those with sulfa allergy.
- **Alternative:** ceftriaxone 2 g IM/IV once daily × 10–14 days (less clinical experience than with PCN regimens).
- Doxycycline not recommended.
- Some experts recommend benzathine PCN G 2.4 million units every week for 1–3 doses after completion of IV PCN regimen.

AZITHROMYCIN
- Avoid macrolides, resistance documented.

FOLLOW-UP
Assessing "Cure" After Treatment
- Resolution of clinical Sx and appropriate serologic response (decline in nontreponemal titer) are best measures of therapeutic response.
- Errors in *Bicillin* formulation (use of benzathine penicillin G/procaine penicillin G rather than benzathine penicillin G) have led to inadequate treatment of syphilis cases and FDA alert.
- Serofast reponse = reactive treponemal test <1:8 after successful Rx, occurs in 15%–20%, does not represent Rx failure.

Primary/Secondary Syphilis
- RPR (or other nontreponemal test titer) at 3, 6, 9, 12, 24 mos; 4-fold decline from baseline titer 6 mos after therapy expected. Treatment failure requires LP and retreatment with 3 weekly doses of benzathine PCN G if LP is negative.

Latent Syphilis and Neurosyphilis
- RPR (or other nontreponemal test titer) at 6, 12, 18, 24 mos; 4-fold decline from initially high baseline titer (>1:32) at 12–24 mos after therapy expected.
- If follow-up RPR (or other nontreponemal test titer) fails to decline as above, or declines then rises, evaluate for reinfection and for neurosyphilis, then retreat.
- Neurosyphilis: repeat LP every 6 mos until cell count normal. Consider retreatment if cell count has not decreased after 6 mos or if not entirely normal after 2 yrs.

SELECTED REFERENCES
Workowski KA, Berman S; Centers for Disease Control and Prevention. Sexually transmitted diseases treatment guidelines, 2010 *MMWR Recomm Rep*, 2010; 59: 1–110.
Comments: Guidelines recommend LP, ocular slit-lamp, and otologic exam for those with neurologic or ophthalmic signs or symptoms. LP not recommended for CD4 <350, RPR >1:32, unless neurologic signs/Sx present.

Kaplan JE, Benson C, Holmes KH, et al. Guidelines for prevention and treatment of opportunistic infections in HIV-infected adults and adolescents: recommendations from CDC, the National Institutes of Health, and HIV Medicine Association of the Infectious Diseases Society of America. *MMWR Recomm Rep*, 2009; 58: 1–207.

Comments: CSF exam recommended in patients with neuro/ophtho signs or Sx, active tertiary syphilis, treatment failure, and late-latent syphilis. Some specialists recommend CSF exam for all HIV+ patients with syphilis, regardless of stage, particularly if CD4 <350 and RPR 1:32.

Ghanem KG, Moore RD, Rompalo AM, Erbelding EJ, Zenilman JM, Gebo KA. Antiretroviral therapy is associated with reduced serologic failure rates for syphilis among HIV-infected patients. *Clin Infect Dis*, 2008; 47: 258–65.

Comments: In this study of 231 cases of syphilis, CD4 <200 at time of syphilis Dx associated with 2.5-fold increased risk of serologic failure. Receipt of ART associated with 60% reduction in rate of serologic failure independent of concomitant CD4 response.

Ghanem KG. Evaluation and management of syphilis in the HIV-infected patient. *Curr Infect Dis Rep*, 2010; 12: 140–6.

Comments: Review emphasizes frequency of Dx early symptomatic neurosyphilis in HIV+ patients. Supports CSF exam in those with low CD4 ≤350 and high titer ≥1:32.

Ghanem KG, Moore RD, Rompalo AM, Erbelding EJ, Zenilman JM, Gebo KA. Neurosyphilis in a clinical cohort of HIV-1-infected patients. *AIDS*, 2008; 22: 1145–51.

Comments: In this study of 41 HIV+ patients with neurosyphilis, risk factors included CD4 <350 at time of syphilis Dx, a RPR titer >1:128, and male sex. Use of ART before syphilis infection reduced odds of neurosyphilis by 65%. 63% of cases presented with early neurosyphilis, and median time to neurosyphilis Dx was 9 mos.

Stoner BP. Current controversies in the management of adult syphilis. *Clin Infect Dis*, 2007; 44 Suppl 3: S130–46.

Comments: Summarizes current controversies in syphilis management and current evidence bases for addressing them.

Marra CM, Maxwell CL, Smith SL, et al. Cerebrospinal fluid abnormalities in patients with syphilis: association with clinical and laboratory features. *J Infect Dis*, 2004; 189: 369–76.

Comments: In clinical series of 326 patients with syphilis referred for LP, RPR titer >1:32, HIV+, CD4 <350 all independently associated with neurosyphilis.

TUBERCULOSIS, LATENT

Timothy R. Sterling, MD

PATHOGENS
- *M. tuberculosis.*
- 1/3 of world's population infected with *M. tuberculosis.*

CLINICAL
- TB risk in HIV+ person as high as 40% after recent exposure to active case.
- Risk of TB 10% per year in PPD+/HIV+ persons.
- ART decreases TB risk in PPD+/HIV+ by 80%, but risk still higher than in HIV-negatives.
- INH in conjunction with ART effective in decreasing TB risk.

DIAGNOSIS
- All HIV+ persons should have baseline tuberculin skin test (TST) or interferon gamma release assay (IGRA). Repeat annually thereafter if at increased risk of TB exposure.
- IGRA: *QuantiFERON-TB Gold*, *QuantiFERON-TB Gold In-tube*, and *T.SPOT.TB* are FDA-approved for Dx of TB infection and disease, but cannot distinguish between the two. Decreased sensitivity in HIV+ persons, particularly when CD4 < 200.
- Indications for treatment of latent infection (TLI): >5 mm induration on TST, positive IGRA, or close contact to an active case (regardless of TST status or prior treatment for latent infection).
- Exclude active TB before TLI. Obtain CXR if TST or IGRA skin test +; sputum AFB smear and Cx if CXR abnormal and/or patient symptomatic. HIV+ persons can be asymptomatic, which can make detection of TB difficult.
- Anergy testing with TST not indicated (not reliable in HIV+ persons).

TREATMENT
Adults
- **Preferred:** INH 5 mg/kg (300-mg max) PO once daily × 9 mos. Pyridoxine (vitamin B6) 50 mg once daily may decrease neuropathy risk.

- **Alternative:** RIF 10 mg/kg (600-mg max) once daily × 4 mos. For persons who are contacts of INH-resistant, RIF-susceptible TB. Limited data on effectiveness and tolerability. Caution in HIV-infected individuals, in whom risk of undiagnosed active TB is higher. DO NOT treat active TB with RIF alone.
- Short-course RIF + pyrazinamide (PZA) contraindicated due to risk of severe hepatotoxicity and death.
- Short-course INH + rifapentine not recommended in pts on PI- and NNRTI-based ARVs.
- RIF interactions: PIs and NNRTIs, methadone, oral contraceptives, anticoagulants, steroids, etc.

Children
- **Preferred:** INH 10–20 mg/kg (300-mg max) PO once daily × 9 mos. Pyridoxine generally not necessary.

Monitoring for Toxicity
- INH: baseline LFTs in patients at increased risk of hepatotoxicity (HIV+, known liver disease, alcoholics, pregnant or <3 mos postpartum).

FOLLOW-UP
- Completion rates of TLI generally poor (30%–60%). Encourage adherence given high risk of progression to active TB.
- Cource of TLI does not provide adequate protection in HIV+ patients if there is subsequent exposure to active TB case; another course is indicated.

SELECTED REFERENCES

Panel on Antiretroviral Guidelines for Adults and Adolescents. Guidelines for the use of antiretroviral agents in HIV-1-infected adults and adolescents. Department of Health and Human Services; January 1, 2011; 1–166. http://aidsinfo.nih.gov/content-files/AdultandAdolescentGL.pdf. Accessed July 17, 2011.
Comments: Sensitivity of TST and IGRA low, particularly in HIV+-patients with CD4 <200. Patients with a negative TST or IGRA when CD4 <200 should have test repeated when CD4 >200.

World Health Organization. Guidelines for intensified tuberculosis case-finding and isoniazid preventive therapy for people living with HIV in resource-constrained settings. World Health Organization; 2011; 1–187. http://whqlibdoc.who.int/publications/2011/9789241500708_eng.pdf. Accessed Juy 17, 2011.
Comments: In resource-constrained settings, HIV+ adults and adolescents should be screened for TB with a clinical algorithm, and those who do not report any one of the symptoms of current cough, fever, weight loss, or night sweats are unlikely to have active TB and should be offered INH. Persons with any one of these 4 Sx should be evaluated for TB and other diseases.

Mazurek GH et al: Updated guidelines for using Interferon Gamma Release Assays to detect Mycobacterium tuberculosis infection - United States, 2010. *MMWR Recomm Rep* 59: 1, 2010 June 25.
Comments: Updated CDC guidelines for use of *QuantiFERON-TB Gold, QuantiFERON-TB Gold In-tube,* and *T.SPOT.TB.*

Kaplan JE, Benson C, Holmes KH, et al. Guidelines for prevention and treatment of opportunistic infections in HIV-infected adults and adolescents: recommendations from CDC, the National Institutes of Health, and the HIV Medicine Association of the Infectious Diseases Society of America. *MMWR Recomm Rep,* 2009; 58: 1–207.
Comments: Recommendations from CDC, the NIH, and the HIV Medicine Association of the IDSA. Includes TB infection and disease.

Golub JE, Pronyk P, Mohapi L, et al. Isoniazid preventive therapy, HAART and tuberculosis risk in HIV-infected adults in South Africa: a prospective cohort. *AIDS,* 2009; 23: 631–6.
Comments: Benefit of INH + ART.

Sterling TR. New approaches to the treatment of latent tuberculosis. *Semin Respir Crit Care Med,* 2008; 29: 532–41.
Comments: Review of current therapy for latent infection.

Pai M, Zwerling A, Menzies D. Systematic review: T-cell-based assays for the diagnosis of latent tuberculosis infection: an update. *Ann Intern Med,* 2008; 149: 177–84.
Comments: Excellent review of IGRAs (interferon gamma release assays).

TUBERCULOSIS, ACTIVE

Timothy R. Sterling, MD

PATHOGENS
- *M. tuberculosis* (**M. tb**).
- *M. bovis*.

CLINICAL
- Hx: cough >2 wks, fever, night sweats, weight loss, hemoptysis, SOB, chest pain.
- CXR: upper lobe infiltrate classic (may be cavitary); atypical presentations in children or HIV+ adults; lymphadenopathy.
- Clinical and radiographic manifestations may be atypical in HIV+ persons, especially with low CD4 count: lower-lobe infiltrates, adenopathy alone, and even normal CXR.
- Extrapulmonary disease more common in HIV+ patients, especially with low CD4 counts.
- TB often subclinical in HIV+ patients, particularly with low CD4. Disease can be "unmasked" on ART.
- IRIS may result in worsening of TB symptoms on TB and HIV treatment.

DIAGNOSIS
- Characteristic symptoms (see previous Clinical section).
- **Sputum AFB smear:** 50% sensitive. Lower sensitivity in HIV+ patients.
- **AFB Cx:** 80% sensitive.
- **Nucleic acid amplification (NAA) tests:** sensitive, specific for sputum AFB smear +; less sensitive for smear-negative sputum (negative NAA does not exclude TB if sputum AFB smear-negative); expensive; also low sensitivity for nonrespiratory specimens.
- **Interferon-gamma release assays (IGRAs):** *QuantiFERON-TB Gold In-tube* and *T.SPOT. TB* now FDA-approved. Limited data in HIV+; *T.SPOT.TB* probably more sensitive than *QuantiFERON-TB Gold In-tube* in HIV+. Does not distinguish between *M. tb* infection and TB disease.
- New tests not yet FDA-approved but endorsed by WHO:
  - **Line-probe assays:** (e.g., *MTBDRplus* and *MTBDRsl* by Hain Lifescience) can detect *M. tb* in Cx or directly in clinical specimens; can also detect genotypic mutations associated with resistance: INH, RIF, injectable agents, FQ.
  - *GeneXpert MTB/RIF*: test can detect *M.tb* and RIF resistance directly in clinical specimens in approximately 2 hr.

TREATMENT
Adults
- INH 5 mg/kg (300-mg max) + RIF 10 mg/kg (600-mg max) + PZA 15–30 mg/kg (2-g max) + EMB 15–25 mg/kg (1.6-g max) + pyridoxine (vitamin B6) 50 mg—all PO once daily × 8 wks, then INH + RIF (same doses PO once daily); see below for duration.
- Can use RFB in place of RIF in persons on PIs, NNRTIs, methadone. Dose adjustments necessary (see specific ART module for drug dosing recommendations).
- Check drug susceptibilities; treat with at least 2 drugs to which isolate is susceptible.
- Rx duration determined by site of disease, response to therapy. Pulmonary and most extrapulmonary: 6 mos (except if at high risk for relapse—see Follow-up section); CNS: 12 mos; bone/joint: 9–12 mos.
- Refer to health department so patient can receive directly observed therapy (DOT).
- Dosing less frequent than daily is possible if via DOT.
- RIF 10 mg/kg (600-mg max) can be given with EFV (see p. 277) (standard 600-mg dose; may need to increase to 800 mg, especially if patient weighs >60 kg).

Children
- INH 10–15 mg/kg (300-mg max) + RIF 10–20 mg/kg (600-mg max) + PZA 15–30 mg/kg (2-g max) + EMB 15–20 mg/kg (1-g max)—all PO once daily.
- Use EMB only if can monitor visual acuity (e.g., >8 yrs) or drug resistance strongly suspected.
- Can use RFB in place of RIF in persons on HIV PIs, NNRTI. Dose adjustments necessary.
- Check drug susceptibilities; treat with at least 2 drugs to which isolate is susceptible.
- Rx duration determined by site of disease, response to therapy.
- Refer to health department so patient can receive DOT.

- Dosing less frequent than daily is possible if via DOT.

Isolation

- Respiratory isolation for cough >2 wks + abnormal CXR.
- Can discontinue if 3 sputa (expectorated or induced) are smear-negative. However, if high suspicion of active TB, start treatment.
- If smear + or on Rx, can discontinue isolation after 2 wks of Rx plus clinical improvement, plus AFB smear-negative (3 sputum specimens).

General Treatment Issues

- Refer all cases to local health department for treatment and contact investigation.
- DOT preferred for both adults and children.
- Caution regarding drug interactions, toxicity, paradoxical worsening (IRIS). Consult expert.
- If HIV+ and CD4 <100, give daily TB treatment for 1st 60 days, then no less frequent than 3 ×/wk.
- When to start ART in relation to starting TB therapy (2011 DHHS Guidelines):
  - If already on ART at time of TB diagnosis, continue ART and start TB Rx.
  - If not on ART, timing of initiation depends on CD4 count:
    - CD4 <200: start ART within 2–4 wks of TB Rx.
    - CD4 200–500: start ART within 2–4 wks, or at least within 8 wks, of TB Rx.
    - CD4 >500: start ART within 8 wks of TB Rx.

FOLLOW-UP

- Patients should be followed by health department while on therapy. Seen monthly for signs/Sx of toxicity, and sputum Cx to document negative Cx. Generally not followed after completion of therapy, but should return if signs/Sx of TB recur.
- Based on ATS/CDC/IDSA Guidelines (Blumberg). Includes a new recommendation to extend treatment to 9 mos if cavitary disease plus Cx + after 2 mos of Rx.

SELECTED REFERENCES

Centers for Disease Control and Prevention. Managing drug interactions in the treatment of HIV-related tuberculosis. *http://www.cdc.gov/tb/publications/guidelines/TB_HIV_Drugs/default.htm.* Accessed July 17, 2011.
Comments: Most current recommendations re: drug-drug interactions and dose adjustments. Web site is updated regularly.

Sterling TR, Pham PA, Chaisson RE. HIV infection-related tuberculosis: clinical manifestations and treatment. *Clin Infect Dis*, 2010; 50 Suppl 3; S223–30.
Comments: Update on clinical manifestations, treatment issues, and drug interactions.

Panel on Antiretroviral Guidelines for Adults and Adolescents. Guidelines for the use of antiretroviral agents in HIV-1-infected adults and adolescents. Department of Health and Human Services; January 1, 2011; 1–166. http://aidsinfo.nih.gov/contentfiles/AdultandAdolescentGL.pdf. Accessed July 17, 2011.
Comments: Most recent recommendations regarding timing of ART in relation to anti-TB therapy, as well as drug-drug interactions. Have not incorporated the most recent updates from CROI 2011.

Abdool Karim SS, Naidoo K, Grobler A, et al. Timing of initiation of antiretroviral drugs during tuberculosis therapy. *N Engl J Med*, 2010; 362: 697–706.
Comments: Initiating ART during TB treatment decreased risk of death by 56% compared to waiting until after completion of anti-TB Rx. Benefit of starting within 4 wks (vs 8–12 wks) of TB Rx start seen only among patients with CD4 <50

Blanc FX, Sok T, Laureillard D, et al. The CAMELIA trial: CAMbodian early vs. late introduction of antiretrovirals (CAMELIA) trial. Paper presented at: Late Breaker Session B-1, XVIII IAS Conference; July 22, 2010; Vienna, Austria.
Comments: Among persons with low CD4 (median 25), risk of death was 34% lower in persons starting ART within 2 wks of anti-TB therapy compared to persons starting ART 8 wks after anti-TB therapy.

Havlir D, Ive P, Kendall M, et al. International randomized trial of immediate vs early ART in HIV+ patients treated for TB: ACTG 5221 STRIDE study. Paper presented at: Conference on Retroviruses and Opportunistic Infections; February 28, 2011; Boston, MA.
Comments: Primary endpoint was death or new AIDS-defining event among persons starting ART within 2 wks vs 8–12 wks after starting anti-TB Rx. Benefit of starting at 2 seen only among persons with CD4 <50. IRIS risk high.

Boehme CC, Nabeta P, Hillemann D, et al. Rapid molecular detection of tuberculosis and rifampin resistance. *N Engl J Med*, 2010; 363: 1005–15.
Comments: Performing test once was 98% sensitive for smear-positive pulmonary TB and 73% sensitive for smear-negative TB; performing 3 tests increased sensitivity to 90% for smear-negative disease. Detection of rifampin resistance was 98% sensitive and specific.

Mazurek GH, Jereb J, Vernon A, et al. Updated guidelines for using interferon gamma release assays to detect *Mycobacterium tuberculosis* infection - United States, 2010. *MMWR Recomm Rep*, 2010; 59: 1–25.
Comments: Updated CDC guidelines for use of *QuantiFERON-TB Gold, QuantiFERON-TB Gold In-tube*, and *T.SPOT.TB*.

Maartens G, Wilkinson RJ. Tuberculosis. *Lancet,* 2007; 370: 2030–43.
Comments: Thorough review of TB.

Havlir DV, Getahun H, Sanne I, Nunn P. Opportunities and challenges for HIV care in overlapping HIV and TB epidemics. *JAMA*, 2008; 300: 423–30.
Comments: Recent review of TB/HIV issues.

CANDIDIASIS, ESOPHAGEAL

Michael Melia, MD and Amita Gupta, MD, MHS

PATHOGENS
- *Candida albicans.*
- *Candida glabrata.*
- *Candida tropicalis.*
- *Candida parapsilosis.*
- *Candida krusei.*
- *Candida lusitaniae.*

CLINICAL
- Generally seen in patients with CD4 <100; AIDS-defining illness.
- Sx: retrosternal pain or discomfort, dysphagia and/or odynophagia, usually without fever.
- Occurs in 20%–40% of all AIDS patients.
- Candidiasis is most common cause of esophageal candidiasis (EC) with HIV infection, but CMV, HSV, and aphthous ulcerations can cause similar Sx.
- Most common cause is *C. albicans.* While there is increasing recognition of non-albicans *Candida* spp. with azole-resistance especially *C. glabrata*, as cause of treatment-refractory EC, most isolates with azole resistance are found in patients with extensive prior azole exposure.
- Approximately half of recurrent cases are caused by same strain of *Candida.*
- Refractory EC arises in 4%–5% of HIV+ patients who have CD4 <50 and multiple prior exposures to azole antifungals. Treatment failure defined as EC that persists after 7–14 days of usually appropriate therapy.
- Development of systemic candidiasis due to EC unusual in HIV+ patients.
- IRIS not reported in association with mucosal candidiasis.

DIAGNOSIS
- Dx typically presumptive based on symptoms of retrosternal pain, dysphagia and/or odynophagia, with the presence of oropharyngeal candidiasis on exam.
- Endoscopy indicated for unusual presentations or lack of response to azole within several days.
- Endoscopy: Superficial esophageal mucosal ulcerations with white plaques, biopsy findings or microscopy from brush samples.
- Wet mount microscopy or histopathology useful for evaluation of yeast and/or pseudohyphae. Fungal cx of esophageal lesions rarely required but allows identification of infecting species and resistance testing, especially if poor response to azole therapy. Cx of limited use in Dx of oral candidiasis due to colonization.
- Resistance testing for *Candida* spp. has been standardized, with defined breakpoints for fluconazole, itraconazole, and flucytosine (5-FC).
- Less resistance now seen in the HAART era to fluconazole (45% → 10%) and itraconazole (37% → 7%) among oropharyngeal isolates of *Candida* spp.

TREATMENT
First-line (Preferred) Therapy
- Fluconazole 200–400 mg/day PO or 400 mg/day IV.
- Itraconazole 200 mg/day PO (oral soln preferred) or IV.
- IV azoles may be needed for patients w/ severe dysphagia/odynophagia.
- Empiric trial of fluconazole (prior to endoscopy) indicated if HIV+, CD4<200, oropharyngeal thrush, and/or esophageal symptoms.
- Fluconazole superior to ketoconazole, itraconazole capsules, and 5-FC.
- Always review for drug-drug interactions prior to prescribing any azole.
- All therapy should be continued for 14–21 days.

Second-line (Alternate) Therapy
- Itraconazole oral soln 200 mg/day PO is the agent of choice for clinical fluconazole failures, as up to 80% respond.
- Posaconazole 400 mg PO twice daily.
- Voriconazole 200 mg PO or IV twice daily.
- Caspofungin 70 mg IV × 1 then 50 mg IV once daily, or micafungin 150 mg once daily or anidulafungin 200 mg IV once daily.
- Amphotericin B (AmB) 0.6 (0.3–0.7) mg/kg IV once daily.
- Lipid amphotericin 3–5 mg/kg IV once daily.
- Review for drug-drug interactions prior to prescribing any antifungal.
- All therapy should be continued for 14–21 days.

Resistant or Refractory Candidiasis
- Itraconazole soln effective in 55%–80% of patients who have inadequate responses to fluconazole.
- Voriconazole as effective as fluconazole and can be tried for fluconazole failures, but associated with more adverse events.
- Posaconazole 400 mg PO twice-daily × 28 days effective in 75% of patients who have inadequate response to azoles, but given broader antifungal spectrum and cost, use for EC should be limited to this setting only.
- Caspofungin or amphotericin should be limited to patients with Cx-confirmed fluconazole-resistant candidiasis or clinical failure with fluconazole and itraconazole.
- Little data on other echinocandins (anidulafungin, micafungin), but should be effective, although echinocandins are associated with higher relapse rates than fluconazole.
- Amphotericin lipid formulations or AmB also usually effective.

Prophylaxis
- Primary prophylaxis not recommended due to cost, lack of attributable morbidity, potential for development of resistance, drug interactions, and efficacy of therapy for acute disease.
- Consider chronic (secondary) prophylaxis with daily or thrice-weekly fluconazole (100–200 mg) for patients with recurrent esophagitis (at least 3 episodes per year).
- For patients with recurrent EC refractory to fluconazole, secondary prophylaxis with an effective agent (e.g., voriconazole or posaconazole) should be continued until immune reconstitution occurs with ART because of high relapse rates off treatment.
- Best approach to prophylaxis by far is immune reconstitution with ART.

FOLLOW-UP
- 85%–90% respond within 7–14 days.
- Endoscopy for Bx and Cx required after failure of empiric antifungal therapy to look for other causes of esophagitis.
- If not responding: can increase fluconazole dose as some *Candida* spp. Have intermediate MIC to fluconazole and respond to higher dose, or use alternative azole (itraconazole, voriconazole, or posaconazole) or IV therapy (caspofungin, amphotericin).
- ART important to reduce risk of disease occurrence, relapse.
- No specific data on discontinuation of secondary (chronic maintenance) if instituted, but based on other OI experience, consider discontinuation when CD4>200 on ART.
- Oral azoles can be associated with nausea, vomiting, diarrhea, and transaminase elevations. Consider monitoring if on azole therapy >3 wks.

OTHER INFORMATION
- Pregnant patients should not be treated with azoles or echinocandins.
- Neonates born to women on chronic AmB should be evaluated for renal failure and hypokalemia.
- IRIS not reported in association with mucosal candidiasis.

SELECTED REFERENCES

Pappas PG, Kauffman CA, Andes D, et al. Clinical practice guidelines for the management of candidiasis: 2009 update by the Infectious Diseases Society of America. *Clin Infect Dis*, 2009; 48: 503–35.

Comments: Evidence-based, systematic literature review regarding the management of all manifestations of candidiasis, including oropharyngeal and esophageal. Oral fluconazole is the agent of choice for EC; IV medications (fluconazole, amphotericin, echinocandin) should be reserved for persons unable to tolerate oral medications.

Kaplan JE, Benson CA, Holmes KH, et al. Guidelines for prevention and treatment of opportunistic infections in HIV-infected adults and adolescents: recommendations from CDC, the National Institutes of Health, and the HIV Medicine Association of the Infectious Diseases Society of America. *MMWR Recomm Rep*, 2009; 58: 1–206.

Comments: US guidelines regarding use of azoles for prophylaxis of esophageal candidiasis with strength of evidence rating.

CANDIDIASIS, OROPHARYNGEAL

Amita Gupta, MD, MHS

PATHOGENS
- *Candida albicans*: common commensal in human mouth, colon, and vagina. Most common cause of oropharyngeal candidiasis (OPC).
- Other *Candida* spp. can cause OPC, including *C. tropicalis*, *C. glabrata*, and *C. krusei*. Some species may not respond as well to standard therapy.

CLINICAL
- Characterized by white pseudomembranous painless plaques that are easily scraped off ("thrush") of buccal, pharyngeal, or tongue areas, and/or erythematous mucosal patches, or angular cheilitis.
- Risk factors include CD4 <250, recent ABx, diabetes mellitus, and steroid use.
- Recurrent disease caused by same strain of *Candida* in ~50%.
- Sx can include oral pain and altered taste perception but many patients are asymptomatic. Retrosternal dysphagia or odynophagia suggest esophageal involvement and should trigger clinicians to use systemic therapy rather than topical antifungals.
- DDx includes oral hairy leukoplakia. Erythematous mucosal patches of candidiasis can be confused with oral HSV and aphthous ulcerations. White coated tongue without buccal or palate lesions less likely to be thrush.
- Indication for initiation of PCP prophylaxis and ART.

DIAGNOSIS
- Dx usually made based on clinical appearance.
- Microscopic examination with KOH prep useful for evaluation of yeast and/or pseudohyphae.
- Fungal Cx of mucosal lesions allows identification of infecting *Candida* spp. and enables resistance testing if response to therapy is poor. Cx not useful for Dx, however, as positive Cx may be due to colonization.
- Resistance testing for yeasts has been standardized with CLSI M27-A2 methodology with defined breakpoints for *Candida* spp. to fluconazole, itraconazole, and 5-FC.
- Significant decline in resistance to fluconazole and itraconazole in HAART era.

TREATMENT
Acute Disease: Preferred Therapy
- Clotrimazole: troche 10 mg PO 5×/day for 7–14 days after clinical improvement (dissolve in mouth).
- Nystatin: 500,000 U PO 5×/day swish and swallow for 7–14 days after clinical improvement.
- Fluconazole: 100 mg PO once daily × 7–14 days.
- Miconazole: mucoadhesive tab PO once daily.

Acute Disease: Alternative Therapy
- Fluconazole: 100–200 mg PO once daily × 7–14 days after clinical improvement.
- Itraconazole (liquid or capsule): 200 mg/day PO (swish and swallow liquid formulation) × 7–14 days after clinical improvement.
- AmB oral suspension (100 mg/mL): 1 mL PO 4 times a day swish and swallow × 7–14 days after clinical improvement. No longer commercially available in US but can be made by a compounding pharmacy.
- AmB: 0.3 mg/kg per day IV × 7–14 days after clinical improvement.
- Caspofungin: 50 mg/day IV × 7–14 days after clinical improvement.
- Posaconazole: oral soln 400 mg PO twice daily × 1 day then once daily, but given broad spectrum and high cost, not recommended for this indication (though listed in 2009 CDC OI guidelines).

Suppression: Preferred Therapy

- Not generally recommended. Considerations for suppressive therapy should include severity and frequency of relapse, presence of esophagitis, cost, drug-drug interactions, risk of azole resistance, and potential for pregnancy.
- **Preferred:** fluconazole 100 mg PO once daily or 200 mg PO 3 × weekly.
- **Alternative:** itraconazole (liquid or capsule) 200 mg PO once daily. Liquid (swish and swallow) preferred as it provides topical therapy and higher systemic levels.
- Patients without esophagitis can sometimes be suppressed with chronic topical therapy (e.g., clotrimazole). Less convenient, but decreased risk of azole resistance.
- ART is most effective treatment for recurrent OPC.

OTHER INFORMATION

- Pregnant patients should not be treated with azoles. Echinocandins, clotrimazole and nystatin are category C in pregnancy.
- Tea tree oil has *in vitro* activity against *Candida* spp., even those resistant to azoles.
- *In vitro* azole resistance associated with prolonged prior azole exposure, CD4 <50.
- IRIS not reported in association with OPC.

SELECTED REFERENCES

Kaplan JE, Benson CA, Holmes KH, et al. Guidelines for prevention and treatment of opportunistic infections in HIV-infected adults and adolescents: recommendations from CDC, the National Institutes of Health, and the HIV Medicine Association of the Infectious Diseases Society of America. *MMWR Recomm Rep*, 2009; 58: 1–206.
Comments: US guidelines regarding use of antifungals for oropharyngeal candidiasis with strength of evidence rating.

Egusa H, Soysa NS, Ellepola AN, Yatani H, Samaranayake LP. Oral candidosis in HIV-infected patients. *Curr HIV Res*, 2008; 6: 485–99.
Comments: General review.

CANDIDIASIS, VULVOVAGINAL

Barbara E. Wilgus, MSN, CRNP

PATHOGENS

- *Candida albicans.*
- *Candida glabrata.*
- Other non-*albicans Candida* spp.

CLINICAL

- Symptomatic vulvovaginal candidiasis more frequent in HIV+ women and correlates with degree of immunodeficiency.
- 5%–10% of immunocompetent women have recurrent episodes, defined as >4 episodes/yr.
- Uncomplicated vulvovaginal candidiasis affects 90% of HIV-infected women; occurs at higher CD4 counts than other forms of candidiasis.
- Among HIV-infected women, severity, frequency, duration, and response to standard therapy may be altered with advanced immunosuppression.
- 80% caused by *C. albicans.*
- 10%–20% caused by *C. glabrata* or other non-*albicans* spp.
- Sx: pruritis, discharge, vulvar burning, external dysuria, erythema, and labial swelling. Vulvovaginal candidiasis associated with increased cell-associated and cell-free HIV RNA in cervicovaginal secretions.
- Possibility of increased viral shedding in presence of concomitant candidiasis associated with increase in concentration of leukocytes in vagina.

DIAGNOSIS

- Microscopic examination of vaginal discharge with 10% KOH or Gram stain demonstrates presence of yeast or pseudohyphae.
- Vaginal fungal Cx may be useful to demonstrate presence of non-*albicans* spp. or resistant strains.
- *Candida* may also be identified on cytologic specimens.

TREATMENT
Principles of Therapy
- Should be treated similarly in HIV+ and HIV-negative women.
- Patients with recurrent candidiasis may benefit from long-term prophylactic therapy with fluconazole 150 mg PO weekly × 6 mos or topical clotrimazole 200 mg twice weekly.
- Oil-based suppositories and creams have adverse effect on latex condoms, which could cause condom failure.
- Treatment of sex partners generally not necessary, as not acquired through sexual intercourse (see Follow-up below).

Topical Therapy
- Miconazole: 2% cream 5 g intravaginally once-daily × 7 days, or one 100-mg vaginal suppository once-daily × 7 days, or one 200-mg vaginal suppository once-daily × 3 days.
- Butoconazole: 2% cream 5 g intravaginally once daily × 3 days, or 2% cream 5 g (Butoconazole 1-sustained release) as single intravaginal application.
- Clotrimazole: 1% cream 5 g intravaginally once daily × 7–14 days, or one 100-mg vaginal tab once daily × 7 days, or two 100-mg vaginal tabs once daily × 3 days, or one 500-mg vaginal tab as single application.
- Nystatin: one 100,000-unit vaginal tab once-daily × 14 days.
- Terconazole: 0.4% cream 5 g intravaginally once daily × 7 days, or 0.8% cream 5 g intravaginally once-daily × 3 days, or one 80-mg vaginal suppository once-daily × 3 days.
- Tioconazole: 6.5% ointment 5 g intravaginally as single application.

Systemic Therapy
- Fluconazole: 150 mg PO as single dose.

FOLLOW-UP
- Test of cure generally unnecessary if asymptomatic after treatment.
- Consider fungal Cx to identify strain if persistent Sx after treatment.
- Treatment of sex partners not recommended, but may be considered in women who have recurrent infection.
- A minority of male sex partners may have balantitis. Treat with topical antifungal agents.

SELECTED REFERENCES
Johnson LF, Lewis DA. The effect of genital tract infections on HIV-1 shedding in the genital tract: a systematic review and meta-analysis. *Sex Transm Dis*, 2008; 35: 946–59.
Comments: Good overview of impact of all genital tract infections on HIV viral shedding.

Workowski KA, Berman SM, Centers for Disease Control and Prevention. Sexually transmitted diseases treatment guidelines, 2010. *MMWR Recomm Rep*, 2010; 59: 1–110.
Comments: Included in CDC guidelines even though non-STD, comprehensive review of Dx and Rx, 2010 is most recent CDC update.

COCCIDIOIDOMYCOSIS

Amita Gupta, MD, MHS

PATHOGENS
- *Coccidioides immitis.*
- *Coccidioides posadasii.*
- Dimorphic fungi existing as mycelial form in nature and as endosporulating spherule in tissue.
- *Coccidioides* spp. endemic in central CA, southern AZ, southern NM, west TX, northern Mexico, and parts of Central and South America.
- Oganism lives in soil. Arthroconidia inhaled, then convert to spherules within 48 hrs.

CLINICAL
- Vast majority of cases due to inhalation of soil or dust containing the fungus. Most cases are among residents in endemic areas but sporadic cases have been Dx'd outside those areas and may be from reactivation of prior infection.
- Immunocompetent hosts: asymptomatic pulmonary disease most common; can cause acute or subacute pneumonia or extrapulmonary disease, most often affecting meninges, skin, or bones.

- HIV+ patients: spectrum varies, including positive serology without clinical disease; pulmonary disease such as diffuse reticulonodular infiltrates presenting with fever, dyspnea, and night sweats (like PCP); focal pulmonary involvement presenting like community-acquired pneumonia (most common with CD4 >250), or disseminated disease or meningitis (CSF typically with low glucose, high protein, lymphocytic pleocytosis). Disseminated disease includes fever, lymphadenopathy, skin nodules or ulcers, hepatitis, or peritonitis. Bone/joint lesions can occur but rare. Fever, weight loss without any clear organ involvement also described.
- Can occur as primary disease or reactivation of latent infection. Most cases identified within endemic areas appear to be due to recent acquisition. Clinically, outcome does not appear to vary on basis of whether infection acute or reactivation disease.
- No person-to-person spread by respiratory route.
- Risk factors for active disease in HIV+ patients include CD4 <250 and Dx of AIDS. Risk for disseminated disease also elevated in pregnant women and Filipino, black, and Hispanic patients.
- Prevention efforts limited to advising patients to avoid exposure to disturbed soil such as work on excavation sites or during dust storms in endemic areas.
- DDx (pulmonary disease): PCP, cryptococcosis, histoplasmosis, TB, nontuberculous mycobacterial infection, *Pseudomonas aeruginosa*, *Nocardia* spp., and *Rhodococcus equi*.
- Continues to be relatively common cause of death in highly endemic areas, but ART has decreased incidence.
- Prospective study in endemic region found that nearly 25% of those with CD4 <250 developed coccidiomycosis within 3.5 yrs of follow-up.

DIAGNOSIS

- Dx usually based on serology. Obtain complement-fixing (CF) antibodies associated with IgG response. Elevated CF titers associated with poor prognosis and are measured serially to follow response to Rx.
- Serology negative in up to 30% of HIV+ patients; higher likelihood of negative serology in those with low CD4.
- Wet mount smear of sputum, BAL fluid, or pus and histopathology of affected tissues with identification of coccidioidal spherules can assist in rapid Dx. Cytological staining with Papinicolau and Gomori methenamine stains preferred staining methods. KOH 10% not useful.
- Cx should be obtained of sputum or affected tissues. Lab should be notified of suspicion for coccidioidomycosis so that appropriate precautions can be taken to avoid infection of lab workers.
- Unlike other pathogenic, endemic fungi, organism often isolated within <5 days even when plated on routine bacteriologic medium (except in blood and CSF culture lower yield (CSF Cx+ less than 30% in those with meningitis).
- Tube precipitin antibodies (not generally available) associated with IgM response found in recent or relapsing infection. Enzyme immunoassay also available for IgM and IgG measurement but interpretation uncertain. Skin testing with coccidioidin (spherulin) in endemic areas not predictive of disease and no longer available. Routine screening with serologic assays not recommended. Prophylactic therapy not recommended.
- Histopathlogy of involved tissue with typical spherule can be helpful.

TREATMENT

Initial Management of Severe Nonmeningeal Disease (Diffuse Pulmonary or Severe Extrathoracic Disseminated Disease)

- **First line:** AmB 0.7–1.0 mg/kg/day IV; lipid formulations of AmB 4–6 mg/kg/day. Continue until patient clinically stable or improved, usually 2 wks, then therapy switched to oral azole.
- **Second line:** fluconazole 400–800 mg PO once daily; itraconazole 200 mg PO twice daily (liquid formulation preferred; see authors' comments); ketoconazole 400 mg PO once daily.
- Some specialists add triazole to AmB and continue triazole once AmB is stopped.

Initial Management of Mild to Moderate Nonmeningeal Disease

- **First line:** fluconazole 400–800 mg PO once daily; itraconazole 200 mg PO twice daily (liquid formulation preferred).
- **Second line:** ketoconazole 400 mg PO once daily; AmB 0.5–0.7 mg/kg/day IV; lipid formulations of AmB 3–5 mg/kg/day (limited data).

Meningeal Disease

- **First line:** fluconazole 400–800 mg PO once daily. Some experts advocate higher doses of 1200 mg PO once daily.

- **Second line:** itraconazole 200 mg PO 3 times a day × 3 days then 200 mg PO twice daily (liquid formulation preferred); intrathecal AmB 0.01–1.0 mg once daily to once weekly when triazole antifungals not effective. Start at lowest dose and increase as tolerated.
- Some clinicians combine a PO azole with intrathecal amphotericin.
- Newer azoles such as voriconazole and posaconazole have good CNS activity and appear to be effective based on limited data. Drug interactions also a concern. Recommend expert consultation if these drugs being considered.

Chronic Maintenance Therapy
- **First line:** fluconazole 400 mg PO once daily; itraconazole 200 mg PO twice daily (liquid formulation preferred).
- **Second line:** ketoconazole 400 mg PO once daily.
- **Discontinuation of maintenance therapy:** not currently recommended for meningitis, diffuse pulmonary disease, or disseminated nonmeningeal disease. Relapse after discontinuation reported despite immune reconstitution. Patients with focal coccidioidal pneumonia who have responded to antifungal therapy at low risk for recurrence if CD4 >250 and on ART. Reasonable to D/C therapy after 12 mos of continued monitoring with serial CXRs and serology.

Other Treatment Considerations
- AmB treatment of choice in pregnancy. Azoles should not be used. Monitor neonate for renal dysfuntion and hypokalemia.
- Surgical debridement may be required for severe focal disease.
- Primary prophylaxis generally not recommended. However some specialists consider fluconazole 400 mg or itraconazole 200 mg PO twice daily in HIV+ patient who is asymptomatic but has positive IgM or IgG and CD4 <250; D/C if CD4 >250 for 6 mos on ART.
- Decreased incidence of symptomatic coccidioidomycosis in HAART era.
- Complications in meningitis form such as hydrocephalus, cerebral infarction, vasculitic infarctions, and arachnoiditis can occur; treatments directed at these complications may be necessary.

Follow-up
- **Pulmonary disease:** response to therapy should be monitored with serial physical exam, CXR or CT, serial fungal sputum CX, and CF antibodies in serum.
- **Extrapulmonary disease:** response to therapy should be monitored with serial physical exam, imaging if appropriate, CF antibodies.
- **Meningeal disease:** as above, plus CSF antibodies.
- Obtain **CF antibody titers** every 6–12 wks to guide response to therapy. Lag in response may occur in 1st 1–2 mos.
- Initiate **ART**, as cellular immune function is critical in control of coccidioidomycosis. IRIS possible but not reported in published literature.
- **Management of treatment failure on fluconazole or itraconazole:** may benefit from newer azoles, voriconazole, or posaconazole, but limited data. Consider combining triazole with amphotericin.

Selected References

Kaplan JE, Benson CA, Holmes KH, et al. Guidelines for prevention and treatment of opportunistic infections in HIV-infected adults and adolescents: recommendations from CDC, the National Institutes of Health, and the HIV Medicine Association of the Infectious Diseases Society of America. *MMWR Recomm Rep*, 2009; 58: 1–206.
Comments: US guidelines regarding prevention of active coccidioidomycosis in HIV-infected persons.

Johnson RH, Einstein HE. Coccidioidal meningitis. *Clin Infect Dis*, 2006; 42: 103–7.
Comments: Good clinical review of coccidioidal meningitis.

Ampel NM. Coccidioidomycosis in persons infected with HIV type 1. *Clin Infect Dis*, 2005; 41: 1174–8.
Comments: Good clinical review of coccidioidomycosis in HIV infected persons.

CRYPTOCOCCAL MENINGITIS

Amita Gupta, MD, MHS

Pathogens
- *Cryptococcus neoformans* var. *neoformans* (serotypes A and D).

- *Cryptococcus neoformans* var. *gattii* (serotypes B and C, rare in HIV).
- *Cryptococcus neoformans* var. *grubii* (has been used to designate serotype A).
- Yeast-like round fungus, 5–10 μm with polysaccharide capsule.
- Epidemiology: found worldwide in soil; major OI in sub-saharan Africa, Thailand, India. In US, pre-HAART era 5%–8% of HIV+ patients developed cryptococcosis. Dramatically reduced incidence in HAART era.

CLINICAL

- Infection via inhalation of fungus. Most common clinical syndrome in HIV is meningitis or meningoencephalitis. Less common pulmonary presentation with pneumonia can occur (focal infiltrates, nodules, or rarely, cavitary lesions accompanied by low grade fever). Most patients with meningitis have no history of pneumonia and usually have CD4 <100.
- Less commonly can disseminate to other organs (skin, bone, prostate, eye). Skin lesions resembling molluscum contagiosum can occur in the setting of disseminated cryptococcosis.
- Sx of cryptococcal meningitis include gradually increasing headache with low-grade fever (subacute meningitis). However, may also present without fever, with seizure, confusion, lethargy, progressive dementia, fever without localizing signs, or bizarre behavior. Evidence of meningeal irritation often absent.
- Reported mortality rate of meningitis 6%–25%.
- CNS mass lesions or cryptococcomas usually accompanied by meningitis. Neck stiffness and photophobia only in 25%–33% patients.
- Elevated intracranial pressure (>200 mm H_2O) common and may be accompanied by evidence of cerebral edema: blurred vision, diplopia, hearing loss, severe headaches, confusion, and papilledema.
- Hydrocephalus can occur in more indolent cases and may require placement of CSF shunt.
- Patients who initiate ART are at risk for cryptococcal IRIS (either unmasking type or exacerbation of partly treated disease). Presentations can be atypical, such as lymphadenitis.

DIAGNOSIS

- Cx for fungus: sputum, skin Bx, blood, and CSF. Blood Cx + in 50%–70% with meningitis.
- Serum cryptococcal antigen (CrAg) positive in >99% of HIV+ patients with cryptococcal meningitis, less often with isolated pulmonary disease.
- CSF CrAg important tool to diagnose meningeal disease but can be negative in nonmeningeal cryptococcosis.
- Patients with evidence of pulmonary or systemic cryptococcosis by CrAg or Cx should undergo LP to rule out meningitis. Patients with focal signs or evidence of cerebral edema should have a head CT or MRI prior to LP to assure no mass effect or risk of herniation.
- CSF evaluation should include: opening pressure (up to 75% have >200 mm, fungal Cx, CrAg, glucose, protein, cell count and differential. CSF typically shows mild increase in protein, low-normal glucose, pleocytosis with lymphocytes, although some patients have no cells, which can be associated with more severe disease. CSF CrAg and fungal Cx positive in >95%. India ink less sensitive (60%–80%).
- Pulmonary: positive sputum Cx or serum CrAg, clinical, and CXR/CT findings.
- In US, routine screening of asymptomatic patients with serum CrAg not recommended.

TREATMENT

Mild to Moderate Pulmonary Disease or Nonmeningeal Cryptococcosis

- **First line:** fluconazole 400 mg (6 mg/kg) PO once daily × 6–12 mos. Consider stopping maintenance fluconazole after 1 year of treatment for HIV patients on ART with CD4 >100 and cryptococcal antigen titer.

Severe Pulmonary Disease or Nonmeningeal Cryptococcosis

- Treat as CNS disease. Refer to cryptococcal meningitis treatment.

Cryptococcal Meningitis: Induction/Consolidation

- **First line:** AmB 0.7–1 mg/kg/day IV OR lipid amphotericin formulation 4–6 mg/kg/day IV (consider for patients with renal dysfunction or at high risk for renal failure) ± 5-FC 100 mg/kg/day PO divided over 4 doses × 2 wks until CSF sterile, then fluconazole 400 mg/day × 8 wks. Addition of 5-FC associated with more rapid sterilization and decreased risk for subsequent relapse but often not well tolerated; monitor CBC and 5-FC levels.

- **Second line:** (1) AmB 0.7–1 mg/kg/day IV, liposomal amphotericin (3–4 mg/kg/day IV up to 6 mg/kg), or amphotericin B lipid complex (ABLC) (5 mg/kg/day IV) for 4–6 wks without 5-FC; (2) AmB 0.7 mg/kg/day plus fluconazole 800 mg/day for 2 wks, then fluconazole 800 mg/day PO for minimum of 8 wks; (3) fluconazole (>800 mg/day; 1200 mg/day favored) plus 5-FC (100 mg/kg/day PO) 6 wks; (4) fluconazole 800–2000 mg/day po 10–12 wks (fluconazole >1200 mg/day recommended if used without 5-FC).

Cryptococcal Meningitis: Maintenance
- **First line:** fluconazole 200 mg PO once daily.
- **Second line:** itraconazole 200 mg PO twice daily (TDM recommended); AmB 1 mg/kg/wk. Intermittent amphotericin therapy associated with higher rate of relapse and greater toxicity compared to fluconazole.
- Initiate ART 2–10 wks after starting antifungal therapy as it may improve immunology control and decrease risk of IRIS and rates of relapse. See Follow-up section below.
- Some experts recommend ART only after CSF has been sterilized.

Cerebral Cryptococcomas
- Induction therapy: AmB 0.7–1 mg/kg/day IV, liposomal amphotericin 3–4 mg/kg/day IV, or ABLC 5 mg/kg/day IV + 5-FC 100 mg/kg/day PO in 4 divided doses × >6 wks.
- Consolidation and maintenance therapy: fluconazole 400–800 mg/day PO × 6–18 mos.
- Adjunctive therapies: Corticosteroids for mass effect and edema. Surgery may be considered.

Elevated Intracranial Pressure (ICP)
- Elevated ICP is most common cause of death or neurologic sequelae with cryptococcal meningitis, and should be managed aggressively.
- If ICP >250 mm and signs of cerebral edema present, do daily LP to reduce pressure until patient is improved. One approach is to remove vol of CSF that halves opening pressure (typically 20–30 mL).
- If clinical signs of cerebral edema do not improve after about 2 wks of daily LPs, consider placement of lumbar drain or VP shunt.
- Patients with hydrocephalus may or may not have increased ICP and rarely have cerebral edema.
- Corticosteroids, mannitol, and acetazolamide not recommended.

Primary Prevention
- Primary antifungal prophylaxis for cryptococcosis is not routinely recommended in HIV-infected patients in the United States and Europe, but areas with limited HAART availability, high levels of antiretroviral drug resistance, and a high burden of disease might consider it or a preemptive strategy with serum cryptococcal antigen testing for asymptomatic antigenemia.

FOLLOW-UP

Discontinuation of Maintenance Therapy
- In pre-HAART era, risk of relapse 4% on maintenance therapy but up to 37%–60% in those who discontinued therapy.
- Consider discontinuing suppressive therapy during HAART in patients with a CD4 cell count >100 cells/mL and an undetectable or very low HIV RNA level sustained for ≥3 months (minimum of 12 months of antifungal therapy) (B-II); consider reinstitution of maintenance therapy if the CD4 cell count decreases to >100 cells/mL (B-III).

Toxicity
- Monitor for treatment related toxicity on biweekly schedule during induction phase and every other wk on consolidation phase.
- 5-FC: severe colitis, leukopenia, thrombocytopenia, rash, or hepatitis. Dosage should be reduced for cytopenias or colitis and levels monitored to limit toxicity. Addition of 5-FC to AmB provides only marginal benefit at most. 5-FC may be held if toxicity encountered that cannot be controlled with dosing changes.
- Azoles: liver toxicity.
- AmB: electrolyte imbalances, renal insufficiency, anemia, acute infusion-related toxicity and may require close monitoring. Liposomal formulation less toxic.

Diagnosis of Relapse
- Perform fungal Cx. Serum CrAg not reliable to evaluate patients for relapse of cryptococcal disease. If convalescence CSF CrAg titer available for comparison, an increase in titer of 2 dilutions suggests relapse.

- Fungal Cx may help differentiate between relapse and IRIS. IRIS after initiation of ART can include worsening meningitis with elevated ICP, lymphadenitis, sterile abscess, or cavitation of pulmonary lesions.
- Treatment failure defined as either lack of clinical improvement after 2 wks of appropriate therapy or relapse after initial response (positive CSF Cx and/or compatible clinical picture with rising CSF CrAg). Optimal therapy not defined. If started on fluconazole switch to AmB ±5-FC. Consider liposomal amphotericin or higher doses of fluconazole or addition of 5-FC (see p. 202).

Other Follow-up Issues

- After initial 2 wks of treatment, repeat LP should be performed to ensure organism has been cleared from CSF. Positive Cx at 2 wks predictive of future relapse and associated with less favorable outcomes.
- When to start ART in setting of cryptococcal meningitis unknown. Some data from US with small number of cases (ACTG 5164) favor early ART, but data from Uganda suggest increased mortality with early initiation (within 2 wks of Dx). 2009 OI guidelines suggest delaying initiation at least until completion of induction of therapy, especially with elevated ICP.
- IRIS can occur in up to 30%. With severe symptoms, consider cocorticosteroids.

OTHER INFORMATION

- Antifungal resistance testing should be limited to patients with multiple recurrences or disease in setting of adherence to standard therapy, as fluconazole or amphotericin resistance is rare.

SELECTED REFERENCES

Huston SM, Mody CH. Cryptococcosis: an emerging respiratory mycosis. *Clin Chest Med*, 2009; 30: 253–64, vi.
Comments: Review of cryptococcosis, including in HIV+ patients.

Bicanic T, Meintjes G, Rebe K, et al. Immune reconstitution inflammatory syndrome in HIV-associated cryptococcal meningitis: a prospective study. *J Acquir Immune Defic Syndr*, 2009; 51: 130–134.
Comments: 65 patients who started ART median of 47 days after Dx of cryptococcal meningitis. No increase in mortality in those who developed IRIS vs those who did not, in contrast to some abstracts presented at CROI 2008 and 2009, where IRIS was associated with higher mortality.

Kaplan JE, Benson CA, Holmes KH, et al. Guidelines for prevention and treatment of opportunistic infections in HIV-infected adults and adolescents: recommendations from CDC, the National Institutes of Health, and the HIV Medicine Association of the Infectious Diseases Society of America. *MMWR Recomm Rep*, 2009; 58: 1–206.
Comments: National guidelines for prevention of OIs, including cryptococcal meningitis, and recommendations regarding discontinuation of secondary prophylaxis.

Perfect JR, Dismukes WE, Dromer F, et al, Clinical Practice Guidelines for the Management of Cryptococcal Disease: 2010 Update by the Infectious Diseases Society of America; Clin Infect Dis; 2010; Vol. 50
Comment: IDSA guidelines for management of cryptococcus both in HIV+ and HIV-negative individuals.

Sloan D, Dlamini S, Paul N, Dedicoat M. Treatment of acute cryptococcal meningitis in HIV infected adults, with an emphasis on resource-limited settings. *Cochrane Database Syst Rev*, 2008; CD005647.
Comments: Systematic review. No studies suitable for inclusion in the review compared AmB with fluconazole in resource-limited settings (RLS); therefore, authors unable to recommend either treatment as superior. Optimal dosing of AmB remains unclear. Liposomal amphotericin associated with less adverse events than AmB and may be useful in selected patients where resources allow. 5-FC in combination with AmB leads to faster and increased sterilization of CSF compared to AmB alone, and authors argue that 5-FC should be more readily available in RLS.

HISTOPLASMOSIS

Amita Gupta, MD, MHS

PATHOGENS

- *Histoplasma capsulatum* is a dimorphic fungus. At 37°C or in human tissue, grows as a small oval yeast, 2–5 μm in diameter. Grows as a mycelium in nature.
- Primarily intracellular pathogen infecting macrophages and causing granulomatous inflammation.
- Soil-based fungus that thrives in moist, acidic soil w/ a high nitrogen content (rich in droppings from birds and bats). Old abandoned buildings and caves can contain high levels.

- In US, endemic in Ohio and Mississippi River valleys. Also endemic in areas of Central and South America with microfoci in eastern US, southern Europe, Africa, S and SE Asia.
- Most cases sporadic but occasionally occur in outbreaks.

CLINICAL
- Most patients either have no Sx or mild pulmonary complaints and go undetected.
- Organism establishes infection after inhalation. Hematogenous dissemination leads to involvement of other organ systems.
- Can occur after new infection or reactivation of latent disease.
- Clinical syndromes in immunocompetent patients: acute or chronic pulmonary disease, chronic meningitis or focal brain lesions, granulomatous mediastinitis, fibrosing mediastinitis, pericarditis, erythema nodosum, and indolent disseminated disease.
- For patients with CD4 >300, often limited to respiratory tract. Pneumonia is most common manifestation, atypical with patchy or diffuse reticulonodular infiltrates (with or without hilar or mediastinal lymphadenopathy) and can progress to ARDS.
- Disseminated disease occurs in 3%–5% of AIDS patients living in endemic areas of the US.
- HIV+ patients at increased risk of dissemination (most common at CD4 <150): fever, chills, weight loss, hepatosplenomegaly, bone marrow infiltration/suppression, lymphadenopathy, pulmonary infiltrates, meningitis or focal CNS lesions, skin lesions, adrenal insufficiency, and oral and/or GI tract ulcerations. IRIS has been described.
- In US, HIV-associated FUO associated with disseminated histo in 7% of cases. IRIS uncommonly reported, but can occur in association with ART and should be considered in the DDx of patients with worsening of disease on appropriate antifungal therapy who have recently started ART.

DIAGNOSIS
- Rapid Dx sometimes accomplished by careful evaluation of buffy coat smear of peripheral blood, Gomori methenamine silver, or periodic acid-Schiff stains of bone marrow or involved tissue.
- Dx testing should include blood Cx (lysis-centrifugation system with incubation for 21–28 days) or Cx of bone marrow or BAL fluid.
- Sensitivity of *Histoplasma* antigen (Ag) testing in AIDS patients w/ disseminated histo is 97% for urine and 79% for blood. Increasing titers in serum or urine are useful in diagnosing relapse. CSF Ag helpful in Dx of meningitis. Ag test insensitive in indolent or localized disease. *H. capsulatum* Ag detection: MiraVista Diagnostics (866-647-2847).
- Ag cross-reactions can be seen with blastomycosis, coccidioidomycosis, penicilliosis, paracoccidioidomycosis, and African histoplasmosis.
- Diffuse pulmonary infiltrates due to disseminated histo can be Dx'd in BAL by Gomori methenamine silver, Giemsa stain, or with *Histoplasma* Ag (sensitivity ~70%). BAL Cx detects about 89% of cases.
- CXR in disseminated histo may show diffuse reticulonodular infiltrates, focal infiltrates, or may be normal.
- Serology not helpful in AIDS but may be helpful in patients with intact immune responses, consistent clinical presentation, and epidemiologic risk, but takes 4–8 wks to develop, so not helpful for rapid Dx.

TREATMENT
Acute Pulmonary Disease (High CD4)
- Acute pulmonary histoplasmosis in HIV+ patients with intact immunity (i.e., CD4 >300) should be managed as in immunocompetent hosts.

Initial Therapy of Moderate-to-Severe Disseminated Disease
- **Preferred:** liposomal amphotericin 3.0 mg/kg/day IV for >14 days (or until clinically improved) (see Follow-up section on p. 48).
- AmB 0.7 mg/kg/day IV for >14 days (or until clinically improved).
- Initial IV therapy continued until patient becomes afebrile, can take oral medications, and does not require circulatory or ventilatory support or IV fluids or nutrition. This is followed with a regimen recommended for initial therapy of mild disease.

Initial Therapy for Mild Nonmeningeal Disease
- **Preferred:** itraconazole (oral soln) 200 mg PO 3 ×/day × 3 days then 200 mg PO twice daily.
- Itraconazole capsules 200 mg PO 3 ×/day × 3 days then 200 mg PO twice daily.

- AmB to total dose of 35 mg/kg given over 2–4 mos.
- Fluconazole not recommended as standard treatment and should only be used in patients who cannot tolerate itraconazole or who cannot achieve adequate blood levels. Patients treated with fluconazole should be monitored carefully for relapse.

Initial Therapy for Meningeal Disease
- Liposomal amphotericin 5 mg/kg/day × 4–6 wks.
- AmB 0.7–1 mg/kg/day to complete 35 mg/kg over 3–4 mos.

Chronic Maintenance Therapy for Nonmeningeal Disease
- **Preferred:** itraconazole (oral soln) 200 mg PO twice daily.
- AmB 50 mg IV once or twice weekly.
- Fluconazole not recommended as standard treatment and should only be used in patients who cannot tolerate itraconazole or who cannot achieve adequate blood levels. Patients who are treated with fluconazole should be monitored carefully for relapse.
- Itraconazole levels recommended to ensure adequate absorption.
- Duration of therapy: >12 mos.

Chronic Maintenance for Meningeal Disease
- **Preferred:** itraconazole 200 mg PO 2–3 ×/day (oral soln preferred) for >12 mos and until resolution of abnormal CSF findings.
- See Follow-up for information about discontinuation of maintenance therapy.

FOLLOW-UP
- Monitor *Histoplasma* Ag (serum or urine) every 3–6 mos during therapy. Rise in level suggestive of relapse.
- Discontinuation of maintenance therapy may be safe if patients on stable ART >6 mos with CD4 >150, serum Ag <2 units, and have completed induction and minimum of 12 mos of maintenance antifungal therapy. Resume if CD4 <150.
- Serum itaconazole levels should be obtained at least once as absorption can be erratic; should be >1 mcg/mL (drawn as trough level >7 days on current regimen).
- In a secondary analysis of a small study, induction therapy with liposomal amphotericin associated with reduced mortality at day 17 (3/22 vs 1/51; P = 0.04) but not at later time points, and caused less toxicity compared to AmB.

PREVENTION
- Patients with CD4 <150 and residing in *H. capsulatum*-endemic areas should avoid high-risk activities (creating dust when working with surface soil or working with soil contaminated with bird droppings; cleaning chicken coops; cleaning, remodeling, or demolishing old buildings; and spelunking).
- Prophylaxis with itraconazole (200 mg PO once daily) may be considered if CD4 <150 and high-risk occupational exposures or living in areas with >10 cases of histoplasmosis per 100 patient-years. D/C primary prophylaxis if CD4>150 for 6 mos on ART.

SELECTED REFERENCES

Kauffman CA. Histoplasmosis. *Clin Chest Med*, 2009; 30: 217–25, v.
Comments: Comprehensive review of organism and management.

Kaplan JE, Benson CA, Holmes KH, et al. Guidelines for prevention and treatment of opportunistic infections in HIV-infected adults and adolescents: recommendations from CDC, the National Institutes of Health, and the HIV Medicine Association of the Infectious Diseases Society of America. *MMWR Recomm Rep*, 2009; 58: 1–206.
Comments: Prevention and treatment guidelines that include specific discussion of histoplasmosis.

Wheat LJ, Freifeld AG, Kleiman MB, et al. Clinical practice guidelines for the management of patients with histoplasmosis: 2007 update by the Infectious Diseases Society of America. *Clin Infect Dis*, 2007; 45: 807–25.
Comments: Describes management of all forms of histoplasmosis, including in HIV+ patients.

Breton G, Adle-Biassette H, Therby A, et al. Immune reconstitution inflammatory syndrome in HIV-infected patients with disseminated histoplasmosis. *AIDS*, 2006; 20: 119–21.
Comments: Four HIV-1-infected patients presented with unusual clinical manifestations in the course of disseminated histoplasmosis, including liver abscesses, compressive lymphadenitis, intestinal obstruction, uveitis, and arthritis within a median of 45 days after initiation of ART.

PNEUMOCYSTIS PNEUMONIA

Noah Lechtzin, MD, MHS

PATHOGENS
- *Pneumocystis jiroveci* or *jirovecii* (formerly *P. carinii*), a fungal organism previously classified as a protozoan.
- Ubiquitous organism, respiratory transmission.
- Active cases due to both reactivation of old and acquisition of new infection.

CLINICAL
- Incidence peaked 1987–1988, with subsequent decrease due to prophylaxis and ART.
- Occurs when CD4 <200; risk increases with decreasing CD4 count.
- Hx: gradual/subacute onset of cough (usually nonproductive), dyspnea, fever in most patients. Chills, fatigue, chest pain, weight loss less common.
- PE: fever, normal lung exam in ~50%. May have crackles and/or rhonchi.
- Extrapulmonary involvement rare but can occur.
- Hypoxemia and low DLCO common. Oxygen saturation may be normal at rest, but decreases with exercise.

DIAGNOSIS
- CXR: diffuse interstitial and/or alveolar infiltrates. 25% are normal with early disease.
- CXR findings variable; can have lobar infiltrates, nodules, masses, dense infiltrates, blebs, spontaneous pneumothorax, and possibly pleural effusions.
- Induced sputum diagnostic in 60%; BAL diagnostic in >90%.
- Elevated LDH common but nonspecific.
- Molecular-based diagnostic tests on sputum or oral washings hold promise. Real time PCR has high sensitivity and specificity but does not differentiate colonization from infection (Arcenas 2006).
- Definitive Dx (by sputum or BAL) preferred over presumptive Dx, as presentation similar for other OIs, toxicity common during 3-wk treatment course, and adjunctive corticosteroids may exacerbate other conditions.

TREATMENT

Initial Therapy
- **Preferred:** TMP-SMX 5 mg/kg (of TMP component) q8h × 21 days.
- **Alternative:** clindamycin 600 mg q8h and primaquine 15–30 mg once daily × 21 days.
- **Alternative:** dapsone 100 mg once daily and TMP 5 mg/kg q8h × 21 days (mild-to-moderate PCP only).
- **Alternative:** atovaquone 750 mg 3 ×/day × 21 days (mild-to-moderate PCP only).
- **Alternative:** pentamidine 4 mg/kg/day IV (high rate of side effects: ARF, hypotension, pancreatitis, hypo- and hyperglycemia, and electrolyte abnormalities).
- Regimens 1–4 can be given orally. Side effects including rash, anemia, hyperkalemia are common. Check G6PD before using dapsone and primaquine.
- Resistance to TMP-SMX described, but not clearly correlated with treatment outcome. Approach to patients failing TMP-SMX controversial, as it is treatment of choice, and failure may be due to ARDS rather than resistance.

Adjunctive Therapy
- If PaO_2 <70 mmHg or A-a gradient >35 mmHg add corticosteroids: prednisone 40 mg PO twice daily × 5d, then 40 mg once daily × 5d, then 20 mg once daily × 11d (or IV equivalent).

Prophylaxis
- Indications: CD4 <200 or history of thrush. Consider for CD4% <14 or history of AIDS-defining illness.
- **Preferred:** TMP-SMX, 1 SS or 1 DS tab once daily. Alternative is 1 DS tab 3 ×/wk (1 DS once daily preferred for *Toxoplasma* seropositives with CD4 <100).
- **Alternative:** dapsone 100 mg once daily.
- **Alternative:** pentamidine 300 mg in 6 mL sterile water aerosolized monthly.

- **Alternative:** atovaquone suspension 750 mg twice daily or 1500 mg once daily.
- Discontinue if CD4 >200 × >3 mos on ART.
- Early ART reduces risk of AIDS progression and death in setting of PCP and can be initiated without increasing risk of IRIS.

Infection Control

- Need for isolation of patients from other immunosuppressed patients controversial.

SELECTED REFERENCES

Kaplan JE, Benson CA, Holmes KH, et al. Guidelines for prevention and treatment of opportunistic infections in HIV-infected adults and adolescents: recommendations from CDC, the National Institutes of Health, and the HIV Medicine Association of the Infectious Diseases Society of America. *MMWR Recomm Rep*, 2009; 58: 1–206.
Comments: Expert panel recommendations on prevention and treatment of OIs with grading of evidence and strength of recommendations.

Arcenas RC, Uhl JR, Buckwalter SP, et al. A real-time polymerase chain reaction assay for detection of Pneumocystis from bronchoalveolar lavage fluid. *Diagn Microbiol Infect Dis*, 2006; 54: 169–75.
Comments: Study showing that real time PCR increases the sensitivity of diagnosing PCP by 21% compared to calcofluor-white staining and the assay does not cross react with other pathogens.

Grant PM, Komarow L, Andersen J, et al. Risk factor analyses for immune reconstitution inflammatory syndrome in a randomized study of early vs. deferred ART during an opportunistic infection. *PLoS One*, 2010; 5: e11416.
Comments: Randomized trial demonstrating the initiation of ART early in the treatment of OIs does not increase the incidence of IRIS.

Zolopa A, Andersen J, Powderly W, et al. Early antiretroviral therapy reduces AIDS progression/death in individuals with acute opportunistic infections: a multicenter randomized strategy trial. *PLoS One*, 2009; 4: e5575. Epub 2009 May 18.
Comments: Starting ART early after initiation of OI treatment decreases the risk of AIDS progression and death.

Opportunistic Infections: Parasitic

CRYPTOSPORIDIOSIS

Lisa A. Spacek, MD, PhD and Khalil G. Ghanem, MD, PhD

PATHOGENS

- *Cryptosporidium*: intracellular protozoan parasite. Most common species infecting humans are *C. hominis*, *C. parvum*, and *C. meleagridis*.
- Sporulated oocysts (4–6 μ in diameter) are ingested, then excyst and attach to intestinal epithelium; trophozoites mature to meronts, which release merozoites leading to zygote formation; oocysts then released through feces into environment.
- In immunocompromised patients, parasites develop intracellularly throughout GI tract, within epithelial cells of biliary tree and pancreatic ducts. Infection causes loss of villi, crypt hyperplasia, and reduction in brush border enzyme activity.
- Environmental oocysts infectious when shed, small in size, can survive for at least 6 mos (if kept moist), and are resistant to chlorination. Sensitive to dessication, hydrogen peroxide, ozone, and UV radiation.
- Person-to-person transmission among family members and close contacts tends to occur because infectious dose is small (as few as 10 oocysts); zoonotic and food-borne (raw oysters) transmission; most outbreak cases water-borne, as in Milwaukee, Wisconsin (1993).

CLINICAL

- Most common cause of chronic diarrhea in severely immunosuppressed (CD4 <100). Accounts for 10%–20% of diarrheal episodes.
- Incubation period 1–2 wks.
- Median time from exposure to Sx ~ 13 days in patients w/ AIDS.
- Sx: frequent, foul-smelling, watery (scant in some cases), nonbloody, noninflammatory diarrhea; occasional crampy abdominal pain; occasional low-grade fever; N and V. Weight loss and nutrient malabsorption may accompany diarrhea.
- DDx: Microsporidia, *Cyclospora, Isospora*, MAC, *Giardia, Entamoeba*, and *Clostridium difficile*.
- Other manifestations: acalculous cholecystitis (chronic carriage in gallbladder may make eradication difficult), sclerosing cholangitis, and pancreatitis due to papillary stenosis; sinusitis and tracheitis described; reactive arthritis; pulmonary infection.

DIAGNOSIS

- Stool/duodenal aspirate/bile smears; concentration techniques (e.g., formalin ether or formalin-ethyl acetate methods) should be performed to increase sensitivity.
- Direct immunofluorescence using monoclonal antibodies offers highest sensitivity and specificity.
- Modified Kinyoun's acid-fast stain for differential staining; oocysts stain red. Giemsa stain (purple oocysts) may not distinguish from yeast forms.
- For profuse diarrhea, single stool specimen usually adequate. Duodenal Bx rarely needed.
- Commercial serology (EIA), stool IFA used in outbreak settings where large volumes of studies are performed and results needed promptly; PCR of research interest.
- Ultrasound evaluates bile ducts and gallbladder. ERCP for visualization and Bx.

TREATMENT

Art

- ART with immune restoration to a CD4 >100 is mainstay of treatment.
- PIs may confer benefit due to *in vitro* and *in vivo* anti-cryptosporidial activity.

Antiparasitics

- Nitazoxanide 0.5–1.0 g PO twice daily with food × 2 wks.
- Data do NOT support the use of paromomycin for cryptosporidiosis.

Symptomatic RX

- Diet: high fiber and low fat; frequent small meals; avoid caffeine and lactose.
- Antiperistaltics: loperamide 4 mg PO × 1, then 2 mg PO prn, up to 16 mg/day; atropine/diphenoxylate 1–2 tabs PO 3–4 times daily prn; deodorized tincture of opium (DTO) 0.3–1 mL PO 4 times daily prn.

Prevention
- Use bottled water (filtered through 1 μ filter) or boil water for 3 min.
- Avoid exposure to feces, farm animals, domestic pets with diarrhea.
- Wear gloves and wash hands after potential exposure; i.e., handling pets, diapering, gardening.

SELECTED REFERENCES

O'Connor RM, Shaffie R, Kang G, Ward HD. Cryptosporidiosis in patients with HIV/AIDS. *AIDS*, 2011; 25: 549–60.
Comments: Immune reconstitution with ART is mainstay of therapy. PIs may have some anticryptosporidial activity. Nitazoxanide is the only drug with anticryptosporidial efficacy approved by FDA in immunocompetent patients.

Huppmann AR, Orenstein JM. Opportunistic disorders of the gastrointestinal tract in the age of highly active antiretroviral therapy. *Hum Pathol*, 2010; 41: 1777–87.
Comments: Broad review includes discussion of cryptosporidiosis. Figures include Giemsa stain of small round intracellular and extracytoplasmic cryptosporidia.

Yoder JS, Harral C, Beach MJ; Centers for Disease Control and Prevention. Cryptosporidiosis surveillance – United States, 2006–2008. *MMWR Surveill Summ*, 2010; 59: 1–14.
Comments: Due to increased risk of transmission from early summer to early fall, immunocompromised patients are advised to avoid exposure to chlorine-resistant cryptosporidia in settings of communal swimming.

Rossignol JF. Cryptosporidium and Giardia: treatment options and prospects for new drugs. *Exp Parasitol*, 2010; 124: 45–53. Epub 2009 Jul 24.
Comments: Review of literature focuses on history of cryptosporidiosis and includes detailed discussion of drug treatment.

Kaplan JE, Benson, CA, Holmes, KH, et al. Guidelines for prevention and treatment of opportunistic infections in HIV-infected adults and adolescents: recommendations from CDC, the National Institutes of Health, and the HIV Medicine Association of the Infectious Diseases Society of America. *MMWR Recomm Rep*, 2009; 58: 1–206.
Comments: Guidelines for OI prevention and treatment released April 10, 2009.

Abubakar I, Aliyu SH, Arumugam C, Hunter PR, Usman NK. Prevention and treatment of cryptosporidiosis in immunocompromised patients. *Cochrane Database Syst Rev*, 2007: CD004932.
Comments: Seven trials involving 169 patients, including 130 adults with AIDS in 5 studies. Although data showed no reduction in duration or frequency of diarrhea for nitazoxanide or paramomycin vs placebo, due to efficacy of nitazoxanide seen in immunocompetent children, its use is recommended in AIDS patients.

MICROSPORIDIOSIS

Lisa A. Spacek, MD, PhD and Khalil G. Ghanem, MD, PhD

PATHOGENS
- Microsporidia are protists related to fungi, not parasites.
- Five genera (*Enterocytozoon*, *Encephalitozoon*, *Septata*, *Pleistophora*, and *Nosema*), as well as unclassified microsporidial organisms may be associated with human disease. The 1st two genera listed are the most frequently encountered.
- Sources of infection and modes of transmission unclear, likely zoonotic and/or waterborne.
- Spores are quite resistant to environmental conditions and can remain infectious for several years, particularly if protected from desiccation.

CLINICAL
- Causes diarrhea, encephalitis, ocular infection, sinusitis, myositis, and disseminated infection in patients with advanced immunodeficiency (CD4 <100).
- *Enterocytozoon bieneusi*: most common species seen in HIV/AIDS; almost exclusively infects the epithelium of the small bowel and causes malabsorption, diarrhea, and cholangitis; present in 7%–50% of HIV+ patients with CD4 < 100 and unexplained chronic diarrhea.
- 3 spp., *Encephalitozoon hellem*, *Encephalitozoon cuniculi*, and *Encephalitozoon intestinalis*, may disseminate by infecting macrophages.

DIAGNOSIS
- Dx: morphological demonstration of organisms by light or electron microscopic examination of clinical specimens (e.g., stool, duodenal aspirate, urine, sputum, nasal discharge, bronchoalveolar lavage fluid, conjunctival discharge).
- Modified trichrome stain produces differential contrast between spores and debris. IFA also available; PCR is research tool.

- Using chromotrope staining, spores of *E. bieneusi* measure 0.9 × 1.5 μm ovoid and refractile; larger spores of *S. intestinalis* and *Encephalitozoon* spp. measure 1.0–1.5 × 2.5–3.0 μm, and polarize brighter than those of *E. bieneusi*.
- Organisms may be visible on Gram's or Giemsa stain or with chemofluorescent agents (e.g., Calcofluor white).

TREATMENT

General Guidelines
- Most effective therapy is immune reconstitution with ART.

Enterocytozoon bieneusi
- No specific therapeutic agent available for Rx.
- Preferred therapy: fumagillin 20 mg PO 3 times daily × 2 wks (not available in US). TNP-470, a synthetic analog of fumagillin (not available in US).
- Alternative therapy: nitazoxanide 1000 mg PO twice-daily with food × 60 days.

Encephalitozoon spp.
- Preferred therapy: albendazole 400 mg PO twice-daily, continue until CD4 >200 for >6 mos after ART initiated.
- Alternative therapy: itraconazole 400 mg PO once-daily PLUS albendazole 400 mg PO twice-daily for disseminated disease.

Other Microsporidia
- Based on case reports; no RCTs available.
- *Vittaforma corneae*, *Pleistophora* spp., and *Septata intestinalis* have been treated successfully w/ albendazole 400 mg PO twice daily.

FOLLOW-UP
- Without immune reconstitution (ART), patients likely to relapse.
- Albendazole 400 mg PO twice daily as maintenance therapy for *E. intestinalis* and other susceptible microsporidia may be effective until immune reconstitution is achieved.
- AVOID albendazole in pregnant women: embryotoxic and teratogenic in animals.
- Reports suggest that most patients can be taken off maintenance therapy once CD4 >100.

SELECTED REFERENCES

Sokolova OI, Demyanov AV, Bowers LC, et al. Emerging microsporidia infections in Russian HIV-infected patients. *J Clin Microbiol*, 2011; 49: 2102–8.
Comments: Case-control study of HIV+ patients with diarrhea. Microsporidia were identified in stool specimens by histochemistry and PCR in 30 (18.9%) of 159. Those diagnosed with microsporidia were more likely to exhibit CD4 ≤100 (OR, 3.2; 95% CI, 1.2–7.8) and weight loss >10% of baseline (OR, 3.0; 95% CI, 1.1–8.2).

Huppmann AR, Orenstein JM. Opportunistic disorders of the gastrointestinal tract in the age of highly active antiretroviral therapy. *Hum Pathol*, 2010; 41: 1777–87.
Comments: Broad review includes discussion of microsporidiosis.

Viriyavejakul P, Nintasen R, Punsawad C, Chaisri U, Punpoowong B, Riganti M. High prevalence of Microsporidium infection in HIV-infected patients. *Southeast Asian J Trop Med Public Health*, 2009; 40: 223–8.
Comments: Microsporidium most common enteric OI (81%) in 64 HIV+ Thais.

Kaplan JE, Benson CA, Holmes KH, et al. Guidelines for prevention and treatment of opportunistic infections in HIV-infected adults and adolescents: recommendations from CDC, the National Institutes of Health, and the HIV Medicine Association of the Infectious Diseases Society of America. *MMWR Recomm Rep*, 2009; 58: 17–9.
Comments: Most effective therapy is ART with immune reconstitution. Rx of *Enterocytozoon bieneusi* based on limited data, and fumagillin and TNP-470 are not available for systematic use in the US. In other species, albendazole is preferred initial Rx.

SCABIES

Khalil G. Ghanem, MD, PhD

PATHOGENS
- *Sarcoptes scabiei* var. *hominis*, a mite that burrows and reproduces under skin and is an obligate parasite.
- Transmission by direct skin-to-skin contact often clustered in households.

- Live mites may survive and be transmitted from dust or bedding for up to 3 days; Sx may take 3–5 wks to develop.

CLINICAL

- Can occur with or without HIV infection or at any CD4 count, but more severe with HIV infection, especially with lower CD4 counts.
- **Classic presentation:** clusters of pinpoint to pinhead sized papules topped by crusts with excoriation; burrows occasionally visible; preferential locations: interdigital webspaces, wrists, antecubital fossae, anterior axillary fold, periareolar, periumbilical, flanks, scrotum (nodules), and lateral aspects of feet. Pruritus intense and more pronounced at night.
- Crusted or "Norwegian" scabies: most frequently described in debilitated or immunocompromised persons (AIDS); widespread crusted, hyperkeratotic papules and plaques, heavy mite burden, and highly contagious.
- Intense hypersensitivity reaction in skin to mite, eggs, and feces is basis of pruritic eruption.
- Secondary skin findings may lead to consideration of alternative diagnoses: eczema; secondary bacterial infection (either impetigo or cellulitis) commonly described in crusted scabies.
- Cross-reactivity with antigens of household mites (storage mite, household mite) may cause persistent reactions after therapy.

DIAGNOSIS

- **Presumptive:** characteristic skin findings or observed response to specific scabicidal therapy.
- **Definitive:** visualization of mite, eggs, or feces packets (scybala) in skin scrapings (mineral oil prep) or on skin Bx (latter rarely required).

TREATMENT

General Considerations

- Wash bedding and affected clothing in hot water at time of treatment or avoid contact with it for 72 hrs to prevent reinfection.
- Mites may persist under fingernails after Rx; close nail clipping recommended with crusted scabies, both to minimize self-injury from scratching and improve scabicidal effect.
- Institutionalized or hospitalized patients with crusted scabies should be isolated; caretakers and other close contacts may need prophylactic scabicidal treatment.
- Pregnant or lactating women should be treated with permethrin.
- Repeat treatments or combination treatments (ivermectin along with up to 6 weekly applications of topical scabicides) may be required for crusted scabies.
- Some experts have recommended retreatment 7–10 days after initial Rx if Sx persist or recur; others recommend repeat Rx only if live mites observed.
- Sexual and close personal contacts with exposure to index case within past month should be referred for exam and Rx.

Topical and Systemic Therapy

- **Permethrin:** 5% cream applied to all areas of body from neck down, wash off after 8–14 hrs; single application results in 97.8% cure (preferred therapy) and more effective than lindane or crotamiton. Consider repeating treatment if symptomatic after 7–10 days.
- **Lindane:** 1%, 1-oz lotion or 30 g cream, applied to all areas of body from neck down and washed off after 8 hrs. FDA advises use only if other options fail or not tolerated.
- **Ivermectin:** 200 g/kg PO × 2 doses at 2-wk interval (not FDA-licensed for this indication) results in 95% cure rate (70% after single dose).
- **Crotamiton:** 10% lotion or cream: apply to entire body from chin down; reapply in 24 hrs, then bathe in 48 hrs.

FOLLOW-UP

- Sx may persist for up to 2 wks following Rx; longer persistence may be due to failure or reinfection.

SELECTED REFERENCES

Leone PA. Scabies and pediculosis pubis: an update of treatment regimens and general review. *Clin Infect Dis*, 2007; 44 Suppl 3: S153–9.

Comments: Overview of recently compiled evidence for treatment of these infestations.

Chouela E, Abeldaño A, Pellerano G, Hernández MI. Diagnosis and treatment of scabies: a practical guide. *Am J Clin Dermatol*, 2002; 3: 9–18.

Comments: Summary of clinical presentation and scabicidal therapeutic options.

TOXOPLASMOSIS

Lisa A. Spacek, MD, PhD and Khalil G. Ghanem, M, PhD

DIAGNOSIS

PATHOGENS
- *Toxoplasma gondii*, an obligate intracellular protozoan.
- Environmental exposure to oocysts (cat feces) or food exposure (undercooked meat containing tissue cysts) leads to human infection.
- Infection lifelong; disease due to reactivation of latent tissue cysts.
- No transmission by person-to-person contact.

CLINICAL
- Most frequent CNS OI in many HIV settings, occurring with CD4 <100.
- Headache, confusion, focal neurologic signs, ± seizures, cranial nerve deficits, rapid mental status decline if lesions hemorrhagic.
- PE: fever, focal motor deficits, ataxia, tremor, altered mental status.
- Primary infection may cause acute cerebral or disseminated disease. Retinochoroiditis and, pneumonia are rare.
- DDx (CNS lesions): primary CNS lymphoma (PCNSL), PML, other malignancy, nocardiosis, tuberculoma, cryptococcoma, syphilitic gumma, *Trypanosoma cruzi* if patient from endemic area (i.e., rural Brazil, Argentina, Chile).

DIAGNOSIS
- Contrast-enhancing mass lesion(s) on MRI or CT; CSF examination rarely helpful in confirming diagnosis, but may be useful in ruling out other CNS processes.
- Positive anti-*Toxoplasma* IgG defines those at risk, low risk of disease if IgG-negative. Check IgG at time of HIV Dx to detect latent infection.
- Rx based upon clinical and radiographic findings; objective response to Rx establishes presumptive diagnosis.
- Brain Bx indicated if no response to Rx.
- If etiology of CNS lesions remains unclear based upon lab/imaging findings, use PET or SPECT scanning and CSF EBV PCR to r/o PCNSL.

TREATMENT
General Principles
- ART with effective immune reconstitution.
- Relapse or side effects may limit success of induction or maintenance therapy; relapse occurs in up to 20%–30% of patients on long-term therapy; interventions to support adherence may be beneficial.
- Corticosteroids (dexamethasone 4 mg PO/IV q6hr) often used if mass effect or significant edema. Discontinue as soon as possible.
- Anticonvulsants indicated for patients with seizures, but not given prophylactically.

Initial Therapy (6 wks or More, if Disease Extensive)
- Pyrimethamine 200 mg PO × 1 loading dose, then 50 mg (<60 kg) to 75 mg (≥60 kg) PO once-daily PLUS sulfadiazine 1000 mg (<60 kg) to 1500 mg (≥60 kg) PO q6h PLUS leucovorin 10–25 mg PO once-daily.
- Alternative: pyrimethamine 200 mg PO loading dose, then 50–75 mg PO once-daily PLUS clindamycin 600 mg IV or PO q6h PLUS leucovorin 10–25 mg PO once-daily.
- Alternative: pyrimethamine + leucovorin (above doses) PLUS azithro 900–1200 mg PO once-daily.
- Alternative: pyrimethamine + leucovorin (above doses) PLUS atovaquone 1500 mg PO twice-daily with food.
- Alternative: TMP-SMX (5 mg/kg TMP and 25 mg/kg SMX) IV or PO twice-daily.
- Alternative: atovaquone 1500 mg PO twice-daily with food PLUS sulfadiazine 1000–1500 mg PO q6h.

Chronic Maintenance
- Preferred: pyrimethamine 25–50 mg PO once-daily PLUS sulfadiazine 2000–4000 mg/day in 2–4 divided doses PLUS leucovorin 10–25 mg PO once-daily.
- Alternative: clindamycin 600 mg PO q8h PLUS pyrimethamine PLUS leucovorin (above doses). Add Rx for PCP prophylaxis.

- Alternative: atovaquone 750 mg PO q6–12h ± [(pyrimethamine PLUS leucovorin) or sulfadiazine 2000–4000 mg PO once-daily].
- Maintenance therapy can be discontinued after completion of initial Rx without signs and Sx with CD4 >200 for >6 mos in response to ART.

Prophylaxis

- Indicated if anti-*Toxoplasma* IgG + and CD4 <100. Re-test IgG-negative patients on PCP prophylaxis that is not active against toxoplasmosis once CD4 <100.
- **Preferred:** TMP-SMX 1 DS once daily.
- **Alternative:** dapsone 50 mg once daily + pyrimethamine 50 mg weekly + leucovorin 25 mg weekly.
- **Alternative:** atovoquone 1500 mg once daily ± pyrimethamine 25 mg once daily + leucovorin 10 mg once daily.
- Discontinue primary prophylaxis when CD4 >200 × >3 mos on ART.
- *Toxoplasma* IgG-negative patients should be counseled to avoid exposure: no raw/undercooked meat, strict handwashing with meat preparation or gardening, avoid changing cat litter.

Non-CNS Toxoplasmosis

- Limited treatment data on non-CNS disease in HIV; therefore, pulmonary, ocular, or proven disease in other organ system should be treated with regimens proven to be effective in CNS.

SELECTED REFERENCES

Adurthi S, Mahadevan A, Bantwal R, et al. Utility of molecular and serodiagnostic tools in cerebral toxoplasmosis with and without tuberculous meningitis in AIDS patients: a study from South India. *Ann Indian Acad Neurol*, 2010; 13: 263–70.
Comments: Study of autopsy-based data, 11 of 17 (65%) cases of tuberculous meningitis were co-infected with *T. gondii*.

Mesquita RT, Ziegler AP, Hiramoto RM, Vidal JE, Pereira-Chioccola VL. Real-time quantitative PCR in cerebral toxoplasmosis diagnosis of Brazilian human immunodeficiency virus-infected patients. *J Med Microbiol*, 2010; 59: 641–7. Epub 2010 Feb 11.
Comments: Report on real-time quantitative PCR for blood and CSF samples based on two primer sets: B1Tg and RETg. Sensitivities were 86% and 98%, respectively. Specificities were 97% and 88.8%, respectively.

Kaplan JE, Benson CA, Holmes KH, et al. Guidelines for prevention and treatment of opportunistic infections in HIV-infected adults and adolescents: recommendations from CDC, the National Institues of Health, and the HIV Medicine Association of the Infectious Diseases Society of America. *MMWR Recomm Rep*, 2009; 58: 61–3.
Comments: Pre-ART, 12-month risk of toxoplasmosis in *Toxoplasma* seropositive AIDS patients was 33%. Baseline testing for IgG identifies those with latent toxo. Prophylaxis TMP/SMX same as PCP. Preferred Rx for encephalitis is combination pyrimethamin + sulfadiazine + leucovorin.

Lago EG, Conrado GS, Piccoli CS, Carvalho RL, Bender AL. *Toxoplasma gondii* antibody profile in HIV-infected pregnant women and the risk of congenital toxoplasmosis. *Eur J Clin Microbiol Infect Dis*, 2009; 28: 345–51. Epub 2008 Oct 15.
Comments: High *T. gondii*-specific IgG values much more frequent among HIV+ pregnant women, but no increased risk of maternal-fetal transmission of toxoplasmosis.

Dedicoat M, Livesley N. Management of toxoplasmic encephalitis in HIV-infected adults (with an emphasis on resource-poor settings). *Cochrane Database Syst Rev*, 2006; 3: CD005420.
Comments: In this systematic review, TMP-SMX was found to be an effective alternative therapy for toxoplasmosis in resource-poor settings where preferred regimens not available.

Opportunistic Infections: Viral

CMV, GASTROINTESTINAL

Lisa A. Spacek, MD, PhD and Khalil G. Ghanem, MD, PhD

PATHOGENS
- A member of the Beta *herpesviridae*, double-stranded DNA virus; up to 60%–100% seroprevalence. Most infections asymptomatic, virus shed in absence of Sx. Severe disease seen in fetus, AIDS, and immunosuppressed.
- Transmitted vertically, sexually, or by close contact (family members, daycare) via blood, tears, saliva, breast milk, urine, cervical secretions, and semen.
- Establishes permanent latent infection in host.
- Both primary and secondary infections (reactivation of latent infection or reinfection with another strain) occur. Most cases in immunosuppressed adults tend to be reactivation.

CLINICAL
- In HIV, CD4 usually <50. GI tract is 2nd most common site of disease after eye.
- In AIDS, esophagitis accounts for 5%–10% of CMV disease, with fever and odynophagia; also causes gastritis, gastric ulcers, duodenitis, duodenal ulcers, enteritis, and mesenteric vasculitis.
- In AIDS, colitis accounts for 5%–10% of CMV disease, with fever, weight loss, abdominal pain, hematochezia, and diarrhea (guaiac + stool and fecal leukocytes). Complications include perforation and hemorrhage; most common finding is a mild, patchy colitis including vasculitis.
- CMV in GI tract should prompt ophthalmologic exam for CMV retinitis.
- Median survival after Dx is <10 mos without ART.
- Begin ART for immune reconstitution.

DIAGNOSIS
- **Esophagitis:** endoscopy with Bx required in patients w/ odynophagia or dysphagia who fail to respond to empiric antifungal therapy.
- **Colitis:** colonoscopic Bx when stool studies non-diagnostic; Bx necessary even if mucosa appears normal. Stool Cx for CMV not helpful.
- CMV GI disease defined by clinical Sx, findings of macroscopic mucosal lesions on endoscopy, and demonstration of CMV in Bx specimen. Intranuclear "owl's eye" inclusions have surrounding halo and marginated chromatin.
- Tests to detect viremia (e.g., PCR or CMV antigenemia) not shown to predict active disease or recurrence. CMV VL has poor positive predictive value, but reasonable negative predictive value for disease.
- Treatment of viremia in absence of organ system involvement not recommended.

TREATMENT
Antiviral Therapy
- Valganciclovir 900 mg PO twice daily w/ food × 3–4 wks (if GI symptoms don't interfere with meds); most data are in HIV+ w/ retinitis.
- If patient unable to swallow, choice of GCV (5 mg/kg IV twice daily × 3–4 wks) vs foscarnet (FOS) (60 mg/kg q8h or 90 mg/kg q12h × 3–4 wks) according to toxicity profile of each drug.
- Recent data indicate disappearance of CMV inclusion bodies after 3 wks and complete healing after 6 wks of therapy.
- No available data on the use of cidofovir (CDV) for CMV GI tract disease.
- Initiate or optimize ART. Chronic maintenance CMV therapy not recommended, may consider for relapse.

Antiviral Resistance
- Drug resistance occurs after prolonged periods of antiviral therapy, when treatment is interrupted or given at suboptimal doses, and with persistent high-level viral replication.
- Combination IV ganciclovir and IV foscarnet therapy may be attempted if monotherapy fails.
- Mutations in UL97 gene confer variable resistance to GCV. Combined mutations in UL97 and UL54 confer high-level resistance to GCV and cross-resistance to CDV. Less commonly, UL54 mutation may confer GCV-FOS cross-resistance.

SELECTED REFERENCES

Kaplan JE, Benson CA, Holmes KH, et al. Guidelines for prevention and treatment of opportunistic infections in HIV-infected adults and adolescents: recommendations from CDC, the National Institutes of Health, and the HIV Medicine Association of the Infectious Diseases Society of America. *MMWR Recomm Rep*, 2009; 58: 1–206.
Comments: Updated OI treatment guidelines.

Reddy N, Wilcox CM. Diagnosis and management of cytomegalovirus infections in the GI tract. *Expert Rev Gastroenterol Hepatol*, 2007; 1: 287–94.
Comments: Review of CMV GI disease for HIV-infected and transplant population.

Wohl DA, Zeng D, Stewart P, et al. Cytomegalovirus viremia, mortality, and end-organ disease among patients with AIDS receiving potent antiretroviral therapies. *J Acquir Immune Defic Syndr*, 2005; 38: 538–44.
Comments: Prospective study of 187 AIDS patients, CMV seropositive without CMV disease, evaluated for development of CMV disease and viremia with plasma CMV DNA PCR and whole blood CMV hybrid capture. Detectable plasma CMV DNA PCR predicted death after adjusting for HIV RNA and CD4 count, but neither assay associated with CMV disease.

CMV, NEUROLOGIC

Paul G. Auwaerter, MD

PATHOGENS
- Cytomegalovirus.

CLINICAL
- CMV disease afflicts up to 40% in untreated AIDS. CMV seroprevalence 50%–80%, >90% in active MSM. CNS disease seen only in immune suppressed, HIV CD4 <50–100.
- CMV CNS disease uncommon: pathological evidence in >30% (autopsy series), but <2% with clinical neurological disorders.
- Typically a progressive encephalopathy, usually in patient w/ Hx of prior CMV disease (e.g., retinitis). Acute onset, rapid progression helps distinguish from HIV encephalitis or PML.
- CMV encephalitis subsets: **diffuse** (decreased memory with dementia-like presentations, attention, motor/sensory/CN deficits, ataxia ± fever and often confused with HIV-related dementia), **ventriculoencephalitis** (radiculopathy, CN deficits, nystagmus less neurocognitive features presenting in more aggressive fashion), **mass lesion** (focal deficits relating to mass).
- **CMV polyradiculitis:** presents as back pain, sciatica, paresthesia, sphincter dysfunction, distal sensory loss, ascending paralysis. May appear Guillain-Barré–like with lower extremity weakness or include urinary retention/loss of bowel function. Transverse myelitis presentation w/ para- or quadraplegia, sensory deficits. DDx includes HSV-2, VZV.
- CMV viremia may occur in absence of end-organ disease.
- Clinical disease usually a consequence of CMV reactivation.

DIAGNOSIS
- **CMV encephalitis:** periventricular enhancement (ventriculitis) or diffuse hyperintense T2 images on MRI. Dx based on clinical presentation, imaging studies and CSF PCR (sensitivity 62%–100%, specificity 89%–100%). Brain Bx: CMV inclusions ("owl's eye") or CMV+ stains. Bx not typically performed given usual brainstem or periventricular locations of disease.
- **CMV polyradiculomyelitis:** MRI may show enhancement of cauda equina or meninges. Positive CSF CMV PCR.
- **CSF studies:** findings often nonspecific. Low glucose and/or PMN pleocytosis seen with encephalitis (ventriculoencephalitis > diffuse) and polyradiculomyelitis.
- **CSF CMV viral Cx:** insensitive, but 100% specific if positive. Role of quantitative CMV PCR (blood) less clear, but high/rising levels may correlate with increased incidence of end-organ disease.
- CMV retinitis may occur concomitantly in up to 30% of patients. Ophthalmological examination of all patients recommended.

TREATMENT
General Principles
- Treatment recommendations based on studies of CMV retinitis and colitis given lack of controlled studies on CNS CMV infection.

DIAGNOSIS

CMV Encephalitis/Polyradiculomyelitis: Primary Induction

- **Preferred:** ganciclovir (GCV) 5 mg/kg IV q12h.
- **Alternative:** foscarnet (FOS) 90 mg/kg IV q12h.
- Decision to use GCV or FOS based upon hematologic and renal aspects of patient.
- Combination GCV + FOS (above doses) used by some, unclear if superior response (one open-label trial showed 94 days median survival vs 42 days historical control) (Anduze-Faris) to monotherapy and regimen poorly tolerated. Due to poor prognosis, combination therapy typically employed by Johns Hopkins Neurology ID service.
- **Alternative:** cidofovir (CDV) 5 mg/kg IV qwk × 2wks, then dose q2wks. Note: CSF penetration of CDV not well studied.
- Usual induction duration: 2 wks.
- Immune reconstitution with ART should be concomitant goal.
- Guideline (Kaplan) warns that although no data exist that IRIS worsens CMV neurologic infections.

CMV Encephalitis/Radiculomyelitis: Post-Induction

- **Preferred:** valganciclovir 900 mg PO twice daily.
- **Alternative:** GCV 5 mg/kg/day IV.
- **Alternative:** FOS 90–120 mg/kg/day IV.
- **Alternative:** if using combination therapy, valganciclovir 900 mg PO twice daily + FOS 90 mg/kg/day IV.
- Usual duration of therapy is 3–6 wks if immune reconstitution occurs. Otherwise long-term maintenance therapy recommended with profound immune suppression to reduce risk of relapse. Regimen for maintenance unclear but valganciclovir 900 mg once or twice daily preferred due to oral route.
- Oral GCV rarely used because valganciclovir has superior bioavailability.

FOLLOW-UP

Encephalitis

- CMV progression despite monotherapy: consider combination therapy GCV + FOS (above dosing). Progression despite combination therapy: consider CDV.
- GCV resistance well described, and may occur even in previously untreated patients.
- Generally poor prognosis for patients w/ AIDS and CNS CMV. Neurological sequelae common, and existing deficits at time of treatment initiation may not reverse.

Radiculopathy

- Radiculopathy tends to improve within 2–3 wks.
- In severe cases, primary induction/maintenance dosing may need to be continued beyond 6 wks until sufficient clinical response noted. Role of serial CMV PCR testing unclear as to guiding intensity/duration of therapy.

SELECTED REFERENCES

Silva CA, Oliveira AC, Vilas-Boas L, Fink MC, Pannuti CS, Vidal JE. Neurologic cytomegalovirus complications in patients with AIDS: retrospective review of 13 cases and review of the literature. *Rev Inst Med Trop Sao Paulo*, 2010; 52: 305–10.
Comments: Review of 13 patients Dx'd between 2004 and 2008 found that only 4 (31%) were on ART but 8 (62%) had CMV neurological disease as presenting OI. In this group, most presented with diffuse encephalitis (7, 62%), then poly-radiculopathy (7), rhomboencephalitis (1) and ventriculo-encephalitis, although some presentations included multiple presentations types. Mean CD4 was 13 and overall mortality 38%. Variety of treatment regimens used, but no conclusions could be reached regarding their use. Similar to pre-HAART era, 30% of patients present with concomitant CMV retinitis. Authors recommend routine optho exams in all patients with CMV neurological disease. No patients experienced RIS.

Kaplan JE, Benson CA, Holmes KH, et al. Guidelines for prevention and treatment of opportunistic infections in HIV-infected adults and adolescents: recommendations from CDC, the National Institutes of Health, and the HIV Medicine Association of the Infectious Diseases Society of America. *MMWR Recomm Rep*, 2009; 58: 1–206.
Comments: Guideline gives moderately weighted recommendations for combination therapy at outset (rated BII), but also acknowledges significant toxicities with this approach.

Griffiths P. Cytomegalovirus infection of the central nervous system. *Herpes*, 2004; 11 Suppl 2: 95A–104A.
Comments: Author suggests reserving FOS only for GCV-resistant cases due nephrotoxicity concerns or GCV intolerance.

Whitley RJ, Jacobson MA, Friedberg DN, et al. Guidelines for the treatment of cytomegalovirus diseases in patients with AIDS in the era of potent antiretroviral therapy: recommendations of an international panel. International AIDS Society-USA. *Arch Intern Med*, 1998; 158: 957–69.

Comments: Document that serves as basis for suggested therapies. Though little data other than case series exist for neurological CMV disease, extrapolation from CMV retinitis and GI studies not unreasonable given excellent penetration of both GCV (24%–67% of serum level) and FOS (13%–68%) into the CSF.

CMV RETINITIS

James P. Dunn, MD

PATHOGENS

- A member of the Beta *herpesviridae*, double-stranded DNA virus; up to 60%–100% seroprevalence. Most infections asymptomatic, virus shed in absence of Sx. Severe disease seen in fetus, AIDS, and immunosuppressed.
- Transmitted vertically, sexually, or by close contact (family members, daycare) via blood, tears, saliva, breast milk, urine, cervical secretions, and semen.
- Establishes permanent latent infection in host.
- Both primary and secondary infections (reactivation of latent infection or reinfection with another strain) occur. Most cases in immunosuppressed adults tend to be reactivation.

CLINICAL

- CMV retinitis (CMV-R) occurred in ~30% AIDS patients pre-HAART, now ~5% or less in HAART era.
- Most common cause of visual loss in AIDS and most common ocular disease; major cause of impaired quality of life. Retinitis comprises 80%–90% of end-organ CMV disease.
- Median survival after Dx w/ CMV-R 8.5–12 mos in pre-HAART era.
- Sx: (1) often none (15%–50% asymptomatic); (2) floaters, photopsias, blind spots, distortion (blind spots % distortion especially if macula involved); (3) no pain, redness, photophobia.
- Bilateral involvement at time of Dx in 35%. 50% w/ unilateral retinitis develop contralateral involvement within 6 mos if untreated.
- Causes of visual loss: central macular (foveal) necrosis (irreversible); optic neuritis (occasionally reversible); macular edema (occasionally reversible); retinal detachment (surgically treatable). Greater risk in eyes with larger lesions and with lesions involving vitreous base anteriorly. 50% will have detachment in >1 eye at 1 yr after Dx of CMV-R without immune recovery; 33% of eyes will suffer detachment. In HAART era, detachment rate has decreased, but remains similar among those with CD4 <50. Cataract and macular edema are most common causes of visual loss in patients with immune recovery uveitis.
- Clinical course: relentless progression of retinitis in untreated patients: 24 μm/day (range 0–164).

DIAGNOSIS

- Location of retinitis: Zone 1 (posterior, often visible with direct ophthalmoscopy) within 1500 μm (~1 disc diameter) of optic disc or 3000 μm of fovea; considered immediately vision-threatening. Zone 2 (peripheral to Zone 1 but posterior to Zone 3) not considered immediately vision-threatening; direct ophthalmoscopy in well-dilated pupil can image retina into mid-periphery of Zone 2. Zone 3 (anterior to imaginary circle connecting ampulla of vortex veins).
- Spectrum of clinical findings: (1) fulminant/granular retinitis: hemorrhagic retinal necrosis, often with perivascular sheathing (may be present in retina away from area of necrosis); rarely mis-Dx'd; (2) indolent/granular retinitis: minimal or no hemorrhage and no perivascular sheathing; more commonly misdiagnosed; (3) mixed features can be present; (4) dry, granular-appearing border characteristic; (5) lesions may be single or multiple, unilateral, or bilateral; (6) full-thickness retinal necrosis with irreversible loss of function in affected tissue; (7) mild anterior chamber and vitreous inflammatory reaction usually present; fine keratic precipitates typical; no posterior synechiae.
- DDx: acute retinal necrosis (HSV or VZV), progressive outer retinal necrosis (VZV), toxoplasmosis, syphilis, cotton-wool spots, metastatic *Candida* or other fungal endophthalmitis, intraocular lymphoma, tuberculosis.

- Dx: made clinically, confirmatory tests rarely necessary. CMV PCR from vitreous, blood, other sources not in widespread clinical use, but vitreous PCR occasionally helpful in distinguishing CMV-R from necrotizing herpetic retinitis or toxoplasmosis. CMV VL: not used, uncertain significance.
- Sensitivity testing: not yet in widespread use; resistant CMV uncommon at time of Dx but reported to occur at rate of 0.25/person-year in pre-HAART era, similar for GCV and FOS; rate is lower in era of HAART, perhaps due to more potent anti-CMV therapy.

TREATMENT
General Principles
- **Induction-maintenance**: induction: higher or more frequent doses of drug given initially with systemic therapy for 2–3 wks; maintenance (2° prophylaxis): lower or less frequent chronic suppressive doses continued indefinitely to prevent relapse.
- Choice of treatment based on location of retinitis, patient preference, overall general health.
- IV GCV and FOS now rarely used because of need for permanent indwelling catheter and availability of safer options (valganciclovir).
- Systemic GCV shown in randomized clinical trial to reduce risk of KS in patients with CMV-R. Systemic anti-CMV therapy in persistently immunocompromised patients increases survival.
- Zone 1 lesions in patients without immune recovery are best candidates for GCV implant. Small Zone 2 or Zone 3 lesions may respond to ART alone, but concurrent valGCV therapy for up to 6 mos recommended.
- Additional anti-CMV Rx may decrease risk of immune recovery uveitis and may have systemic benefits. Relapse after cessation of therapy is certain in patients not on ART: average within 4 wks.
- Clinical features of treated retinitis: sharp demarcation between necrotic and uninvolved retina; variable pigmentation of necrotic retina; lipid or calcification may be present and should not be confused with active retinitis.

Systemic Therapy
- **IV GCV** (FDA-approved): induction: 5 mg/kg twice daily × 2 wks; maintenance: 5 mg/kg once daily. Side effects: reversible bone marrow suppression (especially leukopenia and anemia), GI (nausea, diarrhea), requires indwelling central venous catheter for daily infusions.
- **Oral GCV** (FDA-approved for maintenance therapy only after 3-wk IV induction therapy completed): 1 g PO 3 times a day. Side effects: similar to IV GCV but no catheter-related complications. Due to large pill burden, use has been replaced by valganciclovir.
- **Valganciclovir** (FDA-approved): valine ester (prodrug) of GCV gives comparable serum levels to IV GCV. Induction: 900 mg PO twice daily × 3 wks; maintenance: 900 mg orally PO once daily. Side effects: similar to IV GCV but no catheter-related complications.
- **Foscarnet (FOS)** (FDA-approved): induction 90 mg/kg IV q12h × 2 wks then maintenance 90–120 mg/kg IV once daily. Efficacy similar to IV GCV. Side effects: reversible nephrotoxicity (dose adjustment required), nausea, hypocalcemia, genital ulcerations, catheter-related infections (including sepsis). Use of FOS now generally limited to patients with bone marrow suppression, unable to tolerate GCV implant surgery, and/or evidence of resistance to GCV. In pre-HAART era, survival in patients treated with FOS longer than with IV GCV (12.6 vs 8.5 mos), possibly due to weak antiretroviral effect of FOS. Probably no enhanced survival benefit of FOS vs GCV in patients concurrently treated with ART.
- **Cidofovir (CDV)** (FDA-approved): induction: 5 mg/kg IV qwk × 2 wks then maintenance: 5 mg/kg IV q2 wks. Avoids need for permanent IV catheter. Side effects: nephrotoxicity (drug given with probenecid and saline hydration before and after CDV infusion), which is usually but not always reversible, cessation of CDV usually required; probenecid toxicity (rash, malaise); uveitis—may be severe, with loss of vision due to ocular hypotony (more common with repeated infusions, usually responds to topical corticosteroids and cessation of CDV therapy). Efficacy: comparable to GCV implant in randomized clinical trial.

Local Therapy
- **GCV ocular implant** (FDA-approved): 4.5 mg sustained-release pellet of GCV surgically placed into vitreous cavity through pars plana incision. Provides constant drug levels × ~8 mos. Intravitreous GCV levels 4-fold higher than IV GCV: faster, more sustained response. Rapid loss of anti-CMV effect when implant exhausted of drug. Planned exchange of implant

sometimes recommended in patients with advanced Zone 1 disease not on ART. Side effects: requires surgery, cataract, endophthalmitis (approximately 0.5%/surgery), vitreous hemorrhage, retinal detachment, no systemic anti-CMV effect. Implant usually given with systemic anti-CMV therapy (e.g., valganciclovir) to reduce risk of contralateral CMV-R (2° prophylaxis) or extraocular CMV and perhaps to improve survival.

- **Intravitreous injections** (non-FDA-approved): sometimes used to obtain rapid intraocular drug levels in eyes with Zone 1 disease prior to more definitive therapy. Usually not sole therapy as inconvenient, provides no protection against contralateral or extraocular CMV infection. May allow control of retinitis during times when patient unable to tolerate systemic therapy because of illness or toxicity. Dosages: GCV 2 mg/0.1 mL 1–2 ×/wk; FOS 2.4 mg/0.1 mL 1–2 ×/wk. Side effects: infection, retinal detachment, vitreous hemorrhage, cataract. Note: intravitreous CDV is toxic to the eye (inflammation and hypotony) and should not be used.

Relapse

- Clinical features of relapse or progression: increased border opacification ("smoldering retinitis"); expansion of previously inactive border of retinitis; appearance of new lesions in same or fellow eye; progression may occur without visible border opacification.
- Careful monitoring of retinitis with serial retinal photographs is most effective means of determining active vs inactive disease.
- Effect of progression on vision is function of location: small progression in Zone 1 disease may cause severe visual loss; occurs within 48–121 days in patients not treated with ART (depending on criteria used to define relapse).
- Hemorrhage alone not an indication of relapse.
- Causes: nonadherence to therapy; poor intraocular drug availability; antiviral resistance (occurred at a rate of ~0.25/person-year with systemic therapy in pre-HAART era, but much lower now).
- Resistance: (1) UL97 mutations: low-grade GCV resistance. Results in decreased phosphorylation of GCV (required for cellular antiviral effect uptake). May respond to GCV implant; usually responds to CDV or FOS (neither requires phosphorylation by viral enzymes). (2) UL54 mutations: high-grade GCV resistance. Results in failure to impair CMV DNA polymerase. Often causes resistance to GCV implant and CDV. (3) Mutations causing FOS resistance less well studied and more difficult to identify.

Treatment of Relapse (or Progression)

- Option: reinduction with same drug.
- Higher dose of maintenance therapy (e.g., FOS 120 vs 90 mg/kg/day) after reinduction.
- Change to different drug (e.g., CDV instead of GCV; use of GCV implant).
- Combination therapy (e.g., GCV + FOS); may be more effective but also more toxic.
- Most effective means of treating or preventing relapse is immune recovery with ART.
- Response to treatment: relapse-free intervals become progressively shorter.

Impact of ART

- Reduced incidence of CMV-R and other ocular infection: 75%–85% reduction in incidence of CMV-R in several studies.
- ART alone may control CMV-R: occasional finding of inactive or regressing CMV-R in patients treated with ART but no specific anti-CMV therapy.
- Not recommended as sole therapy due to: (1) risk of spread of retinitis to fovea or optic nerve before immune recovery occurs in patients with Zone 1 disease; (2) increased risk of immune recovery uveitis among patients with inadequate treatment of CMV-R then started on ART; (3) benefit of systemic anti-CMV therapy on survival among immunocompromised patients.
- Use of ART associated with fewer ocular complications in patients with CMV-R and lower risks of retinal detachment and vision loss.
- Immune recovery uveitis (IRU): syndrome of vitritis and other sequelae of increased intraocular inflammation (± cystoid macular edema [CME], epiretinal membranes) in patients with CMV-R who have been treated with ART. More common in eyes with larger area of retinal involvement, in less aggressively treated eyes, and in eyes of patients treated with IV CDV. Dx: clinical examination, fluorescein angiography, optical coherence tomography. Rx: 50% of patients with CME respond to oral or periocular corticosteroids. Relapse of retinitis in patients treated with corticosteroids rare. May respond to valganciclovir.

- Cessation of anti-CMV therapy: chronic maintenance can be safely discontinued in patients with immune recovery (CD4 >100 × >3–6 mos). Resume maintenance if CD4 declines to <75. Best candidates are those who are ART-naïve at time of Dx, show good immune recovery, and are adherent to ART regimen. Patients with immune recovery have relapse rate of 0.03/person-yr and require regular ophthalmic follow-up (recommended q3 mos).

OTHER INFORMATION
- Most newly Dx'd CMV-R now found in ART-experienced patients.
- ART reduces ocular morbidity associated with CMV-R, especially in patients with immune recovery but to a lesser extent even in nonresponders.
- Progression of CMV-R can occur even in patients with excellent response to ART (0.03/person-yr), so regular ophthalmic monitoring is indicated.

SELECTED REFERENCES

Guidelines for Prevention and Treatment of Opportunistic Infections in HIV-Infected Adults and Adolescents. MMWR Recomm Rep. 2009 Sep 4; 58(RR-11): 1–166.
Comment: Updated OI treatment guidelines.

Otiti-Sengeri J, Meenken C, van den Horn GJ, Kempen JH. Ocular immune reconstitution inflammatory syndromes. *Curr Opin HIV AIDS*, 2008; 3: 432–7.
Comments: Review of immune recovery uveitis (IRU) summarizes risk factors (in addition to improved immunity itself, a low CD4 count at time of initiation of ART, and involvement of a larger proportion of retina), effect on vision and morbidity, and current treatment. A precise definition of IRU remains lacking.

Holland GN. AIDS and ophthalmology: the first quarter century. *Am J Ophthalmol*, 2008; 145: 397–408.
Comments: Reviews evolution of CMV-R from preterminal manifestation of AIDS to chronic, manageable disease with numerous complications. Points of emphasis include retinal detachment, immune recovery uveitis, and visual disturbances (reduced contrast sensitivity, altered color vision, visual field abnormalities) that can occur in HIV+ patients even without infectious retinopathy.

Jabs DA, Van Natta ML, Holbrook JT, et al. Longitudinal study of the ocular complications of AIDS: 1. Ocular diagnoses at enrollment. *Ophthalmology*, 2007; 114: 780–6.
Comments: Large cohort of patients with AIDS in HAART era shows substantial decline in incidence of CMV retinitis compared to pre-HAART era. Incidence of CMV retinitis estimated from retrospective data was 5.60/100 person-yrs. Of 360 patients with CMV-R, over 75% had preexisting CMV-R.

Jabs DA, Van Natta ML, Holbrook JT, et al. Longitudinal study of the ocular complications of AIDS: 2. Ocular examination results at enrollment. *Ophthalmology*, 2007; 114: 787–93.
Comments: In HAART era, CMV-R and other ocular OIs are associated with intraocular inflammation, structural ocular complications, and visual impairment. Patients with newly diagnosed CMV-R have eye examination findings similar to those in pre-HAART era.

HEPATITIS A

Christopher J. Hoffmann, MD, MPH

PATHOGEN
- Hepatitis A virus (HAV): nonenveloped, icosahedral, positive-stranded RNA virus.
- Spread via fecal-oral route; more prevalent in low- and middle-income countries.
- Transmission through contaminated food and water and some sexual practices (oral-anal and digital-anal sex).
- Pathogenesis from robust HAV-specific CD8+ T-cell, NK T-cell, and IFN response leading to hepatocyte destruction.

CLINICAL
- Avg. incubation period 30 days (range 15–50); illness begins in symptomatic patients with abrupt onset of malaise, N/V, anorexia, fevers, hepatomegaly, and RUQ pain followed by icteris and pruritis. Rash and leukocytoclastic vasculitis may occur.
- ALT usually >1000 IU/dL but lower in HIV+ than HIV-negative; alk phos elevated in HIV+, up to 1000 IU/dL. Total bilirubin (>10 common) and direct bilirubin elevated (ALT peak precedes bili elevation).

- Typically acute, self-limited illness with resolution of Sx in 4 wks and normalization of ALT in 8–12 wks.
- Fulminant hepatic failure rare (1/100); occurs more commonly in patients with underlying liver disease, particularly HCV.
- Chronic infection does not occur, but serum viremia and fecal shedding persist longer in HIV+ (viremia may last up to 36 wks and fecal shedding >15 wks).

DIAGNOSIS

- Anti-HAV IgM diagnostic of acute infection, remains + for 4–6 mos; total HAV Ab useful for evidence of past exposure or immunization.
- Other lab abnormalities include nonspecific elevations of ESR, CRP, and increased immunoglobulins.

TREATMENT

Management of Acute or Fulminant Hepatitis

- Usually self limited. Treatment supportive. No pathogen-specific Rx available.
- ART management during acute HAV not well studied. Some providers stop ART until ALT normalizes, while others continue ART. Stopping ART may have its own risks for reasons unrelated to hepatitis as well as increase in risk of liver disease (SMART study) and resistance. Thus, it is prudent to follow 2 or 3 ALT measurements before deciding. If ALT stable or declining, continue ART. If ALT high and rapidly rising, consider discontinuation.
- Patients with fulminant hepatitis require aggressive supportive therapy, and should be transferred to center capable of performing liver transplantation. ART should generally be stopped.

PREVENTION

- Prevent exposure with good hygiene, proper food preparation, and avoidance of unboiled water and uncooked foods from HAV-endemic areas.
- Hepatitis A vaccination should be offered to all at higher risk for HAV infection or of fulminant hepatic failure (international travelers, IDUs, MSM, homeless, HCV or HBV coinfected, chronic liver disease). In addition, consider revaccination after CD4 recovery, as preservation of immunity uncertain even with previous vaccination or exposure. In low-income settings, most people are exposed to HAV early in life and have immunity.
- **Hepatitis A vaccine**: used in patients over 2 years old. Recommended dose for adults 1 mL IM followed by a booster dose in 6–12 mos (consider 3 dose schedule (0, 1, 6 mos) for improved vaccine response; 88% vs 72% seroconversion).
- **Combined hepatitis A/B vaccine** (*Twinrix*): contains 720 ELU of HAV antigen and 20 mcg of HBV antigen. Recommended dose: 3 doses (1 mL each) given on a 0, 1, and 6-month schedule.
- Response to vaccination lower with HIV, especially CD4 (<200) and higher HIV viremia (>1000), but vaccine should still be given, if indicated.
- Follow-up vaccination 1 month later with assessment of Ab response (HAV titer >20 lU/mL). Non-responders should be vaccinated (delay revaccination until CD4 >200).
- **Post-exposure prophylaxis:** if exposed and unvaccinated, efficacy of immune globulin (IG) for prevention of HAV infection well documented. ACIP recommends administration of single IM dose of 0.02 mL/kg as soon as possible but not more than 2 wks after last exposure. Persons who have received at least 1 dose of hepatitis A vaccine at least 1 month before exposure do not need IG.

SELECTED REFERENCES

Launay O, Grabar S, Gordien E, et al. Immunological efficacy of a three-dose schedule of hepatitis A vaccine in HIV-infected adults: HEPAVAC study. *J Acquir Immune Defic Syndr*, 2008; 49: 272–5.
Comments: RCT of 2- vs 3-dose schedule for HAV vaccine. Greater seroconversion with 3 dose, median CD4 350.

Rezende G, Roque-Afonso AM, Samuel D, et al. Viral and clinical factors associated with the fulminant course of hepatitis A infection. *Hepatology*, 2003; 38: 613–8.
Comments: Reviews factors associated with fulminant hepatic failure in patients infected with HAV.

Ida S, Tachikawa N, Nakajima A, et al. Influence of human immunodeficiency virus type 1 infection on acute hepatitis A virus infection. *Clin Infect Dis*, 2002; 34: 379–85.
Comments: Comparison of acute HAV in HIV+ and HIV-negative patients.

HEPATITIS B

Christopher J. Hoffmann, MD, MPH

PATHOGENS
- Hepatitis B virus (HBV): enveloped DNA virus with surface antigen surrounding nucleocapsid made up of core protein, viral genome, and polymerase protein. Maintains persistence in hepatocytes with covalently closed circular (ccc) DNA.

CLINICAL

ACUTE HEPATITIS B
- Acute infection rare in US (3/100,000 person-yrs). Risk factors: unprotected sex, sharing IDU needles, maternal to fetal, piercing and tattoo with unsterile equipment, and lack of vaccination.
- After exposure, average incubation period 45–160 days before Sx. Subclinical in most patients. In patients with Sx: malaise, anorexia, loss of taste for food and cigarettes, aches, arthralgias, and low-grade fever followed by jaundice. Fulminant and fatal <1%.
- Extrahepatic manifestations: PAN, membranous nephropathy, aplastic anemia, erythema multiforme, and serum sickness.

CHRONIC HEPATITIS B
- Chronic hepatitis B (CHB; defined by persistence of HBsAg >6 mos) common among HIV+ patients because of shared modes of transmission and increased progression from acute to CHB with HIV coinfection. Approx. 10% of HIV+ patients coinfected with HBV in US, Europe, and Australia.
- Approximately 5% of HIV-negative adults progress from acute to chronic infection vs 25% of HIV+ adults.
- HIV alters natural Hx of CHB, leading to higher HBV DNA levels, higher likelihood of HBeAg persistence, lower rates of treatment response, and more rapid emergence of resistance to therapy.
- With CHB monoinfection, 25% develop chronic active hepatitis, with progression to cirrhosis in 15%–30%. Hepatocellular carcinoma (HCC) usually occurs after cirrhosis but can also occur without cirrhosis. Among HIV-HBV coinfected, progression to liver disease and death from liver disease occurs more frequently than in CHB monoinfected patients.
- ALT flares during ART can occur for multiple reasons: (1) ART-related hepatotoxicity: usually asymptomatic and spontaneously resolving elevation occurring in 1st 6 mos of ART, but can be life threatening. (2) IRIS: immune response to HBV antigens in liver. May lead to severe hepatitis. Usually occurs in 1st 6 mos. (3) ALT flares as part of natural Hx of CHB, may herald seroconversion from HBeAg to anti-HBe. Occurs at any time, usually among HBeAg+. (4) HBV reactivation after suppression with an anti-HBV agent when agent is withdrawn or with development of resistance (2–12 wks after stopping therapy). (5) Reactivation of HBV with waning immunity.
- CHB does not affect HIV progression (CD4 decline, etc.) or ART response (HIV suppression or CD4 increase).
- Occult hepatitis B defined by presence of HBV DNA (usually <10^5 c/mL) in absence of HBsAg. It is more common in HIV+ patients and is associated with lower CD4 count. Occult HBV can be transmitted but clinical impact unclear.

DIAGNOSIS
- **Acute hepatitis:** detection of anti-HBc IgM with or without HBsAg with appropriate clinical picture. (Both anti-HBc IgM and HBsAg may also be present during chronic infection; clinical picture important.) HBV DNA and HBeAg also present.
- **Recovery from acute HBV infection:** disappearance of HBV DNA, seroconversion of HBeAg to anti-HBe and HBsAg to anti-HBs.
- **Resolved HBV infection:** presence of anti-HBs and anti-HBc. However, anti-HBs detectability wanes with time, anti-HBc persists. Immunity to HBV infection after vaccination indicated by presence of anti-HBs only.
- **Chronic HBV infection:** carrier state defined as persistence of HBsAg >6 mos. If positive, check for high-level HBV replication with HBeAg and HBV DNA.

- **Occult HBV:** HBV DNA present, no detectable HBsAg, HBeAg, or anti-HBs. Anti-HBc may be present.
- Check HBV DNA if (1) HBsAg+, (2) HBsAg-negative with unexplained elevation in ALT, (3) anti-HBc+ with negative HBsAb and HBsAg.
- HBsAg: marker of viral replication and infectiousness. HBeAg: marker of high-level replication and enhanced infectiousness. Absence of both and presence of anti-HBs and anti-HBe, suggests immunologic control (but may still have HBV cccDNA in hepatocytes).
- Liver Bx for evaluation of HBV not usually necessary, though Bx may support decision to delay therapy in coinfected patients.
- Test for HAV, HCV, and HDV to rule out superinfection with other hepatitis viruses.

TREATMENT

Goals of Therapy

- Prevent progression of fibrosis and development of cirrhosis or HCC by suppressing HBV replication.
- Seroconversion from HBeAg+ to anti-HBe and establishment of effective immune control.
- Suppression of HBV DNA; however, therapy does not eradicate cccHBV in hepatocytes.

Criteria for Starting Therapy (Among HIV+)

- HBsAg+ and HBeAg+ and liver disease (ALT >2x ULN or necroinflammation on liver Bx).
- HBsAg+ and HBeAg-and HBV DNA >10^4 c/mL (2000 IU/mL) and evidence of liver inflammation (ALT > ULN or fibrosis on biopsy).
- Use HBV-active ART if ART indicated: dual therapy with TDF/FTC is optimal.
- ART using HBV-active agents (e.g., TDF/FTC + 3rd agent) now indicated in all coinfected patients when HBV therapy required.
- If TDF not tolerated, use entecavir with 3TC or FTC.
- If no ART needed, consider telbivudine (low barrier to resistance) or pegylated interferon (peg-IFN) (if HBV genotype A or B), though often preferable and easier to treat HIV and HBV regardless of ART indications.

Monitoring Therapy

- Routinely assess HBV DNA, ALT, and HBeAg (if + at start of Rx).
- HBV DNA level should decline gradually on effective therapy, without development of resistance. Usually HBV DNA rapidly declines several logs, becoming undetectable within 6–12 mos.
- Consider adding entecavir for patient on TDF + either FTC or 3TC with persistently detectable HBV DNA. However, no RCTs have evaluated this approach.

Criteria for Stopping Therapy

- Peg-IFN: HBeAg+ × 16 wks (goal of HBe seroconversion); HBeAg-negative × 12 mos.
- All therapy: after seroconversion from HBeAg+ to anti-HBe if anti-HBe persists >6 mos.
- NRTIs: indefinite therapy may be needed if no seroconversion, risk of HBV flare if HBV therapy stopped. Monitor closely if Rx stopped with ALT, HBV DNA levels.

HBV Therapies

- **TDF:** (active against HIV and HBV) 300 mg once daily: potent (avg. decrease in HBV DNA 5 log), including those with 3TC resistance. Low rates of resistance reported.
- **3TC:** (active against HIV and HBV) 100 mg once daily for HBV, 300 mg once daily for HIV. At 12 mos, most have decreased ALT and negative HBV DNA. Resistance develops rapidly w/ monotherapy: 50% in 2 yrs, 90% at 4 yrs. Cross-resistance with entecavir, telbivudine, FTC.
- **FTC:** (active against HIV and HBV) 200 mg/day: limited clinical experience but activity appears similar to 3TC. Also coformulated with TDF.
- **Entecavir:** (HBV active, partial HIV RT inhibitor, may select for M184V HIV mutation) 0.5 mg PO once daily (for 3TC-naïve patients) or 1 mg PO once daily (for 3TC-refractory patients) on empty stomach. Potent agent. Cross-resistance with FTC, 3TC, telbivudine.
- **Adefovir (ADF):** (active only against HBV at 10 mg/day) 10 mg once daily (with or without 3TC). Less potent than TDF or entecavir.
- **Telbivudine:** (active only against HBV). Less potent than TDF or entecavir with low barrier to resistance.
- **Peg-IFN:** 180 mcg/wk: minimal experience with HBV, but probably equally effective as IFN-alfa and better tolerated. Good option for HBV genotype A, low HBV DNA, elevated ALT, and when ART not desired (uncommon scenario).

Treatment Categories

- HBV and HIV Rx in 3TC naïve: include TDF/FTC in ART regimen. Adding FTC to TDF for Rx of HBV may increase potency and delay TDF resistance, but no data yet on TDF/FTC for HBV.
- HBV and HIV Rx in 3TC naive but not able to use TDF (renal disease): include FTC or 3TC with ART and add entecavir.
- HBV and HIV Rx in 3TC-experienced with possible HBV resistance to 3TC: continue 3TC or FTC and add TDF.
- HIV Rx only: Avoid, as it would require use of non-recommended ART regimens. Use Rx effective for both HIV and HBV (consider TDF/FTC backbone).
- HBV Rx only: treatment of both HIV and HBV preferred because of simplicity of treating both infections. If treating only HBV, consider peg-IFN (especially if genotype A, low HBV DNA, and high ALT). ADF is option but limited potency. Resistance develops rapidly with telbivudine. Others have HIV activity and select for HIV resistance if non-suppressive of HIV (TDF, FTC, 3TC, possibly entecavir).

Use of ART in HIV-HBV Coinfected Patients

- Increased survival among HIV+ patients with ART has led to increased benefit of treatment of HBV; however, goal of HBV treatment is avoidance of cirrhosis rather than viral eradication.
- Reactivation of HBV following immune reconstitution with ART also described, monitor ALT in coinfected patients early after initiating ART.
- Initiate ART with drugs active against HIV and HBV (TDF + either FTC or 3TC + 3rd agent) if either HIV or HBV therapy required, regardless of CD4 count (DHHS 2008 recommendation).

Other Recommendations for Chronic HBV Coinfection

- Advise abstinence from alcohol.
- Vaccinate against HAV.
- Monitor ALT regularly (q3 mos) and HBV DNA if not current Rx candidate.
- HCC screening q6–12 mos with AFP and US. Most important if patient in high-risk group (age >45 yrs, cirrhosis, or family history of HCC). Note that unlike HCV, HBV can cause HCC in the absence of cirrhosis. Optimal HCC screening in HIV unknown. For now, follow HIV-negative guidelines.
- Transplantation an option for ESLD. HBV infection rate high in transplanted liver but risk of cirrhosis reduced with HBV immune globulin and antivirals.

Prevention

- Vaccination indicated for all HIV+ individuals negative for anti-HBs and HBsAg. Unclear whether HIV+ patients with only positive anti-HBc benefit from immunization; evidence of lack of amnestic response among these individuals, suggesting that vaccination necessary to achieve HBV immunity.
- Vaccination response best with HIV RNA <50 and CD4 >200. Defer vaccination until CD4 >200 or check titers after vaccination at lower CD4 count.
- Dose schedule: 0 mos, 1 mo (1–2 mos), and 6 mos (6–12 mos). If vaccination schedule interrupted, complete 3 doses as if no interruption occurred (unnecessary to restart).
- Alternative dosing schedules have been studied in other populations to achieve higher rates of completing series (0, 7 days, 21 days, and 12 mo; 0, 1 mo, 2 mos, and 12 mos). However, rates of completion similar to standard schedule and limited data available for accelerated schedules among HIV+ populations.
- For highest risk transmission groups, check anti-HBs soon after completing series (within 6 mos). If titer <10 IU/L, repeat 3 dose series with double-dose vaccine.

SELECTED REFERENCES

Joshi D, O'Grady J, Dieterich D, Gazzard B, Agarwal K. Increasing burden of liver disease in patients with HIV infection. *Lancet*, 2011; 377: 1198–209.
Comments: Comprehensive review of issues of liver disease among people living with HIV. Includes overview of HBV treatment.

Thio CL. Hepatitis B and human immunodeficiency virus coinfection. *Hepatology*, 2009; 49(5 Suppl): S138–S45.
Comments: Clear review of current literature on management of HBV among HIV co-infected individuals.

Matthews GV, Seaberg E, Dore GJ, et al. Combination HBV therapy is linked to greater HBV DNA suppression in a cohort of lamivudine-experienced HIV/HBV coinfected individuals. *AIDS*, 2009; 23: 1707–15.
Comments: Cohort study with finding that combined TDF + 3TC or FTC had better HBV DNA suppression than TDF alone, even in 3TC treatment experienced pts.

HEPATITIS C

Christopher J. Hoffmann, MD, MPH

PATHOGENS

- Hepatitis C virus (HCV): small, enveloped, single-stranded RNA virus of the family *Flaviviridae* spread primarily by contact with blood and blood products.

CLINICAL

- HIV/HCV coinfection common in US and Europe due to shared routes of transmission. In US 30% of HIV+ patients are coinfected, with highest rates among IDUs (nearly 95%). HCV is 10× more infectious from needlestick than HIV. Coinfection uncommon in most of Africa.
- After exposure, HIV+ patients more likely to progress to chronic HCV infection (>80%) especially patients with low CD4 counts. They also have higher HCV RNA levels and are more likely to progress to liver disease fibrosis (7–26 vs 23–38 yrs) and cirrhosis than with HCV alone. Lower CD4 count associated with increased fibrosis.
- End-stage liver disease (ESLD) is common cause of mortality in HIV+ patients, especially HCV coinfected. Sustained virologic response (SVR) to HCV therapy lower than with HCV infection alone.
- Effect of HCV on HIV progression unclear.
- Extrahepatic manifestations of HCV: porphyria cutanea tarda, lichen planus, arthralgias, fatigue, mixed cryoglobulinemia (cutaneous and renal disease), and splenic lymphoma.

DIAGNOSIS

- HCV EIA (Ab) for screening; sensitivity and specificity 99% with 3rd-generation assay. All HIV+ patients should be tested in high HCV prevalence regions (such as US).
- False negatives (1%–5% among all HIV+ patients, 15% among IDUs) justify RNA testing in high-risk patients with negative EIA (IDU, low CD4, unexplained high ALT). False negatives also occur during acute infection before seroconversion.
- False positives common in Africa, where prevalence of HCV generally very low.
- Positive EIA should be followed with HCV RNA, which indicates current infection.
- Detectable HCV RNA should be followed with HCV genotype to determine treatment approach and to predict treatment response.
- Liver Bx useful to determine stage of disease and to assess need for therapy, but not always necessary. Serum tests (e.g., *FibroSure*) may be useful if they suggest either cirrhosis or no liver disease; intermediate results less informative. Imaging can help to assess for cirrhosis but has limited sensitivity. Patients not candidates for treatment because of minimal fibrosis should be re-evaluated q2–3 yrs (with Bx or noninvasive means).
- ALT fluctuates during natural Hx and does not reflect disease activity or prognosis.

TREATMENT

General Considerations

- Reduce hepatic risks: vaccinate against HAV and HBV if nonimmune, counsel on abstinence from alcohol and IDU, enroll in IDU treatment and/or methadone maintenance when appropriate, manage psychiatric comorbidities, start ART if patient meets criteria for therapy.
- Educate on HCV transmission modes: blood, shared IDU needles and "works"; anal sex.
- If HCV untreated, screen annually for HCC in high-risk (men, age >45, cirrhotics, patients with HBV coinfection) with AFP and US or CT if high risk.
- Treatment indications: detectable HCV RNA, stable HIV infection, portal or bridging fibrosis or worse liver histology (on Bx or non-invasive testing). Consider treatment even in minimal fibrosis because of accelerated liver disease in HIV-HCV co-infected.
- Treatment contraindications: decompensated liver disease, pregnancy (if on treatment, use contraceptives and 2 forms of birth control until 6 mos after completion of therapy due to risk

of fetal loss and teratogenicity). Drug use and psychiatric disease not contraindications, but patients need to be carefully evaluated and may need extra support.

- Decompensated liver disease (portal hypertension, coagulopathy, ascites, encephalopathy) increase mortality with peg-IFN. Consider evaluation for orthotopic liver transplantation.
- Liver fibrosis score improves with SVR.
- Peg-IFN + RBV is standard for treatment of HCV infection.
- Serine protease inhibitors (boceprevir and telaprevir) are available for treatment of genotype 1 HCV (have in vivo and in vitro activity against genotype 2, but no clinical trials. No activity against genotype 3 or 4). Other protease inhibitors (PIs) and direct antiviral agents are in development that will have activity against wider range of genotypes.

Response to Treatment (for HCV-HIV Coinfection)

- Better response: genotypes 2 and 3 vs 1 and 4; lower HCV RNA ($<$600,000 IU/mL), white race, younger age, elevated ALT at treatment start, IL28B CC genotype.
- RVR (rapid virologic response): negative HCV RNA at wk 4 of treatment.
- eRVR (extended rapid virologic response): negative HCV RNA at wk 4 and wk 12.
- EVR (early virologic response): negative HCV RNA at wk 12 or reduction of HCV RNA by $>$2 log.
- SVR (sustained virologic response): negative HCV RNA $\geq$24 wks after end of treatment.
- SVR genotype 1 with peg-IFN + RBV + PI (HIV-negative): 53%–69%.
- SVR genotype 1 and 4 with peg-IFN + RBV: 14%–46%.
- SVR genoype 2 and 3 with peg-IFN + RBV: 24%–71%.

Acute infection

- If acute HCV Dx'd, repeat HCV RNA assay at 8–12 wks postexposure. If HCV RNA persistently detectable, treat with peg-IFN alfa for 24 wks (see below for dosing). Early treatment after acute infection increases probability of SVR.

Treatment Naïve: Genotype 1 (Using Serine Protease Inhibitor)

- Telaprevir (TVR) 750 mg PO 3 ×/day (when used with EFV, increase dose to 1125 mg PO 3 ×/day) + peg-IFN alfa-2a 180 mcg SQ qwk + RBV 800–1200 mg/day PO (weight based: 1000 mg ≤75 kg; 1200 mg >75 kg) in divided doses.
- Duration: TVR + peg-IFN + RBV dosed for 12 wks followed by peg-IFN + RBV for **12 wks** if eRVR or **36 wks** if no eRVR.
- Boceprevir (BOC) 800 mg PO 3 ×/day (take with food) + peg-IFN alfa-2b 1.5 mcg/kg SQ qwk + RBV 800–1200 mg/day PO (weight based: 800 mg <65 kg; 1000 mg 65–85 kg; 1200 mg 85–105 kg; 1400 mg >105 kg) in divided doses.
- Duration: start with 4 wks peg-IFN + RBV, add BOC at wk 4. Continue with BOC + peg-IFN + RBV for **24 wks** if HCV RNA undetectable after 4 wks of BOC. If HCV RNA detectable after 4 wks of BOC, treat with total of **24 wks** with BOC + peg-IFN + RBV, then continue **20 wks** more with peg-IFN + RBV.

Treatment-experienced Patients Without SVR: Genotype 1 (using serine protease inhibitor)

- Past failure of conventional (3 ×/wk) IFN (± RBV) does not preclude response to peg-IFN + RBV (retreat with peg-IFN + RBV).
- TVR 750 mg PO 3 ×/day (when used with EFV increase dose to 1125 mg PO 3 ×/day) + peg-IFN alfa-2a 180 mcg SQ qwk + RBV 800–1200 mg/day PO (weight based: 1000 mg ≤75 kg; 1200 mg >75 kg) in divided doses.
- Duration: TRV + peg-IFN + RBV dosed for 12 wks followed by peg-IFN + RBV for 36 wks.
- BOC 800 mg PO 3 ×/day + peg-IFN alfa-2b 1.5 mcg/kg SQ qwk + RBV 800–1200 mg/day PO (weight based: 800 mg <65 kg; 1000 mg 65–85 kg; 1200 mg 85–105 kg; 1400 mg >105 kg) in divided doses.
- Duration: start with 4 wks peg-IFN + RBV, at wk 4, add BOC. Continue with BOC + peg-IFN + RBV for 32 wks if HCV RNA undetectable after 4 wks of BOC. If HCV RNA detectable after 4 wks of BOC, treat with total of 44 wks with BOC + peg-IFN + RBV.

Treatment Naïve: Genotype 1 or 4 (Without Serine Protease Inhibitor)

- Peg-IFN alfa-2a 180 mcg SQ qwk + RBV 800–1200 mg/day PO (weight based: 1000 mg ≤75 kg; 1200 mg >75 kg) in divided doses.
- Peg-IFN alfa-2b 1.5 mcg/kg SQ qwk + RBV 800–1400 mg/day PO (weight based: 800 mg <65 kg; 1000 mg 65–85 kg; 1200 mg 85–105 kg; 1400 mg >105 kg) in divided doses.

- Peg-IFN alfa-2a and alfa-2b have similar efficacy in HIV+ patients.
- Duration: 12 wks if no EVR; 24 wks if EVR but HCV RNA still detectable at 24 wks; 48 wks if RVR or HCV RNA undetectable at 12 wks; 72 wks if EVR but with detectable HCV RNA at 12 wks and HCV RNA undetectable at 24 wks (can consider 24 wks if RVR).

Treatment Naïve: Genotypes 2, 3

- Peg-IFN alfa-2a 180 mcg SQ qwk + RBV 800–1200 (weight based: 1000 mg ≤75kg; 1200 mg >75 kg) mg/day PO in divided doses.
- Peg-IFN alfa-2b 1.5 mcg/kg SQ qwk + RBV 800–1200 mg/day PO (weight based: 1,000 mg ≤75 kg; 1200 mg >75 kg).
- Peg-IFN alfa-2a and alfa-2b have similar efficacy in HIV+ patients.
- Duration: 12 wks if no EVR; 24 wks if EVR but HCV RNA detectable at 12 wks and HCV RNA still detectable at 24 wks; 24 wks if RVR (can consider 12–16 wks with RVR); 48 wks if EVR but HCV RNA detectable at 12 wks and HCV RNA undetectable at 24 wks.

Treatment-experienced Patients Without SVR: Genotypes 1,2,3,4 (not Using Serine Protease Inhibitor)

- Past failure of conventional (3 ×/wk) IFN (± RBV) does not preclude response to peg-IFN + RBV (retreat with peg-IFN + RBV); past failure with peg-IFN + RBV suggests low chance of success with repeat treatment.
- Among HIV-negative non-responders, prolonged low-dose IFN does not slow fibrosis.

Use of ART During HCV Therapy

- ART-associated hepatotoxicity may be reduced by treating HCV first.
- NVP has high risk of hepatotoxicity, consider alternative.
- RBV increases toxicity of ddI: avoid combination.
- Anemia common with RBV + AZT: avoid AZT or use with careful monitoring and erythropoietin (EPO) if necessary.
- ABC may decrease SVR, especially with higher HCV RNA and lower RBV dose, consider another agent.
- ATV/r, EFV, RAL, ENF may be co-administered with telaprevir.

Laboratory Monitoring

- CBC, ALT at 2, 4 wks, and qmo. TSH q3–6 mos. Neuropsych eval qmo.
- Human chorionic gonadotropin (HCG) qmo in women.
- CD4 q12 wks. Absolute CD4 usually declines approximately 60% or 100–200 cells while CD4% often rises 3%. Decline in CD4 count does not appear to affect OI risk and should not prompt change in therapy.

Management of Adverse Events

- Anemia (from RBV, peg-IFN, BOC, or TRV): if Hgb <10 g/dL, decrease RBV (by 200 mg at a time); stop RBV if Hgb <8.5 and support with epoeitin alfa (40K IU SQ qwk).
- Severe neutropenia (from peg-IFN): support with G-CSF (5 mcg/day SQ until ANC >1000).
- Depression: consider SSRI (optimally start before starting HCV therapy).

SELECTED REFERENCES

Laguno M, Cifuentes C, Murillas J, et al. Randomized trial comparing pegylated interferon alpha-2b versus pegylated interferon alpha-2a, both plus ribavirin, to treat chronic hepatitis C in human immunodeficiency virus patients. *Hepatology*, 2009; 49: 22–31.
Comments: RCT among HIV+ patients demonstrating similar SVR 24 wks after completing treatment with peg-IFN alfa 2a and 2b (46% vs 42%).

Pawlotsky JM. The results of phase III clinical trials with telaprevir and boceprevir presented at the liver meeting 2010: a new standard of care for hepatitis C virus genotype 1 infection, but with issues still pending. *Gastroenterology*, 2011; 140: 746–54.
Comments: Review of clinical trials, dosing, and side effects of telaprevir and boceprevir.

Ghany MG, Strader DB, Thomas DL, Seeff LB; American Association for the Study of Liver Disease. Diagnosis, management, and treatment of hepatitis C: an update. *Hepatology*, 2009; 49: 1335–74.
Comments: AASLD Practice Guidelines for HCV management.

Bacon BR, Gordon SC, Lawitz E, et al. Boceprevir for previously treated chronic HCV genotype 1 infection. *N Engl J Med*, 2011; 364: 1207–17.
Comments: Phase III product registration trial for boceprevir in patients with relapsed HCV.

Poordad F, McCone J Jr, Bacon BR, et al. Boceprevir for untreated chronic HCV genotype 1 infection. *N Engl J Med*, 2011; 364: 1195–206.
Comments: Phase III product registration trial for boceprevir in treatment naïve patients.

HERPES SIMPLEX

Lisa A. Spacek, MD, PhD and Khalil G. Ghanem, MD, PhD

DIAGNOSIS

PATHOGENS

- HSV-1 and HSV-2 are double-stranded enveloped DNA viruses.
- Chronic herpesvirus infection establishes latency in sensory ganglia of nerves innervating site of initial mucocutaneous infection.
- Prevalence of both HSV-1 or HSV-2 infection as high as 80% in HIV+ persons.
- Activates HIV replication and enhances sexual transmission of HIV.

CLINICAL

- **HSV-1:** orolabial ulcers, herpetic whitlow (felon), stomatitis, keratitis, anogenital ulcerations, proctitis, esophagitis, tracheobronchitis/pneumonitis, retinal necrosis, encephalitis, transverse myelitis, disseminated infection.
- **HSV-2:** ulcerative anogenital disease and proctitis more common than with HSV-1, though clinical syndromes overlap extensively; meningitis, lumbosacral radiculitis.
- **Genital herpes:** grouped vesicles on erythematous base ("dew drops on rose petal"); "atypical" presentations (erythema, itching, tingling, shallow or linear erosions) also common.
- **DDx of genital ulcers:** syphilis, chancroid, Behçet's disease, herpes zoster, lymphogranuloma venereum, granuloma inguinale, leishmaniasis, blastomycosis, mucocutaneous manifestation of inflammatory bowel disease, idiopathic ulcers.
- **DDx of orolabial ulcers:** aphthous ulcers, Behçet's disease, histoplasmosis.
- **DDx of perianal herpes/proctitis:** similar to genital ulcer disease; also consider HPV-associated anal lesions, gonorrhea, and chlamydia.
- **HSV retinitis:** as acute retinal necrosis can led to rapid vision loss.

DIAGNOSIS

- PCR most sensitive; can discriminate HSV-1/2; gold standard for Dx of HSV encephalitis.
- Viral Cx from lesion confirms Dx; isolates should be typed, HSV-1/2. Low sensitivity in setting of recurrence, lesions in healing phase, or after initiation of antiviral Rx.
- Skin Bx: may be useful with atypical lesions; antigen detection by HSV-1/2 DFA staining diagnostic.
- Chronic infection diagnosed by type-specific serologic testing.
- "Tzanck prep" of lesion scrapings may demonstrate multinucleated giant cells (60% sensitive for infection with Herpesviridae family), not sensitive or specific for HSV.

TREATMENT

General Principles

- HIV+ patients with preserved immune function may be managed similarly to HIV-negative patients; those with low CD4 may benefit from higher dose of antivirals and/or longer duration of therapy.
- Extend duration of therapy for all clinical episodes if lesion healing incomplete after the term stated; consider possibility of drug resistance.
- Bacterial superinfection may complicate genital outbreaks causing perineal cellulitis, requiring antibacterial as well as more aggressive antiviral therapy.
- Higher rates of asymptomatic HSV shedding in immunosuppressed HIV+ persons (compared to HIV-negative).
- Consistent use of latex condoms reduces HSV-2 acquisition.

Orolabial Lesions and Initial or Recurrent Genital HSV

- **Acyclovir (ACV):** 400 mg PO 3 times daily.
- **Valacyclovir:** 1 g PO twice daily.
- **Famciclovir:** 500 mg PO twice daily.

Severe Mucocutaneous HSV

- **ACV:** 5–10 mg/kg IV q8h continue until clinical improvement observed. Then change to PO therapy until lesions completely healed.

ACV-Resistant Mucocutaneous HSV

- Thymidine kinase-deficient mutations most frequent cause of acyclovir resistance; cross-resistant to valacyclovir and famciclovir. Consider viral resistance testing when clinically significant disease progresses or persists despite therapy.

- FOS 80–120 mg/kg/day IV in 2–3 divided doses until clinical response.
- Topical trifluridine, CDV, and imiquimod. Treat 21–28 days or more. Topical preparations can be prepared by compounding IV CDV and ophthalmic trifluridine.

HSV Encephalitis

- ACV 10 mg/kg IV q8h × 21 days.
- Monitor renal function 1–2 × per wk and dose-adjust prn. TTP/HUS reported on high-dose valacyclovir (8 gm/day), but not reported at doses used for Rx of HSV.

Suppressive Therapy in HIV

- **ACV:** 400 mg PO twice daily.
- **Valcyclovir:** 500 mg PO twice daily.
- **Famiciclovir:** 500 mg PO twice daily (500–1000 mg PO once daily often used).
- Suppressive therapy indicated if frequent or severe recurrences of genital herpes.

SELECTED REFERENCES

Tanton C, Weiss HA, Le Goff J, et al. Correlates of HIV-1 genital shedding in Tanzanian women. *PLoS One*, 2011; 6: e17480. **Comments:** Nested study of HIV+ women enrolled in a randomized, controlled study of HSV suppressive Rx detected cervico-vaginal HIV-1 RNA at 52.0% of 971 visits among 482 women, which was independently associated with HSV DNA detection.

Baeten JM, Lingappa J, Beck I, et al. Herpes simplex virus type 2 suppressive therapy with acyclovir or valacyclovir does not select for specific HIV-1 resistance in HIV-1/HSV-2 dually infected persons. *J Infect Dis*, 2011; 203: 117–21. **Comments:** Prospective testing for HIV-1 genotypic resistance at RT codon 75 in plasma from 168 HIV+ persons from Botswana, Kenya, Peru, and the United States taking daily ACV or valacyclovir for 8 wks to 24 mos did NOT detect V75I (95% CI, 0%–2.2%).

Workowski KA, Berman S; Centers for Disease Control and Prevention. Sexually transmitted diseases treatment guidelines, 2010. *MMWR Recomm Rep*, 2010; 59: 20–5. **Comments:** Suppressive Rx can reduce recurrences by 70%–80%, safety and efficacy documented.

Hayes R, Watson-Jones D, Celum C, van de Wijgert J, Wasserheit J. Treatment of sexually transmitted infections for HIV prevention: end of the road or new beginning? *AIDS*, 2010; 24 Suppl 4: S15–26. **Comments:** Despite lack of evidence to support reduced HIV transmission (1 of 9 trials showed effect), article argues that Rx of curable STIs is cheap, simple, effective, and an essential component of community HIV control programs.

Kim HN, Wang J, Hughes J, et al. Effect of acyclovir on HIV-1 set point among herpes simplex virus type 2-seropositive persons during early HIV-1 infection. *J Infect Dis*, 2010; 202: 734–8. **Comments:** Study of 76 HIV+ seroconverters enrolled in placebo-controlled trial of acyclovir (400 mg bid) for the prevention of HIV acquisition in HSV-2-seropositive persons, found no difference in VL or CD4 for ACV vs placebo. Development of V75I was not observed.

Celum C, Wald A, Lingappa JR, et al. Acyclovir and transmission of HIV-1 from persons infected with HIV-1 and HSV-2. *N Engl J Med*, 2010; 362: 427–39. **Comments:** A randomized, placebo-controlled trial of suppressive Rx for HSV-2 (ACV 400 mg PO twice daily) in couples in which only one of the partners was seropositive for HIV-1 (CD4 ≥250), co-infected with HSV-2, and was not taking ART studied HIV-1 transmission. Of 132 HIV-1 seroconversions, 84 were linked within couples by viral sequencing: 41 in the acyclovir group and 43 in the placebo group (HR, 0.9; 95% CI, 0.6–1.4).

Kaplan JE, Benson CA, Holmes KH, et al. Guidelines for prevention and treatment of opportunistic infections in HIV-infected adults and adolescents: recommendations from CDC, the National Institutes of Health, and the HIV Medicine Association of the Infectious Diseases Society of America. *MMWR Recomm Rep*, 2009; 58: 61–63. **Comments:** HSV infects the majority of HIV+ patients, laboratory confirmation of dx recommended, suppressive Rx (valacyclovir 500 mg q day) reduced HSV-2 transmission by 50%.

HERPES ZOSTER

Lisa A. Spacek, MD, PhD and Khalil G. Ghanem, MD, PhD

PATHOGENS

- Varicella zoster virus (VZV), an enveloped double-stranded DNA virus, member of *Herpesviridae* family; establishes lifelong latency after initial infection.
- Primary infection (varicella) usually acquired by respiratory droplet; acquisition from reactivation zoster less common; contact with vesicle/ulcer (zoster), disseminated disease (zoster), or pneumonitis (varicella or disseminated zoster).

CLINICAL

- Primary varicella infection ("chicken pox") usually occurs in early life within community-based outbreaks; significantly less common since widespread adoption of VZV immunization for children.
- Recurrent infection (herpes zoster [HZ] or dermatomal zoster) occurs later; highest risk in elderly or immunocompromised, including HIV/AIDS, where risk is >15-fold higher than age-matched controls.
- Other clinical manifestations: disseminated (nondermatomal) zoster, acute or chronic encephalitis, transverse myelitis, cerebellar ataxia (especially following acute infection), cerebral angiitis, aseptic meningitis, acute retinal necrosis, progressive outer retinal necrosis, and pneumonitis.
- Zoster-associated pain syndromes: major morbidity of HZ; acute neuritis and zoster-associated neuralgia.
- Greater risk of HZ events and HZ complications with CD4 <200; case reports and clinical series suggest risk of HZ may increase shortly after ART initiation as immune restoration occurs. After 4–16 wks on ART, risk of HZ increased 2- to 4-fold from baseline.
- Immunocompromise associated with prolonged clinical course, recurrent or chronic lesions, multiple dermatomes, and verrucous or nodular lesions.

DIAGNOSIS

- Characteristic rash (either of primary varicella or HZ) usually leads to clinical Dx without need for additional testing. Lesions may be atypical with advanced immune suppression requiring Tzanck, Bx, or Cx.
- Tzanck prep of lesion scrapings may demonstrate multinucleated giant cells (60% sensitive for infection with *Herpesviridae* family).
- Skin Bx: may be especially useful with atypical lesions; VZV DFA stain diagnostic.
- PCR from lesion exudate or from CSF (in encephalitis, may be positive with HZ reactivation/meningitis) highly sensitive and specific.
- Cx from lesion also confirmatory; reduced sensitivity if antiviral therapy initiated; rarely useful to support early medical decision making.

TREATMENT

Dermatomal Herpes Zoster

- **Valacyclovir:** 1 g PO 3 ×/day × 7–10 days.
- **Famciclovir:** 500 mg PO 3 ×/day × 7–10 days.
- **ACV:** 800 mg PO 5 ×/day × 7–10 days.
- Effective in immune competent patients only if initiated within 72 hr; for immune suppressed, treat unless lesions crusted.
- Use of adjunct corticosteroids for HZ of equivocal benefit in immunocompetent hosts for preventing zoster-associated neuralgia; not recommended in HIV infection.

Severe Infection (CNS, Ocular, Disseminated)

- **ACV:** 10 mg/kg IV q8h × 14–21 days.
- Consider Rx for severe infection whenever clinical diagnosis of zoster likely + altered mental status or visual Sx while definitive Dx pursued.

Suspected ACV Resistance

- Relatively infrequent event, risk of occurrence increases when immunocompromised hosts are on prolonged ACV (or other nucleoside) therapy.
- **Foscarnet:** 40 mg/kg IV q8h or 60 mg/kg IV q12h.
- Consider ACV resistance and viral susceptibility testing when new lesions evolve on high-dose ACV therapy.

Pain Control and Adjunct Measures

- Pain control, in addition to antiviral therapy, is among primary clinical goals in HZ management and is frequently suboptimal, both for acute neuritis and zoster-associated neuralgia. Tricyclic antidepressant (TCA) started within 48 hrs reduced occurrence of postherpetic neuralgia (PHN).
- Narcotics may be most useful for pain of acute episode; for chronic HN, controlled-release oxycodone (up to 60 mg daily) or morphone (up to 240 mg daily).

- Adjunct for chronic pain: gabapentin: start 100–300 mg qhs or 100 mg 3 times daliy, then titrate by 100 mg 3 ×/day as tolerated to reach 1800–3600 mg daily target; lidocaine patch 5% (lidoderm): use up to 12h daily, up to 3 patches; TCAs: amitriptyline 25 mg at bedtime for 3 mo within 48 hr of rash onset.
- Options to try in refractory patients: capsaicin 0.025%–0.075% cream 4 ×/day, nerve blocks, spinal cord stimulation, intrathecal methylprednisolone.
- Use of adjunct corticosteroids for HZ of equivocal benefit in immunocompetent hosts for preventing PHN; not recommended in HIV infection.

Prevention and Prophylaxis
- Chronic suppressive antiviral therapy may be warranted in persons with multiple or severe HZ events while at elevated risk (low CD4 or during period of immune restoration with ART).
- Period of infectiousness: primary or disseminated varicella—48 hrs prior to lesion onset until lesions crusted or dry; for HZ, significant exposure would require direct lesion contact during early eruption (48 hrs).
- Precautions: airborne and contact isolation in healthcare facility for primary varicella; standard precautions for HZ. Staff who are VZV-susceptible should not care for patients with primary varicella or HZ.
- **Postexposure prophylaxis:** if exposure to primary or disseminated VZV in person with no history of chickenpox and/or negative anti-varicella IgG, varicella zoster immune globulin (VZIG) indicated, ideally within 48 hrs (up to 96 hrs): 500 units IM (4 125 unit vials) for patients 30–40 kg and 625 units IM (one 625 unit vial × 1 vial) for patients >40 kg.
- **Varicella vaccination:** consensus panel recommendations for giving live viral vaccine (*Varivax*) to HIV+ children if age-specific CD4 15%–24%; 2-dose series starting at 12 mos, at least 3 mos apart. If rash evolves, skin should be covered and contact with immunocompromised adults in household restricted. Adolescents and adults without natural immunity should be vaccinated if CD4 >200.
- **Herpes zoster vaccination:** single dose of HZ vaccine (*zostavax*) approved for use in older nonimmunocompromised adults >60 years to prevent zoster.
- Per ACIP recommendations: zoster vaccine should not be administered to persons with AIDS or other clinical manifestations of HIV, including persons with CD4 counts <200 or CD4 % <15.

Primary Infection: Varicella
- Normal adult: Rx within 24 hr onset of exanthem for efficacy. ACV 800 mg PO 5 ×/day × 5 days.
- Varicella pneumonia: ACV 10–12 mg/kg q8h, or valacyclovir 1 g PO 3 ×/day or famciclovir 500 mg PO 3 ×/day, all for 7–10 days.

SELECTED REFERENCES

Kaplan JE, Benson CA, Holmes KH, et al. Guidelines for prevention and treatment of opportunistic infections in HIV-infected adults and adolescents: recommendations from CDC, the National Institutes of Health, and the HIV Medicine Association of the Infectious Diseases Society of America. *MMWR Recomm Rep*, 2009; 58: 64–66.
Comments: Updates OI guidelines include discussion of necrotizing retinopathy. Both acute retinal necrosis (ARN) and progressive outer retinal necrosis (PORN) are associated with vision loss.

Birlea M, Arendt G, Orhan E, et al. Subclinical reactivation of varicella zoster virus in all stages of HIV infection. *J Neurol Sci*, 2011; 304: 22–4.
Comments: Serologic study of 200 paired serum and CSF samples from 180 HIV+ patients, 28 (16%) had CSF VSV antibodies. In CNS VZV infection, CSF may be VZV DNA–, but VZV Ab+; therefore, test for VZV DNA, anti-VZV IgG and IgM Abs.

Newsome SD, Nath A. Varicella-zoster virus vasculopathy and central nervous system immune reconstitution inflammatory syndrome with human immunodeficiency virus infection treated with steroids. *J Neurovirol*, 2009; 15: 288–91.
Comments: Case report of VZV vasculopathy describes CNS-IRIS in a HIV+ patient whose condition deteriorated after corticosteroids were withdrawn, then recovered on reinstitution of IV methylprenisolone. Patient required prolonged steroid Rx including high-dose IV steroids followed by prednisone taper.

Harpaz R, Ortega-Sanchez IR, Seward JF; Advisory Committee on Immunization Practices (ACIP) Centers for Disease Control and Prevention. Prevention of herpes zoster: recommendations of the Advisory Committee on Immunization Practices (ACIP). *MMWR Recomm Rep*, 2008; 57: 1–30.
Comments: Comprehensive review of zoster and current vaccine recommendations. Guidelines suggest zoster vaccine not be administered to persons with AIDS or other clinical manifestations of HIV, including CD4 <200 or CD4 % <15%.

Kimberlin DW, Whitley RJ. Varicella-zoster vaccine for the prevention of herpes zoster. *N Engl J Med*, 2007; 356: 1338–43.
Comments: Review of VZV pathophysiology and vaccine indications.

PROGRESSIVE MULTIFOCAL LEUKOENCEPHALOPATHY (PML)

Scott Newsome, DO and Jeffrey Rumbaugh, MD, PhD

DIAGNOSIS

PATHOGENS

- Caused by JC virus, a double-stranded DNA polyomavirus. JC virus infection leads to destruction of oligodendrocytes in susceptible individuals.
- JC virus present in >70% of human population and is typically asymptomatic, although it can reactivate and cause PML in immunosuppressed host (i.e., HIV, post-organ transplant, etc.) and in patients with autoimmune disorders on immunomodulating therapies (i.e., natalizumab, rituximab).
- Virus resides in extraneural reservoirs such as lymphoid tissue, kidney, and bone marrow.
- Primarily affects white matter of brain, but can involve deep gray matter structures and rarely spinal cord.

CLINICAL

- Demyelinating disease of CNS. Areas of demyelination are monofocal or multifocal and can occur in any region of brain. Posterior regions of brain and posterior fossa structures (i.e., brainstem and cerebellum) commonly involved. Myelopathy rare.
- Affects patients with immunosuppression due to HIV and other causes. Most patients have advanced AIDS, though can sometimes present with higher CD4 counts. Was associated with poor prognosis before ART.
- Presenting Sx: subacute onset of focal neurological deficits (classic triad of hemiparesis, visual field deficit, and cognitive dysfunction).
- Other Sx: gait disorders, brainstem signs, sensory, and language disturbances. Focal seizures in 10%.
- Higher mortality with CD4 <100.
- Favorable prognostic features: younger age, presenting manifestation of AIDS, CD4 >300, low JC virus DNA load at baseline, contrast-enhancement on MRI, ART-naïve, neurologic improvement on ART.
- Though ART is treatment of choice, PML may progress or appear after initiating ART due to IRIS.
- Even with ART, mortality still approximately 50% within 1st year of Sx onset.

DIAGNOSIS

- MRI with and without contrast: subcortical white matter hyperintense areas on T-2 weighted images and fluid attenuated inversion recovery (FLAIR) sequences. T-1 weighted images reveal hypointense lesions that typically do not enhance but can do so in 5%–10% of cases. Mass effect and edema can rarely be seen in setting of PML-IRIS.
- Enhancing MRI lesions may occur on ART in context of IRIS.
- HIV dementia can be differentiated from PML by its symmetrical appearance and involvement of periventricular and deep white matter areas. Also, U-fiber involvement commonly seen in PML and not HIV dementia.
- CSF valuable to exclude other OIs and to obtain CSF JC virus PCR: moderate sensitivity, high specificity. Higher CSF levels of JC virus associated with poorer prognosis.
- Brain Bx: multifocal demyelination, hyperchromatic and enlarged oligodendrocytes, and enlarged bizarre astrocytes. EM: JC virus in oligodendrocytes.

TREATMENT

Medications

- Most effective therapy is ART, which prolongs survival and decreases neurologic deficits when effective immune reconstitution achieved.
- MRI lesions may get worse after beginning ART because of IRIS. For severe cases of PML-IRIS, steroids have been used with varying success. Further studies needed to specifically evaluate potential role of steroids in PML-IRIS.
- Interferon (IFN) alfa studied in an open-label trial, with delayed progression and slightly prolonged survival; some patients showed marked improvement. MRI showed lesion regression in 4 patients, but did not correlate with clinical remission.
- Topotecan at dose of 0.3 gm/m^2/day to maximum dose of 0.6 mg/m^2/day showed decreased lesion size and prolonged survival, but small study size. Most frequent side effects were hematologic (anemia, thrombocytopenia, and neutropenia).

- Cytosine arabinoside (ARA-C) administered IV or intrathecally did not affect overall prognosis or neurologic status.
- Cidofovir (CDV) not effective in treatment of PML; can cause nephrotoxicity and ocular hypotonia.
- CMX001 (1-O-hexadecyloxypropyl-cidofovir) inhibits JCV replication *in vitro*.
- 5HT2A receptor antagonists (chlorpromazine, clozapine, mirtazapine) decrease replication of JC virus in vitro; no adequate clinical studies available. Other medications studied include atypical antipsychotics (ziprasidone, olanzapine, risperidone).
- *In vitro* screening suggests that the antimalarial drug, mefloquine, could be an effective therapy for PML by an unknown mechanism. A randomized, rater-blinded human study to determine mefloquine's usefulness in PML was stopped prematurely after interim analysis demonstrated no benefit.

FOLLOW-UP
Common Practice
- Reassess MRI 1 mo after beginning therapy to look for improvement or progression.
- Monitor virological serology (i.e., CD4 count and VL) while on ART to assess for immune reconstitution.

SELECTED REFERENCES

Tan K, Roda R, Ostrow L, McArthur J, Nath A. PML-IRIS in patients with HIV infection: clinical manifestation and treatment with steroids. *Neurology*, 2009; 72: 1458–64.
Comments: Some patients with PML-IRIS may derive benefit from steroid treatment; however, controlled trials are needed.

Cettomai D, McArthur J. Mirtazapine use in human immunodeficiency virus-infected patients with progressive multifocal leukoencephalopathy. *Arch Neurol*, 2009; 66: 255–8.
Comments: Mirtazapine may be useful for treating PML in combination with ART; however, a clinical trial is warranted.

Clifford DB, Yiannoutsos C, Glicksman M, et al. HAART improves prognosis in HIV-associated progressive multifocal leukoencephalopathy. *Neurology*, 1999; 52: 623–5.
Comments: ART improves prognosis in PML, correlated with viral load reduction.

Guidelines for Prevention and Treatment of Opportunistic Infections in HIV-Infected Adults and Adolescents. MMWR Recomm Rep. 2009 Sep 4; 58(RR-11): 1–166.
Comments: Latest OI Guidelines.

Musculoskeletal Complications

AVASCULAR NECROSIS

Todd T. Brown, MD, PhD

PATHOGENESIS
- In general population, ethanol use and glucorticoid use account for 90% of cases. Other associated conditions include lupus, sickle cell disease, organ transplantation, antiphospholipid antibodies, trauma, radiation.
- In HIV+ patients, incidence is 100× that of general population. Asymptomatic disease found in 6%.
- Risk factors include low CD4 nadir, prior AIDS-defining illness, dyslipidemia, and traditional risk factors. Majority of patients exposed to glucocorticoids or megestrol.
- Direct role of ART controversial. Pharmacologic inhibition of CYP3A4 may increase exogenous glucocorticoid exposure.
- Exact pathogenesis is uncertain. Above risk factors may predispose to compromised local blood flow.

CLINICAL
- Hip involvement most common (>75% cases). Knee, ankle, shoulder, small bones of hands and feet also reported.
- Multiple sites (including contralateral side) affected in >40%.
- Pain with weight bearing or motion is the most common Sx. For AVN of the hip, pain can be in groin, thigh, or buttocks. In more advanced cases, pain can occur at rest and at night.
- Asymptomatic disease is common and most remain pain free.

DIAGNOSIS
- Evaluation begins with plain films (anterior-posterior and frog-leg views for hip). Findings may include changes in density and sclerosis. Subchondral lucency (crescent sign) indicates subchondral collapse. Sensitivity of plain films limited, especially in mild disease.
- MRI is most sensitive diagnostic tool. It may show border between healthy and diseased bone or linear area of vascular granulation tissue (double line sign). In hip, greater involvement of joint surface (>50%) associated with worse Sx and poorer prognosis, including collapse.

TREATMENT

Treatments
- Nonsurgical therapy including analgesia, physical therapy to strengthen surrounding muscle, and limitation of weight bearing may be appropriate in mild cases, particularly if <15% of joint involved.
- Small, short-term clinical trials of bisphosphonates (alendronate 70 mg weekly) have shown promising results and anti-resorptive therapy may be beneficial in selected patients. Long-term efficacy and safety not established. Bisphosphonate therapy has been associated with osteonecrosis of jaw, although mechanism unclear.
- Surgical treatment may include core decompression, osteotomy of necrotic bone, or joint replacement. Success of joint replacement for osteonecrosis may be less than for other conditions.

SELECTED REFERENCES

Cardozo JB, Andrade DM, Santiago MB. The use of bisphosphonate in the treatment of avascular necrosis: a systematic review. *Clin Rheumatol*, 2008; 27: 685–8.
Comments: Review of the use of bisphosphonates in AVN.

Miller KD, Masur H, Jones EC, Joe GO, et al. High prevalence of osteonecrosis of the femoral head in HIV-infected adults. *Ann Int. Med*, 2002 Jul 2; 137(1): 17–25.

Morse CG, Mican JM, Jones EC, et al. The incidence and natural history of osteonecrosis in HIV-infected adults. *Clin Infect Dis*, 2007; 44: 739–48.
Comments: Recent follow-up to previous NIH study (Miller, *Ann Int Med*, 2002) which initially showed 4.5% prevalence of asymptomatic osteonecrosis in 339 patients. Over 7 years of follow-up, 1.5% of those without osteoncrosis developed disease (2/5 cases symptomatic). 4/18 of the original asymptomatic cases required hip replacement.

Mary-Krause M, Billaud E, Poizot-Martin I, et al. Risk factors for osteonecrosis in HIV-infected patients: impact of treatment with combination antiretroviral therapy. *AIDS*, 2006; 20: 1627–35.
Comments: Well-done study implicating ART in pathogenesis of osteonecrosis. Compared to untreated patients, relative risk of osteonecrosis 2.5 (95% CI 1.2–5.9) for those treated with ART <12 mos and 5.1 (95% CI, 2.1–12.6) for those treated for >60 mos.

Gutiérrez F, Padilla S, Masiá M, et al. Osteonecrosis in patients infected with HIV: clinical epidemiology and natural history in a large case series from Spain. *J Acquir Immune Defic Syndr*, 2006; 42: 286–92.
Comments: Documents significant disability in half of patients with symptomatic osteonecrosis. Location at hip and male gender associated with less favorable outcomes.

Lai KA, Shen WJ, Yang CY, et al. The use of alendronate to prevent early collapse of the femoral head in patients with nontraumatic osteonecrosis. A randomized clinical study. *J Bone Joint Surg Am*, 2005; 87: 2155–9.
Comments: One of a few clinical trials of bisphosphonates for osteonecrosis. Alendronate 70 mg weekly associated with improved Sx and reduced progression to collapse compared to control group.

MUSCLE DISORDERS

Christopher P. Eckstein, MD and Michael Levy, MD, PhD

CLINICAL

- Most common cause of weakness and disability with AIDS is muscle atrophy and wasting from nutritional deficiency and repeated infections.
- Three most common primary muscle disorders in HIV are HIV myopathy, idiopathic polymyositis, and myopathy due to toxicity from NRTIs. Less common primary muscle disorders include lymphoma, inclusion body myositis, and infections such as toxoplasmosis.
- Myalgias, muscle tenderness, and weakness of the proximal muscles are common features of all primary muscle disorders in HIV. Inclusion body myositis spreads to include distal muscles as well.
- Differentiating among the many etiologies of primary muscle disorders is difficult. Empiric treatment and retrograde Dx is common.
- Infectious causes of myopathy must be ruled out before empiric immunosuppression. These include pyomyositis by *S. aureus* (90% of cases) and *Toxoplasma*. Pyomyositis usually presents with localized tenderness and swelling more than weakness; toxoplasmosis presents insidiously with diffuse muscle wasting and weakness similar to noninfectious etiologies.
- Secondary causes of muscle weakness and tenderness include rhabdomyolysis, involvement in non-Hodgkin lymphoma, cocaine abuse, trauma, and seizures. These can present in all stages of HIV infection.

DIAGNOSIS

- Evaluate for general systemic features such as fever, arthralgias, or rash, including thorough neurological examination with detailed evaluation of involved muscles to look for localized muscle infections.
- CD4 count does not correlate with HIV myopathy but is low in infectious myopathies.
- Reflexes usually preserved in primary myopathy. Involvement of reflexes suggests an additional neuropathy (decreased reflexes) or spinal cord dysfunction (increased reflexes).
- Serum CPK elevated >10× normal in HIV myopathy and in several of other etiologies. Follow CPK levels to monitor resolution. Aldolase does not add additional information. Lactate occasionally elevated and usually follows CPK levels.
- In both HIV myopathy and polymyositis, EMG reveals increased insertional activity, fibrillations, and polyphasic potentials. In NRTI-associated myopathy, EMG may show mild myopathic changes or may be normal.
- Muscle Bx may reveal pathology. Bx with HIV myopathy and polymyositis shows CD8+ T lymphocytes in endomysium. Evidence of HIV viral infection of muscle tissue rare in HIV myopathy. NRTI-associated myopathy usually unremarkable except in cases involving high doses of AZT, which can cause mitochondrial myopathy with "ragged-red" fibers. Intracellular cysts containing *T. gondii* confirms Dx of toxoplasmosis.
- Compile complete drug Hx, including use of AZT, illicit drugs, and statins.

TREATMENT

Medical and Surgical

- **Pyomyositis:** broad spectrum ABx ± surgical drainage may be needed.
- **HIV myopathy/idiopathic polymyositis:** long-term corticosteroids, dose 1 mg/kg/day with gradual taper if CD4 <200. Alternative: IVIG 0.4 mg/kg/day × 5 days on monthly basis.
- **NRTI-associated myopathy:** discontinue NRTI and follow CPK levels. If levels do not return to normal within 1–2 mos, HIV myopathy or polymyositis should be suspected. For NRTI-

associated myopathy, NSAIDs may provide symptomatic relief and carnitine may prevent development of myopathy if administered concurrently with NRTI.
- **Rhabdomyolysis:** stop offending agent; IV hydration to prevent renal failure.
- **HIV-associated wasting:** see Wasting p. 98.
- **Toxoplasmosis:** primary regimen is combination of pyrimethamine (200-mg loading dose followed by 50–75 mg daily) plus sulfadiazine (4–6 g daily). Patients with sulfa intolerance can substitute clindamycin (600 mg 4 times daily) for sulfadiazine. Leucovorin or folic acid will prevent bone marrow toxicity from pyrimethamine.

FOLLOW-UP
Routine Clinical Monitoring
- Monitor CPK monthly during treatment of muscle disorders.
- Muscle strength examination. May use dynamometer: gives objective values on weakened muscles.
- Monitor renal function with high CPK and during IVIG therapy.
- Corticosteroid therapy: monitor for complications, including OIs. Use OI prophylaxis based on CD4 count.
- Discontinue therapy when asymptomatic and CPK normal for >3 mos.
- Taper steroids slowly over 1–2 mos.

SELECTED REFERENCES
Pongrantz D. Therapeutic options in autoimmune inflammatory myopathies (dermatomyositis, polymyositis, inclusion body myositis). *J Neurol*, 2006; 253 Supplement 5: v64–5.
Comments: Review of treatment of inflammatory muscle disorders.

Authier FJ, Chariot P, Gherardi RK. Skeletal muscle involvement in human immunodeficiency virus (HIV)-infected patients in the era of highly active antiretroviral therapy (HAART). *Muscle Nerve*, 2005; 32: 247–60.
Comments: Review article describing muscle disorders in HIV infection.

Reveille JD. Rheumatologic complications of HIV infection. *Best Pract Res Clin Rheumatol*, 2006; 20: 1159–79.
Comments: Review of systemic complications associated with HIV, including myopathies.

Biviji AA, Paiment GD, Steinbach LS. Musculoskeletal manifestations of human immunodeficiency virus infection; *J Am Acad Orthop Surg*, 2002; 10: 312–20.
Comments: Review of pyomyositis.

OSTEOPOROSIS

Todd T. Brown, MD, PhD

CLINICAL
- Osteoporosis in HIV+ patients 3–4× more common than in general population.
- Increased prevalence may be due in part to high prevalence of risk factors, including low body weight, hypogonadism, smoking, alcohol use, steroid use.
- Role of ART unclear. ART initiation associated with 2%–6% loss in bone mineral density (BMD) in 1st 12–24 mos in multiple studies. Unclear if due to medication effect or by-product of viral suppression and/or immune reconstitution. Longitudinal studies of treated HIV+ patients generally show stable BMD over time.
- TDF associated with ~1%–2% larger decrease in BMD with ART initiation vs ABC and d4T. Magnitude of TDF effect confirmed in PrEP studies in HIV-negative MSMs. Etiology and clinical consequences not clearly established.
- Certain PIs also associated with lower BMD in HIV+ persons initiating ART, including ATV/r.
- BMD explains approximately 50% of fracture risk in general population, perhaps less in HIV+ patients. Bone quality also important but difficult to assess.
- Fracture risk in HIV+ patients 30%–80% increased vs HIV-negative populations, though data limited.

DIAGNOSIS
- Dual energy X-ray absorptiometry (DEXA) of hip and spine used to assess BMD.
- Osteoporosis defined as T-score <−2.5 (i.e., BMD >2.5 standard deviations lower than a young, gender-matched control population).

- Osteopenia defined as T-score between −1 and −2.5.
- Definitions using T-scores created for postmenopausal women, later validated in older men (>50 yrs). For younger populations, Z-score (number of SD lower than age, and gender-matched population) should be used. Z-score ≤−2 is considered abnormal.
- In general population, fracture risk increases ~2 × for each SD decrease in BMD.
- Given high prevalence of osteoporosis and emerging evidence of increased risk of fracture in HIV+ patients, DEXA screening should be considered in all post-menopausal women and men ≥50 yrs, especially in presence of other risk factors including gonadal dysfunction, low body weight, steroid use, hepatitis C, smoking, heavy alcohol use.

TREATMENT
Secondary Cause Evaluation
- Lab evaluation for significant osteopenia or osteoporosis: PTH, calcium, fractional excretion of phosphate ([urine phosphate × serum creatinine]/[serum phosphate × urine creatinine] × 100), TSH, free testosterone (men), and 25-OH vitamin D.
- In selected cases, consider celiac disease, multiple myeloma, idiopathic hypercalciuria, and Cushing's syndrome.

Nonpharmacologic Therapy
- Calcium 1200–1500 mg/day plus vitamin D 400–800 IU/day.
- Weight-bearing exercise (30 mins at least 3 day/wk).
- Cessation of heavy alcohol use and smoking.

Pharmacologic Therapy
- Consider drug treatment for those with T-score ≤−2.5 or fragility fracture. For osteopenia, consider therapy in those with 10-yr hip fracture probability ≥3% or 10-year all major osteoporosis-related fracture ≥20% based on FRAX model (www.shef.ac.uk/FRAX/) according to US National Osteoporosis Foundation Guidelines.
- If no treatment, repeat DEXA in 1–2 years.
- Bisphosphonates considered first line and have been shown to safe and efficacious to increase BMD in HIV+ patients. Alendronate [70 mg qwk] available in generic form. Annual IV zoledronate [5 mg qyr] useful if PO therapy not tolerated. Duration of therapy unclear. Other bisphosphonates can be used but have not been tested in HIV+ populations (risedronate [35 mg qwk], ibandronate [150 mg qmo]).
- Raloxifene (60 mg once daily) is reasonable alternative in postmenopausal women if bisphosphonates not tolerated.
- Teriparatide (parathyroid hormone analog) stimulates new bone formation and should be considered in those not responsive to bisphosphonates (20 mcg once daily SQ). A course of 18–24 mos without concomitant bisphosphonates is recommended. Has not been specifically evaluated in HIV+ patients.

SELECTED REFERENCES
McComsey GA, Kendall MA, Tebas P, et al. Alendronate with calcium and vitamin D supplementation is safe and effective for the treatment of decreased bone mineral density in HIV. *AIDS*, 2007; 21: 2473–82.
Comments: ACTG RCT of alendronate in HIV+ patient demonstrating safety and efficacy.

Brown TT, Qaqish RB. Antiretroviral therapy and the prevalence of osteopenia and osteoporosis: a meta-analytic review. *AIDS*, 2006; 20: 2165–74.
Comments: Meta-analysis of cross-sectional studies regarding prevalence of osteoporosis and reduced BMD. Limitations of existing literature discussed.

McComsey GA, Tebas P, Shane E, et al. Bone disease in HIV infection: a practical review and recommendations for HIV care providers. *Clin Infect Dis*. 2010; 51: 937–46.
Comments: Recent recommendations regarding evaluation and management of osteoporosis in HIV+ patients.

Triant VA, Brown TT, Lee H, Grinspoon SK. Fracture prevalence among human immunodeficiency virus (HIV)-infected versus non-HIV-infected patients in a large U.S. healthcare system. *J Clin Endocrinol Metab*. 2008; 93: 3499–504.
Comments: Large administrative database study showing higher prevalence of spine, hip, and wrist fractures among HIV+ vs. HIV-negative patients.

Gallant JE, Staszewski S, Pozniak AL, et al. Efficacy and safety of tenofovir DF vs stavudine in combination therapy in antiretroviral-naïve patients: a 3-year randomized trial. *JAMA*, 2004; 292: 191–201.
Comments: Randomized trial in treatment-naïve patients found mild decreases in BMD with ART initiation, more pronounced with TDF. Subsequent studies of treatment-naïve patients using other regimen have had similar findings.

DIAGNOSIS

CARDIAC MANIFESTATIONS OF HIV INFECTIONS

Christopher J. Hoffman, MD, MPH and Paul G. Auwaerter, MD

PATHOGENS

- Cytomegalovirus: myocarditis.
- *Cryptococcus neoformans*: myocarditis, pericarditis.
- Epstein-Barr virus: myocarditis (rare).
- Herpes simplex virus: myocarditis.
- HHV-8: associated with pulmonary hypertension. KS-related pericardial effusion, cardiac tumors.
- *Mycobacterium* spp.: pericarditis, myocarditis (TB>>MAC).
- *Staphylococcus* spp.: endocarditis, purulent pericarditis.
- *Streptococcus pneumoniae*: purulent pericarditis.
- *Toxoplasma gondii*: myocarditis.
- Enterovirus (coxsackie, echovirus): myocarditis, pericarditis.
- *Nocardia* spp.: pericarditis.
- *Histoplasma capsulatum*: pericarditis.
- *Cryptococcus neoformans*: pericarditis.

CLINICAL

- **Cardiovascular malignancy:** KS may cause cardiac tumors, pericardial lesions but usually clinically silent. Lymphoma rare.
- **Dilated cardiomyopathy:** generally defined as <50% EF on echo with LV dilation. Affected 30%–40% of AIDS patients pre-HAART, now est. 3%–15%. May present with CHF, palpitations/arrythmia, syncope. Sudden death rare.
- **Endocarditis:** HIV infection and low CD4 count have been both associated with increased risk of infective endocarditis (mostly occurs among IDUs). Common organisms: *S. aureus* and *Streptococcus viridans*. Most patients have similar presentations and survival, although 30% increased mortality in end-stage AIDS vs matched asymptomatic HIV+ patients.
- **Myocarditis:** most causes undefined, direct role of HIV unclear. OI found in <20% (see Pathogens section above), along with occasional coxsackie virus, EBV, CMV cases. Noninfectious causes may include hypersensitivity/drug reactions (AZT), cocaine, thyrotoxicosis.
- **Pericardial effusion:** common (~11%) in untreated AIDS patients, lower on ART. Most small, etiology unknown. Identifiable causes include TB, pyogenic bacteria, *Nocardia*, and primary effusion body lymphoma. Presence in AIDS equates with median survival 6 mos.
- **Pericarditis:** may cause tamponade, bodes poor prognosis. Causes: mycobacterial > pyogenic > lymphoma > KS > viral > fungal.
- **Pulmonary hypertension:** surprisingly common, 1/200 incidence including RV hypertrophy/dilation. Causes include recurrent bronchopulmonary infections, IDU, thromboembolic disease, cirrhosis. Association with HHV-8 defined. Common Sx include cough, chest pain, fatigue, and hemoptysis.
- **Coronary heart disease (CHD):** HIV leads to a proinflammatory state and endothelial dysfunction increasing risk for CHD (data especially strong among patients with treatment interruption). ABC implicated with increased MI risk (doubles MI risk among high-risk group). Rates of CHD, atherosclerosis may be increased with some PIs (see Lipodystrophy, p. 11, Hyperlipidemia, p. 3). Other CAD risks: tobacco, HTN, low HDL-C, diabetes mellitus, age, family history, and obesity.
- Pre-HAART autopsy series: cardiac lesions identified in 25%–75% of patients with AIDS. Cases of myocarditis >80% undefined etiology.

DIAGNOSIS

- **CHF:** obtain echo, ECG, TSH. Brain natriuretic peptide (BNP) may assist with clinical assessment. Role of myocardial Bx not defined, consider selectively. Consider evaluation for CAD (ischemic cardiomyopathy).

- **Pericardial effusion:** obtain echo, consider pericardiocentesis with hemodynamic compromise or if concerned about active infection.
- **Arrhythmia:** baseline ECG for QTc prolongation, Holter monitor, electrolytes, magnesium. Consider echo to look for structural heart disease. Survey medications for likely causes (pentamidine most famous, associated with torsade de pointes) or drug interactions (PIs, digoxin, etc.).
- **Pulmonary HTN:** Doppler evaluation of right-sided pressures by echo, but right heart catheterization remains gold standard. R/O secondary causes (LV dysfunction, hypoxemia, COPD). CT angiography now preferred for PE evaluation, although VQ scanning or angiography occasionally necessary in some cases, especially chronic PE.
- **Coronary artery disease:** stress testing, coronary angiography, lipid panel, glucose tolerance testing.

TREATMENT
CHF
- No clear documented benefit of ART.
- Rapid onset bodes poor prognosis: >50% mortality over 6–12 mos.
- Consider D/C of cardiotoxic drugs (e.g., AZT), drug and alcohol cessation, optimize BP control.
- Asymptomatic: ACE inhibitors (e.g., start lisinopril 2.5–5.0 mg once daily PO, titrate to 20–40 mg/day).
- Sx (dyspnea, fatigue): ACE inhibitor/ARB + daily diuretic (furosemide 20–40 mg PO, bumetanide 0.5–1.0 mg PO, titrate to dry weight); add beta-blocker when not vol overloaded (carvedilol 3.125–25 mg twice daily target or metoprolol 6.25 mg twice daily, 50 mg twice daily target or metoprolol XL 12.5 mg once daily, to 100 mg once daily target).
- Spironolactone 25 mg PO once daily titrate to 3 ×/day yields mortality benefit for advanced CHF; consider eplerenone 25–50 mg once daily (potential for drug interaction with PIs) for those intolerant of spironolactone.
- Digoxin 0.125–0.25 mg PO once daily. May help reduce hospitalizations, but no mortality benefit.

Pericardial Disease
- Attempts at aspiration ± pericardial Bx generally driven by hemodynamic issues and need to obtain diagnosis.
- Effect of ART on pericardial effusions not known.
- Chronic inflammation may cause constriction, requiring surgical stripping of pericardium.

Pulmonary Hypertension
- Obtain specialty consultation.
- Oxygen supplementation to correct hypoxemia.
- Diuretics may help reduce right-sided vol overload, but use with caution; avoid reduced preload can cause hypotension.
- Anticoagulation may be used even without documented emboli as use improves long-term outcomes.
- If acute pulmonary vasoreactivity documented, calcium channel blockers or other vasodilators may give favorable longer-term benefit.
- Severe pulmonary HTN: consider prostacyclin (epoprostenol) by continuous IV infusion.
- ART may improve pulmonary hypertension.

Coronary Artery Disease
- Risk factor modification: stop smoking, increase exercise, control glucose and BP, continue ART; switch from ABC (unclear association seen some but not all studies) or drugs causing dyslipidemia and/or insulin resistance if possible.
- ASA, lipid-lowering therapy (if on PI use atorvastatin, rosuvastatin; pravastatin safe with all PIs except DRV, but less effective), beta-blockers.

SELECTED REFERENCES
Aberg JA. Cardiovascular complications in HIV management: past, present, and future. *J Acquir Immune Defic Syndr,* 2009; 50: 54–64.
Comments: Review of coronary artery disease and HIV.

D:A:D Study Group, Sabin CA, Worm SW, et al. Use of nucleoside reverse transcriptase inhibitors and risk of myocardial infarction in HIV-infected patients enrolled in the D:A:D study: a multi-cohort collaboration. *Lancet,* 2008; 371: 1417–26.

Comments: Analysis of multisite cohort of relationship between antiretroviral agents and myocardial infarction. Risk was increased with both ABC and ddI. Other studies have failed to find an association.

Limsukon A, Saeed AI, Ramasamy V, et al. HIV-related pulmonary hypertension. *Mt Sinai J Med,* 2006; 73: 1037–44.
Comments: Estimated 0.5% of HIV+ patients may develop pulmonary HTN. Significantly symptomatic patients experience considerable mortality (47%–70% 1-year mortality).

Magnani JW, Dec GW. Myocarditis: current trends in diagnosis and treatment. *Circulation,* 2006; 113: 876–90.
Comments: Symptomatic, conservative treatment suggested, as corticosteroids seem to have little role for lymphocytic myocarditis. HIV-related myocarditis has poorer prognosis than lymphocytic myocarditis in HIV-negative patients.

Gebo KA, Burkey MD, Lucas GM, et al. Incidence of, risk factors for, clinical presentation, and 1-year outcomes of infective endocarditis in an urban HIV cohort. *J Acquir Immune Defic Syndr,* 2006; 43: 426–32.
Comments: Most HIV+ patients with endocarditis are intravenous drug users. Age >40 associated with worse outcome.

Hunt SA, Abraham WT, Chin MH, et al. ACC/AHA 2005 guideline update for the diagnosis and management of chronic heart failure in the adult: a report of the American College of Cardiology/American Heart Association Task Force on Practice Guidelines (Writing Committee to Update the 2001 Guidelines for the Evaluation and Management of Heart Failure): developed in collaboration with the American College of Chest Physicians and the International Society for Heart and Lung Transplantation: endorsed by the Heart Rhythm Society. *Circulation,* 2005; 112: e154–235.
Comments: Current treatment guidelines for heart failure.

DIAGNOSIS

Dermatologic

FOLLICULITIS

Spyridon S. Marinopoulos, MD

PATHOGENS
- *Staphylococcus aureus* (most common in HIV- and non-HIV-related folliculitis).
- *Pityrosporum ovale* (aka *Malassezia furfur*).
- *Demodex folliculorum*.
- None: eosinophilic folliculitis.
- HSV.
- *Micrococcus*.
- *Pseudomonas*.
- *Trichophyton*.
- Gram-negative rods (*Klebsiella, Enterobacter, Proteus*).
- Community-acquired methicillin-resistance *Staph. aureus* (CA-MRSA).

CLINICAL
- **Eosinophilic folliculitis:** more common in advanced HIV w/ CD4 typically <250. Hx: severe pruritus w/ lesions over face, neck, upper trunk, upper arms. Spares palms, soles and digital web spaces. Chronic, waxing/waning course. PE: multiple erythematous and edematous (urticarial) papules of follicular distribution w/ a few lesions topped by pustules or crusts. Usually affects upper trunk but also face (especially forehead), neck and upper arms. Scratching causes excoriated papules, crusts, bleeding, scarring, and (in dark-skinned patients) secondary hyperpigmentation. Repeated trauma induces development of prurigo nodularis.
- **Papular urticaria:** pruritic, skin-colored or erythematous, nonfollicular papules. Similar in appearance to insect bites and in distribution to eosinophilic folliculitis. Histology: nonspecific.
- ***Pityrosporum (Malassezia) folliculitis:*** multiple small, monomorphic follicular-centered papules and pustules affecting upper trunk, arms, occasionally face. Very pruritic. Histology: *pityrosporum* spores within follicular lumen.
- ***Demodex* folliculitis:** papular eruption on head, neck, trunk, and arms. Histology: presence of mites.
- **Staphylococcal folliculitis:** isolated, follicular-centered pustules. Eventual formation of bullae/honey-colored crusts w/erythema, edema, and exudate. Most common type in HIV+ patients. Consider CA-MRSA if periumbilical folliculitis or superficial folliculitis arising in areas not typically affected by MSSA, such as the chest, flanks, and scrotum.
- **HSV folliculitis:** vesiculopustular eruption often from autoinoculation after shaving through HSV lesion on lip/mouth. Usually affects face/beard area. HIV+ patients may present w/ necrotizing folliculitis manifesting as 0.2–1.0 cm papules w/ firm central crusts. Bx may be required for Dx.
- ***Pseudomonas* ("hot tub") folliculitis:** multiple pruritic, round, edematous/erythematous lesions w/ central papule/pustule. Acquired from hot tubs, whirlpools, heated swimming pools contaminated w/ *Pseudomonas*. Lesions appear on trunk ± extremities 6–72 hr post exposure and resolve spontaneously in 7–10 days.
- **Gram-negative (non-*Pseudomonas*) folliculitis:** most often presents as sudden exacerbation in patients on long-term ABx for acne as a result of Gram-negative bacterial overgrowth.
- **Predisposing factors:** friction, perspiration, occlusion (clothing, adhesives), shaving, depilatories, preexisting dermatitis, reduced host resistance (DM, hypogammaglobulinemia, chronic granulomatous disease, meds: systemic corticosteroids or cytotoxic agents), *Staph* nasal carriage, skin injuries/wounds/abscess, exposure to precipitants (mineral oils, tars, cutting oils, paraffin-based ointment).

DIAGNOSIS
- Skin Bx w/ special stains for fungi and bacteria as well as Gram stain and KOH prep of pustule contents should be performed whenever possible.

- **Eosinophilic folliculitis:** elevated serum IgE. Peripheral eosinophilia (25%–50% of patients). CD4 <250. Skin Bx: follicular spongiosis with infiltration and destruction of follicular wall by eosinophils, folliculocentric inflammation. Micro: bacteria, yeasts or mites are usually not seen.
- **Other:** skin scraping to r/o scabies (*Sarcoptes scabiei*). Gram stain and Cx to r/o bacterial folliculitis. KOH stain to r/o fungal or *Pityrosporum* folliculitis. Tzanck smear and viral Cx to r/o HSV.
- **Superficial folliculitis:** small (1–2 mm) erythematous papules/pustules at openings of hair follicles. Not assoc w/ systemic Sx; heals without scarring.
- **Deep folliculitis:** red, swollen, tender, nodular/pustular follicle-centered masses. Involving entire hair follicle; appears as red, swollen nodules/pustules deeper and larger than in superficial folliculitis.
- **DDx:** eosinophilic folliculitis, infectious folliculitis (fungal: *Pityrosporum/Trichophyton*; bacterial: *Staph/Pseudomonas*/other Gram-negatives; parasitic: *Demodex*; viral: HSV), papular urticaria, acne, keratosis pilaris, drug eruption, scabies, insect bites, follicular eczema, pustular psoriasis, subcorneal pustular dermatosis.

TREATMENT
Topical
- **Eosinophilic folliculitis:** preferred: topical corticosteroids—usually mid-to-high potency, i.e., fluocinonide 0.05% or betamethasone 0.1%. May decrease inflammation and temporize Sx. On face/sensitive body sites, start w/ lower potency, i.e., hydrocortisone (HC) 1%, and escalate prn.
- **Alternative:** 5% permethrin cream, apply to affected area qhs × 7 days or until decreased pruritus/lesions, then 1–2 ×/wk.
- ***Demodex* folliculitis:** 5% permethrin cream, apply to affected area qhs × 7 days. Alternative: metronidazole 0.75%–1% lotion, cream, gel qhs × 4–8 wk.
- ***Pityrosporum* (*Malassezia*) folliculitis:** 2% ketoconazole cream or shampoo, apply to affected area twice daily.
- ***Staphylococcal* folliculitis:** chlorhexidine gluconate (*Hibiclens*) washes + topical 2% mupirocin to affected areas. If recurrent, eliminate nasal carriage: mupirocin 2% to nares twice daily × 5–7 days. May repeat q3mos if no resolution. Family members may be nasal carriers; consider Rx'ing. Local skin care and topical ABx can be used first line, especially if infection superficial. If area involved widespread or deep infection present, use PO ABx (see below).
- **Gram-negative folliculitis:** (1) *Pseudomonas* folliculitis: acetic acid 5% compresses × 20 min 2–4 ×/day effective for Sx relief. (2) Gram-negative (non-*Pseudomonas*) folliculitis: D/C PO ABx (tetracycline [TCN], minocycline, etc.) for acne and use benzoyl peroxide wash twice daily + systemic regimen.
- **Fungal folliculitis:** broad-spectrum topical antifungals may be used first line in superficial cases, with PO antifungals reserved for persistent/deep infection.
- **All cases:** topical antipruritic medications such as menthol-containing lotions, pramoxine, or doxepin 5% cream may help control pruritus. May safely treat folliculitis w/ topical corticosteroids and cetirizine while awaiting Bx or Cx results. If results positive, treat specific etiology.

Systemic
- **Eosinophilic folliculitis:** ART may result in improvement by restoring immune function, but may also cause flare-up during the immune reconstitution period.
  - Cetirizine 20–40 mg PO once daily in divided doses (preferred, has anti-eosinophil effect) or hydroxyzine 25–50 mg PO qhs.
  - Metronidazole 250 mg PO 3 ×/day × 3–4 wk completely cleared lesions in one small study.
  - Itraconazole 200 mg PO once daily × 4 wk; if no/inadequate response, retreat w/ itraconazole 300–400 mg once daily × 4 wk.
  - Severe disease: isotretinoin 0.5 mg/kg PO twice daily × 4–6 wks.
  - Severe, acute disease: prednisone (>0.5 mg/kg/day) as short course may be used to induce rapid remission. Relatively contraindicated in immunocompromised population, use as last resort.
- ***Pityrosporum* (*Malassezia*) folliculitis:** itraconazole 200 mg PO once daily × 4 wks.
- **Staphylococcal folliculitis (MSSA):** dicloxacillin 500 mg PO 4 ×/day × 7–10 days. PCN allergy: clindamycin 300 mg PO 3 ×/day × 7–10 days or doxycycline 100 mg PO twice daily × 14 days or azithro 500 mg, then 250 mg once daily × 4 days or clarithromycin 500 mg PO twice daily × 7–10 days.

- **Staphylococcal folliculitis (CA-MRSA):** TMP/SMX DS PO twice daily × 7–10 days or clindamycin 300 mg PO 3 ×/day × 7–10 days or doxycycline 100 mg PO twice daily × 14 days or minocycline 100 mg PO twice daily × 14 days (if abscess present, Cx pus and modify treatment based on sensitivities).
- **HSV folliculitis:** ACV 400 mg PO 3 ×/day or valacyclovir 500 mg PO twice daily or famciclovir 125 mg PO twice daily × 5 days.
- **Gram-negative folliculitis:** (1) *Pseudomonas* folliculitis: not first line, use only if persistent/immunosuppressed-ciprofloxacin 500 or 750 mg PO twice daily × 7–10 days. (2) Gram-negative (non-*Pseudomonas*) folliculitis: isotretinoin 0.5–1.0 mg/kg PO twice daily × 4–6 mos effective. Alternative: PO ABx based on C and S of predominant organisms, usually TMP/SMX DS PO twice daily or amox/clav 250–500 mg PO 3 ×/day.

Phototherapy

- **Eosinophilic folliculitis:** UVB or PUVA (psoralen + ultraviolet A) × 3–6 wks. Generally effective.

SELECTED REFERENCES

Avdic E, Cosgrove SE. Management and control strategies for community-associated methicillin-resistant *Staphylococcus aureus*. *Expert Opin Pharmacother*, 2008; 9: 1463–79.
Comments: Review of management and therapeutic options for the treatment of CA-MRSA. Optimal therapy for CA-MRSA infections not fully elucidated. CA-MRSA usually susceptible to variety of oral non-beta-lactam ABx, such as TMP/SMX, clindamycin, tetracyclines, and linezolid.

Sztramko R, Katz K, Antoniou T, et al. Community-associated methicillin-resistant *Staphylococcus aureus* infections in men who have sex with men: a case series. *Can J Infect Dis Med Microbiol*, 2007; 18: 257–61.
Comments: Case series of 17 CA-MRSA infected homosexual men, 12 (71%) of whom were HIV+. Most common clinical presentation was abscess (35%), followed by furuncle (17%), folliculitis (17%), cellulitis (17%), and sinusitis (12%). Majority resistant to ciprofloxacin (92%) and levofloxacin (77%). All isolates susceptible to TMP/SMX, rifampin, linezolid, gentamicin, and clindamycin, and majority (80%) susceptible to tetracycline.

Parker SR, Parker DC, McCall CO. Eosinophilic folliculitis in HIV-infected women: case series and review. *Am J Clin Dermatol*, 2006; 7: 193–200.
Comments: Retrospective chart review of 6 HIV+ women with eosinophilic folliculitis and review of literature. Authors found that eosinophilic folliculitis in women may predominantly affect face and mimic acne excoriee and concluded that HIV-associated eosinophilic folliculitis should be considered in DDx of chronic, pruritic, papular facial eruptions in females.

Osborne GE, Taylor C, Fuller LC. The management of HIV-related skin disease. Part II: neoplasms and inflammatory disorders. *Int J STD AIDS*, 2003; 14: 235–40.
Comments: Review of pruritic papular and follicular eruptions in HIV+ patients, including eosinophilic pustular folliculitis, itchy folliculitis, *Pityrosporum* folliculitis, and *Demodex* folliculitis.

Gelfand JM, Rudikoff D. Evaluation and treatment of itching in HIV-infected patients. *Mt Sinai J Med*, 2001; 68: 298–308.
Comments: Review of causes of pruritus in HIV+ patients, including eosinophilic and bacterial folliculitis. *S. aureus* is common cause of folliculitis.

MOLLUSCUM CONTAGIOSUM

David J. Kouba, MD, PhD

PATHOGENS

- Molluscum contagiosum virus, types I-IV, double-stranded DNA poxvirus with worldwide distribution.
- Narrow cell tropism, replicates in human keratinocyte of epidermis; uses microtubule cytoskeleton within cytoplasm of eukaryotic cells.

CLINICAL

- Lesion: epidermal, flesh-colored, 2–5 mm, firm papule with umbilicated center. Asymptomatic, may be pruritic or tender. Giant molluscum >5mm in diameter, coalescent, ulcerating and fungating.
- Incubation: 2–7 wks. In immunocompetent host, infection self-limited, re-infection common. In immunocompromised, infection is not self-limited.
- Transmission: person-to-person, auto-inoculation, fomites: shared bath, gym equipment, tattooing.

- Location: in AIDS patients, lesions commonly found on face/neck (beard area) or may be disseminated. Lesions may spread within plaques of atopic dermatitis. Trunk, limbs, and eyelids; spares palms and soles. Sexually transmitted infection, lesions in anogenital and intracrural sites.

DIAGNOSIS
- Dx: based on gross appearance. Bx with histopathology is definitive.
- Histopathology: hyaline bodies, molluscum, or Henderson-Patterson bodies, visible in cytoplasm of epithelium, basement membrane remains intact.
- Rapid Dx curette a lesion and smear on glass slide to see characteristic cytoplasmic inclusions on H and E. Special stains are not necessary.
- DDx in immunosuppressed host: disseminated cryptococcosis, histoplasmosis.
- DDx in all patients: warts, nevi, papular granuloma annulare, pyogenic granuloma.

TREATMENT
Uncomplicated Molluscum
- ART with immune restoration resolves lesions.
- Uncomplicated molluscum primarily a cosmetic problem. No permanent cure, but can be easily controlled with local destructive methods and immunomodulatory agents.
- Local destructive methods: curettage, cryotherapy, electrocauterization, KOH soln, trichloroacetic acid (TCA), cantharidin (blister beetle extract), photodynamic therapy (PDT), or 0.5% podophyllotoxin cream should all be considered first-line agents.
- Immunomodulatory agents: imiquimod cream 5%: apply 3 nights/wk. If no irritation results, frequency of administration can be increased to qhs. This can be used as secondary, adjunct to destructive measures.
- Treat while disease limited to avoid spread.

Giant Molluscum
- Very difficult to treat; recalcitrant to all known therapies, with exception of ART and immune restoration.
- Various destructive modalities such as TCA, PDT, and aggressive curettage should be attempted in conjunction with topical immunomodulatory therapy.
- Report of paclitaxel, chemotherapy targeting host cell microtubule cytoskeleton and disruption of MCV lifecycle, not FDA-approved (*Top HIV Med*, 2010).

FOLLOW-UP
- Localized, stable infections should be followed every 3–6 mos.
- Giant molluscum should be routinely debulked/treated to prevent progression/relapse.

SELECTED REFERENCES
Osei-Sekyere B, Karstaedt AS. Immune reconstitution inflammatory syndrome involving the skin. *Clin Exp Dermatol*, 2010; 35: 477–81.
Comments: Cohort study conducted in Soweto, South Africa of 59 ART-naïve patients (med. CD4 60), 30 patients (51%) developed new skin lesions after median of 8 wks (range, 3–24 wks) on ART.

Sadick N, Sorhaindo L. A comparative split-face study of cryosurgery and trichloroacetic acid 100% peels in the treatment of HIV-associated disseminated facial molluscum contagiosum. *Cutis*, 2009; 83: 299–302.
Comments: A comparative split-face study of 20 HIV+ patients with disseminated facial molluscum contagiosum lesions found trichloroacetic acid significantly more effective than cryosurgery (90% vs 55% reduction in lesions) after 2 treatments at 4-wk intervals.

Sisneros SC. Recalcitrant giant molluscum contagiosum in a patient with advanced HIV disease—eradication of disease with paclitaxel. *Top HIV Med*, 2010; 18: 169–72.
Comments: Case report of extensive, ulcerating giant molluscum contagiosum treated with paclitaxel, a chemotherapeutic agent that targets microtubule cytoskeleton and causes apoptosis. CD4 increased from 23 to 59 after 3 mos of ART, then low-dose IV paclitaxel (100 mg/m²) was started. Lesions cleared after initial dose of paclitaxel. Treatment included 4 cycles q21d.

De Carvalho VO, Cruz CR, Noronha L, et al. An inflammatory reaction surrounding molluscum contagiosum as possible manifestation of immune reconstitution inflammatory syndrome in HIV infection. *Pediatr Dermatol*, 2010; 27: 631–4.
Comments: Case study of MCV-associated IRIS described in child with AIDS.

Sen S, Goswami, BK, Karjyi N, et al. Disfiguring molluscum contagiosum in a HIV+ patient responding to antiretroviral therapy. *Indian J Dermatol*, 2009; 54: 180–2.
Comments: Case report of patient w/ AIDS (CD4 58), presenting with numerous lesions on face and neck and large plaque of molluscum contagiosum on scalp, started on ART with resolution of lesions and residual scarring.

SEBORRHEA

Spyridon S. Marinopoulos, MD

PATHOGENS
- *Pityrosporum* spp. (aka *Malassezia*) possible fungal pathogen (controversial).

CLINICAL
- Chronic skin inflammation. More prevalent in HIV (up to 83% incidence) than general population (~3% incidence). More prevalent and severe w/ HIV progression.
- Hx: itching, redness, flaking, skin irritation. PE: erythematous patches/plaques w/ overlying yellow, greasy scales and crusts. Typically symmetrical affecting areas of higher sebaceous gland concentration. Commonly see on: hairy areas of head (scalp, scalp margin, eyebrows/lashes, mustache, beard), forehead, malar area, nasolabial folds, external ear canals, retroauricular creases. Also may affect the chest (presternal area), back and intertriginous areas (axillae, navel, groin, inframammary, anogenital).
- In mild cases, flaking dandruff may be only manifestation. More severe cases present w/ erythematous plaques associated w/ thicker/yellowish powdery or oily scale eventually progressing to erythroderma.
- Disease associations: HIV, Parkinson's, mood disorders, chronic alcoholic pancreatitis, HCV, various cancers, some genetic disorders, dermatologic conditions (rosacea, blepharitis, acne vulgaris, pityriasis versicolor, *Pityrosporum* folliculitis).
- DDx: atopic dermatitis, contact dermatitis, psoriasis, rosacea, superficial fungal infections.

DIAGNOSIS
- Clinical Dx based on characteristic features.
- Skin Bx: characteristic in HIV patients but rarely necessary.
- KOH prep to r/o tinea.

TREATMENT

General Principles
- Use dandruff shampoo, topical antifungals, and/or topical corticosteroids first line × 4 wks.
- If ineffective, may try more potent topical steroid, but limit use to 2 additional wks.
- If again ineffective, escalate to PO antifungals and consider referral to derm for definitive Dx.
- Refer to dermatology if Dx in doubt or no response to Rx or if PO isotretinoin contemplated.

Topical
- **Preferred:** ciclopirox gel 0.77% to affected area twice daily × 4 wks or (if scalp affected) ciclopirox 1% shampoo twice weekly × 4 wks (3 days between applications).
- **Preferred:** ketoconazole 2% cream or shampoo twice daily × 4 wks or until clear; may require weekly maintenance.
- **Alternative:** miconazole 2% cream once or twice daily × 4 wks.
- **Alternative:** terbinafine 1% soln once daily × 4 wks effective for scalp seborrhea.
- **Alternative:** metronidazole 1% gel twice daily × 8 wks.
- **Persistent pruritus:** add topical steroid i.e., 1% HC cream. If no effect, use betamethasone or triamcinolone 0.1% or fluocinonide or FS Shampoo (0.01% fluocinolone).
- **Note:** topical steroids alone may be effective, but generally used as adjunct to topical antifungals to avoid long-term steroid effects.
- Zinc pyrithione 1%–2% shampoo (keratolytic + antifungal activity) or tar/coal tar shampoo or selenium sulphide shampoo 2.5% once daily or qod. HIV-associated seborrhea may not respond to sulphur-containing soaps and creams.
- Sodium sulfacetamide/sulfur lotions applied twice daily.
- Pimecrolimus 1% cream twice daily × 4 wks effective for facial seborrhea.

Systemic
- **Note:** use systemic Rx if lesions widespread or refractory to topical Rx.
- **Preferred:** ketoconazole 200 mg PO once daily × 7–14 days.
- **Alternative:** itraconazole 200 mg PO once daily × 7 days.
- **Alternative:** terbinafine 250 mg PO once daily × 4 wk.

- Severe case refractory to other Rx: isotretinoin 0.1–0.3 mg/kg once daily × 4 wks effective (acts by reducing sebum production). Side effects dictate cautious use. Teratogenic, counsel patients on an effective form of contraception.
- Phototherapy (UVB) tiw until complete clearing or to max 8 wks effective in some patients with severe disease.

SELECTED REFERENCES

Nnoruka EN, Chukwuka JC, Anisuiba B. Correlation of mucocutaneous manifestations of HIV/AIDS infection with CD4 counts and disease progression. *Int J Dermatol*, 2007; 46 Suppl 2: 14–8.

Comments: Nigerian study seeking to identify and correlate mucocutaneous disorders to CD4 count and total lymphocyte count in HIV/AIDS patients. Seborrheic dermatitis occurred at CD4 >200 and was an early skin manifestation of HIV.

Gupta AK, Bluhm R. Seborrheic dermatitis. *J Eur Acad Dermatol Venereol*, 2004; 18: 13–26.

Comments: Excellent review.

Gastrointestinal and Hepatobiliary

CHOLANGIOPATHY, HIV

Andrea L. Cox, MD, PhD and Christopher J. Hoffmann, MD, MPH

PATHOGENS
- *Cryptosporidium parvum* (most common).
- Microsporidia.
- Cytomegalovirus (CMV).
- *Cyclospora cayetanensis*.
- *Giardia lamblia*.

CLINICAL
- Syndrome of biliary obstruction resulting from infection-associated strictures of the biliary tract. Typically occurs in patients with advanced HIV disease (CD4 <50). 4 sub-classifications:
  - Papillary strictures/stenosis (10%).
  - Sclerosing cholangitis-like (20%).
  - Papillary stenosis with sclerosing cholangitis (50%–60%).
  - Extra-hepatic strictures (rare).
- Sx: RUQ pain (90%) often sharp and radiating to back (especially if strictures present). Fever (50%), low grade if present. Diarrhea common due to small bowel involvement with infectious agent.
- Signs: LFTs suggest cholestasis: mild increase in ALT/AST (2–3 × ULN), total bili usually <2 × ULN (jaundice rare but can be present), alk phos 5–10 × ULN. LFTs normal in 20%.
- Large intrahepatic ducts most commonly involved; *Cryptosporidium* and CMV are usual pathogens in such cases.
- Idiopathic in ~20% of cases.

DIAGNOSIS
- Established with ERCP. Sensitivity of ultrasound (US) is 75%–97%.
- If US positive, ERCP indicated to confirm Dx and treat. If US negative, ERCP if abdominal pain is severe or w/ known CMV or *Cryptosporidium* infection.
- OIs (usually CMV, *Cryptosporidium*, or microsporidium) involved in >50% of cases.

TREATMENT
Papillary Stenosis
- ERCP with sphincterotomy provides relief of Sx, but alk phos often remains high.

Isolated Bile Duct Stricture
- Endoscopic stenting considered for pain management.

Cholangiopathy Without Papillary Stenosis
- Ursodeoxycholic acid (ursodiol 300 mg PO 3 ×/day chronically) used experimentally in HIV cholangiopathy.

ART
- Role of ART in managing cholangiopathy is unclear, but overall survival improved by ART.

Differential Diagnosis
- Viral hepatitis (HAV, HBV, HCV, HDV).
- CMV, HSV, EBV infection.
- Hepatobiliary cryptococcosis.
- Mycobacterial infection of the liver (TB, MAC).
- Fatty infiltration of liver.
- Drug reaction (TMP-SMX, INH, rifampin, ketoconazole, pentamidine, pyrimethamine, dapsone).
- Lymphoma.
- Vanishing bile duct syndrome (associated with high bilirubin).

SELECTED REFERENCES

Zuckerman MJ, Peters J, Fleming RV, et al. Cholangiopathy associated with giardiasis in a patient with human immunodeficiency virus infection. *J Clin Gastroenterol*, 2008; 42: 328–9.
Comments: Report of cholangiopathy associated with *Giardia* infection

Hindupur S, Yeung M, Shroff P, et al. Vanishing bile duct syndrome in a patient with advanced AIDS. *HIV Med*, 2007; 8: 70–2.
Comments: Description of the vanishing bile duct syndrome in HIV.

Ko WF, Cello JP, Rogers SJ, et al. Prognostic factors for the survival of patients with AIDS cholangiopathy. *Am J Gastroenterol*, 2003; 98: 2176–81.
Comments: ART shown to improve survival in patients with AIDS and cholangiopathy. Presence or history of any OIs is associated with a worse outcome.

Forbes A, Blanshard C, Gazzard B. Natural history of AIDS related sclerosing cholangitis: a study of 20 cases. *Gut*, 1993; 34: 116–21.
Comments: All 20 patients in this study had abdominal pain; 11 had diarrhea. Alk. phos. was $>2 \times$ normal in 13, but bilirubin raised in only 3. Thirteen had cryptosporidiosis, 6 had active CMV, 5 had no GI pathogen.

Benhamou Y, Caumes E, Gerosa Y, et al. AIDS-related cholangiopathy. Critical analysis of a prospective series of 26 patients. *Dig Dis Sci*, 1993; 38: 1113–8.
Comments: Demonstrates that large intrahepatic ducts most commonly involved. *C. parvum* and CMV are the usual pathogens in such cases.

DIARRHEA

Lisa A. Spacek, MD, PhD and Khalil G. Ghanem, MD, PhD

PATHOGENS

- **Acute:** *Salmonella, Shigella, Campylobacter, Clostridium difficile, E. coli* (enteroaggregative EAEC), *S. aureus, Vibrio parahemolyticus, Yersinia*, norovirus and other viruses (calicivirus, astrovirus, adenovirus).
- **Chronic:** *Cryptosporidium*, microsporidia, *M. avium* complex (MAC), CMV, *Cyclospora, Giardia*, Isospora, *Entamoeba histolytica, Strongyloides*, HIV enteropathy, and causes of acute diarrhea (especially *Salmonella*).
- CD4 <50: *Cryptosporidium*, microsporidia, CMV, MAC.
- Pathogen-negative, chronic, large-volume diarrhea: KS or lymphoma.
- Noninfectious causes: adverse drug reactions (PIs), inflammatory bowel disease, dietary (milk, sorbitol, caffeine), malabsorption, endocrine disease.

CLINICAL

- Characterized by increase in water content, vol, or frequency of stools.
- Small bowel diarrhea, noninflammatory, watery large vol; colitis, inflammatory, dysentery, fever, tenesmus, cramping, small vol.
- Definitions: acute <14 days; persistent >14 days; chronic >30 days.
- DDx depends on duration, CD4 count, Sx (fever, tenesmus, blood), travel, food ingestion (seafood), ABx use (including OI prophylaxis).
- Acute diarrhea incubation period: <2 h—chemical agents; 2–7 hrs—preformed toxin (*S. aureus, B. cereus*); 8–14 hrs—*C. perfringens*; >14 hrs—most bacterial and viral pathogens.
- 2 major causes of vomiting: viral pathogens and preformed toxins of *S. aureus* and *B. cereus*.
- Bloody diarrhea: *Shigella, Salmonella*, hemorrhagic *E. coli, C. jejuni, E. histolytica*, CMV, KS.
- Fever common: *Shigella, Salmonella*, invasive *E. coli, C. jejuni, Vibrio parahemolyticus* (seafood consumption), CMV.
- Fever less common: *S. aureus, B. cereus, C. perfringens*, enterotoxigenic *E. coli and E. coli* 0157:H7, microsporidia, *Cryptosporidium* (if present, usually low-grade), *C. difficile*.

DIAGNOSIS

- Stool Cx for bacteria; O and P (AFB and trichrome stain for *Cyclospora, Isospora, Cryptosporidium*, and microsporidia). Stool toxin assay for *C. difficile*; EIA for *Giardia*.
- Blood cultures: MAC and *Salmonella*.
- Colonoscopy: CMV (blood antigenemia not good indicator in patients. w/ AIDS); also helps to r/o KS and lymphoma.

- Radiology: usually not helpful; CT scan may be useful to localize affected bowel, directing Bx for CMV.

TREATMENT

Antimicrobials

- Empiric Rx for severe acute diarrhea: consider ciprofloxacin 500 mg PO twice daily + metronidazole 500 mg PO 3 ×/day. Avoid empiric therapy if *E. coli* O157:H7 suspected; may increase toxin production and risk of HUS.

Symptomatic Therapy

- Diet: rehydration; frequent small feedings; low-fat; avoid caffeine and milk products. Use fiber supplements to increase stool bulk.
- If nonbloody and not *C. difficile*, antiperistaltic agents can be used: loperamide 4 mg PO × 1 dose then 2 mg prn, max 16 mg/day OR atropine/diphenoxylate 1–2 PO 3–4 ×/day prn.
- Severe chronic diarrhea: codeine 30 mg PO q4–6h prn; DTO.
- 0.6 mL PO 3–4 ×/day prn.
- No etiology found in 30% of patients w/ AIDS and chronic diarrhea. Diarrhea usually responds to antiperistaltics.

SELECTED REFERENCES

Oldfield EC. Evaluation of chronic diarrhea in patients with human immunodeficiency virus infection. *Rev Gastroenterol Disord*, 2002; 2: 176–88.
Comments: Author summarizes evaluation: after medication side effects ruled out, next step is examination of stool for Cx and O and P. If negative, next step is colonoscopy. Highest yield expected in patients with fever, weight loss, and CD4 <50.

Cohen J, West AB, Bini EJ. Infectious diarrhea in human immunodeficiency virus. *Gastroenterol Clin North Am*, 2001; 30: 637–64.
Comments: Endoscopy has high diagnostic yield when stool tests negative, and better outcomes achieved when pathogens identified. Supports practice of routine colonoscopy in chronic HIV-associated diarrhea.

Guerrant RL, Van Gilder T, Steiner TS, et al. Practice guidelines for the management of infectious diarrhea. *Clin Infect Dis*, 2001; 32: 331–51.
Comments: IDSA treatment guidelines for infectious diarrhea.

GINGIVITIS/PERIODONTITIS

Spyridon S. Marinopoulos, MD

PATHOGENS

- *Gemella morbillorum*.
- *Dialister* spp.
- *Veillonella* spp.
- *Peptostreptococcus micros*.
- *Candida albicans* (more common in HIV with high VL).
- *Porphyromonas gingivalis*.
- *Prevotella intermedia*.
- *Tannerella forsythia*.
- *Actinobacillus actinomycetemcomitans*.
- *Treponema denticola*.
- *Bacteroides forsythus*.
- *Capnocytophaga* spp.
- Spirochetes.
- Gram-negative anaerobes.
- *Eikenella corrodens*.

CLINICAL

- **Gingivitis:** gum bleeding (spontaneous or with minor injury) w/ associated edema/erythema.
- **Linear gingival erythema (HIV gingivitis):** brightly inflamed, erythematous band of marginal and papillary gingiva. Disproportional to amount of visible plaque ± bleeding. Pain not prominent. Not associated w/ CD4. Does not resolve despite periodontal debridement.

- **Necrotizing ulcerative gingivitis (NUG) or HIV-NUG ("trench mouth"):** fetid breath, blunting of interdental papillae, and ulcerative necrotic gingival sloughing with bleeding ± fever/regional LN. Rapid progression. Can evolve into necrotizing ulcerative periodonditis w/destruction of periodontium and bone involvement.
- **Periodontitis:** inflamed gingiva w/ loss of supportive connective tissues. Typically no Sx. PE: bone craters w/ increased gingival pocket (probing) depth and tooth mobility. X-ray may show bone loss.
- **Necrotizing ulcerative periodontitis (NUP) or HIV-NUP:** severely painful gingival tissue, severe loss of periodontal attachment, and alveolar bone destruction w/ eventual necrosis. Rapid progression. Bleeding spontaneous or w/ minor probing. Progresses from NUG. CD4 usually <200. Dx: KS, NHL, CMV.
- **Periodontal abscess:** acute, tender, purulent inflammation in gingival wall of periodontal pocket + fluctuance ± sinus tract ± regional LN ± tender/sensitive adjacent teeth + fever if severe.
- Factors predisposing to poor gingival and periodontal health include HIV, pregnancy (hormonal shifts), smoking, diabetes, leukemia, Down syndrome, other immune/leukocyte disorders (Job's syndrome, leukocyte adhesion deficiencies, Chédiak-Higashi syndrome, Papillon-Lefèvre syndrome, chronic granulomatous disease), exogenous immunosuppression (chemotherapy), head and neck radiation, medications causing gingival hyperplasia (nifedipine and other calcium channel blockers, dilantin, cyclosporin), or xerostomia, etc.
- Gingivitis and periodontitis preventable with oral hygiene and regular dental visits.
- Potential complications: tooth loss, necrotizing stomatitis (noma), sinusitis, cavernous sinus thrombosis, Ludwig's angina, retro/parapharyngeal abscess, osteomyelitis, endocarditis, brain abscess.
- In all patients, including HIV+, gingivitis/periodontitis may represent initial presentation of systemic illness: DM, leukemia, other immunocompromising conditions. Consider medication-induced gingival hyperplasia: phenytoin, nifedipine, cyclosporin, etc.
- HIV+ patients can present with atypical, fulminant disease and require indefinite close follow-up. Unique bacterial flora includes GNRs, enterics, and fungi. Must cover *Candida*.

DIAGNOSIS

- Visual inspection sufficient in most cases.
- X-rays may reveal bone loss.
- Consider Cx/Bx in persistent/resistant cases.

TREATMENT

Topical Therapy

- **Gingivitis/periodontitis:** plaque removal with scaling and root planing (SRP) q3mos effective in most cases w/o need for ABx. Prevention: meticulous hygiene w/brushing, flossing, and regular dental visits.
  - Initiate SRP + home hygiene. Consider antibacterial mouthwash if patients unwilling/ unable to comply w/ home hygiene measures. Assess for response 1–3 mos post Rx.
  - Exceptions to above: fulminant disease or disease caused by *A. actinomycetemcomitans* (Aa), including juvenile and some adult, not responsive to SRP alone and requires post-SRP adjunctive systemic ABx.
  - Chlorhexidine 0.12% oral rinse 15 cc twice daily between dental visits reduces bacterial flora/prevents plaque advancement. May cause tooth staining and promote bacterial resistance w/ prolonged use.
  - Advise smoking cessation.
- **Linear gingival erythema:** plaque removal w/ SRP q3mos + chlorhexidine 0.12% oral rinse 15 cc twice daily indefinitely prevents progression to NUP.
- **Refractory and/or recurrent periodontitis:** recommend Cx prior to Rx. Limited disease: SRP + local-delivery ABx. Extensive disease: SRP + systemic ABx (see next page).
  - Local delivery adjunct to SRP (applied once): minocycline 1-mg microsphere, tetracycline 12.7-mg fiber, doxycycline 10% gel, chlorhexidine 2.5-mg chip.
  - Other Rx: (submicrobial dose) doxycycline hyclate 20 mg PO twice daily × 90 days (up to 9 mos) reduces periodontitis by inhibiting collagenase. Effect small but significant. Useful as adjunct to SRP.
- **Periodontal abscess:** NSAIDs ± weak narcotic opioids for pain control. I and D is primary treatment w/ ABx supportive if systemic Sx (fever, LN, etc.). Refer to dentist within 24 hrs.

Systemic Antibiotics

- Although SRP alone effective in most patients with periodontal disease, strong evidence exists for use of ABx as adjunct to SRP in severe/refractory/aggressive cases.
- **Refractory and/or recurrent periodontitis:** recommend Cx prior to Rx. If sites of disease few, SRP + local-delivery ABx (see previous) If extensive disease, SRP + systemic ABx (below).
- If Cx unavailable and no prior ABx: TCN 250 mg PO q6h OR doxycline/minocycline 200 mg PO × 1 dose then 100 mg PO once daily × 14 days. Alternative: amoxicillin/clavulanate 250–500 mg PO q8h × 10 days. PCN allergy: clindamycin 150–300 mg PO q6h × 7–10 days.
- More aggressive disease: amoxicillin 375 mg + metronidazole 250 mg PO q8h × 7 days. PCN allergy: clindamycin 150–300 mg PO q6h × 10 days very effective. Alternative: metronidazole 500 mg + ciprofloxacin 500 mg PO twice daily × 7 days.
- **Linear gingival erythema:** test for *Candida* and treat if positive; eradication of intraoral *Candida* often results in disappearance of characteristic lesions.
- **ANUG (trench mouth), NUP, HIV-NUG, HIV-NUP:** metronidazole 250 mg + amoxicillin/clavulanate 250 mg PO q8h × 7 days (add nystatin rinses 5 mL 4 ×/day or clotrimazole troches 10 mg 5 ×/day or fluconazole 200 mg PO once daily × 7–14 days given *Candida* overgrowth w/ ABx use). PCN allergy: metronidazole 500 mg PO + ciprofloxacin 500 mg PO q12h × 7 days (with antifungal therapy noted above).
- **Periodontal abscess:** ABx controversial. Use if severe/systemic Sx, always in conjunction w/ I and D. Cover anaerobes. 7-day course typical, but can also treat for 3 days then reassess. Amoxicillin/clavulanate 500 mg PO q8h. PCN allergy: metronidazole 500 mg PO q8h. Rx failure: when possible, obtain Cx and tailor ABx accordingly. Empiric Rx for Rx failure: clindamycin 300 mg PO q6h.

FOLLOW-UP

- **Gingivitia/Periodonitis:** q3mos indefinitely for plaque removal with SRP.
- **Linear Gingival Erythema:** q3mos and use chlorhexidine mouth rinse twice daily indefinitely.
- **NUP:** return in 24 h for observation and additional debridement of necrotic tissues, in 7days for meticulous SRP, q3mos indefinitely.

SELECTED REFERENCES

Feller L, Lemmer J. Necrotizing periodontal diseases in HIV-seropositive subjects: pathogenic mechanisms. *J Int Acad Periodontol*, 2008; 10: 10–5.
Comments: Necrotizing periodontal diseases (NPD) in HIV+ and HIV-negative patients similar with regard to spectrum of periodontopathic bacteria, clinical manifestations, natural course and response to treatment. However, in HIV+ patients, higher prevalence of *Candida* spp. and herpesviruses in subgingival plaque and gingival Bx specimens. In periodontal tissues, spirochetes, activated herpesviruses, *Candida* spp. and HIV can deregulate host innate and adaptive immune responses and stimulate host inflammatory reactions. These factors may explain greater prevalence of NPD in HIV+ patients.

Aas JA, Barbuto SM, Alpagot T, et al. Subgingival plaque microbiota in HIV positive patients. *J Clin Periodontol*, 2007; 34: 189–95.
Comments: Review of predominant bacterial and fungal spp. associated with gingivitis, periodontitis, and linear gingival erythema (LGE), in HIV + subjects

Reznik DA. Oral manifestations of HIV disease. *Top HIV Med*, 2005; 13: 143–8.
Comments: Review of HIV-related oral conditions, including periodontal diseases such as linear gingival erythema and necrotizing ulcerative periodontitis.

Holmstrup P, Glick M. Treatment of periodontal disease in the immunodeficient patient. *Periodontol 2000*, 2002; 28: 190–205.
Comments: Review of therapy of periodontal disease in the immunodeficient patient, including HIV.

Plemons JM, Benton E. Oral manifestations of HIV infection. *Tex Dent J*, 2002; 119: 508–18.
Comments: Review of oral manifestations of HIV, including periodontal diseases.

NAUSEA/VOMITING

Robin McKenzie, MD

CLINICAL

- Often caused by medications: antiretrovirals (especially RTV, other PIs, AZT), high-dose TMP-SMX, macrolides, opiates.

- Prevention or treatment of nausea important to improve adherence to therapy.
- Initiation of ART: nausea greatest in 1st 1–2 wks of ART. Consider prn antiemetic when starting some regimens.
- Nausea/vomiting may be a sign of a life-threatening reaction to ART: ABC hypersensitivity; NVP hepatotoxicity; lactic acidosis (d4T, ddI, AZT); pancreatitis w/ ddI, especially if combined with d4T (contraindicated), ribavirin (RBV; contraindicated), or TDF (reduce dose of ddI).
- Metabolic causes: adrenal insufficiency, uremia, hypercalcemia.
- CNS disease: mass lesions, meningitis.
- GI disease: gastritis, gastroparesis, reflux esophagitis, PUD, lymphoma, KS, hepatobiliary disease (including drug-induced hepatitis), pancreatitis.
- Miscellaneous: opiate withdrawal, pregnancy.

DIAGNOSIS

- Review medications and consider drug-related effects, especially life-threatening conditions (above).
- Check urine or serum HCG if pregnancy a possibility.
- Check lactic acid level if taking NRTI, especially d4T, ddI, AZT.
- Consider measuring liver enzymes, creatinine, electrolytes, calcium, amylase/lipase.
- Consider cosyntropin stimulation test (especially with hyperkalemia, weight loss, eosinophilia, orthostatis/hypotension).
- Consider GI and/or CNS imaging.

TREATMENT

General Principles

- If patient has life-threatening ART-related side effect, stop ART.
- If Sx occurs with initiation of ART, remind patient that they may improve within 1–2 wks and consider offering symptomatic treatment.
- If Sx do not improve significantly or if symptomatic Rx inadequate, consider changing ART.
- Higher doses of RTV associated with more GI Sx than lower doses. In CASTLE study, diarrhea and nausea occurred in 2% and 4% of patients taking ATV/r + TDF/FTC vs 11% and 8% taking LPV/r twice daily + TDF/FTC.
- NRTIs: ddI—take on empty stomach. Others—take w/ or w/o food (may be better tolerated w/ food, especially AZT).
- NNRTIs: EFV—take on empty stomach initially, to decrease CNS side effects. ETR—take w/ food. NVP—take w/ or w/o food. RPV—take with a meal.
- PIs: IDV—take on empty stomach. ATV, DRV/r, LPV/r soln, NFV, RTV, SQV/r, TPV/r—take w/ food. FPV, IDV/r, LPV/r tabs—take w/ or w/o food (may be better tolerated w/ food).

Symptomatic Therapy

- Prochlorperazine: 5–10 mg PO q6–8h prn, 25 mg PR twice daily prn, 5–10 mg IM q3–4h prn.
- Promethazine: 12.5–25 mg PO, PR, or IM q4–6h prn.
- Trimethobenzamide: 300 mg PO, 200 mg PR, 200 mg IM q6–8h prn.
- Metoclopramide: 10 mg PO q6h prn. For ART-associated Sx, consider 10 mg PO 30–60 min before ART.
- Ondansetron: 8 mg PO 3 ×/day.
- Dronabinol: 2.5 mg PO twice daily. If persistent CNS Sx, reduce to 2.5 mg/day. If tolerated, may increase to 10–20 mg/day.
- Lorazepam: 1–3 mg PO q4–6h, max 4 mg/day.
- **Note:** prochlorperazine, promethazine, trimethobenzamide, and metoclopramide can cause sedation and dystonic/extrapyramidal reactions.
- Ondansetron and newer 5-HT3 receptor antagonists are expensive. They are used alone or with dexamethasone for chemotherapy-induced nausea and vomiting.
- Marijuana has appetite-stimulating and antiemetic properties. Medicinal use legal only in CA and AZ.
- Lorazepam and other benzodiazepines (BZDs) used only for anxiety-associated nausea and vomiting, usually w/ chemotherapy.

SELECTED REFERENCES

Hesketh PJ. Chemotherpy-induced nausea and vomiting. *NEJM*, 2008; 358: 2482–94.

Comments: Review article discussing pathophysiology of drug-induced nausea and vomiting and use of drugs for patients receiving chemotherapy.

Scorza K, Williams A, Phillips JD, Shaw J. Evaluation of nausea and vomiting. *American Family Physician*, 2007; 76: 76–84.
Comments: Discussion of causes of nausea and vomiting with recommendations for evaluation and treatment.

PANCREATITIS

Robin McKenzie, MD

PATHOGENS

- Acute HIV infection.
- Cytomegalovirus (CMV).
- *Toxoplasma gondii*.
- *Mycobacterium tuberculosis*.
- *Mycobacterium avium* complex (MAC).
- *Pneumocystis jiroveci*.
- *Cryptosporidium parvum*.

CLINICAL

- Increased incidence in HIV+ patients especially with ddI treatment, previous pancreatitis, or CD4 <200.
- Medications are most frequent cause in HIV+ patients, especially ddI and to lesser extent other "d-drugs" that may cause mitochondrial toxicity w/ lactic acidosis, hepatic steatosis + pancreatitis.
- Increased risk with ddI + certain other drugs: d4T, TDF, RBV, hydroxyurea (HU), pentamidine. (Do not use ddI + d4T in pregnant women and avoid if possible in all patients. Use reduced dose of ddI with TDF.).
- Less common: 3TC (children), IV/aerosolized pentamidine, TMP-SMX, INH, rifampin, corticosteroids, erythromycin, valproic acid (VPA).
- Other causes: hypertriglyceridemia (fasting TG >1000 associated with LPV/r and other PIs), alcohol, gallstones, post-ERCP, HIV (acute HIV infection), OIs (CMV, toxoplasmosis, MAC, TB, PCP, cryptosporidiosis).
- Hx: acute, constant, upper abdominal pain that may radiate to back; nausea ± vomiting. Presentation varies from no symptoms to shock/coma.
- PE: fever, tachycardia, epigastric tenderness. Hemorrhagic discoloration of flanks (Grey-Turner's sign) or periumbilical area (Cullen's sign) in ~1% cases.

DIAGNOSIS

- Increased amylase nonspecific. Common in asymptomatic HIV infection and other conditions: renal insufficiency, intestinal or fallopian tube disease, macroamylasemia, acidosis, various medications. Usually >3 × normal in pancreatitis, but may be normal.
- Increased lipase (>3 × normal) more specific. Mildly increased lipase also common with asymptomatic HIV, renal failure, bowel disease, DKA, macrolipasemia, medications. Lipase remains elevated longer than amylase.
- Contrast-enhanced CT useful to r/o other Dx and stage severity of pancreatitis. Not indicated for mild disease unless Dx uncertain. Necrosis (lack of enhancement) best identified several days after presentation; % glandular necrosis correlates with mortality rate. MRI more sensitive for mild pancreatitis and more specific for categorizing fluid collections as necrosis, abscess, hemorrhage, or pseudocyst but less clinical correlation available with MRI.
- If cause not obvious (medications, EtOH), consider US, MRCP, or endoscopic US to detect gallstones or biliary tract disease. ERCP may be needed to detect/remove gallstones and obtain fluid to stain and Cx for OIs (more likely if CD4 low).
- CT- or US-guided FNA indicated if infected necrosis suspected.

TREATMENT

Initial Therapy

- Stop ddI or other causative medications.
- Give IV fluids (avoid hemoconcentration).
- Control pain (often requires narcotics).

Antibiotics
- Infection probably due to translocation of gut flora. Infection rate proportional to extent of necrosis.
- No prophylactic ABx for mild pancreatitis: may cause superinfection with resistant bacteria and *Candida*.
- For acute, severe pancreatitis (>30% necrosis by CT), previous studies supported use of imipenem 500 mg IV q6h as prophylaxis. More recent trials do not support this recommendation. Use of prophylactic ABx for necrotizing pancreatitis not recommended. Instead, if infection suspected, obtain aspirate for Gram stain and Cx, begin empiric ABx and continue ABx only if Cx positive.
- Infected necrosis usually presents in 2nd or 3rd week. Both sterile and infected necrosis cause abdominal pain, fever, leukocytosis. CT- or US-guided aspiration needed for Dx.
- Choice of ABx for infected necrosis ideally based on Cx results. GI flora (aerobes and anaerobes) often present. ABx with good penetration: carbapenems (imipenem, meropenem, ertapenem, doripenem), FQ (ciprofloxacin, levofloxacin, mosifloxacin), ceftazidime, cefepime, metronidazole, clindamycin, fluconazole. For empiric Rx, consider carbapenem alone or FQ + either metronidazole or clindamycin.
- If OI suspected or Dx'd, see appropriate module for management.

Nutritional Support
- Mild pancreatitis: start clear liquids early and advance diet as tolerated.
- Severe pancreatitis: begin enteral nutrition as soon as possible. NJ feeding usually used, but NG as safe in recent small study (Eatock).
- Give parenteral nutrition only if adequate enteral feeding not tolerated.

FOLLOW-UP

Stage Severity
- Calculate APACHE II score on admission: >8 in HIV-negative patient and >9–14 in HIV+ patient predicts severe course.
- Ranson criteria (see Table 1–2) less predictive in HIV+ patients: >3 in HIV-negative patient and >4 in HIV+ patient suggests severe course.
- Obtain contrast-enhanced CT unless pancreatitis is mild. Necrosis best detected 2–3 days after admission. Necrosis >30% predicts mortality >20%.
- Measure CRP: >21 mg/dL on day 2–4 and >12 end of 1st week predict severe pancreatitis.
- Early deaths (1st 2 wks) primarily due to multisystem organ failure.

Diagnose and Treat Complications
- Later deaths due to local and systemic infection.
- Infected necrosis must be Dx'd (CT-guided aspirate) and drained (percutaneously or surgically). If blood Cxs negative and no evidence of sepsis, drainage may be delayed to allow organization of necrotic area.
- Early ERCP indicated for severe gallstone pancreatitis. Cholecystectomy usually performed before discharge in mild cases or within a few months in complicated cases.

TABLE 1-2. RANSON CRITERIA FOR PANCREATITIS SEVERITY

On admission	At 48 hrs
Age >55 yr	Hct decrease >10%
WBC >16,000/mm³	BUN increase 5 mg/dL
LDH >350 IU/L	Ca <8 mg/dL
AST >250 IU/L	PaO$_2$ <60 mm Hg
Glucose >200 mg/dL	Base deficit >4 mEq/L
	Fluid sequestration >6L

OTHER INFORMATION
- Monitor triglycerides in patients taking PIs.

SELECTED REFERENCES

Frossard JL, Steer ML, Pastor CM. Acute pancreatitis. *Lancet*, 2008; 371: 143–52.
Comments: Since prophylactic ABx have no proven efficacy, authors recommend fine needle aspiration when infection suspected. ABx are stopped if infection not confirmed. Infection usually requires debridement, but surgery is delayed if necrotic tissue is not infected. Abdominal decompression via laparotomy indicated if abdominal pressure high causing an abdominal compartment syndrome.

Martínez E, Milinkovic A, de Lazzari E, et al: Pancreatic toxic effects associated with co-administration of didanosine and tenofovir in HIV-infected adults. *Lancet* 2004; 364: 65–7.
Comments: 10-fold greater risk of pancreatitis with coadministration of TDF and ddI. If TDF and ddI are given together, dose of ddI should be reduced.

Dellinger EP, Tellado JM, Soto NE, et al. Early antibiotic treatment for severe acute necrotizing pancreatitis: a randomized, double-blind, placebo-controlled study. *Ann Surg*, 2007; 245: 674–83.
Comments: This is the second randomized, double-blind, placebo-controlled trial of prophylactic ABx for severe acute pancreatitis. In this trial 50 patients received meropenem and 50 received placebo. As in previous blinded, placebo-controlled study, there was no difference in rate of infection or death.

Gan I, May G, Raboud J, et al. Pancreatitis in HIV infection: predictors of severity. *Am J Gastroenterol*, 2003; 98: 1278–83.
Comments: Retrospective study of 73 HIV+ patients with acute pancreatitis. Mortality and complication rates similar to those of HIV-negative patients, but higher cut-off scores recommended to predict severity in HIV+ patients. APACHE II (>14 points most accurate, >12 more sensitive) was better than Ranson (>4) or Glasgow (>4) for predicting a severe course.

WASTING

Joseph Cofrancesco, Jr., MD, MPH

CLINICAL

- **Wasting:** unintentional weight loss >10%. Many experts act when patients lose >5% weight from baseline: usually loss of muscle (men), loss of muscle and fat (women).
- **Wasting syndrome:** unintentional weight loss >10% plus diarrhea or chronic weakness and documented fever for >30 days.
- Wasting syndrome is an AIDS-defining condition (category C); wasting is evidence of symptomatic HIV infection (category B).
- Must be differentiated from lipoatrophy, which is isolated fat loss (see Lipodystrophy, p. 11). Wasting/weight loss is consequence of AIDS disease progression and OIs, while lipoatrophy often seen in patients on successful ART.
- Less common in HAART era.

DIAGNOSIS

- Rule out OIs or other infections.
- Evaluate for GI problems (diarrhea and malabsorption) and malnutrition; check stool O and P, occult blood, and WBC if there are bowel complaints (at minimum).
- Perform age- and gender-appropriate cancer screening.
- Rule out depression and substance abuse.
- Consider endocrine abnormalities: thyroid disorders, adrenal insufficiency, hypogonadism in men. Check TSH and AM-free testosterone level.
- Differentiate lipoatrophy (fat loss, ART associated) from wasting (muscle ± fat loss from advanced disease).

TREATMENT

General Principles

- Treat identified causes of weight loss.
- Control HIV with ART.
- Treat/prevent OIs.
- Ensure adequate nutrition (use oral supplements prn). Patients with active HIV have increased metabolic demands.
- Encourage exercise program/weight training.
- If no response to the above, consider pharmacologic intervention.

Pharmacological Principles: Men

- If AM total testosterone <400 ng/dL or low free testosterone, consider testosterone supplementation (see below for doses). Supraphysiologic doses (generally with injections) may be necessary for 1st 3 mos in wasted patients. Can also add additional anabolic agent (oxandrolone or nandrolone) for 3 mos. After 3 mos, stop anabolic agent; continue testosterone.
- If not hypogonadal (AM testosterone >400 ng/dL): use anabolic agent (oxandrolone, nandrolone, or rhGH) for 3 mos.
- If no response to above, consider rhGH (can cause/exacerbate glucose intolerance and lipoatrophy).
- If appetite poor, consider appetite stimulant such as megastrol (may exacerbate or precipitate hypogonadism).

Pharmcological Principles: Women

- Anabolic steroid use more controversial given androgenic effects of anabolic steroids. Ensure birth control. Consider oxandrolone OR low dose nandrolone × 3 mos OR rhGH.
- Consider appetite stimulant such as megastrol.

Appetite Stimulants

- Consider in wasting patients, especially with anorexia.
- Megestrol (see p. 151) suspension: 800 mg PO once daily. Excellent appetite stimulant but progesterone-related compound with potential for causing hypoadrenalism and hypogonadism. Most weight gain is fat, not muscle, unless coupled with exercise and/or testosterone/anabolics. Can cause hyperglycemia.
- Dronabinol (see p. 148): 2.5–10 mg PO twice daily 4 ×/day prn. Useful for nausea and anorexia, but most studies fail to demonstrate significant weight gain.
- Anabolic steroids can have appetite-stimulating effect.
- Consider nutrition consult.

Testosterone

- **IM injection:** testosterone enanthate or cypionate: 200 mg IM q2wks (range 50–400 mg IM q1–4wks) for standard testosterone replacement. Titrate to amelioration of Sx and AM testosterone level >400 ng/dL. For greater anabolic effect, use higher doses (200–250 mg IM qwk or 300–400 mg IM q2wks).
- **Gels:** testosterone 1% gel 5–10 g qAM: apply to shoulders, upper arms, abdomen. Titrate to Sx/testosterone levels. (5 g = 50 mg testosterone) Difficult to obtain high levels and therefore anabolic effect with gels; for anabolic effects and supraphysiologic doses, injections generally required.
- **Buccal formulation:** 1 unit placed against gum above incisor tooth q12hrs, with rounded side held in place for 30 seconds for adhesion, rotating alternate sides of the mouth. Delivers replacement doses, not supraphysiologic doses.

Anabolic Steroids

- Oxandrolone: 10 mg PO twice daily or 20 mg PO once daily (consider lower doses in women). May have less androgenic effects.
- Nandrolone decanoate: 50–200 mg IM q2wks.
- Oxymetholone: up to 50 mg PO twice daily. Very potent but less often used, may be more hepatotoxic.

Growth Hormone

- rhGH: 0.1 mg/kg SQ at bedtime or every other day (max 6 mg/day) × 3 mos. Can cause or exacerbate glucose intolerance and lipoatrophy. Can cause fluid retention, hypertension, carpal tunnel syndrome. Expensive.

FOLLOW-UP

- Monitor for LFT abnormalities, polycythemia, clotting factors. Baseline and yearly prostate exam and PSA recommended for men on testosterone.
- After 3 mos, consider stopping anabolic steroids and encouraging continued nutrition and exercise. Slight decrease in weight expected once anabolic agents are stopped.
- Sometimes necessary to repeat 3-mo cycle of anabolic steroids if weight not maintained. If HIV cannot be controlled, longer courses of anabolic agents may be necessary.
- Unclear if chronic testosterone needed in HAART era, but reasonable to switch to replacement doses in topical form for men who were hypogonadal.

SELECTED REFERENCES

Moyle GJ, Daar ES, Gertner JM, et al. Growth hormone improves lean body mass, physical performance, and quality of life in subjects with HIV-associated weight loss or wasting on highly active antiretroviral therapy. *J Acquir Immune Defic Syndr*, 2004; 35: 367–75.

Comments: Large randomized, double-blind, placebo-controlled, multicountry trial demonstrated that rhGH (0.1 mg/kg/days or qod, max 6 mg/days) superior to placebo in increasing work output, weight, and lean body mass (by BIA), with better quality of life scores and decreased fat mass. Better response with once daily than every other day, but like many GH studies, there were significant side effects (especially fluid retention and hyperglycemia) and drop outs. 757 entered study, 646 completed the 12 wks and only 555 had "evaluable" data. By week 177 (open-label extension), only 177 remained.

Tang AM, Forrester J, Spiegelman D, et al. Weight loss and survival in HIV-positive patients in the era of highly active antiretroviral therapy. *J Acquir Immune Defic Syndr*, 2002; 31: 230–6.

Comments: Even in era of HAART, weight loss and wasting remain important predictors of mortality.

Kong A, Edmonds P. Testosterone therapy in HIV wasting syndrome: systematic review and meta-analysis. *Lancet Infect Dis*, 2002; 2: 692–9.

Comments: Meta-analysis showing that testosterone, especially by injection, can increase muscle mass.

Grinspoon S, Corcoran C, Parlman K, et al. Effects of testosterone and progressive resistance training in eugonadal men with AIDS wasting. A randomized, controlled trial. *Ann Intern Med*, 2000; 133: 348–55.

Comments: Supervised exercise can increases muscle mass in eugonadal men with wasting.

APHTHOUS ULCERS

Spyridon S. Marinopoulos, MD

PATHOGENS
- None (idiopathic).
- See DDx below for other conditions causing oral ulcers.

CLINICAL
- Common oral lesions classified by size and duration into minor, major, and herpetiform.
- **Minor:** small (<5 mm) single or multiple tender ulcerations, persist × 7–14 days. Exam: superficial erosions w/ fibrinous covering often surrounded by red halo. Involve mobile mucosa (tongue, floor of mouth, soft palate, and buccal/labial mucosa).
- **Major:** larger painful ulcerations, persist for up to 6 wks, eventually heal w/ scar formation.
- **Herpetiform:** crops of small ulcers that eventually coalesce; may be mistaken for HSV by appearance.
- In HIV-infected individuals, tend to occur more frequently, last longer and may be more painful. Can significantly effect nutritional health in an already at risk population.
- DDx: viral (HSV, CMV, Coxsackie), fungal (*Histoplasma, Cryptococcus, Cryptosporidium, Mucor*), bacterial (TB, syphilis), neoplasm (NHL, KS, squamous cell carcinoma), Behçet's disease, Reiter's syndrome, SLE, bullous pemphigoid, pemphigus vulgaris, dermatitis herpetiformis, Crohn's disease, celiac sprue, pernicious anemia, Sweet's syndrome.
- Predisposing factors: family history, stress (emotional/physical), iron or vitamin deficiencies (folic acid, vitamin B12), allergies, hormonal changes, diet/food hypersensitivity, trauma, immune dysfunction, cyclic neutropenia, sodium lauryl sulfate (toothpaste detergent), celiac sprue, inflammatory bowel disease, pernicious anemia, drugs (NSAIDs, alendronate, nicorandil).

DIAGNOSIS
- Clinical presentation and lesion appearance important. Initial Rx trial w/ topical agents helpful diagnostically. Bx ± Cx for persistent, atypical appearing ulcerations.
- Oral mucosal Bx required for atypical or nonhealing ulcers to exclude possibility of deep fungal infection, viral infection, and neoplasms.
- CBC, iron studies, RBC folate, vitamin B12, serum anti-endomysial/transglutaminase antibody.
- Consider other etiologies (infectious): HSV: Tzanck smear w/ inclusion-bearing giant cells; CMV: multinucleated giant cells; syphilis: +RPR/FTA; cryptosporidiosis, mucormycosis, histoplasmosis: +Bx/Cx.
- Consider other etiologies (noninfectious): Behçet's syndrome: genital ulcers, uveitis, retinitis. Reiter's syndrome: uveitis, conjunctivitis, arthritis, HLA B27+. Crohn's: bloody diarrhea, mucus, GI ulcerations. SLE: malar rash, +ANA. Cyclic neutropenia: periodic fever and neutropenia. Squamous cell ca: +Bx, +LN. Bullous pemphigoid/pemphigus vulgaris: diffuse skin involvement.

TREATMENT

General Principles
- Recommendations represent author's opinion.
- Treatments discussed below apply to idiopathic aphthous ulcers only. Treat underlying condition if present.
- Aphthous ulcers in conjunction w/ Sx of uveitis, conjunctivitis, arthritis, diarrhea, genital ulcerations, or other systemic manifestation should prompt search for systemic autoimmune or inflammatory condition.
- Topical corticosteroids are 1st-line Rx: reduce ulcer duration and pain compared with controls, but no consistent effect on incidence of ulceration.
- Reserve PO steroids and thalidomide for severe cases refractory to topical Rx.
- Goals of Rx: promote ulcer healing, reduce pain, diminish frequency of recurrence while maintaining nutritional intake.

Topical

- Topical corticosteroids: 1st-line Rx. Multiple agents can be used: betamethasone, fluocinonide, fluocinolone, fluticasone, and clobetasol more effective than HC and triamcinolone, but higher risk for adrenocortical suppression and predisposition to candidiasis.
- Triamcinolone acetonide dental paste or fluocinonide dental paste: apply to ulcer 2–3 ×/day × 5 days or clobetasol propionate mouthwash 10 cc × 5 min swish and spit 3 ×/day.
- Dexamethasone elixir: 0.5 mg/5 cc swish and spit 3 ×/day.
- Amlexanox paste: apply 1/4 inch (0.5 cm) topically to ulcer 4 ×/day. Apply following oral hygiene and as soon as possible after noticing symptoms.
- Chlorhexidine: 15 cc oral rinse 0.12% swish and spit × 30 sec twice daily: increases number of ulcer-free days and interval between ulcer development but does not affect incidence/ severity of ulceration.
- Tetracycline: 250-mg capsule, dissolve in 180 cc water, swish and spit 4 ×/day.
- Viscous lidocaine 2%: apply to ulcer w/ cotton swab 4 ×/day prn.
- Triamcinolone injection: may be useful for persistent isolated lesions.
- Miles soln: 60 mg HC, 20 cc mycostatin, 2 g tetracycline, and 120 cc viscous lidocaine (swish and spit). The 2 active ingredients are HC and TCN, but clinical trials have used more potent topical steroids.

Systemic

- Severe cases only: prednisone 60 mg PO once daily × 5–7 days, then d/c. Rx >7 days requires slow taper. Avoid if possible in immunocompromised patients, including HIV.
- Thalidomide 200 mg PO once daily × 4 wks effective in 2/3 of patients w/ resistant aphthous ulcers. Some patients may require thalidomide maintenance dose (200 mg twice a wk).
- Dapsone, colchicine and pentoxifylline have been reported as potentially effective in refractory cases, although randomized controlled trials are lacking.

Miscellaneous

- Brush atraumatically (use small-headed, soft toothbrush). Avoid hard/sharp foods/trauma to oral mucosa.
- Correct iron and vitamin deficiencies.
- Exclude potentially offending foods.
- Consider allergy (patch) testing.
- Suppress ovulation if menses/OCP association.
- D/C potentially causal medications.

SELECTED REFERENCES

Shetty K. Current role of thalidomide in HIV-positive patients with recurrent aphthous ulcerations. *Gen Dent*, 2007; 55: 537–42.
Comments: Current status of thalidomide for treating refractory ulcers in HIV+ patients discussed. Suggestions regarding safe and effective prescribing of thalidomide included.

Scully C. Clinical practice: aphthous ulceration. *NEJM*, 2006; 355: 165–72.
Comments: A clinical practice case discussing aphthous ulceration.

Scully C, Gorsky M, Lozada-Nur F. The diagnosis and management of recurrent aphthous stomatitis: a consensus approach. *J Am Dent Assoc*, 2003; 134: 200–7.
Comments: Review of etiology, pathogenesis, Dx, and management of recurrent aphthous stomatitis. Predisposing factors include vitamin deficiency, stress, food allergies, and HIV infection. Topical corticosteroids remain mainstay for therapy, but immunomodulators now available.

Kerr AR, Ship JA. Management strategies for HIV-associated aphthous stomatitis. *Am J Clin Dermatol*, 2003; 4: 669–80.
Comments: Good review. In HIV+ individuals, aphthous ulcers occur more frequently, last longer, and produce more painful Sx than in immunocompetent persons. In addition, they may be associated with similar ulcerations involving esophagus, rectum, anus, and genitals. Oral mucosal Bx required for nonhealing ulcers to exclude possibility of deep fungal infection, viral infections, and neoplasm. Initial therapy for infrequent RAS recurrences includes OTC topical protective and analgesic products. Initial therapy for frequent RAS outbreaks requires topical anesthetics, binding agents, and corticosteroids. Major RAS and nonhealing minor or herpetiform RAS may require intralesional corticosteroids and systemic prednisone. Second-line immunomodulators for frequent and nonhealing ulcers includes thalidomide.

Zunt SL. Recurrent aphthous stomatitis. *Dermatol Clin*, 2003; 21: 33–9.
Comments: A review of recurrent aphthous stomatitis.

Bruce AJ, Rogers RS. Acute oral ulcers. *Dermatol Clin*, 2003; 21: 1–15.
Comments: A review of acute oral ulcers.

Plemons JM, Benton E. Oral manifestations of HIV infection. *Tex Dent J*, 2002; 119: 508–18.
Comments: A review of oral manifestations of HIV including aphthous ulcers.

SALIVARY GLAND DISORDERS

Raj Sindwani, MD

PATHOGENS
- *Staphylococcus* spp., primarily *Staphylococcus aureus* (sialoadenitis).

CLINICAL
- Parotid gland most commonly involved.
- Bilateral painless enlargement common in HIV population.
- Observe for skin changes, palpate gland (direct and bimanual), assess facial nerve function, intraoral exam (milk gland to express saliva, parapharyngeal space involvement) and assess for cervical lymphadenopathy. Bilateral vs unilateral gland swelling is an important feature.
- Signs suspicious for malignancy include skin changes, unilateral swelling, large cervical lymph nodes, tenderness, and facial nerve weakness.
- Character of fluid expressed from salivary duct (intraoral) should be noted; purulent discharge consistent with sialoadenitis.
- Can be associated with cervical lymphadenopathy. May be neoplastic or diffuse infiltrative lymphocytosis syndrome (DILS) secondary to massive CD8 cell lymphoproliferation.
- Lymphocytic infiltration causes destruction of acinar tissue leading to sialoadenitis and xerostomia.
- Bilateral salivary gland enlargement: vitamin deficiency, malnutrition, bulimia, diabetes, hypothyroidism, obesity, malabsorption (pancreatic insufficiency), cirrhosis, anemia, Sjögren's syndrome (risk of non-Hodgkin lymphoma) and medications (i.e., antihypertensives, catecholamines, iodine-containing compounds).
- Neoplastic etiologies in HIV population include adenoid cystic carcinoma, non-Hodgkin lymphoma, Kaposi sarcoma and mucosa-associated lymphoid tissue (MALT) lymphoma. Parotid most common salivary gland involved with lymphoma, sublingual gland is the least. Other neoplastic etiologies: (1) benign: pleomorphic adenoma, Warthin's tumor, oncocytoma, and monomorphic adenoma; (2) malignant: mucoepidermoid, acinic cell, adenocarcinoma, malignant mixed and squamous cell.
- Unilateral gland enlargement: (1) infectious: acute sialoadenitis (typically *S. aureus*, also pneumococcus, dehydration is risk factor), abscess, mumps, granulomatous sialoadenitis, actinomycosis; (2) noninfectious: sialolithiasis, branchial cleft cyst (type I), uveoparotid fever (syndrome of uveitis, parotitis, and fever), retention cysts.
- Benign lymphoepithelial cyst: most common cause of parotid swelling in HIV+ patient. Originates from lymph nodes within the parotid gland. Represents lymphoid hyperplasia with dilated cystic ducts. 20% bilateral.
- Parotid pseudocysts: secondary to viral inflammation. May appear before patient HIV seroconverts. Usually multiple, multiloculated and bilateral in 80% of cases.
- Etiologies of xerostomia (severe dry mouth related to decreased saliva production): irradiation, chronic sialoadenitis, surgery, Sjögrens, DM, dehydration, debilitation, mental stress, infection, anemia, amyloidosis, and medications.

DIAGNOSIS
- FNA for Dx of solid lesions and monitoring in patients with DILS for development of EBV-associated NHL. FNA sensitivity and specificity of 91% and 98%, respectively.
- CT and MRI useful in setting of neoplasm. Can correlate size/location of lesion. Ultrasound most useful in setting of benign lymphoepithelial cyst. Advantages include simplicity, inexpensive, painless, noninvasive, and no radiation exposure.

- Lab work to consider includes mumps titer, CBC, autoimmune, and Sjögrens profile (ss-A, ss-B, ANA, ESR).

TREATMENT

- Other treatment for sialoadenitis includes rehydration, warm compresses, sialogogues, parotid massage, and oral irrigations. If no improvement after 2–3 days consider CT or U/S to evaluate for abscess.

Surgery

- Procedures used include FNA, cyst aspiration, and parotidectomy.
- Surgery for parotid lesions requires parotidectomy via an incision hidden in skin crease in front of ear. Main risk is facial nerve paralysis.
- Diagnostic and therapeutic procedure for parotid tumors is superficial parotidectomy. Total parotidectomy required with involvement of both superficial and deep lobes.
- Intraoperative facial nerve monitoring available to improve identification of the nerve during surgery and avoid injury.

Sclerotherapy

- Intralesional doxycycline injection useful for growth prevention (in 75%) and even regression (in 25%) in the setting of benign parotid cysts.

Radiotherapy

- Can use in setting of severe facial deformity with benign lymphoepithelial cyst, but risk of secondary malignancy.
- Rarely used as sole modality in the treatment of tumors. Adjuvant radiotherapy offered in some situations.

Medication

- ABx in setting of sialoadenitis, Gram-positive coverage with amoxicillin/clavulanate 500 mg PO 3 times daily (or clindamycin 300 mg PO q6h in PCN-allergic patients) is usually sufficient. May require parenteral ABx if severe.
- ART and oral prednisone in presence of DILS.

Observation

- Option in setting of cyst if patient is asymptomatic and no significant cosmetic deformities.

Cyst Aspiration

- AIDS in Dx.
- Helps resolve aesthetic concerns. May be repeated.

FOLLOW-UP

- Typically only prn if undergoing aspiration for lymphoepithelial cyst.
- Postsurgical follow-up for malignancy more frequent to survey for recurrence, particularly in setting of high-grade lesions.
- Some salivary gland tumors can occur bilaterally.

OTHER INFORMATION

- Timely referral to otolaryngologist if uncertain Dx, suspicion of malignancy, or for surgical management.

SELECTED REFERENCES

Rosso R, Pretolesi F, del Bono V, et al. Benign lymphoepithelial parotid lesions in vertically HIV-infected patients. *AIDS Patient Care STDS*, 2006; 20(8): 536–41.
Comments: Describes use of sonographic and Doppler findings to follow parotid enlargement in HIV+ patients.

Marsot-Dupuch K, Quillard J, Meyohas MC. Head and neck lesions in the immunocompromised host. *Eur Radiol*, 2004; 14 Suppl 3: E155–67.
Comments: Current and complete review of head and neck lesions encountered in HIV+ patients, with section on salivary gland involvement that mostly focuses on benign lymphoepithelial lesions and AIDS-related cysts.

Vargas PA, Mauad T, Bohm GM, Saldiva PH, Almeida OP. Parotid gland involvement in advanced AIDS. *Oral Dis*, 2003; 9(2): 55–61.
Comments: Describes involvement and histological alterations found in parotid glands of 100 patients who died with AIDS.

SINONASAL MALIGNANCIES

Raj Sindwani, MD

PATHOGENS
- HHV-8: also known as Kaposi sarcoma-associated herpesvirus (KSHV), the agent of KS.
- EBV: associated with lymphoma.

CLINICAL
- Malignant tumors of sinonasal tract in general population constitute <1% of all malignancies, and 3% of malignancies in upper respiratory tract.
- Most common sinonasal malignancies in HIV+ and non-HIV+ populations include squamous cell carcinoma (45%–80%), salivary gland carcinoma (5%–15%), and sarcomas (5%). Kaposi sarcoma (KS) and non-Hodgkin lymphoma (NHL) associated with HIV infection.
- **Distribution:** maxillary sinus (63%), nasal cavity (35%), ethmoids (19%), and frontal and sphenoid sinuses (1%–2%).
- **Clinical features:** nasal obstruction, nasal drainage, sinusitis unresponsive to medial therapy, otitis media with effusuion, mass effect on face/orbits, cranial nerve palsies. Complaints often nonspecific and result in delay of Dx. Constitutional Sx may be present as well.
- **KS:** less common than at other sites. May involve any mucosal site of upper aerodigestive tract. Additional Sx include pain and bleeding. Associated with concurrent cutaneous lesions. Similar indolent course.
- **NHL:** occurs 25-60× more frequently in HIV+ patients. Sinonasal site rare. More common extranodal sites include CNS, digestive tract, bone marrow. Often accompanied by constitutional Sx of fever, weight loss, malaise. Highy aggressive.
- **Squamous cell carcinoma (SCC):** can arise in sinonasal tract or nasopharynx. Poor prognosis if orbit or intracranial spread.

DIAGNOSIS
- **Clinical exam:** endoscopic evaluation most reliable. May appear as friable, grayish necrotic lesion (NHL) or red, purple, or black macule or papule of nasal mucosa (KS).
- **Sinus CT:** best to evaluate for bony erosion of tumor. Critical areas include bony orbits, ethmoid roof, and posterior maxillary sinus to evaluate orbital, intracranial, or pterygopalantine fossa invasion. High resolution or thin cuts recommended. Contrast usually not helpful.
- **MRI:** excellent delineation of tumor from surrounding inflamed tissue or secretions and to evaluate intracranial spread.
- **Bx:** primary lesion and any nodal metastasis. Transnasal intraoperative Bx preferred. Evaluate tissue using histopathology and immunohistochemisty stains.
- **DDx:** infectious conditions such as fungal diseases (mucormycosis, aspergillosis, *Alternaria, Bipolaris,* etc.) or TB may mimic malignancy. Bx with search for atypical organisms especially important in this population. Inflammatory nasal polyps and pyogenic granuloma (benign nasal tumor) should also be considered.

TREATMENT
- Combination therapy with en bloc resection and radiotherapy (RT) most common approach for tumors of epithelial origin (SCC). RT improves cure in this region due to difficulty obtaining wide surgical margins. Chemotherapy reserved for palliation. Prophylactic neck dissection rarely performed.
- Minimally invasive endoscopic techniques being used to resect some sinonasal maliganancies in select patients; further study needed.
- **KS:** ART dramatically reduces incidence of KS and sometimes results in resolution of disease. Treatment reserved for symptomatic tumors (severe nasal obstruction or infection, significant bleeding, inpingement on vital structures). Cryotherapy, surgical excision, laser ablation, intralesional, or systemic chemotherapy have all been described.
- **NHL:** aggressive chemotherapy treatment of choice. Regimens include CHOP (cyclophosphamide, doxorubicin, vincristine, prednisone) or EPOCH (etoposide, vincristine, cyclophosphamide, doxorubicin, prednisone). Both regimens often given with rituximab. Nonresponders may require local RT, or rarely surgical resection. Poor prognosis.

FOLLOW-UP
- Epithelial tumors require regular follow-up on monthly basis after treatment to monitor for recurrence.
- Sinonasal KS most often asymptomatic and can be followed on a biannual basis. Symptomatic lesions or disseminated disease should be more frequently monitored for profression.
- NHL requires close monitoring by oncology.

SELECTED REFERENCES

Batra PS, Citardi MJ. Endoscopic management of sinonasal malignancy. *Otolaryngol Clin North Am*, 2006; 3: 619–37.
Comments: Endoscopic techniques being used to treat increasingly complex intranasal pathology, including some sino-nasal neoplasms.

Gurney TA, Murr AH. Otolaryngologic manifestations of human immunodeficiency virus infection. *Otolaryngol Clin North Am*, 2003; 36: 607–24.
Comments: Concise review of common HIV-associated pathology in the head and neck.

SINUSITIS

Raj Sindwani, MD

PATHOGENS
- Bacterial: *Streptococcus pneumoniae, Moraxella catarrhalis, Haemophilus* influenza, *Pseudomonas aeruginosa, Staphylococcus aureus.*
- Fungal: *Aspergillus fumigatus, Cryptococcus neoformans, Pseudallescheria boydii*, zygomycetes.
- Other (rare): *Mycobacteria, Nocardia* spp., CMV, *Acanthoamoeba*, microsporidia.

CLINICAL
- **Prevalence:** up to 68% in HIV+ population.
- Maxillary and ethmoid sinuses most frequently involved; high incidence of sphenoid disease (2 × general population).
- Mucociliary dysfunction plays important role; ciliary transport time is significantly prolonged, especially with CD4 <200.
- Increased atopy (due to polyclonal B-cell activation producing excessive IgE) produces new/ increased allergic symptoms leading to nasal congestion and ostia obstruction.
- **Hx:** nasal drainage, congestion, fever, headache, facial pressure/pain.
- **PE:** fever, mucopurulent nasal or posterior pharyngeal drainage, mucosal congestion. Ominous findings include mucosal ischemia/necrosis, cranial nerve deficits, paraesthesias, proptosis, or meningeal symptoms: suggestive of invasive fungal sinusitis or malignancy. Also consider malignancy.
- Incidence of atypical infections, fungal sinusitis, NHL, KS increase with CD4 <150.

DIAGNOSIS
- Acute bacterial sinusitis usually a clinical Dx based on Sx ± anterior rhinoscopy.
- **Nasal endoscopy:** consider if discharge from middle meatus or sphenoid-ethmoid recess, refractory disease after initial ABx, or mucosal pallor or necrosis suggestive of invasive fungal infection.
- **Transnasal Cx** (bacterial, fungal, AFB) and **Bx** for histopathology with special stains recommended for unusual pathogens, or consider antral tap for diagnostic Dx and therapeutic lavage if refractory to ABx or CD4 <200.
- **Sinus CT:** indicated if fever or headache of unknown origin, persistent findings after appropriate therapy, possible complications, or spread of infection.
- **MRI:** indicated for fungal disease or to evaluate intracranial or orbital involvement.

TREATMENT
Antibiotic Therapy
- **Typical acute and chronic sinusitis:** may be treated (initially) as in general population.
- **Acute sinusitis:** amoxicillin 500 mg PO 3 ×/day reasonable choice for uncomplicated cases (CD4 >200). Other choices include amoxicillin-clavulanate 875 mg PO twice daily or cefuroxime 250 mg PO twice-daily. Treat for minimum of 10–14 days. If unresponsive to

therapy after 3–4 days or CD4 <200 consider endoscopic Cx vs broadening coverage with clindamycin 300 mg PO 3 ×/day (anaerobes) or levofloxacin 500 mg PO once daily (Gram negative, *P. aeruginosa*).

- **Chronic sinusitis** (persistent Sx >12 wks): 6 wks ABx therapy with FQ recommended, get endoscopically guided Cx.
- **Chronic resistant sinusitis:** IV therapy such as antipseudomonal PCN or 3rd-generation cephalosporin with aminoglycoside or quinolone.
- **Prophylaxis:** TMP-SMX prophylaxis reduces occurrence of bacterial sinusitis in HIV+ patients.
- **Fungal sinusitis:** empiric amphotericin B (AmB) (1.0–1.5 mg/kg/day IV) for invasive and noninvasive infection plus surgical debridement pending identification.
- Cx-based treatment for complicated, refractory, chronic, or suspected fungal disease.

Adjuvant Medical Therapy

- **Systemic decongestant therapy:** OTC decongestants may provide some symptomatic relief.
- **Topical nasal decongestant therapy:** oxymetazoline or phenylephrine 2–3 sprays per nostril twice daily × 3 days only to avoid rhinitis medicamentosa.
- **Nasal steroid sprays:** may help chronic symptoms.
- **Antihistamines** (with or without decongestant combination): consider if concomitant allergic rhinitis, second generation less sedating: fexofenadine, loratadine, cetirizine.
- **Mucolytics:** guaifenesin 100–400 mg PO q4h.
- **Saline irrigations:** forceful flow of irrigant through nasal passages useful to clear debris and restore mucosal health.

Surgical Therapy

- Fungal sinusitis requires aggressive surgical debridement of affected tissue.
- Endoscopic sinus surgery can be beneficial for chronic refractory sinusitis by improving sinus ventilation and drainage.
- Surgery also important in management of intraorbital and intracranial complications of sinusitis.
- For revision procedures or extensive sinus disease, surgical navigation systems that aid in anatomical localization during surgery are recommended.

FOLLOW-UP

- Frequent follow-up necessary until complete resolution of disease.
- If Sx not resolving, consider repeat Cx (bacterial, fungal, and AFB), CT imaging, and reconsider DDx.
- Neoplasms such as sinonasal lymphoma and KS should remain in DDx.
- Clinical outcome reflects stage of HIV: acute sinusitis likely to resolve with CD4 >200, chronic sinusitis common with CD4 <200, and risk of life-threatening infections increases with CD4 <50.

OTHER INFORMATION

- Otolaryngology consultation recommended for recurrent/chronic sinusitis or refractory acute infection not responsive to initial medical therapy. Refer if suspect complication of sinusitis (spread of infection) or if suspicious for malignancy.
- Nasal endoscopy and endoscopy-guided sinus Cx often useful to tailor therapy in difficult cases.

SELECTED REFERENCES

Shah AR, Hairston JA, Tami TA. Sinusitis in HIV: microbiology and therapy. *Curr Infect Dis Rep*, 2005; 3: 165–69.
Comments: Discusses diagnostic and therapeutic options for HIV+ patients with rhinosinusitis.

Tami TA. The management of sinusitis in patients infected with the human immunodeficiency virus (HIV). *Ear Nose Throat J*, 1995; 74: 360–3.
Comments: Review of pathophysiology, Dx, and treatment as it applies to otolaryngologist as well as general practitioner.

Hematologic

ANEMIA

Richard D. Moore, MD, MHS

CLINICAL
- Prevalence 1%–10% in asymptomatic HIV, 10%–25% with CD4-defined AIDS, 30%–60% with AIDS-defining illness.
- Hypoproliferative anemia more common than hemolytic anemia.
- Earliest Sx affect functional status: easy fatigue, weakness, exertional dyspnea, slowed cognition (Hgb 10–12).
- Later Sx include rapid heart rate, bounding pulse, dyspnea, severe fatigue, confusion, angina, CHF (Hbg <8–9).
- HIV can directly cause suppression of hematopoietic precursor cells in marrow through inflammatory cytokine suppression, inhibition of endogenous EPO response.
- Low testosterone level can cause anemia.
- Anemia a prognostic factor for worse survival in HIV, but association unlikely to be causal.

TABLE 1-3. CAUSES OF ANEMIA AND ASSOCIATED LABORATORY ABNORMALITIES

Cause	Laboratory
Decreased RBC Production 1. HIV induced 2. Iron deficiency (blood loss, most commonly GI) 3. Neoplasm infiltrating bone marrow (lymphoma, KS, other) 4. Infection in marrow (MAC, MTB, parvovirus B19, CMV, fungal) 5. Drugs (AZT, cancer chemotherapy, interferon-alfa, gancyclovir, pyrimethamine, amphotericin, phenytoin)	Reticulocyte count low. Indirect bilirubin normal. MCV low in iron-deficiency, anemia of chronic disease. MCV high with AZT.
Ineffective RBC Production 1. Folic acid deficiency 2. Vitamin B12 deficiency	Reticulocyte count low. Indirect bilirubin high. MCV high.
RBC Destruction (Hemolysis) 1. Coomb's positive hemolytic anemia 2. TTP 3. DIC 4. Drugs: sulfonamides, oxidant drugs such as dapsone, primaquine with G6PD deficiency, RBV	Reticulocyte count high. Indirect bilirubin high. High LDH, low haptoglobin. Peripheral smear may have fragmented RBCs, spherocytes, schistocytes.

DIAGNOSIS
- Hgb <12 (HCT <36) in women and <13 (HCT <41) in men (WHO criteria).
- Reticulocyte count, indirect bilirubin, MCV can help assess cause.
- **Decreased RBC production:** low reticulocyte count, normal indirect bilirubin, normal MCV, except low in iron deficiency, anemia of chronic disease, high with certain drugs (e.g., AZT). Includes: (1) HIV-induced (pattern of anemia of chronic disease, MCV low-normal; normal Fe stores, but laboratory appearance of iron deficiency anemia with Fe <60 µg/dL, transferrin <300, ferritin <100). (2) Iron-deficiency (Fe <60, transferrin <300, ferritin <80; chronic blood loss, most commonly GI). (3) Neoplasm infiltrating bone marrow (lymphoma, KS). (4) Infection in marrow (MAC, MTb, CMV, fungal). (5) Parvovirus B19 (severe anemia, typically with normal neutrophils and platelets; PCR or DNA dot blot

for parvovirus B19). (6) Drugs (AZT, cancer chemotherapy, interferon-alfa, gancyclovir, pyrimethamine, amphotericin, phenytoin).

- **Ineffective RBC production:** low reticulocyte count, high indirect bilirubin, high MCV. Includes: (1) folic acid deficiency (RBC folate <150–200, GI malabsorption in 20% of AIDS patients) (2) B12 deficiency (serum B12 <125–200, GI malabsorption in 20% of AIDS patients).
- **RBC destruction (hemolysis):** high reticulocyte count, high indirect bilirubin, high LDH, low haptoglobin, peripheral smear may have fragmented RBCs, spherocytes, schistocytes. Includes: (1) Coomb's positive hemolytic anemia. (2) TTP. (3) DIC. (4) Drugs: sulfonamides, oxidant drugs such as dapsone, primaquine with G6PD deficiency, RBV.

TREATMENT
General Principles
- **Iron deficiency:** ferrous sulfate 300 mg 3 ×/day; oral Fe may not correct deficit in setting of EPO use and frequent phlebotomy; consider IV ferric gluconate in sucrose 125 mg (10 cc) in 100 cc 0.9% NaCl infused over 1 hr until total body replacement (5–20 doses). Initial test dose, 2 mL IV (25 mg elemental Fe) in 50 mL NS, over 60 min recommended due to risk of hypersensitively reaction.
- **Folate deficiency:** folate 1–5 mg/day for 1–4 mos.
- **B12 deficiency:** B12 1 mg/day IM × 7 days, then qwk × 4, then monthly until malabsorption resolved.
- **Parvovirus B19:** IVIG 0.4 g/kg/day × 5 days. If relapse in <6 mos, consider 2 g/kg over 2 days. Consider maintenance dosing of 0.4 g/kg q4wks for relapse.
- **Marrow infiltration by tumor or infection:** bone marrow Bx. Treat specific cause (e.g., MAC, M. TB, CMV, fungal).
- **Drug-induced anemia:** for G6PD deficiency and oxidant drugs such as dapsone, primaquine, discontinue drug. Severe methemoglobinemia (in patients without G6PD deficiency) can be treated with IV methylene blue (1 mg/kg).
- **HIV induced:** ART may improve Hgb by 1–2 g/dL over 6 mos. Can use hematopoietic growth factor while waiting for response to ART (see below for dosing). Improvement may be slower with AZT-containing regimens.
- Transfuse only for acute blood loss or severe anemia with potential cardiovascular compromise. Evidence that repeated transfusions may compromise immune system recovery, increase VL.

Hematopoietic Growth Factors
- **Erythropoietin-alfa:** effective when serum EPO level <500 u/mL. Only approved HIV indication is AZT-induced anemia. Do not start growth factors unless Hgb < 10. Start with at 10,000 U SQ qwk or 20,000 U SQ q2wks (based on anemia of chronic kidney disease). If Hgb increase <1g by 4–6 wks, increase dose by 25%–50% qwk.
- Aim for Hgb of 10–12. Decrease dose by 25% increments or decrease frequency of dosing (e.g., to q2wks, then q3wks, etc.) to maintain hemoglobin 10–12. If Hgb approaching 12 g/dL, or increases by more than 1 g/dL in a 2-week period, dose should be reduced by 25%. If Hgb continues to increase, withohold dosing until Hgb decrease, then reinitiate at dose when Hgb < 11 at 25% below previous dose.
- **Darbepoetin-alfa:** erythropoiesis-stimulating protein with longer half-life. Initial dose of 0.45 mcg per kg SQ q2wk (based on studies in anemia of CKD). Increase by 25% if increase in Hgb <1 by 4–6 wks. Decrease frequency of dosing (e.g., to q3–4 wks, etc.) or decrease dose by 25% increments to maintain Hgb 10–12.
- Maintain use of growth factors for at least several mos. Taper dose slowly as tolerated to maintain Hgb 11–12.
- Monitor Hgb q2wks during titration, and no less frequently than q4 wks thereafter.
- Measure Fe before starting therapy. Transferrin saturation should be >20% and ferritin > 100 ng/mL. Maintain adequate Fe stores with Fe supplementation. Inadequate Fe stores most common reason for nonresponse to growth factors.
- Treatment with EPO improves QOL, correlated with Hgb improvement.
- Treatment with weekly darbepoetin-alfa (1 mcg = 200 IU EPO conversion) shown to be as effective as 3 ×/wk EPO for anemia in hemodialysis in HIV+ persons, though EPO now given weekly.

- EPO corrects anemia in HIV/HCV-coinfected patients treated with IFN/RBV, including those taking AZT.
- Complete correction of anemia with EPO in patients with chronic kidney disease increases risk of CV events and death. In cancer patients, shortened survival and increase tumor progression/recurrence. Relevance to HIV unknown, but correction of Hgb to >12.0 g/dL should not be goal of treatment.

OTHER INFORMATION

TABLE 1-4. DIAGNOSIS AND TREATMENT OF ANEMIA

Diagnosis	Laboratory	Treatment
Iron deficiency	Fe <60 ug/dL Transferrin <300 ug/dL; Ferritin <80 ng/mL MCV<80; chronic blood loss, most commonly GI	Ferrous sulfate 300 mg 3 times daily; oral iron may not correct the deficit in setting of EPO use and frequent phlebotomy, consider IV ferric gluconate in sucrose 125 mg (10 cc) in 100 cc 0.9% NaCl infused over 1 hr until total body replacement (5–20 doses). Initial test dose, 2 mL IV (25-mg elemental iron) in 50 mL NS, over 60 min recommended due to risk of hypersensitivity reaction.
Folic acid deficiency	Serum folate <2–4 ng/mL; GI malabsorption in 20% of patients with AIDS	Folate 1–5 mg/day for 1–4 mos
Vitamin B12 deficiency	Serum B12 <125–200 pg/mL; GI malabsorption in 20% of patients with AIDS	Vitamin B12 1 g/day IM for 7 days, then qwk × 4, then monthly until malabsorption resolved
Parvovirus B19	Severe anemia, typically with normal neutrophils and platelets; PCR or DNA dot blot for parvovirus B19	IVIG 0.4 g/kg once-daily over 5 days. If relapse in less than 6 mos, consider 2 g/kg over 2 days. Consider maintenance dosing of 0.4 g/kg q4wks for relapse.
HIV: pattern of anemia of chronic disease	MCV low-normal; normal iron stores, but laboratory appearance of iron deficiency anemia with Fe <60 ug/dL, transferrin <300 ug/dL, ferritin >100 ng/mL	ART; hematopoietic growth factors
Marrow infiltration by tumor or infection	Bone marrow biopsy	Treat specific cause
Drug-induced anemia	MCV >100 with AZT; G6PD deficiency and oxidant drugs such as dapsone, primaquine	Discontinue drug or use hematopoietic growth factors with ARVs; severe methemoglobinemia (in patients without G6PD deficiency) can be treated with IV methylene blue (1 mg/kg)

SELECTED REFERENCES
Sullivan PS, Hanson DL, Brooks JT. Impact on hemoglobin of starting combination antiretroviral therapy with or without zidovudine in anemic HIV-infected patients. *J Acquir Immune Defic Syndr*, 2008; 48: 163–8.
Comments: Longer time to improvement in anemia with AZT-containing ART.

Levine AM, Salvato P, Leitz GJ, et al. Efficacy of epoetin alfa administered every 2 weeks to maintain hemoglobin and quality of life in anemic HIV-infected patients. *AIDS Res Hum Retroviruses*, 2008; 24: 131–9.
Comments: EPO given every 2–4 wks can maintain Hg levels in anemic HIV+ patients. Target Hgb of ≥13 no longer recommeded.

Mocroft A, Ledergerber B, Zilmer K, et al. Short-term clinical disease progression in HIV-1-positive patients taking combination antiretroviral therapy: the EuroSIDA risk-score. *AIDS*, 2007; 21: 1867–75.
Comments: Anemia predictive of clinical disease progression and death independent of other prognostic factors in patients on ART.

Curkendall SM, Richardson JT, Emons MF, et al. Incidence of anaemia among HIV-infected patients treated with highly active antiretroviral therapy. *HIV Med*, 2007; 8: 483–90.
Comments: AZT-containing ART more likely to result in new anemia, or worsen existing anemia.

Singh AK, Szczech L, Tang KL, et al. Correction of anemia with epoetin alfa in chronic kidney disease. *NEJM*, 2006; 355: 2085–98.
Comments: More CV events with no improvement in QOL with target Hgb of >13.5 g/dL by EPO treatment in CKD.

Harris RJ, Sterne JA, Abgrall S, et al. Prognostic importance of anaemia in HIV type-1-infected patients starting antiretroviral therapy: collaborative analysis of prospective cohort studies. *Antivir Ther*, 2008; 13: 959–67.
Comments: Meta-analysis whowing that anemia at ART start prognostic for both short- and long-term prognosis (AIDS and death), even if Hgb normalized in 1st 6 mos.

Mocroft AR, Lifson G, Touloumi, et al. Haemoglobin and anaemia in the SMART study. November 7–11, 2010. 10th International Congress on Drug Therapy in HIV Infection. Glasgow, Abstract P144, in *Journal of the International AIDS Society* 2010; 13(suppl 4): 144.
Comments: Association between decrease in Hgb and interruption of ART suggested effect of VL or inflammation.

NEUTROPENIA

Richard D. Moore, MD, MHS

CLINICAL
- Multiple causes, including HIV infection, inflammatory cytokines, drugs (AZT, GCV, FOS, amphotericin, 5-FC, sulfonamides, pyrimethamine, pentamidine, interferon-alfa), OIs with bone marrow replacement, chemotherapy for malignancy.
- HIV can cause decreased growth of progenitor cell, CFU-GM; decreased endogenous G-CSF.
- Prevalence ranges from 10% in asymptomatic HIV, 40%–50% with AIDS.
- Increased risk of bacterial and fungal infection with absolute neutrophil count (ANC) <750, but absolute risk relatively low. Greatest risk for infection and hospitalization with ANC <500.
- Neutropenia (<1000) not associated with decreased survival in HIV+ women (possibly in men, but not studied).

DIAGNOSIS
- ANC <1000.
- Anemia often present when caused by HIV infection, drugs, or OIs.

TREATMENT
Treatment of Neutropenia
- Assess for reversible causes requiring specific treatment, such as modifying use or dose of causative drug.
- Consider treatment with growth factors for ANC <500 (increased risk, but absolute risk for infection low).
- **G-CSF (filgrastim):** initial dose of 5 mcg/kg (or 300 mcg = 1 cc) SQ once daily; titrate as necessary after 1 wk by adjusting dosing interval to qod, 3 ×/wk, 2 ×/wk. Can also reduce dose (e.g., 150 mcg, 75 mcg, etc.). Goal is to maintain ANC >1000–2000.
- **Prokine (GM-CSF; sargramostim):** initial dose of 250 mcg/m² once daily; titrate as necessary by adjusting dosing interval as with G-CSF.
- Pegylated G-CSF (pegfilgrastim) 6 mg SQ weekly or less.

- Monitor ANC during G-CSF and GM-CSF 1–2 ×/wk.
- Adverse effects of growth factors: pain at injection site, myalgias, bone pain, low-grade fever, fatigue, flu-like symptoms, possible elevated lactic dehydrogenase and alkaline phosphatase. No evidence of adverse effect on HIV replication.
- USPHS/IDSA guidelines: G-CSF and GM-CSF "not routinely indicated" for neutropenic HIV+ patients.
- ART improves neutropenia in women (probably in men, but not studied).

SELECTED REFERENCES

Morishita M, Leanard RC. Pegfilgrastim: a neutrophil mediated granulocyte colony stimulating factor-expanding uses in cancer chemotherapy. *Expert Opin Biol Ther*, 2008; 8: 993–1001.
Comments: Review of pegfilgrastim to treat neutropenia.

Levine AM, Karim R, Mack W, et al. Neutropenia in human immunodeficiency virus infection: data from the women's interagency HIV study. *Arch Intern Med*, 2006; 166: 405–10.
Comments: Treatment with ART without AZT protects against development of neutropenia; ART use and higher CD4 associated with resolution of neutropenia. Neutropenia not associated with decreased survival in HIV+ women.

Meynard JL, Guiguet M, Arsac S, et al. Frequency and risk factors of infectious complications in neutropenic patients infected with HIV. *AIDS*, 1997; 11: 995–8.
Comments: Review of etiology, clinical implications, and treatment of neutropenia of HIV.

THROMBOCYTOPENIA

Richard D. Moore, MD, MHS

CLINICAL
- 1-yr incidence ranges from 1.7% with asymptomatic HIV to 3.1% with CD4-defined AIDS to 8.7% with AIDS-defining illness.
- Increased risk with decreasing CD4, injection drug use, black race, anemia. Other causes include alcohol abuse, sulfonamides, thiazides, folate and vitamin B12 deficiency, IV cocaine.
- Idiopathic thrombocytopenic purpura (ITP) a major cause. Production of autoantibodies against certain platelet antigens (PA-IgG). Antibody-coated platelets removed by macrophages in the spleen.
- Increased risk of bleeding with PLT <10,000–20,000.
- Heparin-induced thrombocytopenia may be more common in HIV-infected than uninfected.

DIAGNOSIS
- Low PLT count, usually with other blood elements normal.
- Bone marrow shows increase in megakaryocytes in response to PLT phagocytosis in ITP. Megakaryocytes may be decreased in HIV-TP without ITP. Other hematologic elements may be normal.
- Bone marrow Bx rarely necessary with isolated thrombocytopenia.

TREATMENT
Antiretroviral Therapy
- HIV-associated thrombocytopenia responds to antiretroviral therapy. Best data with AZT (600 mg/day; sometimes up to 1000 mg/day); however, most ART probably effective.
- Use most appropriate regimen to suppress VL and improve immune status. Consider AZT if no response to initial regimen.

Specific Treatment for ITP
- **Prednisone:** 80%–90% response rate. Initial dose is 1 mg/kg/day or 60–100 mg/day. Unknown whether long-term use may increase risk of HIV progression or fulminant Kaposi sarcoma in men coinfected with HHV-8.
- **Intravenous immune globulin (IVIG):** at 1000 mg/kg × 2 days. Response with significant increase (>100,000) in PLT counts within 24–48 hrs. High cost; reserve for acute bleeding or urgent need for invasive surgical procedure. Acute renal failure secondary to sucrose load reported with some preparations (*Sandoglobulin, Panglobulin, Gammar-P.I.V, and Gammar-I.V.b.*).

- **IV or IM anti-Rh immunoglobulin (anti-D, *WinRho*):** in nonsplenectomized Rh-positive patients produces response. Hemolysis with decrease in hemoglobin of >2 g/dL, fever, and chills seen in 5%–10% of patients.
- Eltrombopag indicated for Rx of ITP in patients at high risk for bleeding who have insufficient response to corticosteroids, IVIG, or splenectomy. Associated with increased risk of portal vein thrombosis in patients with chronic liver disease.
- Splenectomy, if refractory to above. Long-term response in approximately 60% of patients. Risk of infection with encapsulated bacteria after splenectomy (*S. pneumoniae*, *H. influenzae*). Need for pneumococcal vaccine.
- Other treatment modalities, such as dapsone, interferon, vincristine, danazol, low-dose splenic irradiation have shown limited success in ITP.
- For active bleeding, packed RBCs and PLT transfusion plus IVIG (prednisone has slower onset of action than IVIG).

FOLLOW-UP

Relapse

- Even with effective treatment, relapse can occur in 10%–20%. Effective ART may minimize relapse.
- Consider maintenance dose of prednisone, IVIG, or anti-Rh immunoglobulin. Consider eltrombopag.

SELECTED REFERENCES

Thompsoan GR, Lawrence VA, Crawford GE. HIV infection increases the risk of heparin-induced thrombocytopenia. *Clin Infect Dis*, 2007; 45: 1393–6.
Comments: Heparin-induced thrombocytopenia more common in HIV-infected than uninfected.

Scaradavou A. HIV-related thrombocytopenia. *Blood Rev*, 2002; 16: 73–6.
Comments: Review of incidence, mechanism, and treatment of HIV-associated thrombocytopenia.

Arranz Caso JA, Sanchez Mingo C, Garcia Tena J. Effect of highly active antiretroviral therapy on thrombocytopenia in patients with HIV infection. *New Engl J Med*, 1999; 341: 1239–40.
Comments: Important study that demonstrated effectiveness of AART as treatment for thrombocytopenia in HIV.

Cook L, Cooper N. Eltrombopag-a novel approach for the treatment of chronic immune thrombocytopenic purpura: review and safey considerations. *Drug Des Devel Ther*, 2010; 4: 139-45.
Comments: Review of use and safety of eltrombopag. Not specifically studied in HIV+ patients.

Pechère M, Samii K, Hirschel B. HIV-related thrombocytopenia. *New Engl J Med*, 1993; 328: 1785–6.
Comments: Early review of HIV-associated thrombocytopenia and effectiveness of AZT as treatment.

THROMBOTIC THROMBOCYTOPENIC PURPURA

Richard D. Moore, MD, MHS

CLINICAL

- Multisystem disease caused by platelet thrombi in various organs.
- Thrombocytopenia, hemolytic anemia, renal impairment, fever (can be high), and neurologic abnormalities (agitation, disorientation, headache early, late focal deficits, seizure, coma).
- Relatively rare; mortality <10% if recognized and treated early.
- Associated with early and late HIV, malignancy, chemotherapy, pregnancy.
- Drugs associated with TTP: quinine, ticlopidine, cyclosporine.

DIAGNOSIS

- Low platelet count (5000–100,000), hemolytic anemia (causing high indirect bilirubin and high LDH), fragmented RBCs on peripheral smear (schistocytes, spherocytes), azotemia, neurologic dysfunction.
- Low von Willebrand factor-cleaving protease level (<5%–10%) and presence of inhibitor may be demonstrated.

TREATMENT

Treatment of TTP

- Early Dx and urgent treatment required. Mortality rate 60%–80% without treatment.

- Plasma exchange with fresh frozen plasma (FFP) daily until normal PLT count and LDH. Average of 7–16 exchanges may be needed. HIV+ may respond better than HIV-negative to FFP.
- ART use in addition to plasma exchange is beneficial.
- Mild disease may respond to prednisone at 200 mg/day, but plasma exchange needed if no response within 48 hrs. Prednisone can be added if poor response to initial treatment with plasma exchange.
- ASA and dipyridamole not effective if given alone.
- FFP daily until normal platelets and LDH.

FOLLOW-UP

Relapse

- Relapse can occur, usually within 60 days (~10%), but can occur years later.
- Plasma exchange usually effective for relapse.

SELECTED REFERENCES

Novitzky N, Thomson J, Abrahams L, et al. TTP in patients with retroviral infection is highly responsive to plasma infusion therapy. *Br J Haematol*, 2005; 128: 373–9.

Comments: Prospective study. HIV+ patients with TTP responded to FFP faster than HIV-negative patients, and none required apheresis.

Miller RF, Scully M, Cohen H, et al. Thrombotic thrombocytopaenic purpura in HIV-infected patients. *Int J STD AIDS*, 2005; 16: 538–42.

Comments: Benefit of ART in addition to plasma exchange for TTP treatment.

Neurologic

DEMENTIA, HIV-ASSOCIATED

John N. Ratchford, MD and Jeffrey Rumbaugh, MD, PhD

PATHOGENS
- HIV is found in brain in macrophages, microglia, and multinucleated giant cells.
- Neurons injured indirectly when infected cells release noxious substances.

CLINICAL
- **HIV-associate dementia (HAD)** is subacute decline in cognitive function due to HIV.
- Also known as **HIV encephalopathy** or **AIDS-dementia complex.**
- Milder cognitive impairment is called **HIV-associated cognitive/motor complex.** The term **HIV-associated neurocognitive dysfunction (HAND)** is now frequently used and refers to neurocognitive dysfunction of any degree of severity, since severe forms (HAD) are now relatively rare and mild forms much more frequent.
  - Dementia is AIDS-defining illness in 3%.
  - Prevalence 2% for HAD, 12% for mild neurocognitive disorder, and 33% for asymptomatic neurocognitive impairment.
- Risk factors for HAND include Hx of more severe immunosuppression (nadir CD4 <200), so earlier treatment to prevent severe immunosuppression may decrease risk.
- Early Sx: apathy, impaired memory, difficulty with reading and calculation, decreased libido, depressive symptoms, waning interest in work and hobbies causing social withdrawal, occasionally mania or psychosis.
- Later Sx: psychomotor slowing, poor memory, slowed movement. At end stage patients can be mute, bedbound, and incontinent.
- Considered a "subcortical dementia" due to absence of signs like aphasia and apraxia seen in "cortical dementias" like Alzheimer disease.
- Motor symptoms like gait dysfunction, poor balance, and tremor may be present.
- Often accompanied by HIV-related myelopathy or neuropathy.
- Severity rated from 0 to 4: 0–normal, 0.5–subclinical, 1–mild, 2–moderate, 3–severe, 4–end stage.
- When untreated, mean survival ~6 mos.

DIAGNOSIS
- DDx includes PML, CNS toxoplasmosis, primary CNS lymphoma, CMV encephalitis, neurosyphilis, vitamin B12 or thiamine deficiency, delirium, depression, medication/drug effect, or other causes of dementia.
- Differs from delirium in that there is no alteration of consciousness or attention.
- Exam may show frontal release signs, hyperreflexia, and increased tone.
- Consider OI if focal signs or fever present.
- Workup includes brain MRI, neuropsychological testing, serologic testing prn to rule out vitamin deficiency, syphilis.
- MRI usually shows atrophy and ill-defined white matter hyperintensities on T2-weighted scans.
- CSF analysis not essential, but may be needed to rule out OI.
- CSF findings nonspecific: may be acellular or show a lymphocytic pleocytosis; protein elevated in 65%.

TREATMENT

ART
- ART is mainstay of treatment.
- Drugs with greater CNS penetration (including AZT, d4T, 3TC, ABC, NVP, IDV, and LPV/r), are more effective at decreasing CSF VL, but evidence is mixed regarding whether this results in greater clinical benefit.
- IRIS can occasionally be seen following initiation of ART, usually due to PML.
- No other adjunctive treatments have proven to be beneficial.

Non-ART Therapies
- Treatment of comorbid depression, mania, or psychosis may be necessary.
- HAD patients are sensitive to psychoactive medications.

FOLLOW-UP

Common Practice
- Monitor response to ART.
- If neurologic deterioration, perform brain MRI to rule out IRIS or OI.
- Neuropsychological testing can be repeated to evaluate longitudinal change.

SELECTED REFERENCES

Letendre S, Marquie-Beck J, Capparelli E, et al. Validation of the CNS penetration-effectiveness rank for quantifying antiretroviral penetration into the central nervous system. *Arch Neurol*, 2008; 65: 65–70.
Comments: Drugs with higher CNS penetration associated with lower CSF VL.

Heaton RK, Clifford DB, Franklin DR Jr, et al. HIV-associated neurocognitive disorders persists in the era of potent antiretroviral therapy: CHARTER study. *Neurology*, 2010; 75: 2087–96.
Comments: Though HAD is rare, milder forms of HAND are common even among those on ART.

Cysique LA, Vaida F, Letendre S, et al. Dynamics of cognitive change in impaired HIV-positive patients initiating antiretroviral therapy. *Neurology*, 2009; 73: 342–8.
Comments: Neuropsychological improvement peaked 24–36 wks after starting ART; CNS penetration index associated with improvement.

Garvey L, Winston A, Walsh J, et al. Antiretroviral therapy CNS penetration and HIV-1-associated CNS disease. *Neurology*, 2011; 76: 693–700.
Comments: A non-significant association was seen between lower ART CNS penetration effectiveness score and CNS OIs. Lower CNS penetration effectiveness score was associated with higher mortality, though it is unclear whether or not this is a causative association.

NEUROPATHY, PERIPHERAL

Daniel Harrison, MD and Jeffrey Rumbaugh, MD, PhD

PATHOGENS
- HIV can cause distal sensory neuropathy (HIV-DSP).
- HIV productively infects perivascular macrophages in both central and peripheral nervous system (PNS): degree of macrophage activation correlates with Sx.
- HIV DNA demonstrated in perineuronal macrophages in dorsal root ganglia of patients with HIV-associated sensory neuropathy.
- Direct mechanism of neuronal injury may be related to the HIV protein gp120, which can act as modifier of response to inflammatory cytokines.
- HIV, HCV: cause vasculitic neuropathy, but rare.
- VZV: postherpetic neuralgia experienced by some patients.
- Immune-mediated neuropathies (less common): Guillain-Barré Syndrome (GBS) and chronic inflammatory demyelinating neuropathy (CIDP).
- Antiretroviral distal sensory neuropathy (ARV-DSP): can be caused by NRTIs (d4T and ddI). Some studies have also shown neurotoxicity with some PIs (IDV, SQV, and RTV). Exact mechanism of injury unknown but thought to be due to mitochondrial toxicity from dysfunction of mitochondrial oxidative metabolism.
- Higher rates of entrapment neuropathies: ulnar neuropathy at elbows, median neuropathy of hands (carpal tunnel syndrome), peroneal neuropathy in legs.
- Non-HIV-related causes: impaired glucose tolerance, diabetes, vitamin deficiency (B12), alcoholism, thyroid dysfunction, syphilis, other medications (e.g., INH).

CLINICAL
- Risk factors for neuropathy include low CD4 and high VL. Risk factors for progression include low total neuropathy score (TNS), distal epidermal denervation, and white race.
- Patients may not recognize Sx; routine questioning during visits may be necessary.
- HIV-DSP and ARV-DSP can coexist. Difficult to clinically differentiate between the two.

- Pain symmetrical and initially begins in soles of feet. Patients commonly complain of burning, cramping, numbness, and/or paresthesias.
- Consider DDx: neuropathy due to diabetes (which may complicate PI therapy), alcoholism, B12 deficiency, syphilis, thyroid dysfunction, HCV, malnutrition, advanced age, and IDU.
- Patients may be asymptomatic: "silent" peripheral neuropathy found on examination only.
- Progressive neuropathy with motor weakness and absent reflexes: think GBS, which usually occurs at the time of primary infection or HIV seroconversion, or CIPD if more chronic.
- If Sx predominately unilateral, consider entrapment neuropathies.

DIAGNOSIS
- Hx helps differentiate HIV-DSP from ARV-DSP. Obtain information on NRTI and PI use as well as other agents such as HU, INH, and vincristine.
- PE reveals diminished or absent ankle reflexes compared to knees and "stocking" type sensory loss (decreased pain, temp, and vibratory sensation). Distal weakness can be late feature.
- Subjective peripheral neuropathy screen (SPNS) has been widely used to screen for neuropathy. Consists of 3 items assessing for presence of paresthesias, pain, and numbness. Easily and quickly administered at bedside.
- Screen for alcoholism, diabetes (fasting glucose), HCV, B12 deficiency, syphilis, and thyroid dysfunction.
- Electrophysiology studies not necessary except to demonstrate entrapment, polyradiculopathy, and immune-mediated neuropathies.
- Skin Bx shows decrease in epidermal nerve fiber densities, which correlates with clinical and electrophysiologic evidence of neuropathy. Electrophysiology studies evaluate large nerve fibers and may be normal, even when skin Bx shows substantial damage to small nerve fibers.
- MRI lumbosacral spine in patients who present with lower extremity polyradiculopathy.
- Lesions of cervical or thoracic spine can present with Sx suggestive of peripheral neuropathy, usually of lower extremities, but myelopathic examination findings usually present.

TREATMENT
General Principles
- Stop offending NRTIs whenever possible. Consider stopping potentially offending PIs if Hx strongly suggestive. Usually reverses early Sx within 3 mos.
- Control blood sugars if diabetic.
- Stop neurotoxic medications if applicable.
- Avoid alcohol.
- Appropriate nutritional status is key to prevent worsening of neuropathy.
- Fully suppressive ART regimen.
- Ascertain whether pharmacologic intervention necessary.
- Sx may not be completely reversed with any treatment modality in some patients.
- Prior pain modifying therapy: dose at termination and duration.
- Nonpharmacologic measures may be needed to supplement medications, e.g., transcutaneous electrical nerve stimulation (TENS) unit.

Medications
- **Gabapentin:** begin at low doses, increasing gradually as tolerated until pain controlled. Starting dose is 300 mg 3 ×/day. Titrate up slowly until an appropriate threshold dose is reached. Side effects: sedation, fatigue, weight gain.
- **Lamotrigine:** start at 25 mg twice daily and slowly escalate to 100 mg twice daily over 1-mo period to prevent rash, including Stevens-Johnson syndrome. Randomized controlled trial demonstrated efficacy in ARV-DSP.
- **Topiramate:** start at 25 mg once daily and increase by 25 mg qwk to max of 100 mg twice daily. Adverse effects: kidney stones, memory disturbance, and weight loss.
- **Capsaicin:** single application of high dose (640 mcg/cm^2) patch resulted in 12 wks of pain relief in recent controlled trial in painful HIV-DSP. FDA approval for this formulation pending.
- **Amitriptyline and nortriptyline:** qhs may be effective, but did not perform well in clinical studies.
- **Tramadol:** acute treatment with 50 mg twice daily and narcotics reserved for those with excruciating pain.

- **Fentanyl patch:** may start at 25 mcg/hr every 3 days and increase dose if required
  Caution: PIs can increase fentanyl levels.
- **Pregabalin:** approved for painful diabetic neuropathy. Target dose found to be 600 mg/day
  in divided doses. Recently reported randomized controlled trial revealed no superiority to
  placebo in HIV-DSP.
- **Acetyl-l-carnitine:** found to be beneficial in clinical trials for ARV-DSP.
- **Duloxetine:** safety not established in HIV-DSP, no clinical trials underway. Starting dose is
  30 mg once daily, increase up to 60 mg daily. Dose may be increased further if needed.

SELECTED REFERENCES

Simpson D, Brown S, Tobias J, et al. Controlled trial of high-concentration capsaicin patch for treatment of painful
HIV neuropathy. *Neurology*, 2008; 70: 2305–13.
Comments: High-concentration capsaicin patch effective in painful HIV neuropathy.

Zhou L, Kitch DW, Evans SR, et al. Correlates of epidermal nerve fiber densities in HIV-associated distal sensory neuropathy.
Neurology, 2007; 68: 2113–9.
Comment: Epidermal nerve fiber density in HIV patients correlates with clinical and electrophysiologic evidence of
HIV-DSP.

Brew BJ. The peripheral nerve complications of human immunodeficiency virus (HIV) infection. *Muscle Nerve*, 2003;
28: 542–52.
Comments: Epidermal nerve fiber density in HIV patients correlates with clinical and electrophysiologic evidence of
HIV-DSP.

Psychiatric

ANXIETY

Glenn J. Treisman, MD, PhD, Andrew F. Angelino, MD, and Jeffrey Hsu, MD

CLINICAL

- Anxiety is common response to stressful life circumstances, but can also be Sx of anxiety disorder or other underlying disorder (such as major depression).
- Diagnosable anxiety disorders may be present in up to 40% of HIV+ patients, but prevalence of anxiety Sxs (without Dx'd disorder) even higher (up to 72%). Sxs are twice as commonly reported in women vs. men.
- Can be prominent Sx in patients 1st Dx'd with HIV, and in response to progression, such as declining CD4, OIs.
- Diagnostic overlap with other conditions. Greater than 50% of patients with anxiety disorders have comorbid depression. Alcohol dependence also common (especially in women).
- Anxiety symptoms and disorders can increase likelihood of HIV risk behaviors and ART nonadherence. Also, HIV+ patients with panic disorder (PD) and posttraumatic stress disorder (PTSD) experience greater pain intensity and related dysfunction.
- Common medical conditions associated with anxiety Sx include hypoxia, stimulant intoxication, withdrawal from sedative-hypnotics, seizures, hyperthyroidism, pheochromocytoma. Anxiety can also be a side effect of EFV, interferon, or corticosteroid treatment.

DIAGNOSIS

- **Panic disorder (PD):** recurrent, unexpected panic attacks (a discrete period of intense fear or discomfort including >4 of following: palpitations, sweating, trembling, shortness of breath, feeling of choking, chest pain, nausea, dizziness, derealization, fear of losing control or going crazy, fear of dying, paresthesias, chills/hot flushes).
- **Specific phobia:** excessive or unreasonable fear cued by presence or anticipation of an object or situation.
- **Social phobia:** fear of embarrassment in a social situation where person is exposed to scrutiny of others.
- **Obsessive-compulsive disorder (OCD):** obsessions or compulsions that cause marked distress, are time consuming, and interfere with functioning. Obsessions: recurrent, persistent, intrusive thoughts that patient recognizes as unreasonable. Compulsions: repetitive behaviors or mental acts performed in response to an obsession.
- **Generalized anxiety disorder (GAD):** excessive anxiety and worry for >6 mos with >3 of following: restlessness, easily fatigued, difficulty concentrating, irritability, muscle tension, sleep disturbance. Much diagnostic overlap with other conditions.
- **Posttraumatic stress disorder (PTSD):** occurs after a traumatic event that involves serious threat of death or injury. Following present for >1 mo: (1) trauma reexperienced by >1 of following: recurrent memories or dreams of event, reexperiencing event (intrusive "flashbacks"), intense distress at exposure to cues that represent event; (2) avoidance of stimuli associated with event by >3 of following: avoidance of thoughts or feelings associated with event; diminished interest in activities; detachment from others; restricted affect; sense of foreshortened future; (3) increased arousal indicated by >2 of following: insomnia, irritability, poor concentration, hypervigilance, startle response.

TREATMENT

Antidepressants

- Selective serotonin reuptake inhibitors (SSRIs) and selective serotonin and norepinephrine reuptake inhibitors (SNRIs), such as venlafaxine XR and duloxetine, are considered first-line treatment for GAD, PD, social phobia, and OCD.
- SSRIs and SNRIs may be initially activating in anxious patients, so lower dosages should be used initially with slow titration schedule. In most cases, patients will need to be on higher final dosage of medication for Rx of anxiety disorders vs depressive disorders.

- SSRIs and SNRIs may take up to 4 to 6 wks to be effective in controlling anxiety.
- Although FDA indications for treatment of individual anxiety disorders differ among SSRIs, clinical experience shows that all agents are equally efficacious in treating anxiety. Choice of agent depends on side effect profile.
- While benzodiazepines (BZDs) may relieve anxiety symptoms acutely, there are no data to support long-term daily use of BZDs for anxiety disorders, as risk of side effects and dependence generally outweighs short-term benefits. Patients already receiving BZDs may experience worsening anxiety when being tapered off, thus resulting in significant treatment difficulties.
- Tricyclic antidepressants, mirtazapine, and nefazodone are also useful in treating anxiety.
- See Depression (p. 124) for antidepressant dosages, side effects, and drug interactions.

Buspirone
- Non-BZD anxiolytic approved for treatment of GAD.
- Initial dosage is 5 mg 3 ×/day up to total dosage of 60 mg/day in divided doses.
- Side effects: headache, GI distress, dizziness, and parasthesias.
- No clinically significant interactions with ART.
- Often used as augmenting agent in conjunction with SSRIs.
- No abuse potential.
- Well tolerated in HIV+ patients.
- Azoles, macrolides, PIs, DLV, and other CYP3A4 inhibitors may increase buspirone levels. Start with 5 mg 3 ×/day and titrate slowly.
- Phenytoin, phenobarbital, rifamycin, carbamazepine, NVP, EFV, ETR, and other CYP3A4 inducers may decrease buspirone levels. Titrate to effect.

Benzodiazepines
- Can cause seizures and life-threatening withdrawal in dependent patients.
- Usual dosages: diazepam 2–10 mg twice daily; clonazepam 0.25 mg–2 mg twice daily; alprazolam 0.25–1 mg 3 ×/day; oxazepam 10–30 mg 3 ×/day; lorazepam 0.5–1 mg 2–×/day.
- High-potency BZDs more useful for managing symptoms related to PD (e.g., clonazepam, alprazolam, lorazepam).
- Common side effects: sedation, anterograde amnesia, fatigue, and impairment of motor coordination and cognitive function. Concurrent use of BZD with alcohol/other sedatives may increase CNS depression and respiratory failure.
- May cause tolerance and dependence. Should be used judiciously and are best avoided, in patients with alcoholism and substance addiction. Short-acting, high-potency agents (e.g., alprazolam, midazolam) have higher abuse potential.
- More likely to cause delirium in elderly patients and patients with AIDS dementia/cognitive dysfunction; start with lower dosages.
- Alprazolam, clonazepam, midazolam, and triazolam metabolized by CYP3A4; concurrent administration with PIs (especially RTV and possibly EFV) may cause elevated blood levels resulting in increased sedation and respiratory depression.
- Lorazepam, oxazepam, and temazepam not metabolized by CYP3A4; may be safer to use in patients on ART and with liver disease (glucuronidation less affected in liver disease).
- Upon discontinuation of therapy, BZDs should be tapered to avoid withdrawal Sx (rebound anxiety, insomnia, tachycardia, hypertension, seizures).

Atypical Antipsychotics
- Although not specifically approved for treatment of anxiety, low doses of atypical antipsychotics can be used in conjunction with antidepressants to help manage patients who need faster control of anxiety symptoms.
- Usual dosages: olanzapine 2.5–10 mg/day; risperidone 0.25–3 mg/day; quetiapine 25–400 mg/day; ziprasidone 20–80 mg/day in divided doses; aripiprazole 2–10 mg/day.
- Monitor BMI, fasting glucose, triglycerides because of risk of hyperglycemia and hyperlipidemia.
- RTV may decrease olanzapine serum levels and increase risperidone and quetiapine serum levels.

Anticonvulsants
- Not FDA approved for treatment of anxiety, but case reports show GABAergic agents may be useful in relieving Sxs either alone or in conjunction with SSRIs.

- Usual dosages: gabapentin 300–3600 mg/day in divided doses; tiagabine 8–32 mg/day; pregabalin 150–600 mg/day.
- Side effects: sedation and dizziness.
- No interactions with ART.
- Low abuse potential.

Psychotherapy
- Behavioral therapy (exposure, desensitization) is treatment of choice in patients with specific phobias.
- Cognitive-behavioral therapy should be used in conjunction with pharmacologic therapy in treatment of PD, social phobia, GAD, and PTSD.
- OCD poorly responsive to psychotherapy alone. Pharmacologic therapy combined with psychotherapy is treatment of choice.
- Other useful treatment modalities: hypnosis, relaxation therapy, stress management.
- Effective self-help strategies include prayer, meditation, exercise, relaxation techniques, cooking, and walking.

FOLLOW-UP
- No randomized, double-blind, placebo-controlled trials exist examining efficacy of specific pharmacologic agents in partients with comorbid anxiety/HIV. Rx guided by usual clinical practice.
- Treatment with medications unlikely to result in full remission of anxiety disorder in most patients, although most will improve. PD and OCD most difficult to treat.
- Long-term maintenance treatment recommended since Sx remission and relapse common with discontinuation of medications.
- Suicide rate in patients with PD high (20%–40% attempted suicide). Refer to mental health professional/psychiatric admission if suicidal ideation present.

SELECTED REFERENCES

Kemppainen JK, Eller LS, Bunch E, et al. Strategies for self-management of HIV-related anxiety. *AIDS Care*, 2006; 18 (6): 597–607.

Comments: International survey on anxiety self-care management in HIV patients recruited from Norway, Taiwan, and US. Patients rated prayer as being most effective self-management technique in relieving HIV-related anxiety followed by meditation, exercising, using relaxation techniques, cooking, and walking.

Tsao JC, Dobalian A, Naliboff BD. Panic disorder and pain in a national sample of persons living with HIV. *Pain*, 2004; 109: 172–80.

Comments: Supplemental mental health survey of 1489 HIV+ outpatients (subset of HCSUS study sample). Of these patients, 15% met criteria for MDD, 10% for PTSD, 11% for PD. Patients with a psychiatric diagnosis had greater self-reported pain scores than patients without psychiatric disorders. Relative to the other 2 psychiatric disorders, patients with PD reported the highest mean pain scores at 6-mo follow-up and was the only group to report increased pain over time.

Morrison MF, Petitto JM, Ten Have T, et al. Depressive and anxiety disorders in women with HIV infection. *Am J Psychiatry*, 2002; 159: 789–96.

Comments: Examines differences in prevalence of anxiety and depressive disorders between HIV+ and HIV-negative women. HIV+ women scored significantly higher on Hamilton Anxiety Rating Scale than HIV-negative women, although rates of anxiety disorders did not differ significantly between groups.

BIPOLAR DISORDER

Jeffrey Hsu, MD, Andrew F. Angelino, MD, and Glenn J. Treisman, MD, PhD

CLINICAL
- Bipolar affective disorder (BPAD): episodic disorder characterized by extended changes in mood, vital sense, and self-attitude lasting days to weeks or longer.
- Lifetime occurrence of >1 manic or mixed episodes.
- Depressive episodes more common during course of illness but do not need to be present to make Dx of BPAD.

- Lifetime prevalence of BPAD in general population 0.4%–1.6%. Prevalence in HIV+ population unclear but likely to be elevated.
- Equally common in men and women. Mean age of onset of 1st episode is 21.
- Mania in HIV+ patients can either be primary (preexisting BPAD) or secondary (HIV disease).
- Secondary mania (AIDS mania) differs from BPAD in later age of onset and lower occurrence of family or personal history of mood disorder. Typically occurs at later stages of HIV illness and characterized by more irritability, more psychomotor slowing, and increased talkativeness. May be associated with cognitive impairment/dementia and structural brain abnormalities on CT or MRI.
- Common medical conditions mimicking BPAD include cocaine/amphetamine use, steroid treatment, multiple sclerosis, temporal lobe epilepsy, hyperthyroidism, Cushing's syndrome, neurosyphillis, lupus, herpes encephalitis, subcortical dementias, interferon, CNS lesions.
- AIDS mania, described early in epidemic associated with low CD4 and HAD, still may occur in advanced patients.

DIAGNOSIS

- **Manic episode:** distinct period of elevated, expansive or irritable mood lasting >1 wk along with >3 of following: grandiosity, decreased sleep, pressured speech, racing thoughts, distractibility, psychomotor agitation, impulsivity.
- **Mixed episode:** criteria for both manic episode and major depressive episode met during 1-week period.
- **Hypomanic episode:** same criteria as manic episode except elevated mood lasts for >4 days and not severe enough to cause marked impairment or hospitalization. No psychotic features present.
- **BPAD with psychotic features:** presence of mood-congruent hallucinations or delusions.

TREATMENT

General Principles

- BPAD significantly associated with non-adherence to HIV therapy.
- ART may provide protective effect against development of AIDS mania and should be initiated in untreated patients presenting with mania.
- Patients with BPAD usually need life-long maintenance therapy; high risk of recurrence, especially with Hx of multiple episodes.
- Management usually based on lithium or mood-stabilizing anticonvulsant but may also involve antipsychotics/neuroleptics (particularly atypical antipsychotics). Some patients managed on atypical neuroleptics alone.
- Medications with narrow therapeutic index (lithium, valproic acid, carbamazepine) require blood level monitoring but also allow assessment of adherence to therapy.
- Combination therapy with lithium/anticonvulsants and atypical antipsychotics useful for initial treatment of mania. Atypical antipsychotics may sometimes be tapered once acute symptoms resolved.
- Rule out medical causes of new onset mania in patients with no prior history of BPAD, especially in more advanced HIV illness.
- High rate of concurrent alcohol and cocaine dependence. Treat substance use disorder simultaneously.

Lithium Carbonate

- Usual dosage: 300–600 mg twice daily.
- Side effects: polyuria, polydipsia, weight gain, cognitive problems, tremor, sedation, lethargy, impaired coordination, GI distress, hair loss, leukocytosis, acne, edema, hypothyroidism, T-wave abnormalities.
- Renally excreted, no significant metabolic interactions with ART.
- Narrow therapeutic index; monitor blood levels closely. Therapeutic levels 0.5–1.2 mEq/L. Measure blood levels 12 hrs after last dose and check 5 days after dose adjustment.
- Toxicity closely related to serum levels and can occur at therapeutic doses. Signs of toxicity seen at levels >1.5 mEq/L with life-threatening side effects occurring at levels >2.0 mEq/L. Patients with HIV (especially advanced disease) may be more sensitive to toxic effects of lithium.

- Very advanced patients may have sudden unpredictable decreases in lithium clearance leading to toxicity.
- Signs and Sxs of early toxicity: tremor, nausea, diarrhea, blurred vision, vertigo, confusion, increased deep tendon reflexes.
- Signs and Sx of serious toxicity: seizures, coma, cardiac dysrhythmia, permanent neurologic impairment.
- Treatment of lithium toxicity: aggressive hydration, maintenance of electrolyte balance, and hemodialysis if levels >4.0 mEq/L.
- Monitor renal and thyroid function tests and lithium levels q3–6mos. Obtain follow-up ECG in patients with Hx of cardiac disease.

Valproic Acid (VPA)/Divalproex Sodium
- Divalproex almost always favored over VPA due to better GI tolerability.
- Usual dosage: 250–1000 mg twice daily.
- Common side effects: nausea, vomiting, diarrhea, thrombocytopenia, transaminase elevation, sedation, tremor, ataxia, alopecia, weight gain.
- Serious idiosyncratic side effects: hepatic failure, pancreatitis, erythema multiforme.
- Therapeutic serum levels: 50–150 mcg/mL. Check serum levels 12 hrs after last dose.
- Levels may decrease when RTV coadministered. Case report of patient with exacerbated mania with coadministration of LPV/r.
- Check levels and baseline CBC and LFTs at initiation of therapy and monitor q6mos.
- Shown in initial studies to stimulate in vitro viral replication, but not confirmed clinically. Recent reports suggest VPA may play role in eradicating HIV from latent cells.
- Shown to increase AZT concentration in CSF: implications for greater efficacy and/or toxicity.
- May be less effective than lithium for depressive Sx of bipolar disorder.

Lamotrigine
- Start at 25 mg/day × 2 wks, then 50 mg/day × 2 wks, then 100 mg/day. Target dosage 100–200 mg/day. Some patients may need up to 400 mg/day.
- Common side effects: rash, nausea, vomiting, headache, dizziness.
- Serious side effects: Stevens-Johnson syndrome (~0.1%) frequency increased when dose increased quickly.
- Levels may be lower when coadministered with RTV, LPV/r, or carbamezepine.
- Levels higher when coadministered with VPA and doses of both medications must be adjusted.

Other Mood Stabilizers
- **Carbamezepine:** usual dosage 200–1800 mg/day given twice daily. Therapeutic blood level 8–12 mcg/mL. Potent inducer of CYP3A4. Aplastic anemia and agranulocytosis occurs in <1/20,000 patients.
- **Gabapentin:** sometimes used as mood stabilizer but no clear clinical data supporting efficacy. More useful for chronic pain. Usual dosage 600–3600 mg/day given 2–3 ×/day. Mild side effect profile: sedation, dizziness. Minimal drug-drug interactions.
- **Topiramate:** anecdotal case reports suggesting efficacy. More likely to cause weight loss than weight gain. Dosage range 25–250 mg twice daily. Common side effects: sedation, anxiety, ataxia, nervousness.
- **Oxcarbazepine:** usual dosage 300–2400 mg/day given twice daily. Analog of carbamezepine. Improved side effect profile and less likely to cause drug-drug interactions. Not FDA approved for Rx of BPAD, but some open label trials and 1 double-blind placebo trial show efficacy in Rx acute mania.

Atypical Antipsychotics
- Serious side effects of this class: hyperglycemia with ketoacidosis, neuroleptic malignant syndrome, acute dystonia, tardive dyskinesia. All may lead to metabolic syndrome and glucose elevations.
- May be used alone or adjunctively with lithium and anticonvulsants to stabilize acute manic episodes.
- All medications in class may increase risk of metabolic syndrome (weight gain, hyperglycemia, and hyperlipidemia); olanzapine has greatest frequency of weight gain.
- Monitor for extrapyramidal symptoms (EPS) and neuroleptic malignant syndrome (NMS). HIV/AIDS patients at higher risk.

- Few controlled studies exist in literature examining use of these agents in BPAD patients with HIV/AIDS.
- **Olanzapine:** usual dosage 10–20 mg/day. Common side effects: somnolence, constipation, dry mouth, orthostatic hypotension, increased appetite, weight gain, transient LFT elevation, prolactin elevation, hyperlipidemia. No significant drug interactions with ART.
- **Risperidone:** usual dosage 0.25–3 mg twice daily. More likely to cause EPS, dystonia, and prolactin elevation, especially at higher dosages.
- **Zisprasidone:** usual dosage 20–80 mg twice daily. Less sedation and weight gain.
- **Quetiapine:** usual dosage 25–400 mg twice daily. Causes sedation and weight gain.
- **Aripiprazole:** usual dosage 15–30 mg once daily. Lower sedation and weight gain.
- **Paliperidone:** usual dosage 6 mg once-daily. Dosing range 3–12 mg once-daily.
- **Asenapine:** only sublingual administration, requires instruction. Usual dosage 10 mg twice-daily. Start at 5 mg twice-daily when used as adjunctive agent with VPA or lithium.
- **Iloperidone:** usual dosage 6–12 mg twice-daily. Start at 1 mg twice-daily and titrate slowly to avoid orthostatic hypotension. Potential interactions with CYP3A4 and CYP2D6 inhibitors.

Antidepressants

- Lamotrigine or lithium may be particularly useful in patients with bipolar depression.
- If indicated, start antidepressants cautiously and at low doses after patient is on therapeutic dose of mood stabilizer to prevent precipitation of manic episode.
- See Depression section, below, for more information on antidepressant therapy.

Psychotherapy

- Psychotherapy not useful during acute phase. Inpatient hospitalization may be necessary for patients at risk for harm to self or others.
- Supportive psychotherapy important once Sx stabilized with psychotropics.

SELECTED REFERENCES

American Psychiatric Association; Practice Guideline for the Treatment of Patients with HIV/AIDS; American Psychiatric Association; 2000 (Updated Guideline Watch 2006)
Comments: APA Practice Guideline for treating patients with HIV/AIDS and psychiatric disorders. Sections on BPAD and monitoring metabolic abnormalities in patients on atypical antipsychotics and ART.

Archin NM, Cheema M, et al.; Antiretroviral intensification and valproic acid lack sustained effect on residual HIV-1 viremia or resting CD4+ cell infection. PLoS One. 2010 Feb 23; 5(2): e9390.
Comments: VPA added to standard ART resulted in depletion of resting CD4+ T cell infection but effects were not sustained.

Ferrando SJ, Wapenyi K. Psychopharmacological treatment of patients with HIV and AIDS. *Psychiatr Q*, 2002; 73: 33–49.
Comments: Review of psychopharmacologic treatment of mania in HIV+ patients with information about drug-drug interactions.

Spiegel DR, Weller AL, Pennell K, et al.; The successful treatment of mania due to acquired immunodeficiency syndrome
Comments: Case series of 3 patients with secondary mania due to HIV effectively treated with standard doses of ziprasidone.

Walkup JT, Akincigil A, Chakravarty S, et al.: Bipolar Medication Use and Adherence to Antiretroviral Therapy Among Patients With HIV-AIDS and Bipolar Disorder. Psychiatr Serv. 2011 Mar; 62(3): 313–6
Comments: Study showed that patients who had filled bipolar medications the prior month had higher odds of antiretrovirals currently in their possession.

DEPRESSION

Glenn J. Treisman, MD, PhD, Andrew F. Angelino, MD, and Jeffrey Hsu, MD

CLINICAL

- Prevalence of major depressive disorder (MDD) in HIV patients 2–3 × higher than general population; most common psychiatric condition in HIV+ patients. Prevalence of depression 57% in HIV+ patients and 70% in HIV/HCV coinfected patients.
- Lifetime risk of developing MDD 2 × greater in women vs men. Prevalence of MDD in HIV+ women up to 4 × higher than HIV-negative women and 3 × higher than HIV+ men.

- 1st–degree relatives of patients with MDD at greater risk than general population.
- Alcohol, cocaine, or amphetamine dependence may contribute to onset or exacerbation of MDD.
- MDD in HIV patients often under-Dx'd as many Sx similar to Sx of HIV infection or AIDS-related medical complications, e.g., decreased energy, weight loss, insomnia, neurocognitive disturbance.
- Patients with untreated MDD less likely to adhere to medications and keep medical appointments; more likely to engage in high-risk sexual behavior and substance abuse. Untreated depression associated with increased morbidity and mortality in HIV patients.
- Suicide rate in AIDS patients 7 × higher than in general population. Risk for suicide greatest in 1st few mos following initial Dx of HIV and with onset of medical complications of AIDS.

Diagnosis
- MDD: Sx lasting >2 wks with depressed mood and/or anhedonia and >4 of following: appetite changes, sleep changes, psychomotor agitation or retardation, fatigue or loss of energy, worthlessness or guilt, poor concentration, recurrent thoughts of death or suicide. Anhedonia (loss of pleasure) most sensitive and specific diagnostic indicator of depression.
- MDD with psychotic features: major depressive episode with presence of mood-congruent hallucinations and/or delusions.
- Dysthymic disorder: chronically depressed mood >2 yrs with >2 of following: appetite changes, sleep changes, fatigue, low self-esteem, poor concentration, hopelessness.
- Adjustment disorder with depressed mood: development of depressed mood, hopelessness or tearfulness occurring in context of identifiable stressor.
- Medical conditions that can cause depressive Sx include hypothyroidism, hypogonadism, CNS infections or neoplasms, HIV dementia, psychoactive substance use/dependence, medication side effects (especially EFV).
- Common medications causing depressive Sx: EFV, interferon, beta-blockers, steroids.

Treatment
Antidepressant Medications
- All antidepressants have approximately 60% response rate and seem to be equally efficacious. No particular antidepressant shown to be superior for HIV+ patients.
- 90% of depressed patients eventually respond to >1 antidepressant(s) after multiple trials.
- Patients must be on therapeutic dose for >4–6 wks for adequate trial.
- Successful choice of antidepressant depends on favorable side effect profile and drug-drug interactions.
- 50% of patients achieve complete remission on continued antidepressant therapy after 6 mos; up to 75% experience remission within 2 yrs.

Selective Serotonin Reuptake Inhibitors (SSRIs)
- PDR doses usually too low due to trials design.
- Usual dosages: fluoxetine 10–80 mg/day; sertraline 25–200 mg/day; paroxetine 10–60 mg/day; citalopram 10–80 mg/day; escitalopram 10–40 mg/day.
- Common side effects: initial anxiety or agitation, nausea, diarrhea, headaches, sexual dysfunction.
- Most SSRIs inhibit and are metabolized by CYP2D6; use caution when using with other meds metabolized by CYP2D6. RTV documented to increase levels of SSRIs (risk of serotonin syndrome), with exception of escitalopram. Citalopram, escitalopram, and sertraline are weak inhibitors and should be considered with PI-based regimens.
- Discontinuation of SSRIs requires tapering to avoid discontinuation syndrome (dizziness, nausea, insomnia, headaches, diarrhea, myalgias, paresthesias). This is more likely in agents with shorter half-lives, e.g., sertraline, paroxetine, citalopram, escitalopram.

Serotonin-Norepinephrine Reuptake Inhibitors (SNRIs)
- Similar to SSRI drugs but with utility in chronic pain.
- Venlafaxine: 75–375 mg/day in divided doses; side effects: headache, nausea, dizziness.
- Desvelafaxine: 50–100 mg/day once daily: side effects; headache, nausea, dizziness.
- Duloxetine: 60–120 mg/day daily; side effects: nausea, dry mouth, constipation, dizziness.
- Milnacipran: approved for fibromyalgia but not for depression.

Tricyclic Antidepressants (TCAs)

- Must monitor blood levels for toxicity but also useful for therapy.
- Usual dosages: amitriptyline 50–200 mg/day (blood level >120 ng/mL); nortriptyline 50–150 mg/day (50–125 ng/mL); imipramine 50–200 mg/day (>225 ng/mL); desipramine 50–200 mg/day (>125 ng/mL).
- Nortriptyline has best-documented therapeutic blood level.
- Blood levels should be drawn after drug has achieved steady-state levels (usually 5 days) and approximately 12 hrs after last dose.
- After patient at therapeutic dosage, continue to monitor blood levels (2 ×/yr or more frequently with medication changes, worsening of Sxs). Baseline ECG should be obtained prior to treatment in the elderly and patients with prior Hx of cardiac illness.
- Common side effects: dry mouth, blurred vision, orthostatic hypotension, sedation, urinary retention, weight gain.
- Serious side effects: heart block, tachyarrhythmias, delirium, seizures.
- Secondary amines (nortriptyline, desipramine) less anticholinergic and more tolerable than parent compounds (amitriptyline, imipramine).
- Increase in TCA levels possible when coadministered with CYP2D6 inhibitors: SSRIs, PIs (especially RTV). RTV documented to increase DMI levels. Monitor closely for increased TCAs ADR.

Other Antidepressants

- Bupropion: 100–450 mg/day; produces relatively fewer sexual side effects and less sedation; agitation, insomnia, headache, tremor, constipation. Seizure risk 4/1000 patients.
- Mirtazapine: 15–60 mg/day; useful for weight gain and useful in chronic pain; side effects: sedation, weight gain, dizziness.
- Nefazodone: 150–600 mg/day in divided doses; rarely used because of concern over liver toxicity; side effects: headache, dry mouth, nausea, sedation, visual trails, hepatic failure 1/300,000 patient-yrs.
- Selegiline: transdermal patch 6 mg–12 mg/24 hrs; tyramine-restricted diet if dose >6 mg/24 hrs to avoid hypertensive crisis.
- Dehydroepiandrosterone (DHEA): may be useful treatment in patients with dysthymia or subsyndromal MDD.

Adjunctive/Augmenting Medications

- Psychostimulants (dextroamphetamine, methylphenidate): useful in select patients with profound fatigue, but, tolerance develops quickly and may cause weight loss and addiction.
- Atypical antipsychotics (olanzapine, risperidone, ziprasidone, quetiapine, aripiprazole): can be used to augment antidepressant Rx in patients with agitation and/or psychotic Sx; monitor glucose and triglycerides regularly because of increased risk of metabolic abnormalities.
- Other agents commonly used for augmenting antidepressants: lithium, triiodothyronine (T3), buspirone, pindolol, adding another antidepressant with different mechanism of action.
- Testosterone replacement may improve mood in hypogonadal men with Sx of depression.

Psychotherapy

- Combination psychotherapy and medication most effective in treating patients with MDD.
- Psychotherapy is mainstay of treatment in patient with dysthymic disorder or adjustment disorder with depressed mood; little evidence that antidepressants are helpful.
- Types of psychotherapy effective in treating MDD: (1) supportive psychotherapy: therapist helps patient identify innate strengths to improve coping; (2) cognitive-behavioral therapy: therapist focuses on changing self-defeating behaviors and patterns of thinking; (3) interpersonal therapy: therapist helps patient resolve interpersonal conflicts contributing to depression.

FOLLOW-UP

- 50%–85% of patients with MDD will have recurrent episode.
- Risk factors for recurrence include prior Hx of depressive episodes, presence of comorbid psychiatric Dx, presence of comorbid chronic medical Dx, persistent dysthymic symptoms.
- 6–12 mos of maintenance treatment recommended postremission; longer if >1 risk factor for recurrence.
- When discontinuing therapy, taper medication to minimize recurrence and medication discontinuation syndrome (documented in short-acting SSRIs and venlafaxine).

DIAGNOSIS

- Patients should be regularly asked about depressive Sxs and suicidal ideation/intent at follow-up visits and, if present, referred to more intensive psychiatric intervention and/or inpatient admission.

OTHER INFORMATION

- Although both MDD and adjustment disorders can occur in context of life stressors, Dx of MDD more likely in patient with personal or family Hx of mood disorders, comorbid substance abuse, psychotic symptoms, or Hx of suicidal ideation or attempts.
- Rates of comorbid substance dependence high. Rx of substance use disorder should occur concurrently with treatment of depression.
- Patients on ART should be cautioned to avoid ingestion of St. John's wort, an OTC herbal antidepressant that has been associated with decreased serum levels of IDV.

SELECTED REFERENCES

Rabkin JG. HIV and depression: 2008 review and update. *Curr HIV/AIDS Rep*, 2008; 5(4): 163–71.

Comments: People with HIV have increased rates of depression, and depression has a negative impact on outcome and increases mortality. Depression is responsive to treatment and this leads to better outcomes. However, there are numerous confounds in the research related to depression, and these are succinctly and well described in this short but comprehensive review.

Pieper AA, Treisman GJ. Drug treatment of depression in HIV-positive patients: safety considerations. *Drug Saf*, 2005; 28(9): 753–62.

Comments: Review article highlighting prevalence of mood disorders in HIV+ patients, diagnostic considerations, and pharmacologic treatments with section on drug-drug interactions.

Psaros C, Geller PA, Aaron E. The importance of identifying and treating depression in HIV infected, pregnant women: a review. *J Psychosom Obstet Gynaecol*, 2009; 30(4): 275–8.

Comments: Women with pregnancy are at increased risk for depression and HIV increases the risk of depression. Depression has been shown to have numerous negative effects on HIV outcomes, particularly adherence. Numerous evidence based interventions treat depression in pregnant women. This paper briefly reviews the essentials of the problem.

Zarrouf FA, Artz S, Griffith J, Sirbu C, Kommor M. Testosterone and depression: systematic review and meta-analysis. *J Psychiatr Pract*, 2009; 15(4): 289–305.

Comments: This is a meta-analysis of seven studies all showing positive results with mood improvement in patients receiving testosterone (total N = 364). Hypogonadal patients had more improvement and study design and caveats are well described. At present, testosterone therapy is under-appreciated.

Cruess DG, Evans DL, Repetto MJ, et al. Prevalence, diagnosis, and pharmacological treatment of mood disorders in HIV disease. *Biol Psychiatry*, 2003; 54: 307–16.

Comments: Review article highlighting prevalence of mood disorders in HIV+ patients, diagnostic considerations, and pharmacologic treatments with section on drug-drug interactions.

Treisman GJ, Angelino AF. *The Psychiatry of AIDS: A Guide to Diagnosis and Treatment.* Baltimore, MD: The Johns Hopkins University Press; 2004.

Comments: Contains chapter on treating depression complicated by other psychiatric and AIDS-related medical conditions.

INSOMNIA

Glenn J. Treisman, MD, PhD, Andrew F. Angelino, MD, and Jeffrey Hsu, MD

CLINICAL

- Defined as persistent difficulty falling asleep, staying asleep, or non-restorative sleep associated with impaired daytime function.
- Can arise from variety of medical and psychiatric disorders as well as certain drugs and medications.
- Chronic insomnia prevalent in 10%–40% of general population; can be present in >70% of HIV+ patients. Chronic, severe insomnia present in 10%–20% of HIV+ patients.
- More common in women than men (1.5:1) and increases with age.
- Psychiatric conditions that can cause insomnia: mood disorders, anxiety disorders, dementia, delirium, and substance use disorders.

- HIV+ patients can have difficulty with daytime sleepiness, difficulty initiating sleep, nocturnal awakenings, and disrupted sleep architecture that worsens with progression of the disease.
- Insomnia more likely in patients with cognitive impairment or AIDS-defining illness.
- EFV has been well-documented to cause insomnia and other sleep disruptions, especially during early weeks of therapy.
- Cessation of chronic use of alcohol or benzodiazepines (BZDs) will produce insomnia.

DIAGNOSIS

- **Primary insomnia:** difficulty initiating or maintaining sleep for >1 mo. Sleep disturbance not related to another primary sleep disorder, psychiatric disorder, medical disorder, or drug effects.
- **Secondary insomnia:** can be attributed to direct effects of a medication, medical disorder, primary sleep disorder (sleep apnea, disturbances in sleep-wake schedule, restless leg syndrome), or psychiatric disorder.

TREATMENT

Sleep Hygiene

- Maintain regular sleep schedule.
- Maintain dark, quiet, comfortable sleeping environment.
- Exercise in morning or late afternoon.
- Use bed for only sleep and sex.
- Establish regular bedtime routine.
- Avoid caffeine, colas, nicotine, and alcohol near bedtime.
- Avoid large meals near bedtime.
- Avoid daytime naps.
- Limit fluid intake near bedtime.

Benzodiazepines (BZDs)

- BZDs well tolerated and produce pleasant sleep but many patients develop rapid tolerance and become dependent on these agents for sleep.
- BZDs specifically marketed as hypnotics include flurazepam, temazepam, triazolam, quazepam, estazolam.
- Usual dosages: triazolam 0.125–0.5 mg qhs; temazepam 7.5–30 mg qhs; flurazepam 15–30 mg qhs.
- BZDs with longer half-lives (flurazepam, quazepam) less likely to cause rebound insomnia but may cause residual daytime drowsiness. Best used in patients who have difficulty maintaining sleep and who experience early morning awakening.
- BZDs with shorter half-lives (triazolam, lorazepam) more likely to cause rebound insomnia over time but less likely to cause daytime drowsiness and sustained cognitive impairment (important in elderly or demented patients). Tolerance develops quickly.
- Use cautiously in patients. with sleep apnea, COPD, or other respiratory difficulties. Risk of respiratory depression increased with concurrent alcohol use.
- Use sparingly, if at all, in patients with history of alcohol/substance addiction.
- Most BZDs metabolized by CYP3A4 so levels can rise when coadministered with CYP3A4 inhibitors (PIs, DLV, EFV). Exceptions are temazepam, lorazepam, and oxazepam (safer agents to use when ART interactions are a concern).
- BZDs can produce a life-threatening withdrawal syndrome when abruptly discontinued.

Selective Benzodiazepine Receptor Agonists (BZRAs)

- Less likely to lead to dependence and abuse than BZDs.
- Less likely to cause rebound insomnia after discontinuation.
- Tolerance is debated but may occur and cause increased use.
- Zolpidem immediate release 5–10 mg qhs; extended release 6.25–12.5 mg qhs. RTV may increase levels.
- Zaleplon 5–20 mg qhs. Levels may increase with PIs and DLV.
- Eszopiclone 1–3 mg qhs. Increased levels may occur with CYP3A4 inhibitors (RTV, NFV).

Melatonin Receptor Agonist

- No evidence of rebound insomnia or withdrawal symptoms.
- No risk of abuse or dependency.
- No motor or cognitive impairment.
- May be used for long-term management of insomnia.

- Ramelteon 8 mg qhs. Avoid taking with high-fat meal. Avoid use in patients taking fluvoxamine or who have hepatic impairment.

Antihistamines
- Most common sedating antihistamines used for insomnia are diphenhydramine (25–50 mg qhs), hydroxyzine (25–50 mg qhs), and doxylamine (25 mg qhs).
- Anticholinergic side effects such as dry mouth, dizziness, blurred vision are common.
- More likely to cause residual daytime sedation.

Sedating Antidepressants
- Trazodone (25–200 mg qhs) most common antidepressant used for treatment of insomnia.
  - Major side effects of trazodone include postural hypotension and rare priapism (1 in 10,000).
  - Plasma concentrations of trazodone may increase when coadministered with CYP3A4 inhibitors (RTV, IDV).
- Other sedating antidepressants include mirtazapine, amitriptyline, nortriptyline, doxepin, and paroxetine. More commonly used when patient has insomnia as Sx of depressive or anxiety disorder.

Atypical Antipsychotics
- Not FDA approved for insomnia.
- Usual dosages (olanzapine 2.5–10 mg qhs, risperidone 0.25–2 mg qhs, quetiapine 25–300 mg qhs).
- Metabolic abnormalities (weight gain, hyperglycemia, hyperlipidemia) may occur so patients need to be closely monitored.
- Less likely to cause memory problems/cognitive impairment so may be especially useful in patients with AIDS dementia.
- Black box warning regarding usage in elderly patients due to increased risk of death.

Other Agents
- Chloral hydrate 500–1000 mg qhs.
- Tiagabine 2–4 mg qhs.

FOLLOW-UP

Short-term Management of Insomnia
- Whenever possible, identify and manage underlying cause of insomnia (depression, other sleep disorder, medications).
- BZDs ideally used for short-term management of insomnia (1–2 wks) and in conjunction with sleep hygiene and other nonpharmacologic approaches (relaxation, cognitive-behavioral therapy).

Long-term Management of Insomnia
- Long-term treatment of chronic primary insomnia best managed with agents less likely to cause dependence and/or tolerance such as sedating antidepressants, atypical antipsychotics, or ramelteon. Zolpidem (XR) and eszopiclone may be less likely than BZDs to cause dependence with long-term use.
- Need for continued usage of sleep agents should be reassessed every 3–6 mos.

SELECTED REFERENCES

Gallego L, Barreiro P, del Río R, et al. Analyzing sleep abnormalities in HIV-infected patients treated with efavirenz. *Clin Infect Dis*, 2004; 38: 430–2.
Comments: EEG monitoring of small series of HIV-infected patients on EFV showed longer sleep latencies and shorter duration of deep sleep compared to HIV-infected patients not on EFV.

Sateia MJ, Pigeon WR. Identification and management of insomnia. *Med Clin North Am*, 2004; 88: 567–96, vii.
Comments: General review article describing assessment and treatment of patients with insomnia.

Goforth HW, Preud'homme X, Krystal AD. Omonuwa TS, The pharmacologic management of insomnia in patients with HIV. *J Clin Sleep Med*, 2009; 5(3): 251–62.
Comments: Thorough review with a clinical orientation that possibly underestimates the problems with BZDs.

Pulmonary

LYMPHOID INTERSTITIAL PNEUMONITIS

Noah Lechtzin, MD, MHS

PATHOGENS
- No confirmed pathogen; may be associated with Epstein-Barr virus (EBV) infection.

CLINICAL
- Diffuse idiopathic interstitial lung disease; key pathologic finding: polyclonal lymphoid cell infiltrate of alveolar septae.
- Occurs in <1% of HIV+ adults but up to 40% HIV+ children.
- Sx: gradual onset dyspnea, cough, and fever.
- May be asymptomatic, especially adults.
- Less common Sx: weight loss, pleuritic pain, arthralgia.
- PE: basilar crackles; children may have adenopathy and clubbing.
- Approximately 2/3 of cases are indolent but 1/3 progress more rapidly.

DIAGNOSIS
- CXR: bilateral, reticulonodular densities and or small nodules.
- High resolution CT: bilateral ground glass infiltrates and nodules (2–4 mm), occasionally cysts.
- In adults, surgical lung biopsy usually necessary for diagnosis.
- Children may be diagnosed empirically if CXR abnormalities persist >2 mos and no evidence of infectious cause (usually by bronchoscopic exclusion).
- Frequently mimics PCP and may be misdiagnosed clinically.

TREATMENT

Initial Therapy
- Children have been treated with prednisone 2 mg/kg once daily × 2–4 wks followed by taper.
- Adults should receive 1 mg/kg once daily of prednisone × 8–12 wks, followed by taper over 6–8 wks to 0.25 mg/kg.

Duration of Therapy
- Data on treatment limited and optimal duration unknown but 6–12 mos common.
- Some patients require life-long low-dose corticosteroids (e.g., prednisone 0.25 mg/kg once daily).

Adjunctive Therapy
- Case reports of children improving with antiviral therapy (ACV 1500 mg/m^2 daily) directed at EBV.
- May improve with institution of ART.

FOLLOW-UP
- Resolves with 6–12 mos of corticosteroid treatment in some, but others may require lifelong low-dose corticosteroid therapy.
- Obtain serial thoracic CT and pulmonary function tests every 2–3 mos to assess initial response to treatment.
- Decrease frequency of follow-up if disease improves or stabilizes.

SELECTED REFERENCES

Dufour V, Wislez M, Bergot E, et al. Improvement of symptomatic human immunodeficiency virus-related lymphoid interstitial pneumonia in patients receiving highly active antiretroviral therapy. *Clin Infect Dis*, 2003; 36: e127–30.
Comments: Case series of 5 patients with LIP who improved clinically after ART initiated (2 NRTIs + 1 PI). Patients improved in average of 3 mos.

Swigris JJ, Berry GJ, Raffin TA, et al. Lymphoid interstitial pneumonia: a narrative review. *Chest*, 2002; 122: 2150–64.
Comments: Thorough review of LIP in both HIV+ and negative patients. Primarily a disease of elderly in HIV-negative patients, and a disease of HIV+ children.

PNEUMOTHORAX

Joel E. Gallant, MD, MPH and Patrick R. Sosnay, MD

CLINICAL

- Pneumothorax (PTX) defined by air in pleural space, either due to entry from outside chest wall or leakage from lung parenchyma.
- In HIV, occurs most often in setting of *Pneumocystis* pneumonia (PCP). Spontaneous PTX in AIDS patient should prompt work up for PCP.
- PCP-associated PTX independently associated with greater mortality.
- Spontaneous PTX in patients with AIDS can also occur with TB, COPD, pulmonary cryptococcosis, and lymphoid interstitial pneumonitis.
- Iatrogenic causes: central venous line placement, thoracentesis, bronchoscopy.
- Presenting Sx: pleuritic chest pain, dyspnea, cough.
- PE: tachycardia, tachypnea, hypoxia, hyperresonance or decreased breath sounds over one lung field. Some patients may not have any signs or Sx beyond those of pneumonia.
- Higher incidence in males, cigarette smokers, patients on AP prophylaxis, patients w/ pneumatoceles on CXR, injection drug users, patients on mechanical ventilation.

DIAGNOSIS

- CXR line or rim of air seen at apex of lung, beyond which there are no lung markings.
- Dx can be difficult in patients w/ preexisting lung disease, lateral decubitus X-rays or CT can increase yield.
- CT can distinguish PTX from bullous lung disease.
- Size of PTX can be estimated based on rim of air. >2 cm correlates with >50% of hemithorax.

TREATMENT

Asymptomatic/Small Pneumothorax

- Small PTX (<1 cm rim) can be observed in asymptomatic patient.
- Any chest pain or dyspnea requires evaluation.
- PTX in setting of PCP has higher morbidity and mortality; requires inpatient management.
- Treatment with 100% oxygen can speed resolution of small PTX without chest tube.

Symptomatic

- Needle or catheter aspiration less likely to succeed in patients with secondary PTX from underlying lung disease.
- Intercostal tube thoracostomy (chest tube) should be performed by a qualified surgeon, emergency medicine physician, or trained critical care physician.
- Bubbling seen in a containment system is sign of continued air leak and tube should be left in place.
- PTX should be followed with serial CXR.
- Tube can be removed when no air leak on water seal and CXR shows no ongoing PTX.

Persistent Bronchopleural Fistula (BPF)

- Steroids for treatment of PCP have been associated w/ longer time to resolution of PTX.
- Heimlich valve can be adapted to chest tube, which allows outpatient management.
- Medical pleurodesis with talc or tetracycline can be performed at bedside through chest tube as nonoperative means of managing a persistent BPF.
- Lowest recurrence rate w/ surgical pleurodesis/pleurodectomy for persistent BPF.

SELECTED REFERENCES

Henry M, Arnold T, Harvey J, et al. BTS guidelines for the management of spontaneous pneumothorax. *Thorax*, 2003; 58 Suppl 2: ii, 39–52.
Comments: Consensus statement reviewing management of spontaneous PTX.

Vricella LA, Trachiotis GD. Heimlich valve in the management of pneumothorax in patients with advanced AIDS. *Chest*, 2001; 120: 15–8.
Comments: Retrospective description of management with a Heimlich valve.

Tumbarello M, Tacconelli E, Pirronti T, et al. Pneumothorax in HIV-infected patients: role of *Pneumocystis carinii* pneumonia and pulmonary tuberculosis. *Eur Respir J*, 1997; 10: 1332–5.
Comments: Retrospective comparison of HIV+ patients w/ PTX compared to HIV+ patients without PTX. Multivariate analysis done to identify risk factors for pneumothorax.

Renal

NEPHROPATHY, HIV-ASSOCIATED

Lisa A. Spacek, MD, PhD and Eric Nuermberger, MD

PATHOGENS
- HIV infection of renal epithelial cells.

CLINICAL
- HIV-associated nephropathy (HAN) is an AIDS-defining illness and the leading cause of chronic kidney disease and ESRD in HIV.
- Vast predominance in patients of West African ancestry. Other risk factors are low CD4, high VL, and family history of renal disease.
- Manifests as late-stage illness (CD4 <200) or during acute HIV infection.
- Injury of glomerular podocytes results in collapse of glomerulus, collapsing form of focal segmental glomerulosclerosis (FSGS).
- Nephrotic-range proteinuria may be massive and predate renal insufficiency.
- Rapid progression to ESRD without treatment.

DIAGNOSIS
- Other than proteinuria, urinalysis typically bland; nephritic profile suggests other Dx.
- Without Bx, DDx includes: primary FSGS, immune complex glomerulonephritis (GN), GN associated with hepatitis B or C, drug-induced interstitial nephritis, amyloidosis, IgA nephropathy, IDV nephrotoxicity, thrombotic microangiopathy, ATN.
- Renal Bx is gold standard for Dx. Other markers (e.g., proteinuria, CD4, VL) nonspecific.
- Urgent renal Bx indicated by significant proteinuria (>1g/24h), increasing proteinuria, decreasing GFR, or unexplained acute or subacute renal failure.
- Renal ultrasound: echogenic kidneys of normal-to-enlarged size.
- Screening: all patients should have urinalysis and estimation of GFR based on serum creatinine at time of HIV Dx. Black patients or those with CD4 <200, VL >4000, DM, HTN, hepatitis B or C, or family Hx of renal disease should be screened annually.
- Screening: proteinuria >1+ on dipstick, spot urine protein/creatine ratio >300 mg/g or GFR <60 mL/min/1.73 m^2 is indication to quantify proteinuria and consider renal ultrasound, referral to nephrologist and renal Bx.

TREATMENT
Approach to Therapy
- Among treatment options, ART most likely to reverse or stabilize renal dysfunction, prevent progression, and improve long-term renal and patient survival. Should also be considered for dialysis-dependent patients.
- BP should be kept <125/75, with preferential use of ACE-I or ARB since they may reverse proteinuria and renal insufficiency and prevent progression to ESRD.
- Corticosteroids adjunct to ART and ACEi/ARB.
- Early referral to nephrologist highly recommended.

Art
- Initiate ART, regardless of CD4.
- Possible NRTIs: ABC, FTC, 3TC.
- Third agent: EFV, RAL, NVP, MVC, PI/r.
- Avoid potentially nephrotoxic drugs: TDF (glomerular and tubular toxicity), ATV and IDV (nephrolithiasis and interstitial nephritis).
- Monitor renal function closely and dose adjust drugs with renal metabolism (FTC, 3TC, TFV, MVC).

Angiotensin-Converting Enzyme Inhibitors (ACEI) and Angiotensin II Receptor Blockers (ARBS)
- Antiproteinuric and reno-protective properties are independent of antihypertensive effect.
- Reduce rate of progression of proteinuria and nephropathy.
- May cause or exacerbate hyperkalemia.

Corticosteroids
- Observational data suggest corticosteroid therapy can rapidly, but transiently, reverse HAN.
- Prednisone 1 mg/kg (up to 80 mg PO q day) for 2 mo, then tapered over 2–4 mos.
- Exclude OIs before initiating corticosteroids and maintain vigilance for new OIs.

FOLLOW-UP
- Monitor serum creatinine and spot urine protein/creatinine ratio.

SELECTED REFERENCES

Papeta N, Sterken R, Kiryluk K, Kalyesubula R, Gharavi AG. The molecular pathogenesis of HIV-1 associated nephropathy: recent advances. *J Mol Med (Berl)*, 2011; 89(5): 429–36.
Comments: The risk of HIVAN is greatest in populations of African ancestry and is attributable to a genetic variation at the APOL1 locus on chromosome 22.

Estrella MM, Fine DM. Screening for chronic kidney disease in HIV-infected patients. *Adv Chronic Kidney Dis*, 2010; 17: 26–35.
Comments: Review of approach to CKD includes risk assessment (age, race, CKD family Hx, CD4, VL, Hx of cocaine or cigarette use, nephrotoxic meds, and comorbidities—DM, HTN, dyslipidemia, HCV) and screening urinalysis for protein-uria and GRF estimation.

Yahaya I, Uthman AO, Uthman MM. Interventions for HIV-associated nephropathy. *Cochrane Database Syst Rev*, 2009; (4): CD007183.
Comments: Database review of Rx in addition to ART for HIVAN. Steroids and ACEI appear to improve the kidney function of patients in observational studies.

Mocroft A, Kirk O, Reiss P, et al. Estimated glomerular filtration rate, chronic kidney disease and antiretroviral drug use in HIV-positive patients. *AIDS*, 2010; 24: 1667–78.
Comments: In cohort study of 6843 HIV+ patients, 225 progressed to CKD with med. follow-up of 3.7 yrs. Increased rate of CKD associated with TDF (IRR, 1.16; 95% CI 1.0 –1.25), IDV (IRR 1.12; 95% CI 1.06–1.18), and ATV (IRR 1.21, 95% CI 1.09–1.34).

Medapalli RK, He JC, Klotman PE. HIV-associated nephropathy: pathogenesis. *Curr Opin Nephrol Hypertens*, 2011; 20(3): 306–11.
Comments: Review of susceptibility alleles: APOL1, HIVAN1, and HIVAN2, that account for increased risk of HIVAN. Also, discusses mechanisms of podocyte dysfunction, tubular cell apoptosis, and function of renal epithelial cells as separate viral compartment.

Gupta SK, Eustace JA, Winston JA, et al. Guidelines for the management of chronic kidney disease in HIV-infected patients: recommendations of the HIV Medicine Association of the Infectious Diseases Society of America. *Clin Infect Dis*, 2005; 40: 1559–85.
Comments: New HIVMA guidelines on management of chronic kidney disease in HIV-infected patients. Most complete recommendations for Dx and treatment of HAN. Also includes sections on ARV dosing in renal failure, ARV nephrotoxicity, and management of ESRD in HIV+ patients.

DIAGNOSIS

SECTION 2
DRUGS

Analgesics

CAPSAICIN

Paul A. Pham, PharmD and John G. Bartlett, MD

INDICATIONS
FDA
- Diabetic peripheral neuropathy.
- Postherpetic neuralgia.
- Arthritis pain (short-term use).

Non-FDA Approved Uses
- HIV-associated neuropathy.
- Psoriasis.
- Intractable pruritus.
- Neuropathic pain related to local nerve injury.
- Nasal application in cluster headaches.

FORMS TABLE

Brand name (mfr)	Forms†	Cost*
Zostrix and Zostrix HP (other names: Trixaicin, capzacin, capsicum) (Rodlen Labs and generic manufacturers)	Topical cream 0.025% and 0.075% (2-oz. tube)	$16.00 and $20.00
Salonpas Pain Patch (Hisamitsu American Inc.)	Topical patch	$0.86

*Prices represent cost per unit specified, are representative of Average Wholesale Price (AWP).
†Dosage is indicated in mg unless otherwise noted.

USUAL ADULT DOSING
- Neuropathic pain: apply thin film (Zostrix 0.075%) 3–5 ×/day to affected area. Wash hand after use and avoid contact with eyes.
- Onset of action 14–28 days; peak effect 4–6 wks.
- Topical stick may be easier to apply than cream or gel.
- Do not wash area for at least 30 mins after application.
- Do not apply to abraded skin.
- Avoid touching mucous membranes after application.

ADVERSE DRUG REACTIONS
Common
- Local irritation (burning, stinging, erythema).

Occasional
- Cough with inhalation.

DRUG INTERACTIONS
- No known drug interactions.

PHARMACOLOGY
Mechanism
- Local application depletes substance P (pain neurotransmitter) from peripheral sensory neurons, then blocks further synthesis and transport of substance P within the neuron. Substance P is a neurotransmitter responsible for communication of pain and pruritic sensations from the periphery to the central nervous system.

Pharmacokinetic Parameters
- **Absorption:** no significant systemic absorption.

Pregnancy Risk
- Not rated.

Breastfeeding Compatibility
• No data.

COMMENTS
• Effective in treatment of diabetic peripheral neuropathy and postherpetic neuralgia. Disappointing results in HIV-associated neuropathy with high dropout rate and no significant difference in pain score or quality of life vs placebo (Paice). May be useful for treatment of postherpetic neuralgia in HIV-infected patients.

SELECTED REFERENCES
Paice JA, Ferrans CE, Lashley FR, et al. Topical capsaicin in the management of HIV-associated peripheral neuropathy. *J Pain Symptom Manage,* 2000; 19: 45–52.
Comments: This small study randomized 26 patients with HIV-associated PN to capsaicin or placebo for 4 wks. No significant difference in pain score was observed during the study period. In addition, the dropout rate was higher for the capsaicin group (67%) than for the vehicle group (18%) (P = 0.014).

GABAPENTIN

Paul A. Pham, PharmD and John G. Bartlett, MD

DRUGS

INDICATIONS
FDA
• Adjunctive therapy for the treatment of partial seizure with or without secondary generalization.
• Postherpetic neuralgia.
Non-FDA Approved Uses
• Peripheral neuropathy.
• Other neuropathic pain syndrome (dysesthetic pain, trigeminal neuralgia).
FORMS TABLE

Brand name (mfr)	Forms†	Cost*
Neurontin and generic (Parke-Davis and generic manufacturers)	Oral cap 100 mg, 300 mg, 400 mg	$0.53/100 mg cap; $1.33/300 mg cap; $1.60/400 mg cap
	Oral tab 600 mg, 800 mg Oral soln 250 mg/5 mL	$2.53/600 mg tab; $3.03/800 mg tab $9.49: 250 mg/5 mL

*Prices represent cost per unit specified, are representative of Average Wholesale Price (AWP).
†Dosage is indicated in mg unless otherwise noted.

USUAL ADULT DOSING
• 300 mg 3 ×/day (initially); titrate over several days to minimize dizziness and sedation.
• Max dose: 2400–3600 mg/day. For postherpetic neuralgia no additional benefit with doses >1800 mg/day.
ADVERSE DRUG REACTIONS
• Generally well tolerated.
Occasional
• Dizziness and ataxia.
• Somnolence.
• Nausea and vomiting.
• Peripheral edema.
• Weight gain.
Rare
• Nystagmus.
• Rash.
• Tremor.

- Slurred speech.
- Blurry vision.

DRUG INTERACTIONS

- Modest decrease in absorption with *Maalox-TC*.
- Morphine may increase gabapentin concentrations (clinical significance unknown).
- Drugs that causes somnolence (i.e., benzodiazepine, opiate, TCAs) may increase somnolence.

PHARMACOLOGY

Mechanism

- Not known.

Pharmacokinetic Parameters

- **Absorption:** 50%–60% with or without food (bioavailability not dose proportional, with decreased absorption with increasing dose).
- **Metabolism and Excretion:** not metabolized; 80% renal excretion.
- **Protein Binding:** <3%.
- **T$_\frac{1}{2}$:** 5–7 hrs.
- **Distribution:** Vd = 58 L.

Pregnancy Risk

- Category C: fetal toxicity observed at high doses in animal studies. No human data.

Breastfeeding Compatibility

- No data, likely to be excreted into breast milk due to low molecular weight.

DOSING

Dosing for Decreased Hepatic Function

- No data; usual dose likely.

Renal Dosing

- Dosing for GFR of 50–80: usual dose: 300 mg 3 ×/day.
- Dosing for GFR of 10–50: 300 mg twice daily.
- Dosing for GFR of <10: 300 mg once daily.
- Dosing in hemodialysis: 300 mg post-HD.
- Dosing in peritoneal dialysis: no data. Dose reduction likely.
- Dosing in CAVH: no data. Dose reduction likely.

COMMENTS

- Alternative to tricyclic antidepressants in management of peripheral neuropathy. Case series and placebo-controlled trial showing decrease in visual analog pain scale.
- Equivalent to amitriptyline in diabetic neuropathy (*Arch Intern Med,* 1999; 159(16): 1931–7).
- Equivalent to carbamezepine for newly diagnosed partial seizure (*Neurology,* 1998; 51(5): 1282–8), but generally recommended as add-on for partial epilepsy (*Epilepsia,* 2004; 45(5): 410–23).
- Value of monitoring gabapentin blood concentrations not established.
- Does not interfere with metabolism of commonly coadministered antiepileptic drugs.
- False positive readings reported with the *Ames N-Multistix SG* dipstick test for urinary protein (use of more specific sulfosalicylic acid precipitation procedure recommended).

SELECTED REFERENCES

Hahn K, Arendt G, Braun JS, et al. A placebo-controlled trial of gabapentin for painful HIV-associated sensory neuropathies. *J Neurol,* 2004; 251: 1260–6.
Comments: This placebo-controlled study found that gabapentin (1200 mg/day) decreased the pain score by 44.1% and improved the median sleep score by 48.9%.

La Spina I, Porazzi D, Maggiolo F, et al. Gabapentin in painful HIV-related neuropathy: a report of 19 patients, preliminary observations. *Eur J Neurol,* 2001; 8: 71–5.
Comments: In this case series, gabapentin provided significant pain relief in patients with HIV-associated painful sensory neuropathy.

LAMOTRIGINE

Paul A. Pham, PharmD and John G. Bartlett, MD

INDICATIONS
FDA
- Adjunct or conversion to monotherapy for partial seizure.
- Generalized seizure of Lennox-Gastaut syndrome.
- Bipolar disorder.

Non-FDA Approved Uses
- Peripheral neuropathy.

FORMS TABLE

Brand name (mfr)	Forms†	Cost*
Lamictal (GlaxoSmithKline) and generic	Oral tab 25 mg, 100 mg, 150 mg, 200 mg	$5.10/25 mg; $6.12/100 mg; $6.70/150 mg; $7.30/200 mg
	Oral chewable tab 2 mg, 5 mg, 25 mg	$4.57/2, 5 mg; $5.56/25 mg

*Prices represent cost per unit specified, are representative of Average Wholesale Price (AWP).
†Dosage is indicated in mg unless otherwise noted.

USUAL ADULT DOSING
- Neuropathy: start with 50 mg/day; titrate by 50–100 mg q1–2wks up to target dose of 300–400 mg/day (escalation over 6 wks recommended to decrease incidence of rash).
- Seizure (as add-on without valproic acid): 50 mg/day wks 1 and 2; 100 mg/day wks 3 and 4 (in 2 divided doses). Usual maintenance dose: 300–500 mg/day. With valproic acide: reduce lamotrigine dose by 50%.
- Seizure (as add-on with valproic acid): 25 mg qod wks 1 and 2; 25 mg once daily wks 3 and 4. Doses may be increased by 25–50 mg/day q1–2 wks. Usual maintenance dose in patients adding lamotrigine to valproic acid alone ranges from 100–200 mg/day.

ADVERSE DRUG REACTIONS
Common
- Rash. Risk of rash may be increased with concomitant valproate.

Occasional
- Dizziness, ataxia, headache, and somnolence.
- Diplopia.
- Nausea and vomiting.

Rare
- Hyponatremia.
- Hematuria.
- Hypersensitivity reactions (including risk of hepatic and renal failure, DIC, and arthritis).
- Stevens-Johnson syndrome and TEN.
- Aseptic meningitis.

DRUG INTERACTIONS
- Glucuronosyl transferase inducers (i.e., RTV, phenytoin, carbamazepine, and phenobarbital) may decrease lamotrigine serum levels.
- Lamotrigine and valproic acid coadministration resulted in a 25% decrease in valproic acid plasma levels and >2-fold increase in lamotrigine serum levels. Lamotrigine must be given at a reduced dosage (no more than $\frac{1}{2}$ the dose used in patients not receiving valproate).
- LPV/r: lamotrigine serum concentration decreased by 50% with LPV/r coadministration. Monitor for therapeutic efficacy; dose may need to be increased.
- Oral contraceptive may decrease lamotrigine serum levels.

DRUGS

PHARMACOLOGY
Mechanism
- Exact mechanism of action not known but it may inhibit release of glutamate, an excitatory neurotransmitter, via inhibition of voltage-sensitive sodium channels.

Pharmacokinetic Parameters
- **Absorption:** 98% with or without food.
- **Metabolism and Excretion:** metabolized by glucuronic acid conjugation with subsequent renal excretion.
- **Protein Binding:** 55%.
- **$T_{\frac{1}{2}}$:** 32 hrs.
- **Distribution:** Vd = 0.9–1.3 L/kg.

Pregnancy Risk
- Category C: exposure in the 1st trimester may increase the risk of infant being born with a cleft lip or cleft palate.

Breastfeeding Compatibility
- Excreted in breast milk. Manufacturer recommends against use when breastfeeding due to limited clinical experience.

DOSING
Dosing for Decreased Hepatic function
- Decrease dose escalation by 50%–75%.

Renal Dosing
- Dosing for GFR of 10–80: usual dose.
- Dosing for GFR of <10: dose may need to be decreased.
- Dosing in hemodialysis: small amount removed during HD. No supplemental dose needed.
- Dosing in peritoneal dialysis: no data.
- Dosing in hemofiltration: no data.

COMMENTS
- Small prospective placebo-controlled trial demonstrated good clinical efficacy in management for HIV-associated neuropathy. (*Neuropathy,* 2000; 54(11): 2037–8). Larger prospective study confirmed findings but only in patients who were receiving neurotoxic ARTs (Simpson).
- Generally reserved as 3rd-line agent (after tricyclics and gabapentin) since rash may limit its use. Should be discontinued at 1st sign of rash (unless rash not drug related).
- Equivalent to carbamezapine and phenytoin for treatment of partial epilepsy (*Epilepsy Res,* 1999; 37(1): 81–7), but generally recommended as add-on or conversion to monotherapy with refractory partial epilepsy (*Epilepsia,* 2004; 45(5): 410–23).
- Value of TDM has not been established.

SELECTED REFERENCES
Simpson DM, McArthur JC, Olney R, et al. Lamotrigine for HIV-associated painful sensory neuropathies: a placebo-controlled trial. *Neurology,* 2003; 60: 1508–14.
Comments: Mean change from baseline pain score not different between lamotrigine and placebo at end of maintenance phase, but slope of change in pain reflected greater improvement with lamotrigine than with placebo in stratum receiving neurotoxic ARTs (P = 0.004).

METHADONE

Paul A. Pham, PharmD

INDICATIONS
FDA
- Opioid abuse detoxification.
- Treatment of severe pain.

FORMS TABLE

Brand name (mfr)	Forms†	Cost*
Dolophine or generic (Xanodyn Pharmaceuticals, Roxane Laboratories, and various other generic manufacturers)	IV soln for injection 10 mg/mL (20 mL)	$0.85
	Oral soln 5 mg/mL, 10 mg/5 mL, 10 mg/mL	$0.10–0.70 per mL
	Oral tablet 5 mg, 10 mg, 40 mg	$0.10–0.50 per tab

*Prices represent cost per unit specified, are representative of Average Wholesale Price (AWP).
†Dosage is indicated in mg unless otherwise noted.

USUAL ADULT DOSING
- Pain management: dose based on pain severity and opiate tolerance. Usual starting dose for opioid-naïve patients is 2.5–10 mg PO q8–12hrs. Titrate to effect.
- Detoxification: starting dose 20–30 mg once daily; titrate to effect. Larger doses >50–100 mg more effective in curbing use of illicit opioids.
- Equivalent parenteral opioid doses: morphine 10 mg, hydromorphone 1.5 mg, methadone 10 mg.

ADVERSE DRUG REACTIONS
Common
- CNS: lightheadedness, dizziness, sedation, confusion, somnolence.
- GI: nausea, vomiting, constipation.

Occasional
- Respiratory depression (dose dependent and exacerbated with alcohol or benzodiazepine coingestion).

Rare
- CV: cardiac arrest, bradycardia, QTc prolongation, arrhythmia, hypotension.

DRUG INTERACTIONS
General Principles
- Methadone has 2 isomers, R-methadone and S-methadone; only R-methadone active. Dose adjustment generally needed only if R-methadone significantly decreased. Some studies fail to determine effect of interacting drug on specific isomers.
- Methadone is substrate of several CYP450 enzymes (2B6 > 2C19 > 3A4); its metabolism can be induced and/or inhibited by ARVs leading to interactions between ART and methadone; may precipitate Sx of oversedation or withdrawal. Enzyme induction generally takes up to 14 days, and methadone has long half-life, so Sx of withdrawal or sedation may be delayed for up to 2–3 wks.
- In order to prevent any potential interruption in ART due to patient discomfort, clinicians should promptly address withdrawal symptoms and individualize patient's methadone dose when clinically indicated.

DRUG-DRUG INTERACTIONS—See Appendix I, p. 566, for table of drug-drug interactions.
PHARMACOLOGY
Pharmacokinetic Parameters
- **Absorption:** up to 85%.
- **Metabolism and Excretion:** metabolized via CYP2B6>2C19>3A4. Excreted by the kidneys, in the bile, feces, and sweat.
- **Protein Binding:** up to 88%.
- **Cmax, Cmin, and AUC:** correlation between levels and therapeutic efficacy has not been established. Trough of 100 ng/mL has been suggested in methadone for methadone maintenance.
- **T$_{\frac{1}{2}}$:** 22 hrs (up to 48 hrs with repeated dosing). Note that analgesic half-life is shorter than serum half-life.
- **Distribution:** widely distributed (Vd = 3.6 L/kg), crosses placental barrier, brain, liver, kidney, muscles, and lungs. This peripheral accumulation maintains drug release over several days to wks after dosing is stopped.

DRUGS

Pregnancy Risk
- Although physical dependence/withdrawal, intrauterine growth retardation, and respiratory depression have been reported with the use of methadone during pregnancy, benefits of methadone use in pregnant women seeking recovery from opioid addiction may outweigh potential fetal risks.

Breastfeeding Compatibility
- Methadone considered compatible with breastfeeding by American Academy of Pediatrics. Doses up to 80 mg daily can be safely given; transferred amounts to infant are minimal.

DOSING

Dosing for Decreased Hepatic Function
- Usual dose. Half-life may be increased. Titrate to effect.

Renal Dosing
- Dosing for GFR of 10–80: usual dose.
- Dosing for GFR of <10: usual dose. Titrate to effect.
- Dosing in hemodialysis: usual dose. Titrate to effect.
- Dosing in peritoneal dialysis: usual dose. Titrate to effect.
- Dosing in hemofiltration: usual dose. Titrate to effect.

COMMENTS
- Directly observed ART as part of methadone maintenance program may increase adherence.
- Methadone metabolism can be increased or decreased by several ARVs and other HIV-related therapies, which could lead to a reduction on therapeutic effect or increased toxicity (see Drug-Drug Interactions in Appendix 1 on p. 566). Upon discontinuation of EFV or NVP, methadone dose may need to be decreased over the next 2 wks.

SELECTED REFERENCES

Palepu A, Horton NJ, Tibbetts N, et al. Uptake and adherence to highly active antiretroviral therapy among HIV-infected people with alcohol and other substance use problems: the impact of substance abuse treatment. *Addiction,* 2004; 99: 361–8.

Comments: Engagement in substance abuse treatment was independently associated with receiving ARV therapy (adjusted OR; 95% CI: 1.70; 1.03–2.83). However, substance abuse treatment not associated with 30-days adherence or VL suppression.

Umbricht A, Hoover DR, Tucker MJ, et al. Opioid detoxification with buprenorphine, clonidine, or methadone in hospitalized heroin-dependent patients with HIV infection. *Drug Alcohol Depend,* 2003; 69: 263–72.

Comments: Methadone, clonidine, and buprenorphine were effective in decreasing observer- and subject-rated opiate withdrawal scores.

NARCOTIC ANALGESICS

Paul A. Pham, PharmD

INDICATIONS

FDA
- Analgesic.
- Antitussive (codeine).
- Antidiarrheal.
- Premedication or adjunct for anesthesia.

Non-FDA Approved Uses
- Migraine headache.

FORMS TABLE

Brand name (mfr)	Forms†	Cost*
Codeine generic (generic manufacturers)	Oral tablet 15 mg, 30 mg, 60 mg Oral liquid 15 mg/mL	$0.43/15 mg; $0.47/30 mg; $0.86/60 mg $2.76 per carpuject

Brand name (mfr)	Forms†	Cost*
Duragesic patch (Janssen Pharmaceuticals); *Actiq* lozenge (Cephalon) (other generic manufacturers)	Topical patch 12 mcg/hg; 25 mcg/h; 50 mcg/h; 75 mcg/h; 100 mcg/h IV ampule 50 mcg/mL	12 mcg/h: $18.21 per patch; 25 mcg/h: $21.98 per patch; 50 mcg/h: $40.19 per patch; 75 mcg/h: $61.90 per patch; 100 mcg/h: $81.36 per patch $0.41 per 5 mL
Hydrocodone/ acetaminophen (APAP) generics (generic manufacturers)	Oral tablet 5 mg; 7.5 mg; 10 mg (all with 325 mg APAP) Oral liquid (7.5 mg hydrocodone + 325 mg APAP)/15 mL; (10 mg hydrocodone + 325 mg APAP)/15 mL	5/325 mg: $0.54 per tablet; 7.5/325 mg: $0.69 per tablet; 10/325 mg: $0.62 per tablet 7.5/325 mg: $58.12 per 16 oz; 10/325 mg: $149.99 per 16 oz
Dilaudid (Purdue Pharmeceutical and generic manufacturers)	Oral tablet 2 mg; 4 mg; 8 mg IV ampule 1 mg/mL; 2 mg/mL; 4 mg/mL; 10 mg/mL Rectal suppository 3 mg	2 mg: $.0.37 per tab; 4 mg: $0.61 per tab; 8 mg: $1.32 per tab 1 mg/mL: $1.16 per amp; 2 mg/mL: $1.23 per amp; 4 mg/mL: $1.66 per amp; 10 mg/mL: $3.18 per amp $5.38 per suppository
Demerol and generics (generic manufacturers)	Oral tablet 50 mg; 100 mg IV ampule 25 mg/0.5 mL; 50 mg/mL; 100 mg/mL Oral liquid 50 mg/5mL (sold as 500 mL)	50 mg: $0.68 per tablet; 100 mg: $1.30 per tablet 25 mg/0.5 mL: $0.66 per amp; 50 mg/mL: $1.15 per amp; 100 mg/mL: $0.99 per amp 50 mg/5 mL: $0.94 per 5 mL
MS Contin (sustained release) and morphine generics (Purdue Frederick and generic manufacturers)	IV vial 5 mg/mL; 10 mg/mL; 15 mg/mL; 25 mg/mL; 50 mg/mL Oral immediate-release tablet 15 mg; 30 mg Oral sustained-release tablet 15 mg; 30 mg; 60 mg; 100 mg; 200 mg Rectal suppository 10 mg; 20 mg; 30 mg Oral liquid 2 mg/mL; 4 mg/mL; 20 mg/mL	5 mg/mL: $0.78 per 1-mL vial; 10 mg/mL: $0.79 per 1-mL vial; 15 mg/mL: $6.25 per 20-mL vial; 25 mg/mL: $6.04 per 10-mL vial; 50 mg/mL: $23.08 per 50 mL vial 15 mg: $0.18 per tablet; 30 mg: $0.31 per tablet 15 mg: $0.75 per tablet; 30 mg: $1.43 per tablet; 60 mg: $2.79 per tablet; 100 mg: $4.12 per tablet; 200 mg: $7.49 per tablet 10 mg: $4.79 per suppository; 20 mg: $5.83 per suppository; 30 mg: $7.34 per suppository 2 mg/mL: $38.56 per 500 mL; 4 mg/mL: $65.03 per 500 mL; 20 mg/mL: $116.78 per 240 mL

DRUGS

(Continued)

FORMS TABLE (CONT.)

Brand name (mfr)	Forms†	Cost*
Oxycodone; OxyContin (sustained-release) (Purdue Pharmaceuticals and generic manufacturers)	Oral tablet 5 mg; 15 mg; 30 mg	5 mg: $0.48 per tablet; 15 mg: $0.74 per tablet; 30 mg: $1.42 per tablet
	Oral sustained-release tablet 10 mg; 15 mg; 20 mg; 30 mg; 40 mg; 60 mg; 80 mg	$2.01/10 mg; $3.01/15 mg; $3.46/20 mg; $5.44/30 mg; $6.14/40 mg; $9.93/60 mg; $11.55/80 mg
	Oral liquid 1 mg/mL; 20 mg/mL	1 mg/mL: $25.20 per 500 mL; 20 mg/mL: $34.42 for 30 mL
Darvocet (Xanodyne Pharmaceuticals) and generics	Oral tablet 50/325 mg; 100/500 mg; 100/650 mg	50/325 mg: $0.74 per tablet; 100/500 mg: $1.50 per tablet; 100/650 mg: $1.15 per tablet
Methadone (generic manufacturers)	Oral liquid 1 mg/mL; 2 mg/mL; 10 mg/mL	1 mg/mL: $39.88 per 500 mL; 2 mg/mL: $69.07 per 500 mL; 10 mg/mL: $79.87 per 946 mL
	Oral tablet 5 mg; 10 mg; 40 mg	5 mg: $0.08 per tab; 10 mg: $0.15 per tab; 40 mg: $0.33 per tab

*Prices represent cost per unit specified, are representative of Average Wholesale Price (AWP).
†Dosage is indicated in mg unless otherwise noted.

USUAL ADULT DOSING

- Dose must be individualized based on pain severity and opiate tolerance. Initiation of therapy involves titrating dose of an immediate release drug upward to effect (q4–6h), with close monitoring for side effects. Amount of drug used in 24-hr period is then converted to a sustained release form and administered twice daily (*MS Contin, OxyContin*) or fentanyl patch q3 days. Rescue doses of immediate release preparations should be provided.
- Considerable interpatient variability; therefore, important to closely monitor and titrate to effect.
- The following are starting doses of commonly used opiates:
  - Codeine 30–60 mg PO q4–6h.
  - Fentanyl patch 25 mcg/h (see Table 2-1 for morphine equivalent); maintain patch at 48–72 hr intervals. Transdermal fentanyl should be applied to nonirritated and nonirradiated skin on a flat surface of the upper torso. Hair at the application site should be clipped, not shaved.
  - Hydrocodone 5–10 mg PO q4–6h.
  - Hydromorphone 2–4 mg PO q4–6h.
  - Meperidine 50 mg PO q4–6h.
  - Morphine sulfate 20–60 mg PO q4–6h.
  - Oxycodone 5 mg PO q4–6h.
  - Methadone 10 mg PO q8h.
- When switching opioid analgesics, dosage should be converted with consideration to the incomplete cross-tolerance, equianalgesic dose, clinical information, and patient safety. Experts recommend a 30% decrease in the predicted equianalgesic dose (see Table 2-2).

TABLE 2-1. MORPHINE CONVERSION

Oral Morphine per 24 h (mg/day)	Fentanyl Patch Dose (mcg/h)
45–134	25
135–224	50

Oral Morphine per 24 h (mg/day)	Fentanyl Patch Dose (mcg/h)
225–314	75
315–404	100
405–494	125
495–584	150
585–674	175
675–764	200
765–854	225
865–944	250
945–1034	275
1035–1124	300

Note: All opiates should be converted to oral morphine equivalent. The recommended fentanyl patch dose is based on oral morphine requirement for the last 24 hours. Fentanyl is generally not recommended with PIs or DLV. With coadministration, significant fentanyl dose reduction should be considered.

TABLE 2-2. OPIATES EQUIVALENCY TABLE

Generic Name	Equianalgesic Dose (mg)	
	Parenteral	**Oral**
Codeine	120	200
Fentanyl	0.1	N/A
Hydrocodone	N/A	20
Hydromorphone	1.5	6–7.5
Meperidine	75–100	300
Morphine	10	30–40
Oxycodone	N/A	15–30

Note: Equianalgesic dose may differ in opioid-experienced patients and with chronic dosing. For this reason, when switching opioid analgesics, dosage should be converted with consideration of incomplete cross-tolerance; in other words, use 30% less than equianalgesic dose.

ADVERSE DRUG REACTIONS

Common
- CNS: sedation, dizziness, confusion, and disorientation.
- Miosis.
- GI: nausea, vomiting, constipation.
- Euphoria, dysphoria, and hallucinations.

Occasional
- Hypotension, peripheral circulatory collapse, dysrhythmias, cardiac arrest.
- Respiratory depression, bronchoconstriction.
- Increased biliary tract pressure. Incidence may be slightly lower with meperidine but unlikely to be clinically significant.
- Pruritis.
- Flushing, tachycardia, hypotension, and bronchospasm (secondary to histamine release).
- Ileus.

DRUGS

- Physical and psychological dependence.
- Local erythema and pruritis with fentanyl patch.

Rare

- Rash.
- Myoclonus and hyperalgesia (associated with high-dose opiod).
- Seizures (associated with meperidine in patients with renal failure).

DRUG INTERACTIONS

- Antihypertensive agents (beta-blockers and calcium channel blockers): case report of severe hypotension with opiate coadministration. Use with caution with close monitoring of BP.
- CNS depressant (ethanol, barbiturates, benzodiazepines, etc.): additive CNS sedation with coadministration. Use with caution.
- EFV, NVP, and ETR may decrease fentanyl and meperidine serum concentrations. Titrate opiates to effect.
- EFV decreases buprenorphine AUC by 50%, but no withdrawal Sx observed. Use standard doses.
- Rifampin decreases morphine AUC by 27%. Rifamycins and other CY3A4 inducers may also significantly decrease serum level of all opiates. Titrate opiates to effect.
- RTV decreases fentanyl clearance by 67%. All PIs, DLV, and other CYP3A4 inhibitors (macrolides, azoles, etc.) may significantly increase fentanyl serum concentrations. Avoid coadministration.
- RTV decreases meperidine AUC by 67% and increases normeperidine AUC by 47%. Avoid coadministration. Other PIs may increase meperidine serum concentration. All PIs, DLV, and other CYP3A4 inhibitors (macrolides, azoles, etc.) may increase meperidine serum concentrations.
- RTV and LPV/r may increase serum level of codeine, hydrocodone, and oxycodone. Use low dose of opiates with close monitoring. Consider using morphine or hydromorphone. Interaction with other PIs and NNRTIs unlikely.
- RTV (200 mg/day) and ATV/r increases buprenorphine AUC by approximately 56% and 100%, respectively. Monitor for sedation with coadministration.

PHARMACOLOGY

Mechanism

- Mu-receptor agonist; mu-receptors are distributed in the brain, spinal cord, and other tissues. Mu-agonists appear to prevent the release of beta-endorphin, possibly by altering patient's perceived level of pain.

Pharmacokinetic Parameters

- **Absorption:** oral absorption: codeine: well absorbed; fentanyl: absorption temperature dependent. Febrile patients may have increased absorption of fentanyl by ~1/3. Hydromorphone: 62%; meperidine: 57% (from IM site); morphine: 20%–40% (with high variation); oxycodone: 60%–87%; propoxyphene: low bioavailability due to high 1st-pass metabolism.
- **Metabolism and Excretion:** codeine: metabolised via CYP2D6 to morphine; fentanyl: metabolised via CYP3A4 to inactive metabolite then excreted primarily via biliary route; hydrocodone: metabolised via CYP2D6 to hydromorphone; hydromorphone: glucuronidation to inactive metabolite; meperidine: metabolised via CYP2D6 and CYP1A2 to active normeperidine metabolite then excreted in the urine; morphine: glucuronidation to active metabolite then excreted in the urine; oxycodone: metabolised via CYP2D6 then excreted in the urine; propoxyphene metabolized to norpropoxyphene that is excreted in the urine.
- **Protein Binding:** codeine: not protein bound; fentanyl: 86%; meperidine: 65%–80%; morphine: 2%–36%; oxycodone: 45%; propoxyphene: 78%.
- **Cmax, Cmin, and AUC:** Cmax associated with pain relief: codeine: 0.03–0.25 mcg/mL; fentanyl: 0.2–1.2 ng/mL; hydromorphone: 4 ng/mL; meperidine: 0.7 mcg/mL; morphine: 200–300 ng/mL hr (AUC); oxycodone: 15–30 ng/mL; propoxyphene: highly variable.

- $T_{\frac{1}{2}}$: codeine: 3–4 hrs; fentanyl: 1.5–6 hrs; hydrocodone: 3.3–4.4 hrs; hydromorphone: 2–4 hrs; meperidine: 2–7 hrs (active normeperidine metabolite: 15–30 hrs); morphine: 2–4 hrs; oxycodone: 3–4 hrs; propoxyphene: 3.5–15 hrs.
- **Distribution:** widely distributed. Codeine: 2.6 L/kg; fentanyl: 3–6 L/kg; hydromorphone: 1.22 L/kg; meperidine: 3–5 L/kg; morphine: 1–4 L/kg; oxycodone: 2.6 L/kg; oropoxyphene: widely distributed.

Pregnancy Risk
- Category C or Category D if used for prolonged periods or in high doses at term.

Breastfeeding Compatibility
- Excreted in breast milk but concentrations are very low and not likely to affect the infant.

Dosing

Dosing for Decreased Hepatic Function
- Use with close monitoring.

Renal Dosing
- Dosing for GFR of 50–80: usual dose.
- Dosing for GFR of 10–50: morphine, codeine, hydromorphone or oxycodone: use with close monitoring. Fentanyl appears to be safe (usual dose). Hydrocodone, meperidine, and propoxyphenes: no data; use with close monitoring.
- Dosing for GFR of <10: avoid meperidine. Morphine PK not affected but its active metabolite (morphine 6-glucuronide) can accumulate and cause prolonged sedation (avoid). Norpropoxyphene (propoxyphene metabolite) can accumulate (avoid). Codeine and metabolite can accumulate (avoid). Fentanyl appears to be safe (usual dose). Hydrocodone, hydromorphone, and oxycodone: No data; use with caution.
- Dosing in hemodialysis: avoid morphine, codeine. No data for oxycodone. Fentanyl not removed in HD; therefore, no dose adjustment needed (*J Pain Symptom Manage,* 2004; 28(5): 497–504.). Hydrocodone, hydromorphone, and oxycodone: no data.
- Dosing in peritoneal dialysis: no data.
- Dosing in hemofiltration: no data.

Comments
- In methadone-maintained patients, use short-acting narcotics administered at higher doses as often as necessary to relieve pain in addition to maintaining patient on methadone.
- For acute pain, fentanyl and hydromorphone may have a quicker onset of action compared to morphine, but may be associated with higher addiction potential.
- Analgesics given on a fixed dose scheduled around the clock (and not on PRN basis) allows for more consistent pain relief and requires less medication overall.
- If side effects prevent dose escalation or there is a lack of analgesic effect despite dose escalation, another opioid should be tried. Incomplete cross-tolerance between opioids may account for apparent decrease in required dose and side effects when changing switching to an alternative opiate.
- Morphine or hydromorphone are preferred in patients on a PI- and NNRTI-containing ART regimens.

Selected References
Krakowski I, Theobald S, Balp L, et al. [Standards, options and recommendations for the use of medical analgesics for the treatment of pain arising from excess nociception in adults with cancer (update 2002)]. *Bull Cancer,* 2002; 89: 1067–74.

Comments: WHO guidelines on the use of analgesics for the treatment of pain in adults with CA.

Scimeca MM, Savage SR, Portenoy R, et al. Treatment of pain in methadone-maintained patients. *Mt Sinai J Med,* 2000; 67: 412–22.

Comments: Review on management of pain in methadone-maintained patients.

DRUGS

Androgens, Anabolic Steroids, and Drugs for Wasting

DRONABINOL

Paul A. Pham, PharmD and John G. Bartlett, MD

INDICATIONS
FDA
- AIDS-associated anorexia.
- Chemotherapy-induced nausea in patients who failed conventional antiemetic treatments.

FORMS TABLE

Brand name (mfr)	Forms†	Cost*
Marinol (Unimed Pharmaceutical)	Oral caps 2.5 mg; 5 mg; 10 mg	2.5 mg $5.89/cap; 5 mg $12.46/cap; 10 mg $27.07/cap

*Prices represent cost per unit specified, are representative of Average Wholesale Price (AWP).
†Dosage is indicated in mg unless otherwise noted.

USUAL ADULT DOSING
- Anorexia-associated with wasting: 2.5 mg PO twice daily (max 10 mg twice daily).
- Nausea and vomiting: 10 mg twice daily.

ADVERSE DRUG REACTIONS
Occasional
- CNS: "high" with euphoria, paranoia, somnolence, depersonalization, confusion seen in 3%–10% of patients (usually resolves in 1–3 days with continued use. If symptoms are severe or persist, reduce dose to 2.5 mg once daily). Warn patients not to drive, operate machinery, or engage in hazardous activity until established that they are able to tolerate dronabinol and perform these activities safely.
- Doses of 10–20 mg/day are generally well tolerated, but doses >30 mg/day can significantly affect cognitive function.

Rare
- Visual difficulties.
- GI intolerance.
- Central sympathomimetic effects: dizziness, hypotension, tachycardia, vasodilation. Used with caution in patients with cardiac disorders.

DRUG INTERACTIONS
- No significant interaction with IDV and NFV.
- Sympathomimetic agents (cocaine and amphetamines): increased risk of hypertension and tachycardia.
- Anticholinergic drugs (i.e., TCA): increased drowsiness and tachycardia.
- CNS depressant: additive CNS depression.
- EFV: may increase risk of CNS side effect during the 1st 2 wks.
- Pharmacokinetic drug interaction with PIs, NNRTIs, MVC, and RAL unlikely.
- Theophylline: may increase theophylline metabolism with smoking of marijuana.

PHARMACOLOGY
Mechanism
- Synthetic delta-9-tetrahydrocannabinol (delta-9-THC), the active ingredient in marijuana. Exact pharmacologic mechanism of action unknown.

Pharmacokinetic Parameters
- **Absorption:** 90%–95% absorbed. Only 10%–20% of administered dose reach systemic circulation due to high 1st-pass metabolism and lipid solubility.

- **Metabolism and Excretion:** 1st-pass hepatic metabolism and biliary excretion; 10%–15% renal excretion.
- **Protein Binding:** 90%–95%.
- **T$_\frac{1}{2}$:** 2536 hrs.
- **Distribution:** Vd = 10 L/kg; highly distributed into fat; slowly released back into the systemic circulation.

Pregnancy Risk
- Category C: not teratogenic in animal studies. Observational studies suggest that fetal growth may be impaired.

Breastfeeding Compatibility
- Because of its lipophilicity, dronabinol highly concentrated in breastmilk and not recommended for nursing mothers.

DOSING
Dosing for Decreased Hepatic Function
- Usual dose (consider dose reduction in patients with cirrhosis).

Renal Dosing
- No dose adjustment for renal impairment.
- Dosing in hemodialysis: no data; usual dose likely.
- Dosing in peritoneal dialysis: no data; usual dose likely.
- Dosing in hemofiltration: no data.

COMMENTS
- Used for anorexia in patients with wasting syndrome, though not routinely recommended since it leads to only modest weight gain due primarily to increased fat (*J Pain Sympt Man*, 1997; 14:7).
- Higher doses (10 mg twice daily) generally needed to control nausea that has not responded to other antiemetics. Use with caution in patients with schizophrenia, depression, and mania (close psychiatric monitoring recommended) or h/o substance abuse (more prone to abuse).

SELECTED REFERENCES
Struwe M, Kaempfer SH, Geiger CJ, et al. Effect of dronabinol on nutritional status in HIV infection. *Ann Pharmacother*, 1993; 27: 827–31.
Comments: Small double-blind, randomized, placebo-controlled trial that evaluated dronabinol 5 mg twice daily. Trend towards increased in body weight (limited to fat weight).

GROWTH HORMONE, HUMAN

Paul A. Pham, PharmD and John G. Bartlett, MD

INDICATIONS
FDA
- Treatment of HIV-associated wasting or cachexia and failure to thrive.

Non-FDA Approved Uses
- Treatment of HIV-associated fat accumulation (see Lipodystrophy, p. 11).

FORMS TABLE

Brand name (mfr)	Forms†	Cost*
Serostim (Serono Laboratories)	SC vial 4 mg	$221.90 per 4-mg vial
*Prices represent cost per unit specified, are representative of Average Wholesale Price (AWP). †Dosage is indicated in mg unless otherwise noted.		

USUAL ADULT DOSING
- For wasting or cachexia: body weight <35 kg: 0.1 mg/kg SQ at bedtime; 35–45 kg: 4 mg SQ at bedtime; 45–55 kg: 5 mg SQ at bedtime; >55 kg: 6 mg SQ at bedtime.

DRUGS

- Fat accumulation: 3–6 mg once daily to once qod. Optimal dose/dosing schedule unclear (max: 0.1 mg/kg/day or 6 mg/day).
- Use immediately after reconstitution with sterile water; discard unused portion.

ADVERSE DRUG REACTIONS
- ADRs dose-dependent and can be reduced with reduction in dose or number of doses/wk.

Common
- Musculoskeletal discomfort (20%–50%) and increased tissue turgor with swelling of hands and feet (25%). Both usually subside with continued treatment.

Occasional
- Fluid retention and sodium retention with peripheral edema.
- Hypertension.
- Exacerbation of lipoatrophy.
- Insulin resistance/hyperglycemia; exacerbation of diabetes.

Rare
- Flu-like symptoms.
- Rigors.
- Back pain.
- Malaise.
- Carpal tunnel syndrome; d/c if Sx do not resolve with dose reduction.
- Chest pain.
- Nausea.
- Diarrhea.

DRUG INTERACTIONS
- Barbiturates: may prolong elimination half-life of amobarbital.
- Mephenytoin: may increase mephenytoin serum levels.

PHARMACOLOGY
Mechanism
- Produces multiple anabolic and anticatabolic effects.

Pharmacokinetic Parameters
- **Absorption:** bioavailability 70%–90% after SQ injection.
- **Metabolism and Excretion:** cleaved primarily in renal cells to peptides and amino acids; also metabolized in the liver.
- **Cmax, Cmin, and AUC:** AUC = 19.6–40.1 mcg × L/day.
- **T$_{\frac{1}{2}}$:** 3.9–4.3 hrs.
- **Distribution:** Vd = 12 L.

Pregnancy Risk
- Category C: limited data suggest that growth hormone does not transfer across the placenta to fetus.

Breastfeeding Compatibility
- Breastfeeding risk unknown.

DOSING
Renal Dosing
- Dosing for GFR of 50–80: usual dose.
- Dosing for GFR of 10–50: decreased clearance but clinical significance unknown.
- Dosing for GFR of <10: decreased clearance but clinical significance unknown.
- Dosing in hemodialysis, peritoneal dialysis, and hemofiltration: no data.

COMMENTS
- Effective for management of HIV-associated wasting and fat accumulation.
- Benefits include lean body mass, increased body weight, and body fitness.
- Dx and treat conditions associated with weight loss (inadequate nutritional intake, depression, hyperthyroidism, malabsorption, and hypogonadism) before initiating.
- High cost ($21,500 for 12-wk course) limits routine use. Lower maintenance dose and/or treatment only during acute infection can decrease cost.
- Testosterone and/or anabolic steroids are cheaper and better tolerated alternatives for wasting.
- Fat accumulation typically recurs after HGH discontinued.

- Contraindicated in patients with active neoplasia, acute critical illness due to complications following open heart or abdominal surgery, multiple accidental trauma, or acute respiratory failure.
- Growth hormone may play a role in preventing or attenuating rapid weight loss that often occur with acute infections (*Clin Infect Dis,* 2003;36:S69).
- Tesamorelin decreases abdominal fat by a modest 14–18% in HIV pts with lipodystrophy without affecting glucose levels.

SELECTED REFERENCES

Kotler DP, Muurahainen N, Grunfeld C, et al. Effects of growth hormone on abnormal visceral adipose tissue accumulation and dyslipidemia in HIV-infected patients. *J Acquir Immune Defic Syndr,* 2004; 35: 239–52.

Comments: Effects of GH on visceral adipose tissue (VAT) accumulation evaluated in double-blind placebo control trial. From baseline to wk 12, VAT decreased significantly compared with placebo in patients who received GH (4 mg once daily) (–8.6%, P <0.001). Reaccumulation of visceral fat occurred after therapy stopped. Hyperglycemia and high price ($1100–1700/wk) are disadvantages.

Schambelan M, Mulligan K, Grunfeld C, et al. Recombinant human growth hormone in patients with HIV-associated wasting. A randomized, placebo-controlled trial. Serostim Study Group. *Ann Intern Med,* 1996; 125: 873–82.

Comments: Randomized, double-blind, placebo-controlled trial to evaluate HGH in HIV-associated wasting. 178 HIV+ patients with documented weight loss >10% randomized to receive HGH 0.1 mg/kg (6 mg/day) or placebo. HGH resulted in a sustained and statistically significant increase in weight (mean increase ± SD, 1.6 ± 3.7 kg [P <0.001]) and lean body mass (3.0 ± 3.0 kg [P <0.001]), accompanied by decrease in body fat (–1.7 ± 1.7 kg [P <0.001]).

DRUGS

MEGESTROL ACETATE

Paul A. Pham, PharmD and John G. Bartlett, MD

INDICATIONS
FDA
- Appetite stimulant for the treatment of cachexia in patients with HIV or neoplastic disease.

FORMS TABLE

Brand name (mfr)	Forms†	Cost*
Megace ES (Par Pharmaceuticals)	Oral liquid 625 mg/5 mL	$131.28/5 oz
Megestrol acetate (Teva Pharmaceuticals)	Oral tab 20 mg, 40 mg Oral liquid 40 mg/mL	$0.67–1.06/tab $17.99: 400 mg/10 mL

*Prices represent cost per unit specified, are representative of Average Wholesale Price (AWP).
†Dosage is indicated in mg unless otherwise noted.

USUAL ADULT DOSING
- Cachexia: 400–800 mg suspension PO once daily w/ food or *Megace ES* 625 mg PO once daily with or without food.
- *Megace* 800 mg/20 mL = *Megace ES* 625 mg/5 mL.

ADVERSE DRUG REACTIONS
Occasional
- Hypogonadism with prolonged therapy (which may exacerbate wasting).
- Hyperglycemia, including new onset DM.
- Impotence.
- Rash.
- Flatulence.
- Asthenia.
- Diarrhea, nausea, and vomiting.

Rare
- Adrenal insufficiency.
- Carpal tunnel syndrome, thrombosis, edema, vaginal bleeding, and alopecia.
- Hyperpnea, chest pressure, mild increase in blood pressure, dyspnea, and heart failure (with 480–1600 mg/day).
- Osteonecrosis.
- Deep venous thrombosis.
- Cushing's syndrome.

DRUG INTERACTIONS
- Not a substrate, inhibitor, or inducer of CYP3A4, therefore interaction with PIs and NNRTIs unlikely.
- Unboosted IDV: IDV AUC decreased by 28%. Clinical significance unknown. Take IDV on an empty stomach or boost IDV with RTV (IDV/RTV 800/100 mg twice daily).

PHARMACOLOGY

Mechanism
- Inhibits pituitary gonadotropin release.

Pharmacokinetic Parameters
- **Absorption:** absorption >90%.
- **Metabolism and Excretion:** excreted in urine and feces.
- **Cmax, Cmin, and AUC:** 800 mg at steady state. Mean Cmax = 753 ($\pm$ 529) ng/mL. Mean AUC 10,476 ($\pm$ 7788) ng hr per mL.
- $T_{\frac{1}{2}}$: 30 hrs.

Pregnancy Risk
- Category X: contraindicated.

Breastfeeding Compatibility
- Contraindicated.

DOSING

Dosing for Decreased Hepatic Function
- No data.

Renal Dosing
- Dosing for GFR of 50–80: usual dose.
- Dosing for GFR of >50: no data.
- Dosing in hemodialysis, peritoneal dialysis, and CAVH: no data.

COMMENTS
- Weight gain mostly due to fat. May be considered for short-term management of weight loss. Long-term complications: hyperglycemia, adrenal insufficiency, and male hypogonadism, which may further exacerbate weight loss.

SELECTED REFERENCES

Mulligan K, Zackin R, Von Roenn JH, et al. Testosterone supplementation of megestrol therapy does not enhance lean tissue accrual in men with human immunodeficiency virus-associated weight loss: a randomized, double-blind, placebo-controlled, multicenter trial. *J Clin Endocrinol Metab*, 2007; 92: 563–70.

Comments: This randomized, double-blind, placebo-controlled trial evaluated the effect on lean muscle mass gain when testosterone was added to megestrol acetate. Megestrol with or without testosterone resulted in robust increases in weight (median 5.3 and 7.3 kg in megestrol/testosterone and megestrol/placebo, respectively); however lean body mass (3.3 and 3.3 kg) and fat weight (3.0 and 3.8 kg) did not differ significantly. As expected, the trough testosterone concentrations decreased to a greater extent in patients who were not on testosterone.

Batterham MJ, Garsia RA. Comparison of megestrol acetate, nandrolone decanoate and dietary counselling for HIV associated weight loss. *Int J Androl*, 2001; 24: 232–40.

Comments: Small randomized, prospective study comparing nandrolone decanoate, megestrol acetate, or dietary counseling for managing HIV-associated wasting. Percentage of body fat mass increased significantly only in those receiving megestrol (7.77 $\pm$ 4.85%, P = 0.049). Change in weight and percentage body fat mass significantly greater in those receiving megestrol. Long-term complications of megestrol include: hypogonadism in men, hyperglycemia, and adrenal insufficiency.

Mann M, Koller E, Murgo A, et al. Glucocorticoid like activity of megestrol. A summary of Food and Drug Administration experience and a review of the literature. *Arch Intern Med*, 1997; 157: 1651–6.

Comments: FDA reports describe 5 cases of Cushing's syndrome, 12 cases of new-onset diabetes, and 16 cases of adrenal insufficiency identified in association with megestrol therapy.

NANDROLONE

Paul A. Pham, PharmD and John G. Bartlett, MD

INDICATIONS

FDA

• Anemia associated with renal insufficiency (erythropoietin preferred).

Non-FDA Approved Uses

• HIV-associated wasting.

FORMS TABLE

Brand name (mfr)	Forms†	Cost*
Nandrolone (Watson Laboratories)	IM vial 100 mg/mL (2-mL vial); 200 mg/mL (1-mL vial)	$12.25

*Prices represent cost per unit specified, are representative of Average Wholesale Price (AWP).
†Dosage is indicated in mg unless otherwise noted.

USUAL ADULT DOSING

• Wasting (men): 100–200 mg IM q1–2 wk. Consider lower doses or use of other anabolic agents (e.g., oxandrolone) in women: 100 mg IM q2 wk (*Arch Intern Med,* 2005;165(5):578-85). Optimal duration unknown and long-term trials are lacking. Recommend reassessment after 3 mos of use.
• Most recommend use with resistance training for treatment of wasting.
• Anemia: 100–200 mg IM qwk (erythropoietin preferred).

ADVERSE DRUG REACTIONS

Common

• Injection site pain.

Occasional

• Oily skin, hirsutism, and acne, especially in women.
• Priapism.
• Transaminase and alkaline phosphatase elevation.
• Gynecomastia.

Rare

• Irritability/aggression/mood changes (generally seen with higher doses).
• Liver abnormalities, including hepatic necrosis, peliosis hepatitis, hepatocellular carcinoma.

DRUG INTERACTIONS

• Buproprion: may lower seizure threshold with coadministration.
• Warfarin: steroids may cause suppression of clotting factors II, V, VII, and X, and an increase of PT potentiating anticoagulation.

PHARMACOLOGY

Mechanism

• Androgenic-anabolic steroid. Separation of anabolic from androgenic effects is relative, and all anabolic steroids can induce masculinizing effects if sufficient doses are given for prolonged periods.

Pharmacokinetic Parameters

• **Absorption:** IM bioavailability 77%.
• **Metabolism and Excretion:** metabolized in the liver via reduction and oxidation; unchanged nandrolone and its metabolites are excreted in urine.
• $T_{\frac{1}{2}}$: 6–8 days.

Pregnancy Risk

• Category X: contraindicated.

Breastfeeding Compatibility

• Not recommended.

DOSING

Dosing for Decreased Hepatic Function

• No data; use with caution.

DRUGS

Renal Dosing
- Dosing for GFR of 50–80: usual dose.
- Dosing for GFR of <50: no data; usual dose likely.
- Dosing in hemodialysis, peritoneal dialysis, and hemofiltration: no data.

COMMENTS
- Currently not available in US, but generic forms may be available in the future. Nandrolone + progressive resistance training effective in HIV-associated wasting. At lower doses (100 mg q2 wks), nandrolone is preferred over testosterone in women. Advantage of anabolic vs androgenic effect lost at higher doses. Alternatives include oral anabolics (oxandrolone) but much more expensive compared to IM nandrolone.
- Men with HIV-associated wasting should be evaluated for hypogonadism prior to administration of anabolic steroids. If hypogonadal, testosterone replacement is preferred.

SELECTED REFERENCES

Storer TW, Woodhouse LJ, Sattler F, et al. A randomized, placebo-controlled trial of nandrolone decanoate in human immunodeficiency virus-infected men with mild to moderate weight loss with recombinant human growth hormone as active reference treatment. *J Clin Endocrinol Metab*, 2005; 90: 4474–82.

Comments: Placebo-controlled, randomized study to evaluate the effects of nandrolone (150 mg IM biweekly) vs placebo or rhGH (6 mg SC daily) in HIV-associated wasting (patients with 5%–15% weight loss over 6 mos). Nandrolone was associated with a greater increase in LBM ($+1.6 \pm 0.3$ kg) than placebo ($+0.4 \pm 0.3$ kg; P <0.05); however, the change in LBMs with nandrolone was lower but not significantly different from rhGH ($+2.5 \pm 0.3$ kg).

Sattler FR, Jaque SV, Schroeder ET, et al. Effects of pharmacological doses of nandrolone decanoate and progressive resistance training in immunodeficient patients infected with human immunodeficiency virus. *J Clin Endocrinol Metab*, 1999; 84: 1268–76.

Comments: Open label, randomized study to evaluate effects of high-dose nandrolone (600 mg/wk) vs high-dose nandrolone + progressive resistance training in patients with HIV-associated wasting. Total body weight increased significantly in both groups (3.2 ± 2.7 and 4.0 ± 2.0 kg, respectively; P <0.001), with increases due primarily to augmentation of lean tissue. Lean body mass determined by DEXA increased significantly more in nandrolone + resistance training group (3.9 ± 2.3 vs 5.2 ± 5.7 kg, respectively; P = 0.03). Much lower dose (100 mg q1–2 wk) is also effective and generally preferred.

Gold J, High HA, Li Y, et al. Safety and efficacy of nandrolone decanoate for treatment of wasting in patients with HIV infection. *AIDS*, 1996; 10: 745–52.

Comments: Patients with HIV-associated wasting who failed to gain weight after nutritional counseling received nandrolone 100 mg q2 wks for 16 wks in an open-label study. There were significant increases in weight (mean, 0.14 kg per wk; P <0.05) and lean body mass (mean, 3 kg by anthropometry; P <0.005) after 16 wks.

OXANDROLONE

Paul A. Pham, PharmD and John G Bartlett, MD

INDICATIONS
FDA
- Treatment of wasting due to chronic infection, surgery, or severe trauma.

Non-FDA Approved Uses
- Treatment of AIDS-related wasting.

FORMS TABLE

Brand name (mfr)	Forms†	Cost*
Oxandrin (Savient Pharmaceuticals)	Oral tab 2.5 mg	$7.85
	Oral tab 10 mg	$26.62

*Prices represent cost per unit specified, are representative of Average Wholesale Price (AWP).
†Dosage is indicated in mg unless otherwise noted.

USUAL ADULT DOSING
- Treatment of wasting; 15–20 mg/day (up to 40 mg/day) in 2–4 doses; consider using lower doses in women (5–10 mg/day).

ADVERSE DRUG REACTIONS
Occasional
- Virilization (deep voice, acne, clitoral enlargement, and hirsutism in women; acne and increased frequency of erection in men). Some changes irreversible even with drug discontinuation.
- Cholestatic hepatitis; discontinue with abnormal LFTs and jaundice.
- Nausea and vomiting.
- Ankle swelling.
- Depression and insomnia.
- Changes in libido.
- AST/ALT elevation (especially with doses >40 mg).
- LDL elevation (especially with doses >40 mg).
- Decrease in sex hormone-binding globulin, luteinizing hormone, follicle-stimulating hormone, and total and free testosterone levels.

Rare
- Peliosis hepatitis (reversible with discontinuation); may result in intraabdominal hemorrhage or life-threatening hepatic failure.

DRUG INTERACTIONS
- Oral hypoglycemics: may increase activity of oral hypoglycemics.
- Warfarin: may significantly potentiate action of oral anticoagulants.

PHARMACOLOGY
Mechanism
- 17-alpha alkylated synthetic testosterone with a high anabolic-to-androgenic ratio. It increases protein anabolism and decrease protein catabolism.

Pharmacokinetic Parameters
- **Absorption:** 97%.
- **Metabolism and Excretion:** minor liver metabolism. Renal excretion of unchanged drug and metabolites.
- **Protein Binding:** 94%.
- **$T_{\frac{1}{2}}$:** 13 hrs.
- **Distribution:** 0.6 L/kg.

Pregnancy Risk
- Category X: contraindicated.

Breastfeeding Compatibility
- No data.

DOSING
Dosing for Decreased Hepatic Function
- Avoid 17-alpha alkylated synthetic testosterone (i.e., oxandrolone, fluoxymesterone, oxymetholone, methandrostenolone, stanozolol, and methyltestosterone).

Renal Dosing
- Dosing for GFR of 50–80: usual dose.
- Dosing for GFR of 10–50: no data; use with caution due to possible increased water and salt retention. Avoid during nephrotic phase of nephritis.
- Dosing for GFR of <10: no data; use with caution due to possible increased water and salt retention. Avoid during nephrotic phase of nephritis.
- Dosing in hemodialysis, peritoneal dialysis, and hemofiltration: no data.

COMMENTS
- Anabolic steroid. Studies showed modest weight gain associated with increase in lean body mass, physical activity, and appetite (*AIDS*, 1996;10:1657; *AIDS*, 1996:10745). Risk of hepatitis may be higher with synthetic 17-alpha alkylated testosterone but appears to be lower with oxandrolone vs oxymetholone. Oxandrolone is alternative to IM nandrolone but higher cost ($900/mo vs $120/mo). Testosterone preferred for hypogonadal men.

DRUGS

SELECTED REFERENCES

Grunfeld C, Kotler DP, Dobs A, et al. Oxandrolone in the treatment of HIV-associated weight loss in men: a randomized, double-blind, placebo-controlled study. *J Acquir Immune Defic Syndr*, 2006; 41: 304–14.
Comments: Randomized placebo-controlled trial involving 262 patients with HIV wasting (documented 10%–20% weight loss or body mass index ≤20 kg/m) compared 20, 40, or 80 mg of oxandrolone daily to placebo. Body weight increased in the oxandrolone-treated patients was dose-dependent (up to 40 mg/day). However, treatment with oxandrolone was associated with significant decreases in sex hormone-binding globulin, LH, FSH, and total and free testosterone. In addition, significant increase in ALT and LDL was observed in two groups treated with high-dose oxandrolone (40 mg and 80 mg).

Mwamburi DM, Gerrior J, Wilson IB, et al. Comparing megestrol acetate therapy with oxandrolone therapy for HIV-related weight loss: similar results in 2 months. *Clin Infect Dis*, 2004; 38: 895–902.
Comments: Randomized trial comparing megestrol (800 mg/day) or oxandrolone (10 mg twice daily) × 2 mos in patients with weight loss of >5 kg on ART. Mean weight gain in megestrol and oxandrolone arms were 2.8 kg (4.6% of baseline value) and 2.5 kg (3.9% of baseline value), respectively (P = 0.80). Lean body mass accounted for 39% of weight gain in megestrol acetate arm and 56% in oxandrolone arm (P = 0.38). ADRs similar in both groups.

OXYMETHOLONE

Paul A. Pham, PharmD and John G. Bartlett, MD

INDICATIONS

FDA
- Acquired aplastic anemia (only moderately effective; erythropoietin preferred).
- Anemia associated with chronic renal failure.
- Chemotherapy-induced myleosuppression.
- Fanconi's anemia.
- Red cell aplasia.

Non-FDA Approved Uses
- HIV-associated wasting.

FORMS TABLE

Brand name (mfr)	Forms†	Cost*
Anadrol-50 (Unimed Pharmaceuticals)	Oral tab 50 mg	$24.69

*Prices represent cost per unit specified, are representative of Average Wholesale Price (AWP).
†Dosage is indicated in mg unless otherwise noted.

USUAL ADULT DOSING
- Wasting: 1–5 mg/kg/day.
- Monitor LFTs and lipids.
- Contraindicated in patients with breast and prostate cancer, severe liver disease, and nephrosis.

ADVERSE DRUG REACTIONS

Common
- Hepatoxicity (17-alpha alkylated synthetic testosterone, such as oxymetholone, may have higher incidence of hepatoxicity; consider nandrolone or oxandrolone). Up to 43% in patients receiving high doses.
- Hirsutism and male-pattern baldness in women.
- Male-pattern hair loss in postpubertal males.
- Edema.
- Insomnia.
- Muscle cramps.
- Acne, gynecomastia, priapism, excitation.

Occasional
- Peliosis hepatitis (blood filled cyst in liver).
- Cholestatic hepatitis.
- Glucose intolerance.
- Decreased TSH and T4.
- Osteoporosis with prolonged use.
- Increase LDL.

Rare
- Hepatic necrosis.
- Hepatocellular neoplasms.

DRUG INTERACTIONS
- Warfarin: increase in INR.

PHARMACOLOGY
Mechanism
- Androgenic-anabolic steroid that is synthetic derivative of testosterone. Stimulates receptors in organs and tissues to promote growth.

Pharmacokinetic Parameters
- **Absorption:** unknown PK parameters.
- **Metabolism and Excretion:** metabolized in liver via reduction and oxidation; 20%–30% excreted in urine.
- $T_{\frac{1}{2}}$: 1–2 days.

Pregnancy Risk
- Category X: contraindicated. Animal studies show embryo toxicity, fetotoxicity, infertility, and masculinization.

Breastfeeding Compatibility
- Not recommended.

DOSING
Dosing for Decreased Hepatic Function
- Not recommended.

Renal Dosing
- Dosing for GFR of 50–80: usual dose.
- Dosing for GFR of 10–50: no data.
- Dosing for GFR of <10 mL/min: not recommended.
- Dosing in hemodialysis, peritoneal dialysis, and hemofiltration: no data.

COMMENTS
- Alternative anabolic steroids (nandrolone, oxandrolone) should be considered due to higher incidence of hepatoxicity with oxymetholone. Potential concern for additive hepatoxicity with PIs and NNRTIs.

SELECTED REFERENCES
Hengge UR, Stocks K, Faulkner S, et al. Oxymetholone for the treatment of HIV-wasting: a double-blind, randomized, placebo-controlled phase III trial in eugonadal men and women. *HIV Clin Trials*, 2003; 4: 150–63.
Comments: Double-blind, randomized, placebo-controlled trial of 89 HIV+ eugonadal women and men. Patients with HIV-associated wasting received oxymetholone (50 mg twice daily or 3 ×/day) or placebo for 16 wks. Oxymetholone use correlated with increases in body cell mass in twice daily and 3 ×/day groups (3.8 ± 0.4 kg; P <0.0001 and 2.1 ± 0.6 kg; P <0.005 respectively). Hepatotoxicity (ALT, AST, or GGT >5x ULN) was seen in 43%, 25%, and 8% of patients in the 3 ×/day, twice daily, placebo groups, respectively.

TESAMORELIN

Paul A. Pham, PharmD

INDICATIONS
FDA
- Reduction of excess abdominal fat secondary to lipodystrophy in HIV-infected patients.

DRUGS

FORMS TABLE

Brand name (mfr)	Forms†	Cost*
Egrifta (Theratechnologies, Inc.)	SQ vial 1 mg	$39 per 1mg vial

*Prices represent cost per unit specified, are representative of Average Wholesale Price (AWP).
†Dosage is indicated in mg unless otherwise noted.

USUAL ADULT DOSING
- 2 mg SQ once daily.

ADVERSE DRUG REACTIONS
General
- Discontinuations due to adverse reactions occurred in 9.6% treated with tesamorelin (vs 6.8% with placebo).

Common
- Arthralgia (13%) and myalgia (6%).
- Injection site erythema and pruritis (8%–9%).
- Pain in extremity (6%).
- Peripheral edema (6.1% vs 2.3% in placebo).

Occasional
- Paresthesia (4.8% vs 2.3% in placebo).
- Musculoskeletal pain and stiffness (2%).
- Carpal tunnel syndrome (1.5%).
- Nausea and vomiting (3%–4%).
- Pruritis and rash (3%–4%).
- Hyperglycemia (4.5%).

Rare
- Hypertension.
- CK elevation.

DRUG INTERACTIONS
- Does not inhibit CYP450 3A4.
- Anticonvulsants (e.g., phenytoin, phenobarbital, carbamazepine): monitor anticonvulsants concentrations closely with coadministration.
- Cyclosporine: monitor cyclosporine concentrations with coadministration.
- Glucocorticoid: higher glucocorticoid dose may be needed with tesamorelin coadministration.
- Ritonavir: no significant drug-drug interaction.

PHARMACOLOGY
Mechanism
- Tesamorelin, a synthetic analogue of human hypothalamic growth hormone-releasing factor (hGRF), acts on the pituitary cells to stimulate synthesis and release of endogenous growth hormone.

Pharmacokinetic Parameters
- **Absorption:** <4%.
- **Metabolism and Excretion:** no data.
- **Cmax, Cmin, and AUC:** AUC = 852.8 (CV 91.9) pg.h/mL.
- **$T_{\frac{1}{2}}$:** 38 mins.
- **Distribution:** Vd = 10.5 L/kg.

Pregnancy Risk
- Category X: contraindicated.

Breastfeeding Compatibility
- Not recommended.

DOSING
Dosing for Decreased Hepatic Function
- No data.

Renal Dosing
- Dosing for renal impairment: no data; usual dose likely.
- Dosing for hemodialysis, pritoneal dialysis, and hemofiltration: no data.

COMMENTS
- Tesamorelin decreases abdominal fat by a modest 14%–18% in HIV+ patients with lipodystrophy.
- Musculoskeletal adverse effects, local injection site reactions, and cost may prevent routine use of tesamorelin. Reversal of benefits seen with discontinuation of drug. With currently used ARV regimens, most weight gain is due to increased subcutaneous fat rather than lipodystrophy. Expensive.

SELECTED REFERENCES
Egrifta (tesamorelin) for injection. US Food and Drug Administration. November 2010. *www.accessdata.fda.gov/drug-satfda_docs/label/2010/022505s000lbl.pdf*. Accessed August 15, 2011.

Comments: In two randomized placebo-controlled trials, 543 patients received tesamorelin for 26 wks. In both studies, patients treated with tesamorelin experienced greater reductions in abdominal fat (14%–18%) as measured by CT scan compared to placebo.

TESTOSTERONE

Paul A. Pham, PharmD and John G. Bartlett, MD

INDICATIONS

FDA
- Hypogonadism (replacement therapy recommended for men with low or low-normal levels).
- Wasting.
- Hypogonadotropic hypogonadism (congenital or acquired).
- Palliation of inoperable mammary cancer in women.

FORMS TABLE

Brand name (mfr)	Forms†	Cost*
Delatestryl (Savient Pharmaceuticals)	IM vial 100 mg/mL; 200 mg/mL (5-mL vial)	$99.32 per 5-mL vial
Androderm (Watson Pharmaceuticals)	Transdermal patch 2.5 mg; 5 mg	$5.03/2.5 mg 24-hr patch; $10.06/5 mg 24-hr patch
Striant (Columbia Laboratories)	Buccal system 30 mg	$4.31 per 30 mg
Testim (Auxilium Pharmaceuticals)	Topical gel 1% (50 mg)	$10.26/50 mg
Androgel (Unimed Pharmaceuticals)	Topical gel (unit dose) 1% (25 mg; 50 mg) Topical gel (meter dose pump) 1% (12.5 mg)	$9.70 per 25 mg; $9.96 per 50 mg $291.00 per mo supply
Depo-Testosterone (Pfizer)	IM vial 100 mg/mL; 200 mg/mL (10 mL or 1 mL)	$139.37 per 10 mL; $76.68 per 1 mL
Testosterone cypionate (generic manufacturer)	IM vial 200 mg/mL (5 mL)	$23.18 per 200 mg

(Continued)

Brand name (mfr)	Forms†	Cost*
Testosterone enantate (generic manufacturer)	IM vial 200 mg/mL	$16.99 per 200 mg

*Costs (rounded to the nearest dollar) are based on usual adult dosing per day, are representative of Average Wholesale Price (AWP), and are current within the prior three months.
†Dosage is indicated in mg unless otherwise noted.

USUAL ADULT DOSING
- Wasting: 200 mg IM q2 wks; can start with 400 mg IM q2 wks until weight restored. Not recommended for wasting in patients with normal testosterone levels.
- Alternative: 100–200 mg IM qwk to provide less variable levels throughout dosing cycle.
- Hypogonadism: replacement doses: testosterone 100 IM mg/wk or 200 mg IM q2 wks.
- Anabolic steroids (i.e., nandrolone or oxandrolone) preferred for treatment of wasting in eugonadal men.
- IM testosterone offers convenience of weekly or bimonthly administration and is cheaper than other formulations. Pain at injection site and low troughs at end of dosing intervals make topical preparations more attractive.
- **Gels:** *Androgel* (1% gel) or *Testim* (1% gel) 2.5–10 g (equivalent to 25 mg–100 mg) qAM: apply to shoulders, upper arms, abdomen (titrate to testosterone levels). **Patch:** *Androderm* 5-mg patch to back, abdomen, arms; rotate site (associated with more rash compared to gels). **Buccal:** *Striant*, 1 unit (30 mg) placed against gum above incisor tooth q12 hrs (rotating sides of the mouth).

ADVERSE DRUG REACTIONS
Common
- Androgenic effects include acne, flushing, gynecomastia, increased libido, priapism, and edema.
- Women may experience virilization: voice change, hirsutism, and clitoral enlargement.
- Local reactions from patches include pruritus, blistering, erythema, pain.
- With long-term treatment, intrinsic production of testosterone is shut off, which can result in prolonged or worsened hypogonadism after discontinuation.
- Testicular shrinkage.

Occasional
- Aggravation of sleep apnea.
- Salt retention.
- Secondary polycythemia.

Rare
- Possible promotion of KS, breast, or prostate cancer.
- Cholestatic hepatitis.
- Hyperglycemia.

DRUG INTERACTIONS
- Warfarin: INR may be increased.

PHARMACOLOGY
Mechanism
- Binds to androgen receptor, exerting multiple anabolic and androgenic effects (increase protein anabolism and decrease protein catabolism). Can cause retention of phosphorous, potassium, sodium, and nitrogen, and decrease renal excretion of calcium. Increases production of RBCs secondary to erythropoietic factor stimulation.

Pharmacokinetic Parameters
- **Absorption:** cypionate and enanthate esters are absorbed slowly from IM injection sites.
- **Metabolism and Excretion:** hepatic metabolism to 17 ketosteroids; excreted in urine.
- **Protein Binding:** Binding to testosterone-estradiol binding globulin.
- **Cmax, Cmin, and AUC:** mean Cmax: IM: 1200–1500 ng/dL; buccal and transdermal: 900 ng/dL; gel: 500–800 ng/dL.

- **T$_{\frac{1}{2}}$:** 10–100 min.
- **Distribution:** 70–120 L/kg.

Pregnancy Risk

- Category X: contraindicated.

Breastfeeding Compatibility

- Not recommended.

DOSING

Dosing For Decreased Hepatic Function

- Use with caution.

Renal Dosing

- Dosing for GFR of 50–80: usual dose.
- Dosing for GFR of <50: use with caution.
- Dosing in hemodialysis, peritoneal dialysis, and hemofiltration: use with caution.

COMMENTS

- Low testosterone levels have been found in 45% of patients with AIDS and 20%–30% of HIV+ patients without AIDS.
- Because HIV-infected persons may have high levels of sex hormone binding globulin, use of total testosterone in the diagnosis of hypogonadism may underestimate its prevalence. For this reason, free testosterone using a reference methodology (equilbrium dialysis or calculated free testosterone) should be used. "Direct" free testosterone assays using radioimmunoassay are unreliable and should not be used.
- Use free testosterone to guide therapy with goal in the midrange of normal. Testing should be done mid-cylce for those taking injections and at any time of day for those on transdermal preparations.
- Low free testosterone level should be confirmed to establish the Dx of hypogonadism.
- Testosterone circulates primarily bound to plasma proteins (albumin and sex hormone binding globulin [SHBG]), so determination of free testosterone using reliable assay (e.g., equilibrium dialysis) may be needed if alterations in binding proteins are suspected. Alternatively, a free testosterone can be estimated using free androgen index (total testosterone/SHBG).
- Once Dx of hypogonadism established, check LH and FSH distinguish primary (testicular failure) or central (hypothalamic of pituitary dysfunction). Low or inappropriately normal LH and FSH suggestive of central hypogonadism and should prompt further evaluation to establish cause (e.g., prolactin, iron studies, pituitary imaging).
- Supraphysiologic testosterone in eugonodal males with wasting syndrome can result in significant weight gain; however, this must be balanced against long-term risk of high-dose testosterone (reduced HDL cholesterol, hepatotoxicity, increased risk of prostate cancer).
- Secondary topical exposure of testosterone has been reported in children and women. Children and women should avoid contact with unwashed or unclothed application sites in men.

SELECTED REFERENCES

Mulligan K, Zackin R, Von Roenn JH, et al. Testosterone supplementation of megestrol therapy does not enhance lean tissue accrual in men with human immunodeficiency virus-associated weight loss: a randomized, double-blind, placebo-controlled, multicenter trial. *J Clin Endocrinol Metab,* 2007; 92: 563–70.

Comments: Randomized, double-blind, placebo-controlled trial evaluated effect on lean muscle mass gain when testosterone added to megestrol acetate. Megestrol with or without testosterone resulted in robust increases in weight (median 5.3 and 7.3 kg in megestrol/testosterone and megestrol/placebo, respectively); however, lean body mass (3.3 and 3.3 kg) and fat weight (3.0 and 3.8 kg) did not differ significantly. As expected, trough testosterone concentrations decreased to greater extent in patients not on testosterone.

Strawford A, Barbieri T, Van Loan M, et al. Resistance exercise and supraphysiologic androgen therapy in eugonadal men with HIV-related weight loss: a randomized controlled trial. *JAMA,* 1999; 281: 1282–90.

Comments: Double-blind, randomized, placebo-controlled trial to determine whether moderately supraphysiologic androgen regimen, including anabolic steroid (testosterone 100 mg/wk + oxandrolone 20 mg/day), would improve lean body mass in eugonadal men with HIV-related wasting. Lean body mass gain greater in supraphysiologic group compared to placebo. Obvious concern is long-term side effects of high-dose anabolic steroid.

Grinspoon S, Corcoran C, Askari H, et al. Effects of androgen administration in men with the AIDS wasting syndrome. A randomized, double-blind, placebo-controlled trial. *Ann Intern Med,* 1998; 129: 18–26.

DRUGS

Comments: Randomized, double-blind, placebo-controlled study evaluated benefit of physiologic testosterone (300 mg IM q3 wks × 6 mos) in 51 HIV+ hypogonadal men with wasting (>10% of baseline weight). Compared to placebo group, testosterone-treated patients gained more fat-free mass (−0.6 kg and 2.0 kg; P = 0.036), lean body mass (0.0 kg and 1.9 kg; P = 0.041), and muscle mass (−0.8 kg and 2.4 kg; P = 0.005). Patients on testosterone reported improved quality of life (P = 0.04). Hypogonadal men with wasting should be offered physiologic replacement of testosterone.

Coodley GO, Coodley MK. A trial of testosterone therapy for HIV-associated weight loss. *AIDS*, 1997; 11: 1347–52.
Comments: Physiologic testosterone did not significantly increase body weight in HIV-infected patients with CD4 <200 and 5% weight loss in this double-blind placebo controlled trial. In contrast to other trials, this study did not make Dx of hypogonadism, and weight loss was less severe.

THALIDOMIDE

Paul A. Pham, PharmD and John G. Bartlett, MD

INDICATIONS
FDA
- Treatment and prevention of erythema nodosum leprosum (ENL).
- Treatment of multiple myeloma in combination with dexamethasone.

Non-FDA Approved Uses
- Treatment of idiopathic aphthous stomatitis or esophagitis.
- Treatment of HIV-associated wasting.
- Possible other uses: refractory prurigo nodularis and microsporidiosis (unresponsive to albendazole).
- Hypertrophic HSV lesions unresponsive to acyclovir, foscarnet, and cidofovir.

FORMS TABLE

Brand name (mfr)	Forms†	Cost*
Thalomid (Celgene Corporation)	Oral capsule 50 mg; 100 mg; 200 mg	$150.15 per 50 mg cap; $243.73 per 100 mg cap; $277.50 per 200 mg cap

*Prices represent cost per unit specified, are representative of Average Wholesale Price (AWP).
†Dosage is indicated in mg unless otherwise noted.

USUAL ADULT DOSING
- Aphthous ulcer: 200 mg/day, may be increased up to 400 mg/day at wk 4 for nonresponse.
- Wasting: 100 mg/day (higher doses not associated with increased efficacy).
- Controlled by a restricted distribution program know as the System for Thalidomide Education and Prescribing Safety (STEPS); prescribers and pharmacists must register before prescribing and dispensing thalidomide. For more information contact Celgene Corporation at 888-423-5436.
- Hypertrophic HSV lesions: 100 mg twice daily × 8 wks (limited data).

ADVERSE DRUG REACTIONS
Common
- Drowsiness: consider bedtime administration to minimize daytime drowsiness.
- Constipation: 3%–30%.
- Rash: up to 25%–40% of patients; pruritic, erythematous, and macular over back, trunk, and extremities; generally reported 10–14 days after initiation of thalidomide.
- Peripheral neuropathy: up to 15%–50%; irreversible if thalidomide not discontinued. Avoid in patients with baseline peripheral neuropathy.
- Fever.
- Thrombotic events: 22.5% reported with thalidomide + dexamethasone vs 4.9% in patients receiving dexamethasone only.

Occasional
- Leukopenia and neutropenia: D/C if ANC <750.
- Dizziness and headache.

- Mood changes.
- Bitter taste.
- Orthostatic hypotension.
- Nausea.

Rare
- Thrombocytopenia.
- Intermittent "shaking" episode (resembling tremors).

DRUG INTERACTIONS
- Any drugs with potential to interfere with effectiveness of oral contraceptives (i.e., rifampin, rifabutin, RTV, APV, FPV, NVP, DRV) may put patient at risk for pregnancy. Should counsel patients on use of barrier form of contraception to avoid teratogenicity.
- CNS depressants (TCA, benzodiazepine, opiates): additive sedation.
- ddI, d4T: potential for additive peripheral neuropathy.

PHARMACOLOGY
Mechanism
- Numerous anti-inflammatory and immunomodulator properties (including reduction of TNF-alpha production).

Pharmacokinetic Parameters
- **Absorption:** well absorbed.
- **Metabolism and Excretion:** not hepatically metabolized to any large extent; undergoes nonenzymatic hydrolysis in plasma with only small amounts (less than 1%) recovered unchanged in the urine.
- **Protein Binding:** high.
- **Cmax, Cmin, and AUC:** Cmax: 1.7 mcg/mL with 200 mg.
- **$T_{\frac{1}{2}}$:** 5–7 hrs.
- **Distribution:** Vd = 120 L.

Pregnancy Risk
- Category X: teratogenicity well documented. Contraindicated.

Breastfeeding Compatibility
- Contraindicated.

DOSING
Dosing for Decreased Hepatic Function
- No data.

Renal Dosing
- Dosing for GFR of 50–80: usual dose.
- Dosing for GFR of <50: clearance not affected. Usual dose recommended.
- Dosing in hemodialysis: usual dose. No supplement needed.
- Dosing in peritoneal dialysis: no data; usual dose likely.
- Dosing in hemofiltration: no data.

COMMENTS
- Expensive, but highly effective agent for management of idiopathic aphthous ulcers of mouth or esophagus with response rate of 53%–73% between 7–28 days of therapy (*NEJM* 1997, 336:1489, Jacobson).
- Effective for AIDS-associated wasting with mean weight gain of 2.2 kg (Kaplan), but side effects, potential for teratogenicity, and effective alternatives prevent its routine use. Due to serious birth malformations, 2 forms of contraception required for male and female patients treated with thalidomide. Monitor for drug interactions that may decrease oral contraceptive efficacy.

SELECTED REFERENCES

Holmes A et al: Thalidomide therapy for the treatment of hypertrophic herpes simplex virus-related genitalis in HIV-infected individuals. *Clin Infect Dis* 44:e96, 2007 June 1.

Comment: Case reports of treatment success with thalidomide in the treatment of hypertrophic HSV when patients failed valacyclovir, foscarnet, and cidofovir.

Maurer T, Poncelet A, Berger T. Thalidomide treatment for prurigo nodularis in human immunodeficiency virus-infected subjects: efficacy and risk of neuropathy. *Arch Dermatol,* 2004; 140: 845–9.

DRUGS

Comments: In this small open-label trial, thalidomide 100–200 mg PO once daily reduced signs and Sx of refractory prurigo nodularis in HIV+ patients. 1/3 of subjects developed peripheral neuropathy, underscoring importance of careful neurologic assessment.

Kaplan G, Thomas S, Fierer DS, et al. Thalidomide for the treatment of AIDS-associated wasting. *AIDS Res Hum Retroviruses,* 2000; 16(14): 1345–55.

Comments: Significant weight gain observed with thalidomide 100 mg/day (2.2 kg, [33%], P = 0.008 vs placebo) and thalidomide 200 mg/day (1.5 kg [2.5%], P = 0.019 vs placebo).

Jacobson JM, Spritzler J, Fox L, et al. Thalidomide for the treatment of esophageal aphthous ulcers in patients with human immunodeficiency virus infection. National Institute of Allergy and Infectious Disease AIDS Clinical Trials Group. *J Infect Dis,* 1999; 180: 61–7.

Comments: In placebo-controlled trial, thalidomide 200 mg/day × 4 wks resulted in complete resolution of Bx-confirmed esophageal aphthous ulcers in 73% compared to 23% of placebo group (OR 13.8, P = 0.033). Approximately half of weight gain was fat-free mass.

Antimicrobial Agents

ACYCLOVIR

Paul A. Pham, PharmD and John G. Bartlett, MD

INDICATIONS

FDA

- Treatment of initial episode of herpes genitalis in immunocompromised patients.
- Treatment of herpes simplex encephalitis in immunocompetent patients.
- Treatment of herpes zoster.
- Treatment of varicella in immunocompetent patients when started within 24 hrs of onset of typical chickenpox rash (American Academy of Pediatrics does not recommend its use for treatment of uncomplicated chickenpox in healthy children).

FORMS TABLE

Brand name (mfr)	Forms†	Cost*
Zovirax (GSK) and acyclovir (generic manufacturers)	Oral capsule 200 mg	$1.12
	Oral tablet 800 mg	$4.13
	IV vial 500 mg	$20.00
	Oral tablet 400 mg	$1.79
	Topical ointment 5%	$15.20
	Oral suspension 200 mg/5 mL	$137.00 per 16 oz.

*Prices represent cost per unit specified, are representative of Average Wholesale Price (AWP).
†Dosage is indicated in mg unless otherwise noted.

USUAL ADULT DOSING

- Some expert recommends higher doses for patients with AIDS. Valacyclovir or famciclovir generally preferred due to better pharmacokinetic parameter and more convenient dosing.
- Mild HSV labialis: 400 mg PO thrice daily × 7 days.
- Mild genital or perirectal HSV: 400 PO thrice daily × 7 days.
- Severe genital or perirectal HSV: 5–10 mg/kg IV q8h × 7–14 days.
- Mild chickenpox: 800 mg PO 5 ×/day.
- HSV or VZV encephalitis: 10 mg/kg IV q8h.
- Severe chickenpox: 10 mg/kg IV q8h × 7–10 days.
- Severe dermatomal or visceral zoster: 10 mg/kg IV q8h until lesions resolved.
- VZV retinal necrosis: 10 mg/kg IV q8h + IV foscarnet 90 mg/kg IV 12h.

ADVERSE DRUG REACTIONS

General

- Generally very well tolerated.

Occasional

- Irritation and phlebitis at infusion site.
- Nausea and vomiting.
- Rash.
- Renal toxicity (especially crystallization w/ rapid IV infusion, underlying renal disease, and nephrotoxic drugs coadministration).

Rare

- Dizziness, transaminase elevation, pruritis, and headache.
- CNS (especially with high dose in renal failure): agitation, encephalopathy, lethargy, tremor, transient hemiparesis, disorientation, seizures, hallucinations.
- Anemia, neutropenia, hypotension.

DRUG INTERACTIONS

- Meperidine: may increase normeperidine plasma concentration.

DRUGS

- Probenecid: increase in acyclovir levels due to competitive tubular secretion by probenecid; no dose adjustment needed.
- Theophylline: may increase theophylline plasma concentration.

PHARMACOLOGY

Mechanism

- Converted by viral thymidine kinase to active acyclovir monophosphate; cellular enzyme catalase converts acyclovir monophosphate to acyclovir triphosphate, which competitively inhibits viral DNA polymerase.

Pharmacokinetic Parameters

- **Absorption:** 10%–30% bioavailability; decrease absorption with increased dose.
- **Metabolism and Excretion:** only 9%–14% of dose metabolized to inactive metabolite. 45%–79% excreted unchanged in the urine via glomerular filtration and tubular secretion.
- **Protein Binding:** 9%–33%.
- **Cmax, Cmin, and AUC:** 1.2 mcg/mL after 400 mg PO administration; 1.6 mcg/mL after 800 mg PO administration. 9.8 mcg/mL after 5 mg/kg IV administration; 22.9 mcg/mL after 10 mg/kg IV administration.
- **$T_{\frac{1}{2}}$:** 2.5 hrs.
- **Distribution:** high concentration found in kidneys, liver, and intestines. CNS penetration 50% of serum. Also distributed to lung, aqueous humor, tears, muscle, spleen, breast milk, uterine, vaginal mucosa, semen, and amniotic fluid.

Pregnancy Risk

- Category C: not teratogen but potential to cause chromosomal damage at high dose. CDC recommends use of acyclovir for life-threatening disease but does not advocate use for treatment or prophylaxis of genital herpes in pregnancy.

Breastfeeding Compatibility

- Acyclovir is concentrated at high level in breast milk. Because acyclovir has been used in newborns to treat HSV infection without adverse events, the American Academy of Pediatrics considers acyclovir to be safe during breastfeeding.

DOSING

Dosing for Decreased Hepatic Function

- No data. Dose reduction unlikely.

Renal Dosing

- Dosing for GFR of 50–80: 5–10 mg/kg IV q8h; 200–800 mg 5 ×/day.
- Dosing for GFR of 25–50: 5–10 mg/kg q12.
- Dosing for GFR 10–24: 5–10 mg/kg IV q24h; 200–800 mg q8h.
- Dosing for GFR of <10: 2.5–5 mg/kg IV q24h; 200–800 mg q12h.
- Dosing in hemodialysis: 2.5–5 mg/kg IV q24h; dose after HD.
- Dosing in peritoneal dialysis: 2.5–5 mg/kg IV q24h.
- Dosing in hemofiltration: CAVH: 3.5 mg/kg/day; CVVHD: 5–10 mg/kg/day (10 mg/kg/day for zoster and CNS).

COMMENTS

- Well-tolerated oral and parenteral antiviral agent with activity against HSV and VZV. In AIDS patients valacyclovir or famciclovir generally preferred over oral acyclovir due to better pharmacokinetic profiles and more convenient dosing.
- Topical use not effective.
- Monitor for crystalluria in patients receiving large IV doses with dehydration and/or renal insufficiency.

SELECTED REFERENCES

Centers for Disease Control and Prevention, Workowski KA, Berman SM. Sexually transmitted diseases treatment guidelines, 2010. *MMWR Recomm Rep*, 2010; 59.
Comments: STD treatment recommendations.

Spruance SL, Nett R, Marbury T, et al. Acyclovir cream for treatment of herpes simplex labialis: results of two randomized, double-blind, vehicle-controlled, multicenter clinical trials. *Antimicrob Agents Chemother*, 2002; 46: 2238–43.
Comments: These prospective trials involving 1385 patients showed the average duration of episodes was 4. 3 days in treated patients vs 4. 8 days in those given vehicle control (P = 0.007). There was no difference in outcome if treatment

initiated at time of prodrome or with erythema vs treatment during the papule or vesicular stage. Treatment had no effect on evolution of lesions. Many would argue that benefit was marginal: duration of pain was reduced by a mean of only 0.3–0.4 days and duration of the episode reduced by 0.5–0.6 days.

Conant MA, Schacker TW, Murphy RL, et al. Valaciclovir versus aciclovir for herpes simplex virus infection in HIV-infected individuals: two randomized trials. *Int J STD AIDS*, 2002; 13: 12–21.

Comments: Acyclovir as effective as valacyclovir for suppression and episodic treatment of herpes. Most experts now recommend valacyclovir over acyclovir due to better absorption and more convenient dosing schedule.

ADEFOVIR

Paul A. Pham, PharmD and John G. Bartlett, MD

INDICATIONS

FDA

- Chronic hepatitis B (patients w/ clinical evidence of lamivudine-resistant HBV with either compensated or decompensated liver function).

FORMS TABLE

Brand name (mfr)	Forms†	Cost*
Hepsera (Gilead)	PO tab 10 mg	$32.52

*Prices represent cost per unit specified, are representative of Average Wholesale Price (AWP).
†Dosage is indicated in mg unless otherwise noted.

USUAL ADULT DOSING

- 10 mg once daily (with or without food) × 48–92 wks.

ADVERSE DRUG REACTIONS

General

- Generally well tolerated.

Common

- Asthenia.

Occasional

- Nephrotoxicity (w/ underlying renal insufficiency).
- Exacerbation of hepatitis (with discontinuation of therapy or development of HBV resistance).
- Abdominal pain, nausea, vomiting, diarrhea.
- Cough.
- Pruritus.
- Headache.

Rare

- Lactic acidosis, but less likely to occur compared to other NRTIs.
- Fanconi syndrome (reported with large doses).
- Pancreatitis.

DRUG INTERACTIONS

- Ibuprofen increases adefovir AUC by 23%. Drugs that inhibit tubular secretion (i.e., probenecid) may increase adefovir serum level.

Resistance

- In a genotype analysis of an open-label pilot study evaluating the efficacy of adefovir (10 mg q day) in the treatment of lamivudine-resistance HBV infection, adefovir at a suboptimal concentration for (HIV-1) for 12 mos did not result in selection for either adefovir mutations at codons 65 and 70 or any other particular HIV-1 reverse transcriptase resistance in patients with uncontrolled HIV-1 replication (Delaugerre). Larger analysis that includes major and minor viral population with a longer follow-up should be performed before this cross-resistance issue can be settled.

- Another concern regarding adefovir monotherapy for HBV is the potential for the development of adefovir resistant HBV. Thus far, adefovir-resistant HBV has not been detected in approximately 78 wks of follow-up. However, longer follow-up is needed.
- Clinical trials of the various combinations involving interferon, lamivudine, and adefovir are underway, the hope is to prevent the evolution of resistant mutation and improve clinical outcome.

PHARMACOLOGY

Mechanism

- Adefovir diphosphate inhibits HBV DNA polymerase, which results in DNA chain termination after its incorporation into viral DNA.

Pharmacokinetic Parameters

- **Absorption:** 59% (unaffected by food).
- **Metabolism and excretion:** adefovir dipivoxil is converted to adefovir, which is excreted via glomerular filtration and active tubular secretion.
- **Protein binding:** <4%.
- **Cmax, Cmin, and AUC:** 18.4 ± 6.26 ng/mL.
- **$T_{\frac{1}{2}}$:** serum: 1.6. Intracellular (diphosphate): 16 to 18 hours.
- **Distribution:** Vd = 393 ± 75 mL/kg.

Pregnancy Risk

- Category C. Parenteral adefovir, when given at 20 mg/kg (systemic exposure 38 times human), resulted in embryotoxicity and fetal malformations. No human data.

Breastfeeding Compatibility

- No data, not recommended.

DOSING

Dosing for Decreased Hepatic Function

- 10 mg once daily.

Renal Dosing

- Dosing for GFR of 50–80: 10 mg PO once daily.
- Dosing for GFR of 30–49: 10 mg q48h.
- Dosing for GFR 10–29: 10 mg q72hrs.
- Dosing for GFR of <10: no data.
- Dosing in hemodialysis: 10 mg q 7 days following HD.
- Dosing in peritoneal dialysis: no data.
- Dosing in hemofiltration: CVVHD: no data, consider 10 mg q48h.

COMMENTS

- Adefovir is an effective treatment of chronic HBV infection, but entecavir, telbivudine, and tenofovir may be better choices due to higher potency. In HIV-coinfected patients, a concern with the use of low dose adefovir is the potential for the development of cross-resistance with nucleoside analogs and/or future activity of tenofovir. Preliminary data didn't show selection of adefovir mutations. Most HBV experts recommend the use of adefovir (tenofovir preferred) with lamivudine for the treatment of HBV infection.

SELECTED REFERENCES

Sung JJ, Lai JY, Zeuzem S, et al. Lamivudine compared with lamivudine and adefovir dipivoxil for the treatment of HBeAg-positive chronic hepatitis B. *J Hepatol*, 2008; 48: 728–35.
Comments: This double-blind study randomized 150 HBeAg-positive patients to 3TC OR adefovir plus 3TC. At 104 wks, breakthrough HBV DNA (44% vs 19%) and development of resistant mutation (43% vs 15%) was higher in the 3TC monotherapy treated patients. Although ALT normalization was higher in the adefovir + 3TC treated group (34% [19/56] vs 45% (23/51), HBeAg seroconversion was not significantly different between groups.

Peters MG, Andersen J, Lynch P, et al. Randomized controlled study of tenofovir and adefovir in chronic hepatitis B virus and HIV infection: ACTG A5127. *Hepatology*, 2006; 44: 1110–6.
Comments: Fifty-two HIV-HBV coinfected patients were randomized adefovir or tenofovir. At baseline 86% were HBeAg positive and 94% were 3TC resistant. TDF was more potent with a mean time-weighted average change in serum HBV DNA from baseline to wk 48 of −4.44 log(10) copies/mL for TDF and −3.21 log(10) copies/mL for ADV.

Peters MG, Hann HwH, Martin P, et al. Adefovir dipivoxil alone or in combination with lamivudine in patients with lamivudine-resistant chronic hepatitis B. *Gastroenterology*, 2004; 126: 91–101.

Comments: Adefovir monotherapy vs adefovir + lamivudine vs continued lamivudine in patients with chronic hepatitis B with compensated liver disease and lamivudine-resistant hepatitis B virus (HBV) was evaluated. HBV DNA level reduction at wk 48 and normalization of ALT level were comparable in adefovir monotherapy and adefovir plus lamivudine arm. It was not surprising that both adefovir arms had significantly better outcome compared to continued lamivudine monotherapy.

Delaugerre C, Marcelin AG, Thibault V, et al. Human immunodeficiency virus (HIV) type 1 reverse transcriptase resistance mutations in hepatitis B virus (HBV)-HIV-coinfected patients treated for HBV chronic infection once daily with 10 milligrams of adefovir dipivoxil combined with lamivudine. *Antimicrob Agents Chemother*, 2002; 46: 1586–8.

Comments: No selection of ADV resistant mutations was observed in HIV-coinfected patients treated for HBV with low dose ADV (10 mg/day).

ALBENDAZOLE

Paul A. Pham, PharmD and John G. Bartlett, MD

DRUGS

INDICATIONS
FDA
- Neurocysticercosis caused by *Taenia solium*.
- Hydatid disease caused by *Echinococcus granulosus* (tapeworm).

Non-FDA Approved Uses
- Microsporidiosis.
- Trichuriasis.
- Hookworm.
- Toxocariasis.

FORMS TABLE

Brand name (mfr)	Forms†	Cost*
Albenza (GlaxoSmithKline)	Oral tablet 200 mg	$1.58
Eskazole; Zentel (non-US brands) (non-US manufacturer)	Oral tablet 200 mg	n/a (non-US manufacturer)

*Prices represent cost per unit specified, are representative of Average Wholesale Price (AWP).
†Dosage is indicated in mg unless otherwise noted.

USUAL ADULT DOSING
- Microsporidiosis: 400 mg PO twice daily with fatty meals (treat until CD4 count >200).
- Hookworm: 400 mg PO × 1.
- Hydatid disease: 400 mg PO twice daily with meals × 28 days followed by a 14-days drug-free interval for a total of 3 cycles. Note: when medically feasible, surgery is considered treatment of choice.
- Neurocysticercosis: 400 mg PO twice daily with meals for 8–30 days with corticosteroids during the 1st wk of treatment in order to prevent cerebral hypertensive episodes.
- Toxocariasis: 400 mg PO twice daily with meals × 5 days.

ADVERSE DRUG REACTIONS
General
- Generally well tolerated.

Occasional
- Reversible hepatoxicity (monitor LFTs q2 wks).
- GI intolerance: nausea, vomiting, diarrhea, and abdominal pain.

Rare
- Bone marrow suppression (i.e., pancytopenia, aplastic anemia, agranulocytosis, and leukopenia), especially in patients with liver disease, including echinococcosis.
- Dizziness and headache.
- Hypersensitivity reaction.

- Alopecia.
- Increased transaminase levels.

DRUG INTERACTIONS

- Cimetidine: increased albendazole levels in bile and cystic fluid following coadministration with cimetidine (clinical significance unknown).
- Dexamethasone: monitor for albendazole toxicity; dose may need to be decreased. In some case reports trough concentration of albendazole was increased up to 56%.
- Praziquantel: monitor adverse events of albendazole. Dose of albendazole may need to be decreased. In some case reports mean plasma concentration of albendazole was increased up to 50%.
- Theophylline: no reported interaction.

PHARMACOLOGY

Mechanism

- Albendazole causes degenerative alterations in the tegument and intestinal cells of the parasite by inhibiting its polymerization into microtubules; this results in the inability to uptake glucose by the larva and adult stage.

Pharmacokinetic Parameters

- **Absorption:** poor and erratic absorption (enhanced 5-fold with fatty food).
- **Metabolism and Excretion:** hepatic metabolism to active sulfoxide metabolite then excreted by enterohepatic circulation. Metabolites excreted in urine. Only a small amount is found in the feces.
- **Protein Binding:** 70%.
- **Cmax, Cmin, and AUC:** 1.3 mcg/mL after 400-mg PO dose administration.
- **$T_{\frac{1}{2}}$:** 8–9 hrs.
- **Distribution:** distributed in bile, hydatid cyst, and CSF.

Pregnancy Risk

- Category C: teratogenicity demonstrated in laboratory animals. Avoid in 1st trimester of pregnancy.

Breastfeeding Compatibility

- Unknown.

DOSING

Dosing for Decreased Hepatic Function

- No data.

Renal Dosing

- No dose adjustment for renal impairment.
- Dosing in hemodialysis: not removed in hemodialysis. use usual dose.
- Dosing in peritoneal dialysis: no data.
- Dosing in hemofiltration: no data.

COMMENTS

- Well-tolerated oral agent, broad-spectrum antihelminthic.
- An effective agent against microsporidiosis involving *Encephalitozoon intestinalis*. Unfortunately, 80% of HIV-related microsporidiosis is caused by *Enterocytozoon bieneusi*, which has poor response to albendazole. ART is preferred treatment for microsporidiosis.
- Albendazole (400 mg PO × 1) resulted in higher cure rate compared to mebendazole in the treatment of *Ascaris*, hookworm, and *Trichuris*.

SELECTED REFERENCES

Molina JM, Chastang C, Goguel J, et al. Albendazole for treatment and prophylaxis of microsporidiosis due to Encepha-litozoon intestinalis in patients with AIDS: a randomized double-blind controlled trial. *J Infect Dis*, 1998; 177: 1373–7. **Comments:** This small double-blind placebo-controlled trial was conducted to assess the efficacy and safety of albendazole (400 mg PO twice daily for 3 wks) for the treatment of *Encephalitozoon intestinalis* infection in patients with AIDS. Clearance of microsporidia from the intestinal tract was obtained in 4 of 4 patients in the albendazole group versus 0 of 4 in the control group (P = 0.01, one-sided Fisher's exact test) and was associated with significant clinical benefit.

Kelly P, Lungu F, Keane E, et al. Albendazole chemotherapy for treatment of diarrhoea in patients with AIDS in Zambia: a randomised double blind controlled trial. *BMJ*, 1996; 312: 1187–91.

Comments: This was a randomized double-blind placebo-controlled trial of empiric albendazole 800 mg PO twice daily for 2 wks for chronic diarrhea of unknown etiology. Albendazole treated patients had significantly less diarrhea compared to placebo (P <0.0001). In resource-limited countries where the incidence of microsporidium and/or helminthic infections is high, empiric albendazole treatment may be a reasonable therapeutic option.

AMPHOTERICIN B

Paul A. Pham, PharmD and John G. Bartlett, MD

INDICATIONS

FDA

- Aspergillosis.
- Blastomycosis.
- Disseminated candidiasis.
- Leishmaniasis.
- Cryptococcosis.
- Histoplasmosis.
- Cryptococcal meningitis (treatment and suppression).
- Sporotrichosis; mucormycosis; basidiobolomycosis; conidiobolomycosis.
- Coccidioidomycosis.
- Treatment of fungal infections involving the CNS, pulmonary, and urinary tract system.

FORMS TABLE

Brand name (mfr)	Forms†	Cost*
Fungizone and generic (Bristol-Myers Squibb and generic manufacturers)	IV vial 50 mg	$24.50/50-mg vial

*Prices represent cost per unit specified, are representative of Average Wholesale Price (AWP).
†Dosage is indicated in mg unless otherwise noted.

USUAL ADULT DOSING

- Dosing range: 0.3–1.5 mg/kg/day IV (infuse over 2–4 hrs). Oral form no longer commercially available.
- Cryptococcal meningitis: 0.7 mg/kg IV q24h ± flucytosine 25 mg/kg PO q6h × 2 wks, then fluconazole 400 mg PO q24h × 8 wks or until CSF is sterile. Maintenance therapy with fluconazole 200 mg PO q24h.
- *Candida* esophagitis (azole-resistant): 0.3–0.7 mg/kg IV q24h (echinocandins can also be considered).
- Systemic fungal infections: 0.5–1.5 mg/kg/day over 2–4 hrs w/ pre- and posthydration.

ADVERSE DRUG REACTIONS

Common

- Nephrotoxicity: can occur with or without nephrocalcinosis. Reduced with adequate hydration, salt loading (500 cc NS pre- and post-amphotericin B infusion) and avoidance of concurrent nephrotoxic agents.
- Renal tubular acidosis.
- Electrolyte abnormalities: hypokalemia, hypomagnesemia, and hypocalcemia.
- Fever and chills: can be managed with meperidine or hydrocortisone 10–50 mg added to infusion. Alternatively, could premedicate with meperidine or ibuprofen.
- Anemia (normocytic normochromic).
- Phlebitis (improved with the addition of 1000 U heparin to infusion).

Occasional

- Hypotension.
- Nausea and vomiting.
- Metallic taste.
- Headache.

Rare

- Pulmonary reaction (acute dyspnea, hypoxemia, and interstitial infiltrates) when given with leukocyte transfusion.

DRUG INTERACTIONS

- Digoxin: may increase digitalis toxicity secondary to hypokalemia (consider potassium supplementation).
- Diuretics and corticosteroids: may result in additive hypokalemia.
- Nephrotoxic agents (e.g., foscarnet, cidofovir, aminoglycosides, and cyclosporine): may result in additive nephrotoxicity.

RESISTANCE

- Some spp. of *Fusarium oxysporum* and *F. solani* and most spp. of *Pseudallescheria boydii* are resistant.
- *Candida lusitaniae*.

PHARMACOLOGY

Mechanism

- Binds to ergosterol and disrupts fungal cell membrane resulting in leakage of intracellular contents.

Pharmacokinetic Parameters

- **Absorption**: not absorbed from the GI tract.
- **Metabolism and Excretion**: metabolism not fully understood. Undergoes slow renal excretion.
- **Protein Binding**: 90%.
- **Cmax, Cmin, and AUC**: Cmax: 0.5–3.5 mcg/mL after 0.4–0.7 mg/kg IV dose administration.
- **T$_{\frac{1}{2}}$**: 24 hrs (up to 15 days).
- **Distribution**: Vd = 4 L/Kg. Widely distributed in body tissue and fluids such as inflamed pleura, peritoneum, synovium, aqueous humor, vitreous humor, and pericardial fluid. Poor CNS penetration (only 3% of serum concentration is attained in the CSF) but effective in the treatment of cryptococcal meningitis.

Pregnancy Risk

- Category B: Collaborative Perinatal Project identified 9 patients w/ 1st-trimester exposure to amphotericin and found no adverse fetal effect. Animal studies demonstrated amphotericin to be harmless in pregnancy.

Breastfeeding Compatibility

- No data available.

DOSING

Dosing for Decreased Hepatic Function

- No data.

Renal Dosing

- Dosing for GFR of 50–80: usual dose.
- Dosing for GFR of 10–50: usual dose. Consider alternative lipid formulation.
- Dosing for GFR of <10: if ARF reversible, consider alternative lipid formulation.
- Dosing in hemodialysis: usual dose, no supplement needed post HD.
- Dosing in peritoneal dialysis: usual dose.
- Dosing in hemofiltration: no data; usual dose likely.

COMMENTS

- Use is complicated by high rate of infusion and dose-dependent related reactions such as anemia, electrolyte imbalance, and renal failure. A switch to lipid formulation (liposomal amphotericin) generally recommended when serum creatinine elevated to arbitrary threshold (>2.5 used at Johns Hopkins).
- Infusion-related side effects higher than AmBisome and Abelcet but lower than Amphotec. When indicated, alternative agents such as caspofungin may also be considered. Despite lower incidence of nephrotoxicity with lipid formulation, amphotericin B deoxycholate remains drug of choice for treatment of cryptococcal meningitis due to robust clinical data. For other invasive fungal infections, AmBisome and Abelcet generally preferred.

SELECTED REFERENCES

Walsh TJ, Anaissie EJ, Denning DW, et al. Treatment of aspergillosis: clinical practice guidelines of the Infectious Diseases Society of America. *Clin Infect Dis*, 2008; 46: 327–60.

Comments: IDSA guidelines no longer recommend amphotericin B deoxylate for treatment of invasive aspergillosis. AmBisome (3–5 mg/kg/day IV) or Abelcet (5 mg/kg/day IV) can be considered as alternative to voriconazole.

Patterson TF, Kirkpatrick WR, White M, et al. Invasive aspergillosis. Disease spectrum, treatment practices, and outcomes. Aspergillus Study Group. *Medicine* (Baltimore), 2000; 79: 250–60.

Comments: Report of 595 patients with proven or probable invasive aspergillosis. Major risk factors were bone marrow transplantation (32%), hematologic malignancy (29%), solid organ transplants (9%), AIDS (8%), and pulmonary disease (9%). Response to treatment generally poor. Only 25% treated with amphotericin B responded, and mortality rate was 65%. Results better with itraconazole, but these patients were less seriously immunosuppressed so that conclusions regarding relative merits were limited.

Perfect JR, Dismukes WE, Dromer F, et al. Clinical practice guidelines for the management of cryptococcal disease: 2010 update by the Infectious Diseases Society of America. *Clin Infect Dis*, 2010; 50: 291–322.

Comments: The treatment of choice in HIV+ patients with cryptococcal meningitis is induction therapy with amphotericin B (0.7–1 mg/kg/day) + flucytosine (100 mg/kg/day for ≥2 wks) followed by fluconazole (400 mg/day) for a minimum of 10 wks.

van der Horst CM, Saag MS, Cloud GA, et al. Treatment of cryptococcal meningitis associated with the acquired immunodeficiency syndrome. National Institute of Allergy and Infectious Diseases Mycoses Study Group and AIDS Clinical Trials Group. *N Engl J Med*, 1997; 337: 15–21.

Comments: This ACTG trial sets standard of care for management of cryptococcal meningitis in patients with AIDS. Addition of 5-FC to amphotericin resulted in faster CSF sterilization but did not improve clinical outcome.

DRUGS

AMPHOTERICIN, LIPID FORMULATIONS

Paul A. Pham, PharmD and John G. Bartlett, MD

INDICATIONS

FDA

- *AmBisome, Abelcet,* and *Amphotec:* aspergillosis (in patients refractory to or intolerant of amphotericin B deoxycholate).
- *AmBisome:* candidiasis (in patients refractory to or intolerant of amphotericin B deoxycholate).
- *AmBisome:* cryptococcosis, including cryptococcal meningitis (in patients refractory to or intolerant of amphotericin B deoxycholate).
- *AmBisome:* empiric therapy for presumed fungal infection in patients with febrile neutropenia.
- *AmBisome:* visceral leishmaniasis.

FORMS TABLE

Brand name (mfr)	Forms†	Cost*
AmBisome (Fujisawa)	IV vial 50 mg	$188.40
Abelcet (Enzon Inc.)	IV vial 100 mg	$240
Amphotec (Intermune Pharmaceuticals)	IV vial 50 mg; 100 mg	$93.33; $160.00

*Prices represent cost per unit specified, are representative of Average Wholesale Price (AWP).
†Dosage is indicated in mg unless otherwise noted.

USUAL ADULT DOSING

- *AmBisome:* 3–5 mg/kd/day (generally 5 mg/kg/day for most systemic fungal infections).
- *Abelcet:* 5 mg/kg/day.
- *Amphotec:* 3–4 mg/kg.

- Cryptococcal meningitis: *AmBisome* 3–4 mg/kg once daily + 5-FC × ≥2 wks followed by fluconazole (FDA labeled dose for cryptococcal meningitis 6 mg/kg/day) OR *Abelcet* 5 mg/kg + 5-FC × ≥2 wks followed by fluconazole (more limited data). *Amphotec:* no data in the treatment of cryptococcal meningitis and not recommended.
- Empiric treatment of fever in neutropenic patients not responding to antibiotics: *AmBisome* 3 mg/kg once daily. Higher doses (5 mg/kg/day) should be considered with neutropenia >10 days, clinically unstable, and/or evidence of fungal infection.
- Higher doses (up to 10–15 mg/kg/day) have been employed in refractory zygomycotic infections. Limited data support this dosing. Posaconazole may be considered in refractory cases.
- Invasive aspergillosis: 5 mg/kg once daily. Lower doses (3 mg/kg/day) may be considered in clinically stable patients.
- Invasive candidiasis: 5 mg/kg once daily.

ADVERSE DRUG REACTIONS
Occasional
- Chills: 18% in *AmBisome*-treated patients compared to 50% in amphotericin B-treated patients. 53% in *Amphotec*-treated patients compared to 30% amphotericin-treated patients. Infusion-related ADR was higher with *Abelcet* compared to amphotericin.
- Fever (>38): 27% in *Amphotec*-treated patients compared to 16% in amphotericin B-treated patients. 8% in *AmBisome*-treated patients and 10%–20% in *Abelcet*-treated patients compared to up to 40% in amphotericin-treated patients.
- Phlebitis and pain at injection site.
- Creatinine elevation (>2 × baseline) observed in up to 19% in *AmBisome*, 25% in *Amphotec*, 8% in low dose *Abelcet*-treated patients compared to 30%–50% in amphotericin B-treated patients.
- Hypokalemia, hypomagnesemia, hypocalcemia.
- Nausea, vomiting, diarrhea, abdominal pain, metallic taste.
- Hypotension.
- Headache and insomnia.
- Transaminase elevation (>2 × ULN with cumulative dose >2000 mg).
- Increased bilirubin (>1.5 × baseline).
- Anemia.

Rare
- Rash and pruritis.

DRUG INTERACTIONS
- Digoxin: potential increase in digitalis toxicity secondary to amphotericin-induced potassium depletion. Monitor potassium closely with coadministration.
- Nephrotoxic agents (aminoglycosides, cidofovir, foscarnet, and potentially TDF): may result in additive nephrotoxicity.
- Skeletal muscle relaxant: may enhance curariform effect of skeletal muscle relaxants (e.g., tubocurarine) due to hypokalemia. Monitor potassium closely with coadministration.

PHARMACOLOGY
Mechanism
- Polyene agent binds to ergosterol resulting in the disruption of the fungal cell membrane causing leakage of intracellular contents. Lipid formulation designed to reduce binding of amphotericin to mammalian cell membranes, therefore reducing toxicities.

Pharmacokinetic Parameters
- **Absorption:** not absorbed from the GI tract.
- **Metabolism and Excretion:** unknown metabolic pathway with up to 10% renal excretion. Increased uptake by the liver and spleen and decreased renal concentration.
- **Protein Binding:** no data.
- **Cmax, Cmin, and AUC:** Cmax: 3.1 mcg/mL (*Amphotec*); 1.7 mcg/mL (*Abelcet*); 83 mcg/mL (*AmBisome*).
- **$T_{\frac{1}{2}}$:** *AmBisome:* 100–153 hrs; *Abelcet:* 7.2 days; *Amphotec:* 25 hrs.
- **Distribution:** greater Vd compared to conventional amphotericin. Increased uptake by the liver and spleen and decreased kidney concentration.

Pregnancy Risk
- Category B (for all lipid formulation): limited data on use of lipid amphotericin in pregnancy; use should be limited to situations in which benefits outweighs risks.

Breastfeeding Compatibility
- No data.

DOSING

Dosing for Decreased Hepatic Function
- No data.

Renal Dosing
- Dosing for GFR of 10–80: usual dose.
- Dosing for GFR of <10: no data, use with close monitoring of worsening renal function.
- Dosing in hemodialysis: no data. Usual dose likely.
- Dosing in peritoneal dialysis: no data. Usual dose likely.
- Dosing in hemofiltration: no data.

COMMENTS

- Randomized trials showing equivalence with reduced toxicity compared to conventional amphotericin B for aspergillosis, febrile neutropenia, and cryptococcal meningitis. *AmBisome* superior to amphotericin B in treatment of histoplasmosis. For treatment of cryptococcal meningitis, liposomal amphotericin B resulted in faster CSF sterilization with less nephrotoxicity vs standard amphotericin B, but this did not result in improved clinical outcomes.
- Despite high cost of lipid amphotericin formulations, they may be more cost effective due to reduced rates of renal failure and dialysis (*Clin Infect Dis* 2001; 32: 686; 2003; 37: 415).

SELECTED REFERENCES

Perfect JR. Dismukes WE, Dromer F et al. Clinical practice guidelines for the management of cryptococcal disease: 2010 update by the Infectious Diseases Society of America. *Clin Infect Dis*, 2010; 50: 291–322.
Comments: 5-FC + amphotericin B, liposomal amphotericin, or amphotericin lipid complex (× >2 wks) is recommended for treatment of cryptococcal meningitis. Without 5-FC, recommended lipid amphotericin treatment duration is 4–6 wks.

Walsh TJ, Anaissie EJ, Denning DW, et al. Treatment of aspergillosis: clinical practice guidelines of the Infectious Diseases Society of America. *Clin Infect Dis*, 2008; 46: 327–60.
Comments: The IDSA guidelines recommend *AmBisome* (3–5 mg/kg/day IV) or *Abelcet* (5 mg/kg/day IV) as alternatives to voriconazole for treatment of invasive aspergillosis.

Johnson PC, Wheat LJ, Cloud GA, et al. Safety and efficacy of liposomal amphotericin B compared with conventional amphotericin B for induction therapy of histoplasmosis in patients with AIDS. *Ann Intern Med*, 2002; 137(2): 105–9.
Comments: Randomized, double-blind trial that compared liposomal amphotericin 3 mg/kg/day to conventional amphotericin 0.7 mg/kg/day for the treatment of moderate to severe histoplasmosis in 83 HIV+ patients. Clinical success achieved in 14/22 patients (64%) treated with conventional amphotericin B compared with 45/51 patients (88%) receiving liposomal amphotericin B (P = 0.014).

Sobel JD. Practice guidelines for the treatment of fungal infections. For the Mycoses Study Group. Infectious Diseases Society of America. Clin Infect Dis, 2000; 30: 652.
Comments: IDSA guidelines for treatment of fungal infections. ID expert recommendations concerning lipid formulation are: (1) serum creatinine >2.5 mg/dL; (2) most patients with candidiasis, cryptococcosis, and endemic mycosis should not be treated initially with lipid-based amphotericin B preparations; (3) immunocompromised patients with life-threatening infections with aspergillus or zygomycosis—some authorities recommend initiating treatment with lipid-based amphotericin B and others with conventional amphotericin B and switch according to criteria summarized.

Leenders AC, Reiss P, Portegies P, et al. Liposomal amphotericin B (AmBisome) compared with amphotericin B both followed by oral fluconazole in the treatment of AIDS-associated cryptococcal meningitis. *AIDS*, 1997; 11: 1463–71.
Comments: This randomized trial in cryptococcal meningitis demonstrated that liposomal amphotericin B resulted in faster CSF sterilization compared to standard conventional amphotericin B, but this did not result in improved clinical outcomes. Liposomal amphotericin B was clinically equivalent to standard amphotericin and resulted in less nephrotoxicity.

Sharkey PK, Graybill JR, Johnson ES, et al. Amphotericin B lipid complex compared with amphotericin B in the treatment of cryptococcal meningitis in patients with AIDS. *Clin Infect Dis*, 1996; 22: 315–21.

DRUGS

Comments: Clinical improvement occurred in 86% of patients treated with *Abelcet* even though CSF sterilization was achieved in 42% after 2 wks of therapy. This small study suggests that there may be a role for *Abelcet* in the treatment of cryptococcal meningitis, however larger trials need to be conducted.

ATOVAQUONE

Paul A. Pham, PharmD and John G. Bartlett, MD

INDICATIONS

FDA

- Prevention of *Pneumocystis* pneumonia (PCP) in patients who are intolerant to TMP-SMX.
- Oral treatment of mild-to-moderate PCP.
- Atovaquone in combination with proguanil indicated for the prevention and treatment of malaria due to *Plasmodium falciparum* (including chloroquine-resistant strains) in adults and pediatric patients weighing 5–11 kg.

Non-FDA Approved Uses

- Toxoplasmosis treatment alone (limited data with atovaquone 750 mg 4 ×/day).
- Toxoplasmosis treatment in combination with pyrimethamine or sulfadiazine.

FORMS TABLE

Brand name (mfr)	Forms†	Cost*
Mepron (GlaxoSmithKline)	Oral suspension 750 mg/5 mL (210 mL)	$1039.08 per 210 mL (21days supply)
Malarone (atovaquone/ proguanil) (GlaxoSmithKline)	Oral tablet 250 g/100 mg Oral tablet 62.5 mg/25 mg	$7.34 $2.72

*Prices represent cost per unit specified, are representative of Average Wholesale Price (AWP).
†Dosage is indicated in mg unless otherwise noted.

USUAL ADULT DOSING

- Treatment of mild-to-moderate (A-a O$_2$ gradient <46 mmHg and PAO$_2$ >60 mmHg) PCP: 750 mg (5 mL) PO twice daily × 21 days with food.
- PCP prophylaxis 750 mg PO twice daily or 1500 mg PO once daily with food.
- *P. falciparum* treatment: atovaquone/proguanil 4 tabs/day (1000 mg/400 mg) × 3 days with food.
- Malaria prophylaxis: atovaquone/proguanil 1 tab (250 mg/100 mg) once daily with food (beginning 1–2 days before and ending 1 wk after travel).
- Toxoplasmosis (alternative to pyrimethamine + sulfadiazine or clindamycin): atovaquone 1500 mg twice daily with food combined with pyrimethamine 200 mg × 1, then followed by 75 mg/day.

ADVERSE DRUG REACTIONS

General

- Up to 7%–9% discontinued due to side effects with rash accounting for 4% of discontinuations.

Common

- Rash (20%).
- GI intolerance and diarrhea (20%).

Rare

- Stevens-Johnson syndrome reported with malarone (*CID* 2003; 37E5–7).
- Headache.
- Fever.
- Insomnia.
- LFTs elevation and severe hepatitis (atovaquone/proguanil prophylactic use). A single case of hepatic failure requiring liver transplantation has been reported.

DRUG INTERACTIONS

- Atovaquone increased AZT AUC by 31%. Clinical significance unknown. Monitor for AZT ADRs.
- Atovaquone serum levels increased by 70% with food and up to 6-fold with fatty meal.

- ATV/r decreases atovaquone AUC 46%.
- Bactrim: no clinically significant drug interactions.
- EFV decreases atovaquone AUC 75%.
- LPV/r decreased atovaquone AUC 74%.
- Rifabutin decreases atovaquone AUC by 34%.
- Rifampin decreases atovaquone AUC by 50%. Avoid coadministration.
- Tetracycline decreases atovaquone AUC by 40%. Avoid coadministration.

PHARMACOLOGY
Mechanism
- Not well understood but may inhibit mitochondrial electron-transport chain of *Plasmodium falciparum*.

Pharmacokinetic Parameters
- **Absorption**: 47% (liquid formulation) with meals. Significant individual variation in absorption.
- **Metabolism and Excretion**: excreted in the feces; 0.6% renal excretion.
- **Protein Binding**: >99.9%.
- **Cmax, Cmin, and AUC**: Cmax = 24 mcg/mL (suspension).
- **T$_{\frac{1}{2}}$**: 2.2–2.9 days.
- **Distribution**: poor CSF penetration (<1%); Vd = 0.6 L/kg.

Pregnancy Risk
- Category C: not teratogenic in animal studies; no studies in humans.

Breastfeeding Compatibility
- No human data, breast milk excretion in animal studies.

DOSING
Dosing for Decreased Hepatic Function
- No data.

Renal Dosing
- No dose adjustment for renal impairment or dialysis.
- Dosing in hemofiltration: no data.

COMMENTS
- **Pros**: equivalent to dapsone for PCP prophylaxis; Based on CID 33: 1015, 2001 Atovaquone is as effective and better tolerated compared to weekly mefloquine.
- **Cons**: high cost; GI intolerance; needs to be administered with a fatty meal; inferior to TMP/SMX for the treatment of PCP.

SELECTED REFERENCES
Chirgwin K, Hafner R, Leport C, et al. Randomized phase II trial of atovaquone with pyrimethamine or sulfadiazine for treatment of toxoplasmic encephalitis in patients with acquired immunodeficiency syndrome: ACTG 237/ANRS 039 Study. AIDS Clinical Trials Group 237/Agence Nationale de Recherche sur le SIDA, Essai 039. *Clin Infect Dis*, 2002; 34: 1243–50.
Comments: International, noncomparative, randomized phase II trial comparing atovaquone with either pyrimethamine or sulfadiazine for the treatment of toxoplasmosis complicating HIV infection. Atovaquone dose was 1500 mg twice daily, was combined with either pyrimethamine (200 mg × 1 followed by 75 mg/day) or sulfadiazine (1500 mg 4 ×/day). Response rates at 6 wks were 21/28 (75%) in the pyrimethamine and 9/11 (82%) in the sulfadiazine groups, respectively.

El-Sadr WM, Murphy RL, Yurik TM, et al. Atovaquone compared with dapsone for the prevention of *Pneumocystis carinii* pneumonia in patients with HIV infection who cannot tolerate trimethoprim, sulfonamides, or both. Community Program for Clinical Research on AIDS and the AIDS Clinical Trials Group. *N Engl J Med*, 1998; 339: 1889–95.
Comments: Multicenter, open-label, randomized trial comparing once-daily atovaquone (1500 mg suspension) with once daily dapsone (100 mg) for the prevention of PCP in HIV-infected patients who could not tolerate TMP/SMX. Atovaquone was equivalent to dapsone for PCP prevention with 15.7 cases per 100 person-yrs compared to 18.4 cases per 100 person-yrs, respectively. Among patients already on dapsone at baseline, discontinuation rate was higher if they were switched to atovaquone.

Hughes W, Leoung G, Kramer F, et al. Comparison of atovaquone (566C80) with trimethoprim-sulfamethoxazole to treat *Pneumocystis carinii* pneumonia in patients with AIDS. *New Engl J Med*, 1993; 328: 1521–7.
Comments: Prospective, double-blind, multicenter study showing higher failure rates with atovaquone (20% vs 7%) when compared to SMX/TMP in the treatment of PCP.

DRUGS

Kovacs JA. Efficacy of atovaquone in treatment of toxoplasmosis in patients with AIDS. The NIAID-Clinical Center Intramural AIDS Program. *Lancet*, 1992; 340: 637–8.

Comments: Small open-label study involving 8 patients with presumed or biopsy-confirmed toxoplasmosis who were intolerant of or had not responded to standard therapies. Seven patients showed radiographic improvement; the other remained radiographically stable after receiving atovaquone 750 mg 4 ×/day.

AZITHROMYCIN

Paul A. Pham, PharmD and John G. Bartlett, MD

INDICATIONS

FDA

- Treatment and prophylaxis of disseminated *M. avium* complex (MAC) infection (treatment requires coadministration with ethambutol).
- Community-acquired pneumonia (CAP) of mild severity (20%–30% of *S. pneumonia* strains resistant to azithromycin).
- Pharyngitis/tonsillitis; acute bacterial sinusitis.
- Acute bacterial exacerbations of chronic obstructive pulmonary disease (Z-pack and Tri-pack).
- Uncomplicated skin and skin structure infections.
- Urethritis and cervicitis (caused by GC and *C. trachomatis*).
- Genital ulcer disease.

Non-FDA Approved Uses

- Toxoplasmosis (with pyrimethamine).

FORMS TABLE

Brand name (mfr)	Forms†	Cost*
Zithromax and generic azithromycin (Pfizer and generic manufacturers)	PO Z-Pak 6 × 250-mg tabs	$33.36 per pack
	PO Tri-pack 6 × 250-mg tabs	$33.36
	(500 mg × 3days)	$11.12
	PO tablet 250 mg	$15.57; $18.68
	PO tablet 500 mg; 600 mg	$22.24
	IV vial 500 mg	$37.89
	PO powder packet 1 g	$47.08
	PO suspension 100 mg/ 5 mL; 200 mg/5 mL (15 mL)	$67.04
	PO Zmax (SR suspension) 2 g/60 mL	

*Prices represent cost per unit specified, are representative of Average Wholesale Price (AWP).
†Dosage is indicated in mg unless otherwise noted.

USUAL ADULT DOSING

- CAP: *Z-pack* 500 mg 1st day, then 250 mg once daily × 4 days; 500 mg IV once daily or *Zmax* 2 g × 1.
- Acute bacterial sinusitis; acute exacerbations of chronic bronchitis: Tri-pak 500 mg PO daily × 3 days or *Z-pack* 500 mg 1st day, then 250 mg once daily × 4 days or *Zmax* 2 g × 1.
- MAC prophylaxis: 1200 mg (two 600-mg tabs or suspension) qwk.
- MAC treatment: 600 mg once daily + ethambutol 15 mg/kg/day.
- Toxoplasmosis: 900–1200 mg PO once daily + pyrimethamine 200 mg PO × 1, then 50–75 mg PO once daily + leucovorin 10–20 mg once daily × 6 wks, then half dose of each.
- Gonococcal urethritis or cervicitis: 2 g PO × 1 (poor GI tolerability).
- Genital ulcer disease (chancroid) or nongonococcal urethritis (*C. trachomatis*) or cervicitis: 1 g PO × 1.
- Early syphilis: 2 g PO × 1 (poor GI tolerability). High rates of macrolide resistance reported in San Francisco (*CID* 2006; 42: 337).

ADVERSE DRUG REACTIONS

Common

- GI intolerance: diarrhea, nausea, and abdominal pain in up to 14% of patients.

Occasional

- Reversible dose-dependent hearing loss in 5% with mean exposure of 59 g.

Rare

- Erythema multiforme.
- Vaginitis.
- Transaminase elevation.
- Taste/smell perversion and/or loss.
- Exacerbations of myasthenia gravis.

DRUG INTERACTIONS

- Unlike other macrolides, azithromycin does not significantly inhibit CYP3A4.
- Cyclosporin: close monitoring of cyclosporine levels is indicated. Azithromycin did not affect cyclosporine in report of 6 patients.
- Pimozide: avoid concurrent administration due to potential for QTc prolongation and cardiac arrhythmia.
- Theophylline: serum levels of theophylline may be increased. Monitor theophylline levels with coadministration.
- Warfarin: INR may be increased with coadministration. Monitor INR closely.
- No significant interactions with PIs, NNRTIs, RAL, MVC, and ENF.

RESISTANCE

- *S. pneumoniae* resistance increasing (~25%). Resistance may not correlate with clinical failure when macrolides are used to treat ambulatory respiratory tract infections.
- Group A strep resistance increasing. Up to 35% of pharyngeal isolates in children were resistant (*AAC* 2004; 48: 473).
- Breakpoint for *Streptococcus* spp.: <0.5 mcg/mL (sensitive); 1 mcg/mL (intermediate); >2 mcg/mL (resistant).
- Breakpoint for *Haemophilus* spp.: <4 mcg/mL.

PHARMACOLOGY

Mechanism

- Macrolides inhibit protein synthesis by binding to 50S ribosomal subunits, inhibiting translocation of peptidase chain and polypeptide synthesis. The addition of nitrogen at position 9a of the lactone ring gives azithromycin improved resistance to acid degradation, improved tissue penetration, and activity against Gram-negative organisms and a longer elimination half-life.

Pharmacokinetic Parameters

- **Absorption:** 37% absorbed (although food improves tolerability, 600-mg tab and 1-g powder packet may be taken without regard for food).
- **Metabolism and Excretion:** demethylation of 35% of administered dose to inactive metabolites. Up to 10 inactive metabolites identified. Biliary excretion of active drug and inactive metabolites.
- **Protein Binding:** 10%–50% (concentration dependent; the lower the serum levels the higher the protein binding).
- **Cmax, Cmin, and AUC:** 0.4 mcg/mL 2 hr after 500-mg PO dose administration (on day 5 of therapy). 3.63 mcg/mL 1 hr after 500 mg IV administration (on day 5 of therapy).
- **T$_{\frac{1}{2}}$:** serum: 12 hrs; intracellular: 68 hrs.
- **Distribution:** distributed throughout the body. Concentrated intracellularly, resulting in tissue concentration 10–100 × those found in serum. Highly concentrated in fibroblasts and phagocytes. Poor CNS penetration, but good brain tissue concentration (2.63–3.64 mcg/g).

Pregnancy Risk

- Category B: animal studies show no harm to the fetus. No human data available.

Breastfeeding Compatibility

- Accumulates in breast milk. The American Academy of Pediatrics considers erythromycin compatible with breastfeeding. No recommendation has been made for azithromycin.

DRUGS

DOSING

Dosing for Decreased Hepatic Function
• No dose adjustment.

Renal Dosing
• Dosing for GFR of 50–80: usual dose.
• Dosing for GFR of <50: no data, but probably usual dose likely due to high biliary excretion.
• Dosing in hemodialysis: HD: no data, but usual dose likely.
• Dosing in peritoneal dialysis: usual regimen.
• Dosing in hemofiltration: no data.

COMMENTS

• Indicated for MAC prophylaxis and treatment in HIV-infected patients. Clarithromycin may have a slight advantage over azithromycin in terms of MAC Cx clearance. Unlike other macrolides, not likely to interact with PIs and NNRTIs. Significance of rising macrolide-resistance in *S. pneumoniae* (~25% US isolates) of uncertain clinical significance for the treatment of ambulatory respiratory tract infections.

SELECTED REFERENCES

Vergis EN, Indorf A, File TM, et al. Azithromycin vs cefuroxime plus erythromycin for empirical treatment of community-acquired pneumonia in hospitalized patients: a prospective, randomized, multicenter trial. *Arch Intern Med*, 2000; 160: 1294–300.
Comments: Therapeutic trial of antibiotics for CAP showed predictable difference in rate of adverse reactions, especially with erythromycin.

Dunne M, Fessel J, Kumar P, et al. A randomized, double-blind trial comparing azithromycin and clarithromycin in the treatment of disseminated *Mycobacterium avium* infection in patients with human immunodeficiency virus. *Clin Infect Dis*, 2000; 31: 1245–52.
Comments: Large prospective trial showing equivalence between azithromycin and clarithromycin (both with ethambutol) against disseminated MAC infection.

Ward TT, Rimland D, Kauffman C, et al. Randomized, open-label trial of azithromycin plus ethambutol vs. clarithromycin plus ethambutol as therapy for *Mycobacterium avium* complex bacteremia in patients with human immunodeficiency virus infection. Veterans Affairs HIV Research Consortium. *Clin Infect Dis*, 1998; 27: 1278–85.
Comments: Clearance of bacteremia seen at final visit in 37.5% of azithromycin-treated patients and in 85.7% of clarithromycin-treated patients (P = 0.007). Estimated median time to clearance of bacteremia also significantly different between 2 treatment arms: 4.38 wks for clarithromycin recipients vs >16 wks for azithromycin recipients (P = 0.0018), but abatement of Sx and adverse effects were similar in the two groups.

Thorpe EM, Stamm WE, Hook EW, et al. Chlamydial cervicitis and urethritis: single dose treatment compared with doxycycline for seven days in community based practises. *Genitourin Med*, 1996; 72: 93–7.
Comments: Azithromycin has advantage of potential for single-dose observed therapy. A comparative trial with doxycycline for PID showed that azithromycin was significantly better, presumably due to reduced adherence with doxycycline. Doxycycline contraindicated in pregnancy, though azithromycin's safety in pregnancy has not been established; erythromycin has been shown to be safe in pregnancy.

Havlir DV, Dube MP, Sattler FR, et al. Prophylaxis against disseminated *Mycobacterium avium* complex with weekly azithromycin, daily rifabutin, or both. California Collaborative Treatment Group. *N Engl J Med*, 1996; 335: 392–8.
Comments: Therapy of choice for prevention of MAC in HIV+ patients. Convenience of weekly administration and good therapeutic efficacy. Main issue concerns the relative merits of clarithromycin vs azithromycin for MAC prophylaxis. These drugs have not been directly compared, but appear equally effective. Many prefer azithromycin based on convenience of weekly vs twice-daily dosing and cost (AWP $26/wk azithromycin vs $42/wk clarithromycin).

Moran JS, Levine WC. Drugs of choice for the treatment of uncomplicated gonococcal infections. *Clin Infect Dis*, 1995; 20 (suppl 1): S47–65.
Comments: Major reason for interest in use of azithromycin for GC is to permit simultaneous treatment of *C. trachomatis*. Dose required for GC efficacy was associated with GI toxicity and substantial increase in price.

Young LS, Wiviott L, Wu M, et al. Azithromycin for treatment of *Mycobacterium avium-intracellulare* complex infection in patients with AIDS. *Lancet*, 1991; 338: 1107–9.
Comments: Clinical data support use of clarithromycin in combination with ethambutol for the treatment of disseminated MAC; azithromycin is effective alternative to clarithromycin.

CIDOFOVIR

Paul A. Pham, PharmD and John G. Bartlett, MD

INDICATIONS
FDA
- Treatment of CMV retinitis in patients with AIDS.

Non-FDA Approved Uses
- Treatment of CMV colitis and pneumonitis (efficacy not established).

FORMS TABLE

Brand name (mfr)	Forms†	Cost*
Vistide (Gilead Pharmaceuticals)	IV vial 375 mg (75 mg/mL)	$888.00

*Prices represent cost per unit specified, are representative of Average Wholesale Price (AWP).
†Dosage is indicated in mg unless otherwise noted.

USUAL ADULT DOSING
- CMV retinitis-induction: 5 mg/kg IV over 1 hr weekly × 2; maintenance: 5 mg/kg IV over 1 hr q2wks.
- Give probenecid 2 g given 3 hrs prior to cidofovir and 1 g given 2 and 8 hrs after infusion (blocks tubular secretion of cidofovir). Prehydrate with >1L NS immediately before cidofovir infusion; cidofovir is diluted in 100 mL 9% saline.

ADVERSE DRUG REACTIONS
Common
- Dose-dependent nephrotoxicity in ~25% (proteinuria, azotemia, and proximal tubular dysfunction). Increased w/ other nephrotoxins, reduced w/ prehydration and probenecid. Monitor renal function 48 hrs prior to each dose.
- GI intolerance, rash, fever, and chills due to high dose probenecid (reduced by antiemetics, antihistamines, antipyretics, and food intake).

Occasional
- GI intolerance.
- Neutropenia (15%); monitor neutrophil count.
- Metabolic acidosis with Fanconi syndrome: proteinuria, normoglycemic glycosuria, hypophosphatemia, and hypouricemia.

Rare
- Uveitis and ocular hypotony.
- Asthenia.

DRUG INTERACTIONS
- Contraindicated with other nephrotoxic drugs: aminoglycoside, amphotericin B, foscarnet, NSAIDs, and pentamidine. One-wk washout recommended before cidofovir administration. Probenecid inhibits tubular secretion of acyclovir, beta-lactam antibiotics, AZT, and TDF; clinical significance unclear without prolonged coadministration.

PHARMACOLOGY
Mechanism
- Cidofovir converted intracellularly by host enzymes to cidofovir diphosphate, which inhibits viral DNA polymerase.

Pharmacokinetic Parameters
- **Absorption:** n/a.
- **Metabolism and Excretion:** 80%–100% of drug excreted unchanged in urine within 24 hrs.
- **Protein Binding:** low protein binding (0.5%).
- **Cmax, Cmin, and AUC:** 19.6 mcg/mL after 5 mg/kg administration.
- **$T_{\frac{1}{2}}$:** active intracellular metabolite: 17–65 hrs.
- **Distribution:** CSF: limited data; undetectable CSF concentrations in one case report.

Pregnancy Risk
- Category C: carcinogenic, teratogenic, and causes hypospermia in animal studies; no human data available.

DRUGS

Breastfeeding Compatibility
• No data: avoid due to potential for severe toxicity.

DOSING
Dosing for Decreased Hepatic Function
• No data. Usual dose likely.

Renal Dosing
• Dosing for GFR of 55–80: 5 mg/kg.
• Dosing for GFR <55: contraindicated (or with for serum Cr >1.5 mg/dL).
• Dosing in hemodialysis: 52% ± 11% cleared during high-flux hemodialysis. (*Clin Pharm Ther* 1999; 65: 21–8). Dose post-HD.
• Dosing in peritoneal dialysis: not significantly cleared.
• Dosing in hemofiltration: no data.

COMMENTS
• With the availability of ganciclovir ocular implant and oral valganciclovir, cidofovir now considered 2nd- or 3rd-line agent for treatment of CMV retinitis. Advantage of q2wk dosing and activity against ganciclovir-resistant CMV, but nephrotoxicity and probenecid side effects (chills, fever, headache, rash, and nausea in 30%–50% of patients) limit routine use.

SELECTED REFERENCES
Lalezari JP, Holland GN, Kramer F, et al. Randomized, controlled study of the safety and efficacy of intravenous cidofovir for the treatment of relapsing cytomegalovirus retinitis in patients with AIDS. *J Acquir Immune Defic Syndr Hum Retrovirol*, 1998; 17: 339–44.
Comments: Proteinuria and elevations in serum Cr developed in 39% and 24% of participants, respectively. Though effective, cidofovir is not considered a preferred agent for CMV retinitis due to nephrotoxicity and availability of ganciclovir implant. GI side effects of probenecid coadministration have proven frequent and bothersome.

Lalezari J, Schacker T, Feinberg J, et al. A randomized, double-blind, placebo-controlled trial of cidofovir gel for the treatment of acyclovir-unresponsive mucocutaneous herpes simplex virus infection in patients with AIDS. *J Infect Dis*, 1997; 176: 892–8.
Comments: Cidofovir gel not commercially available but can be compounded using the IV formulation. Topical cidofovir offers a therapeutic alternative to patients who are intolerant to foscarnet. Anecdotal reports showing clinical response to topical cidofovir in the treatment of resistant HSV that has failed IV foscarnet.

CIPROFLOXACIN

Paul A. Pham, PharmD and John G. Bartlett, MD

INDICATIONS
FDA
• Uncomplicated UTI (ciprofloxacin XR and ciprofloxacin), complicated UTI (ciprofloxacin).
• Postexposure prophylaxis for inhalation anthrax. CDC recommends as 1st-line agent + 1–2 additional agent(s) with *in vitro* activity.
• Complicated intraabdominal infections (in combination with metronidazole).
• Infectious diarrhea.
• Endocervical and urethral infections caused *N. gonorrhoeae* (Empiric treatment with Fluoroquinolones no longer recommened due to high resistance rates).
• Empiric therapy for neutropenic fever (in combination with piperacillin); typhoid fever.
• Nosocomial pneumonia.
• Prostatitis.
• Acute sinusitis.
• Skin and soft tissue infections; bone and joint infections: (1) bacterial conjunctivitis (ophthalmic ointment); (2) bacterial conjuctivitis and corneal ulcers (ophthalmic soln); (3) acute otitis externa (otic suspension).

Non-FDA Approved Uses
• Tuberculosis, MAC, and other atypical mycobacterial infections (2nd or 3rd line).

FORMS TABLE

Brand name (mfr)	Forms†	Cost*
Cipro and generics (Bayer and generics [Barr Pharmaceuticals, Eon Pharmaceuticals])	Oral tablet 250 mg; 500 mg; 750 mg IV vial 200 mg IV vial 400 mg Oral tablet 100 mg (6 pack) Oral XR tablet 500 mg; 1000 mg	$4.59; $5.37; $5.62 $14.40 $28.80 $13.55 $10.46; $11.91
Ciprodex (Alcon Labs)	Otic suspension 7.5 mL	$126.48
Cipro HC Otic (Alcon Labs)	Otic suspension 10 mL	$126.48
Ciloxan (Alcon Labs)	Topical ophthalmic soln 2.5 mL; 5 mL; 10 mL Topical ophthalmic ointment 3.5 g	$22.30 per 2.5 mL; $66.66 per 5 mL; $90.33 per 10 mL $86.52

*Prices represent cost per unit specified, are representative of Average Wholesale Price (AWP).
†Dosage is indicated in mg unless otherwise noted.

USUAL ADULT DOSING
- Uncomplicated UTI: 250 mg PO twice daily or ciprofloxacin XR 500 mg once daily PO × 3 days.
- Complicated UTI: 500 mg PO twice daily × 7–10 days.
- Nosocomial pneumonia (*P. aeruginosa*): 400 mg IV q8h, then 750 mg PO twice daily × 10–14 days.
- Endocervical and urethral infection caused by N. gonorrhoeae: Fluoroquinolones no longer recommended due to increasing resistance.
- Salmonellosis: 500–750 mg PO twice daily or 400 mg IV twice daily × 7–14 days for mild disease or 4–6 wks for CD4 <200 and/or bacteremia.
- Traveler's diarrhea: 500 mg PO twice daily × 3 days.
- Tuberculosis, MAC, and other atypical mycobacteria: 750 mg PO twice daily.
- Milk or dairy products decreases GI absorption of ciprofloxacin by 36%–47%. Administer ciprofloxacin 2 hrs before dairy products.

ADVERSE DRUG REACTIONS
General
- Generally well tolerated.

Occasional
- GI intolerance: nausea and diarrhea.
- CNS: headache, malaise, insomnia, restlessness, and dizziness.
- *Candida* vaginitis.
- *C. difficile*-associated colitis.

Rare
- Tendon rupture (increased incidence especially seen in patients over age 60, concurrent use of corticosteroids, kidney, heart, and lung transplant recipients).
- Photosensitivity/phototoxicity reaction (can be severe).
- Allergic reactions (fever and rash).
- QTc prolongation.
- Transaminases elevation and rare cases of hepatic failure.
- Peripheral neuropathy.
- Crystalluria.
- Seizure.
- Severe allergic reactions (TEN, Stevens-Johnsons syndrome, allergic pneumonitis, hepatitis, and bone marrow suppression).
- Interstitial nephritis.

DRUGS

Drug-Drug Interactions—See Appendix I, p. 491, for table of drug-drug interactions.

Pharmacology

Mechanism

- Fluoroquinolones inhibits DNA topoisomerases (DNA gyrase and topoisomerase 4) by binding to DNA-enzyme complexes, thereby interfering with bacterial DNA replication and some aspects of transcription, repair, recombination, and transposition.

Pharmacokinetic Parameters

- **Absorption:** 50%–85% absorbed. Not significantly affected by food.
- **Metabolism and Excretion:** 10%–15% of dose is metabolized to desethylene, sulfo, oxo, N-formyl active metabolite. Metabolite and 15%–50% of unchanged drug is excreted in urine by glomerular filtration and tubular secretion. 20%–40% of dose excreted in feces mainly by biliary excretion.
- **Protein Binding:** 13%–43%.
- **Cmax, Cmin, and AUC:** Cmax: 2.5–4.3 mcg/mL after 750 mg PO dose administration and 4.6 mcg/mL after 400 mg IV dose administration.
- **$T_{\frac{1}{2}}$:** 4 hrs.
- **Distribution:** fluoroquinolones are widely distributed to most body fluids and tissues. High concentrations are attained in the kidneys, gallbladder, GYN tissues, liver, lung, prostatic tissue, phagocytic cells, urine, sputum, bile, skin, fat, muscle, bone and cartilage. CNS penetration: 11%–67% with inflamed meninges (consider higher dose for CNS infections 400 mg IV q8h).

Pregnancy Risk

- Category C: in prospective follow-up study conducted by European Network of Teratology Information Services (ENTIS), 666 cases of fluoroquinolone exposure (majority of exposures during 1st trimester) showed congenital malformation rate of 4.8%. From previous epidemiologic data, 4.8% did not exceed the background rate. Animal data demonstrated arthropathy in immature animals with erosions in joint cartilage. Because of animal data and availability of alternative antimicrobial agents, use of fluoroquinolones during pregnancy contraindicated due to concerns about arthropathy.

Breastfeeding Compatibility

- Fluoroquinolones not recommended during breastfeeding due to potential for arthropathy (based on animal data).

Dosing

Dosing for Decreased Hepatic Function

- No data. Usual dose likely.

Renal Dosing

- Dosing for GFR of 50–80: usual dose.
- Dosing for GFR of >30: 0.4 g IV q12h (0.25–0.5 g PO q12h).
- Dosing for GFR <30: 0.4 g IV q24h (0.25–0.5 g PO q12h).
- Dosing for GFR of <10: 0.4 g IV q24h (0.25–0.5 g PO q24h).
- Dosing in hemodialysis: 0.2–0.4 g IV q24h (0.25–0.5 g PO q24h). Give post-HD on days of dialysis.
- Dosing in peritoneal dialysis: 0.2–0.4 g IV q24h (0.25–0.5 g PO q24h).
- Dosing in hemofiltration: CVVH: 200 mg IV q12h; CVVHD: 400 mg q12h.

Comments

- Oral and parenteral fluoroquinolone with best clinical and *in vitro* data for activity against *P. aeruginosa*, but resistance rates have increased over the years. Experience is favorable and extensive for nosocomial pneumonia, osteomyelitis, neutropenic fever, traveler's diarrhea, chronic prostatitis, and UTIs.
- Other fluoroquinolones (e.g., levofloxacin and moxifloxacin) preferred for infections due to *S. pneumoniae*.
- Ciprofloxacin may be used as 3rd- or 4th-line agent for MDR-TB and MAC infections in HIV+ patients (moxifloxacin preferred).
- Like other fluoroquinolones, ciprofloxacin may result in false positive opiate screen (*JAMA* 2001; 286: 3115–9).

SELECTED REFERENCES

Ho PL, Que TL, Chiu SS, et al. Fluoroquinolone and other antimicrobial resistance in invasive pneumococci, Hong Kong, 1995–2001. *Emerg Infect Dis*, 2004; 10: 1250–7.

Comments: In 265 invasive isolates of pneumococci obtained during 1995–2001, prevalence of levofloxacin resistance (MIC ≥8 µg/mL) was 3.8% but increased to 15.2% among PNC-resistant isolates. Resistance to levofloxacin and other fluoroquinolones remains low in the US but is a concern with widespread use.

Centers for Disease Control and Prevention (CDC). Fluoroquinolone-resistance in *Neisseria gonorrhoeae*, Hawaii, 1999, and decreased susceptibility to azithromycin in *N. gonorrhoeae*, Missouri, 1999. *MMWR Morb Mortal Wkly Rep*, 2000; 49: 833–7.

Comments: A review of *N. gonorrhoeae* isolates from health departments in Hawaii showed an increased rate of ciprofloxacin-resistance from 4/290 (1.4%) in 1997 to 22/231 (9.5%) in 1999. This report also showed a cluster of 12 men with gonorrhea had GC isolates showing reduced susceptibility to azithromycin; these strains had a median MIC of 2.0 µg/mL and were susceptible to spectinomycin, ciprofloxacin, and penicillin. Physicians are warned that patients who may have acquired GC in Asia or in Hawaii should be treated with ceftriaxone or cefixime.

Talan DA, Stamm WE, Hooton TM, et al. Comparison of ciprofloxacin (7 days) and trimethoprim-sulfamethoxazole (14 days) for acute uncomplicated pyelonephritis pyelonephritis in women: a randomized trial. *JAMA*, 2000; 283: 1583–90.

Comments: Ciprofloxacin for 7 days was associated with superior bacteriologic and clinical cure rates compared to TMP-SMX given for 14 days. Presumed explanation for differences is escalating resistance of *E. coli* to TMP-SMX. Rate of resistance by *E. coli* to TMP-SMX was 18% vs ciprofloxacin at 0%. There was correlation between *in vitro* sensitivity of *E. coli* and outcome by both Cx and clinical evaluation.

DRUGS

CLARITHROMYCIN

Paul A. Pham, PharmD and John G. Bartlett, MD

INDICATIONS

FDA

- Pharyngitis and tonsillitis.
- Acute maxillary sinusitis.
- Acute bacterial exacerbation of chronic bronchitis.
- Community-acquired pneumonia.
- Acute otitis media.
- Uncomplicated skin and skin structure infections.
- Treatment of disseminated mycobacterial infections due to complex.
- Prophylaxis of *Mycobacterium avium* complex.
- Treatment of active duodenal ulcer associated with *H. pylori* infection (in combination with omeprazole or ranitidine bismuth citrate; amoxicillin and lansoprazole or omeprazole as triple therapy).

Non-FDA Approved Uses

- *Bartonella* infection.

FORMS TABLE

Brand name (mfr)	Forms†	Cost*
Biaxin (Abbott Pharmaceuticals, Ranbaxy Pharmaceuticals)	Oral tablet 250 mg; 500 mg Oral suspension 125 mg/5 mL (50 mL and 100-mL bottle) Oral suspension 250 mg/5 mL (50-mL and 100-mL bottle)	$6.08; $6.87 $25.60 (50-mL bottle); $52.57 (100-mL bottle) $44.28 (50-mL bottle); $100.24 (100-mL bottle)
Biaxin XL (Abbott Pharmaceuticals)	Oral XL tablet 500 mg	$6.51

FORMS TABLE (*Continued*)

Brand name (mfr)	Forms†	Cost*
Clarithromycin (Various generic manufacturers)	Oral tablet 250 mg; 500 mg Oral suspension 125 mg/5 mL (50-mL and 100-mL bottle) Oral suspension 250 mg/5 mL (50-mL and 100-mL bottle)	$4.52 23.70 (50-mL bottle); $48.50 (100-mL bottle) $41.10 (50-mL bottle); $82.91 (100-mL bottle)

*Prices represent cost per unit specified, are representative of Average Wholesale Price (AWP).
†Dosage is indicated in mg unless otherwise noted.

USUAL ADULT DOSING
- MAC prophylaxis: 500 mg PO twice daily (azithromycin 1200 mg weekly preferred).
- MAC treatment: 500 mg PO twice daily or 1000 mg XL once daily (in combination with ethambutol) × 1 yr and treat until immune reconstitution (CD4 >100 × 6 mos).
- Infections due to *H influenzae* and *H. parainfluenzae:* 500 mg twice daily × 7–14 days.
- Community-acquired pneumonia, pharyngitis, tonsillitis, otitis media, and uncomplicated soft tissue infections: 250–500 mg twice daily or 1000 mg XL once daily × 7 days.
- Peptic ulcer disease due to *H. pylori*: 500 mg in combination with PPI and amoxicillin twice daily × 10–14 days.
- Acute bacterial sinusitis: 500 mg twice daily or 1000 mg XL once daily w/ food × 7–14 days.
- Acute exacerbation of chronic bronchitis: 500 mg twice daily or 1000 mg XL once daily with food × 7 days.
- Take clarithromycin XL with food.

ADVERSE DRUG REACTIONS
Occasional
- GI intolerance (diarrhea, nausea, vomiting).
- Metallic taste.
- Transaminases elevation.

Rare
- Headache.
- Reversible hearing loss and tinnitus.
- *C. difficile* colitis.
- Rash.
- Exacerbations of myasthenia gravis.

DRUG INTERACTIONS
- Alfuzosin, ranolazine, pimozide, cisapride, astemizole, and terfenadine: contraindicated.
- Amiodarone: may increase amiodarone serum levels. Monitor closely with proper dose adjustment.
- ATV: ATV AUC increased by 28%. Clarithromycin AUC increased by 94%. QTc prolongation observed with coadministration. 50% of clarithromycin dose recommended when coadministered with ATV. Use azithromycin. Further dose adjustment needed with moderate to severe renal insufficiency and ESRD, no specific dosing guidelines. Consider: CrCl 30–60 mL/min: 250 mg q24h. CrCl <30 mL/min: 250 mg every other day.
- Benzodiazepines (alprazolam, diazepam, midazolam, triazolam): may increase benzodiazepines serum concentrations. Use alternative benzodiazepines (i.e., lorazepam, oxazepam, temazepam).
- Carbamazepine: carbamazepine serum levels increased by 60%. Avoid or use with close monitoring of carbamazepine levels with appropriate dose adjustment.
- Clarithromycin is a substrate and inhibitor of CYP3A4.
- Cyclosporine: may increase cyclosporine serum levels. Monitor closely.
- Digoxin: case reports of digoxin toxicity. Monitor closely with coadministration.
- DRV/r: clarithromycin did not affect DRV AUC, but DRV increases clarithromycin AUC by 57%. Adjust clarithromycin dose according to renal function: CrCl >60 mL/min = 500 mg twice daily; CrCl 30–60 mL/min = 500 mg PO once daily; CrCl <30 mL/min = 250 mg PO once daily. Consider azithromycin.

- EFV: clarithromycin AUC decreased by 39%. Clinical significance unknown. High incidence of rash seen in healthy volunteer receiving this combination. Consider azithromycin.
- Ergot alkaloid: avoid coadministration.
- ETR: clarithromycin AUC decreased 39%, but active OH-clarithromycin increased 21%. ETR AUC increased 42%. Consider azithromycin for MAC infection.
- Fentanyl: may significantly increase fentanyl serum concentrations. Avoid coadministration. Consider morphine.
- FPV: APV AUC increased by 18% (studied with APV). No dose adjustment needed. See RTV for dose adjustment with FPV/r.
- IDV: clarithromycin AUC increased 53% and IDV AUC increased 29%. Reduce clarithromycin dose by 50% in end-stage renal disease.
- Lovastatin and simvastatin: may significantly increase lovastatin and simvastatin serum concentrations. Consider pravastatin with coadministration.
- LPV/r: may increase clarithromycin serum level. Decrease dose of clarithromycin by 50% in ESRD.
- MVC: clarithromycin serum concentrations not affected. MVC may be increased. Dose: MVC 150 mg twice daily.
- NFV: no data.
- NVP: clarithromycin AUC decreased by 29% but 14-hydroxy clarithromycin (active metabolite) AUC increased by 27%. NVP AUC increased by 26%. No dose adjustment needed.
- RAL: interaction unlikely. Use standard dose.
- Rifabutin: clarithromycin AUC decreased by 44% and 14-hydroxy-clarithromycin increased by 57%. 14-hydroxy metabolite has less activity against MAC. Rifabutin AUC increased by 56%. Consider using azithromycin.
- Rifampin: contraindicated.
- RTV: clarithromycin AUC increased by 77%, Cmin increased by 182%. Reduce clarithromycin dose by 50% in end-stage renal disease. Consider using azithromycin.
- SQV: clarithromycin increases SQV AUC by 177% and SQV increases clarithromycin AUC by 45%. See RTV for dose adjustment with SQV/r.
- Tacrolimus, sirolimus, cyclosporine: may significantly increase immunosuppressants serum concentrations. Monitor closely with dose adjustments.
- Theophylline: may increase theophylline serum levels. Monitor serum level with dose adjustment.
- TPV/r: clarithromycin increases TPV AUC by 66% and TPV/r increases clarithromycin AUC by 19%. Adjust clarithromycin dose according to renal function: CrCl >60 mL/min = 500 mg twice daily; CrCl 30–60 mL/min = 500 mg PO once daily; CrCl <30 mL/min = 250 mg PO once daily. Consider azithromycin.
- Warfarin: may increase anticoagulant effect of warfarin. Monitor INR closely.

DRUG-DRUG INTERACTIONS—See Appendix I, p. 492, for table of drug-drug interactions.

RESISTANCE

- *S. pneumoniae* macrolide resistance ~26% but clinical significance unclear (especially with intermediate resistance); treatment failures reported.
- Use of clarithromycin monotherapy for MAC infection in HIV associated with high rates of resistance. Combination therapy (usually with ethambutol ± rifabutin) recommended. Drug sensitivity testing may help guide therapy but clinical significance unclear.
- Clarithromycin resistant *H. pylori* reported in up to 20% of *H.pylori* isolates and is associated with treatment failure.
- Group A strep resistance increasing. Up to 35% of pharyngeal isolates in children were resistant (*AAC* 2004; 48: 473).
- Breakpoint for *Haemophilus* spp.: <8 mcg/mL (sensitive); 16 mcg/mL (intermediate); >32 mcg/mL (resistant).
- Breakpoint for *Streptococcus* spp.: <0.25 mcg/mL (sensitive); 0.5 mcg/mL (intermediate); >1 mcg/mL (resistant).

PHARMACOLOGY

Mechanism

- Macrolides inhibit protein synthesis by binding to 50S ribosomal subunits, inhibiting translocation of peptidase chain and inhibiting polypeptide synthesis. Clarithromycin is methylated at position 6 of the lactone ring; this minimizes acid-catalyzed degradation of clarithromycin.

DRUGS

Pharmacokinetic Parameters
- **Absorption:** 55% absorbed.
- **Metabolism and Excretion:** clarithromycin undergoes extensive 1st-pass metabolism to the active 14-hydroxy metabolite. Both active metabolite and unchanged drug is excreted in urine (38%) and feces (40%).
- **Protein Binding:** 42%–72%.
- **Cmax, Cmin, and AUC:** Cmax: 2–3 mcg/mL after 500 mg PO dose administration.
- **T$_{\frac{1}{2}}$:** 5–7 hrs.
- **Distribution:** clarithromycin and 14-hydroxyclarithromycin has high intracellular concentration, resulting in higher tissue concentration than serum concentration. Poor CNS penetration.

Pregnancy Risk
- Category C: studies in monkeys show growth retardation. Teratogen Information Service in Philadelphia reported the outcome of 34 1st- or 2nd-trimester exposure were similar to those expected in nonexposed population.

Breastfeeding Compatibility
- Excreted into breast milk. The American Academy of Pediatrics considers erythromycin compatible with breastfeeding. Risk to clarithromycin exposure probably minimal.

DOSING

Dosing for Decreased Hepatic Function
- No dose adjustment needed. May require dosage adjustment with concomitant renal dysfunction (*J Clin Pharmacol* 1993; 33: 480).

Renal Dosing
- Dosing for GFR of 50–80: usual dose.
- Dosing for GFR of 10–50: 50% of dose (500 mg q24h) with CrCl <30; especially important with boosted-PI coadministration.
- Dosing for GFR of <10: 0.25–0.5 g q24h.
- Dosing in hemodialysis: 500 mg once daily; on days of dialysis dose post-dialysis.
- Dosing in peritoneal dialysis: no data. Consider 250–500 mg PO q24h.
- Dosing in hemofiltration: no data. Consider 500 mg PO q24h.

COMMENTS

- Clarithromycin important component in treatment of MAC (see p. 23) and other MOTT infections.
- More active than azithromycin against MAC and is preferred macrolide for treatment of disseminated MAC infection, but azithromycin can be considered if intolerant to clarithromycin.
- Weekly azithromycin preferred for MAC prophylaxis because of weekly dosing and lower cost.

SELECTED REFERENCES

Benson CA, Williams PL, Currier JS, et al. A prospective, randomized trial examining the efficacy and safety of clarithromycin in combination with ethambutol, rifabutin, or both for the treatment of disseminated *Mycobacterium avium* complex disease in persons with acquired immunodeficiency syndrome. *Clin Infect Dis*, 2003; 37: 1234–43.
Comments: Safety and efficacy of clarithromycin + ethambutol vs clarithromycin + rifabutin vs clarithromycin + rifabutin + ethambutol was compared in this prospective trial. After 12 wks of treatment, proportion of subjects with complete microbiologic response similar between 3 groups. Subjects in clarithromycin + rifabutin + ethambutol group had improved survival compared with clarithromycin + ethambutol group (HR 0.44; 95% CI, 0.23–0.83).

Dunne M, Fessel J, Kumar P, et al. A randomized, double-blind trial comparing azithromycin and clarithromycin in the treatment of disseminated *Mycobacterium avium* infection in patients with human immunodeficiency virus. *Clin Infect Dis*, 2000; 31: 1245–52.
Comments: Large prospective trial showing equivalency between azithromycin and clarithromycin (both with ethambutol) against disseminated MAC infection.

Ward TT, Rimland D, Kauffman C, et al. Randomized, open-label trial of azithromycin + ethambutol vs clarithromycin + ethambutol as therapy for *Mycobacterium avium* complex bacteremia in patients with human immunodeficiency virus infection. Veterans Affairs HIV Research Consortium. *Clin Infect Dis*, 1998; 27: 1278–85.
Comments: Clearance of bacteremia seen in 37.5% and in 85.7% of azithromycin and clarithromycin-treated patients, respectively (P = 0.007). Estimated median time to clearance of bacteremia was also significantly different between 2 treatment arms: 4.38 wks for clarithromycin vs >16 wks for azithromycin (P = 0.0018), but abatement of Sx and ADR similar in 2 groups.

Pierce M, Crampton S, Henry D, et al. A randomized trial of clarithromycin as prophylaxis against disseminated *Mycobacterium avium* complex infection in patients with advanced acquired immunodeficiency syndrome. *N Engl J Med*, 1996; 335: 384–91.
Comments: Clarithromycin effective in prevention of *M. avium* disease and decreases mortality, but azithromycin preferred due to weekly dosing and lower cost.

Chaisson RE, Benson CA, Dube MP, et al. Clarithromycin therapy for bacteremic *Mycobacterium avium* complex disease. A randomized, double-blind, dose-ranging study in patients with AIDS. AIDS Clinical Trials Group Protocol 157 Study Team. *Ann Intern Med*, 1994; 121: 905–11.
Comments: ACTG trial that provided foundation for current guidelines for treatment of disseminated MAC.

CLINDAMYCIN

Paul A. Pham, PharmD and John G. Bartlett, MD

DRUGS

INDICATIONS
FDA
- Skin and soft tissue infections caused by streptococci, staphylococci, and anaerobes.
- Pelvic infections (endometritis, nongonococcal tubo-ovarian abscess, pelvic cellulitis, and postsurgical vaginal cuff infections).
- *Streptococcus pneumoniae* (empyema, pneumonitis, and lung abscess).
- Septicemia (no longer recommended).
- Intraabdominal infections such as peritonitis and intraabdominal abscess caused by anaerobes (note: IDSA no longer recommends clindamycin due to increased *B. fragilis* resistance rate).
- Acne vulgaris (topical gel).
- Bacterial vaginosis in nonpregnant women (vaginal ovules).

Non-FDA Approved Uses
- PCP in combination with primaquine.
- CNS toxoplasmosis in combination with pyrimethamine and leucovorin.
- Bacterial vaginosis (oral and vaginal ovule).
- Community-acquired MRSA (CA-MRSA) soft tissue infections.
- Osteomyelitis.
- Actinomycosis.
- Acute bacterial sinusitis.
- CA-MRSA pneumonia in combination with vancomycin to reduce toxin production in severe cases.

FORMS TABLE

Brand name (mfr)	Forms†	Cost*
Cleocin (Pfizer)	Oral capsule 150 mg; 300 mg IV vial 300 mg; 600 mg; 900 mg	$1.20; $3.76 $5.06; $9.16; $13.28
Cleocin pediatric soln (Pfizer)	Oral soln 75 mg/5 mL	$61.10 (100 mL)
Cleocin vaginal suppository (Pfizer)	Vaginal ovule suppository 100 mg	$23.51
Cleocin T (Pfizer)	Topical gel 1% (30 g; 60 g) Topical lotion 1% (60 mL)	$62.76; $113.03 $87.33 (60 mL)
Clindamycin (Various generic manufacturers)	Oral capsule 150 mg; 300 mg	$1.15; $3.70

*Prices represent cost per unit specified, are representative of Average Wholesale Price (AWP).
†Dosage is indicated in mg unless otherwise noted.

USUAL ADULT DOSING

- PCP: clindamycin 600 mg IV q6–8h or 300–450 mg PO q6–8h + primaquine 15–30 mg PO once daily (base) ± prednisone (recommended for PO <70) × 21 days.
- CNS toxoplasmosis: clindamycin 600 mg IV q6h or clindamycin 600 mg PO q6h + pyrimethamine 200 mg PO loading dose, then 50–75 mg PO once daily + leucovorin 10–20 mg once daily until immune reconstitution (CD4 >200 on stable ART for 6–12 mos).
- Soft tissue (including CA-MRSA) infections: 300–450 mg PO q6h or 600 mg IV q8h ×14 days then reassess.
- Pelvic inflammatory disease: 900 mg IV q8h (in combination with gentamicin) × 14 days.
- Bacterial vaginosis: 100-mg vaginal suppository at bedtime × 3–7 days.
- Acne: 1–2 applications once daily.
- Osteomyelitis: 600 mg IV q8h × 6–8 wks then reassess.
- Acute bacterial sinusitis: 300 mg PO q6h × 2–3 wks.
- Actinomycosis: 600 mg IV q8h × 2–6 wks, then 300 mg PO q6h × 6–12 mos.
- Capsules should be taken with full glass of water to avoid esophageal irritation.

ADVERSE DRUG REACTIONS

Common

- Diarrhea (without *C. difficile* in 10%–30%).
- GI intolerance: nausea, vomiting, anorexia.

Occasional

- Generalized morbilliform rash.
- *C. difficile* colitis in 6% of patients (clindamycin is most common cause on per patient basis).

Rare

- Stevens-Johnson syndrome.
- Allergic-type reactions (including bronchial asthma) in patients with aspirin hypersensitivity (from tartrazine found in 75- and 150-mg caps).

DRUG INTERACTIONS

- Erythromycin: *in vitro* antagonism. Clinical significance unclear. Avoid coadministration.
- Kaolin-pectin: decreases clindamycin absorption.
- Loperamide and diphenoxylate/atropine: may increase risk of diarrhea and *C. difficile*-associated colitis. Avoid use with clindamycin.
- Nondepolarizing muscle relaxant (pancuronium, tubocurarine): clindamycin may enhance action of nondepolarizing muscle relaxants. Use with caution in patients receiving such agents.

PHARMACOLOGY

Mechanism

- Inhibits protein synthesis by binding to 50S ribosomal subunits, interfering with transpeptidation and early chain termination.

Pharmacokinetic Parameters

- **Absorption:** 90% absorbed.
- **Metabolism and Excretion:** metabolized to sulfoxide and N-dimethyl metabolites. Only 10% is excreted in urine within 24 hrs. Majority excreted as inactive metabolite in feces and bile.
- **Protein Binding:** 85%–94%.
- **Cmin, Cmax, and AUC:** Cmax 10 mcg/mL after 600 mg IV and 2.5 mcg/mL after 150 mg IV and PO dose administration, respectively.
- **$T_{\frac{1}{2}}$:** 2.4 hrs.
- **Distribution:** distributed to many body tissues and fluids including ascites fluid, pleural fluid, synovial fluid.

Pregnancy Risk

- Category B: in surveillance study of Michigan Medicaid recipients, 647 exposures to clindamycin during 1st trimester resulted in 4.8% birth defects. These data do not support an association between clindamycin and congenital effects.

Breastfeeding Compatibility

- Excreted into breast milk. American Academy of Pediatrics considers clindamycin to be safe with breastfeeding.

DOSING

Dosing for Decreased Hepatic Function
- Dose reduction recommended for severe hepatic failure.

Renal Dosing
- No dose adjustment for renal impairment or dialysis.
- Dosing in hemofiltration: some removal during CAVH.

COMMENTS

- Oral and parenteral lincomycins have good activity against anaerobes; increasing resistance with *B. fragilis* makes metronidazole more reliable for intrabdominal infections. On per patient basis, clindamycin is antimicrobial most likely to cause *C. difficile* colitis, but many more patients get diarrhea without *C. difficile* colitis. Prescribe with caution in individuals with h/o colitis. 4 ×/day dosing may limit patient adherence.
- Clindamycin-primaquine is good 2nd-line regimen for PCP in patients who cannot tolerate TMP/SMX. Inferior to pyrimethamine/sulfadiazine for treatment to CNS toxoplasmosis but clindamycin/pyrimethamine can be considered as an alternative treatment regimen in sulfa-allergic patients.
- A 1st-line oral treatment option for CA-MRSA soft tissue infection.

SELECTED REFERENCES

Hasty MB, Klasner A, Kness S, et al. Cutaneous community-associated methicillin-resistant *Staphylococcus aureus* among all skin and soft-tissue infections in two geographically distant pediatric emergency departments. *Acad Emerg Med*, 2007; 14: 35–40.
Comments: Retrospective chart review of 920 children who presented to EDs with skin infections and abscesses. A total 60 cases of CA-MRSA were identified. Sensitivity retained to vancomycin, TMP-SMX, and rifampin. Only two isolates resistant to clindamycin.

Stevens DL, Bisno AL, Chambers HF, et al. Practice guidelines for the diagnosis and management of skin and soft-tissue infections. *Clin Infect Dis*, 2005; 41: 1373–406.
Comments: IDSA guidelines for skin and soft tissue infection. Vancomycin remains the empiric treatment of choice for most severe, suspected CA-MRSA infections, but clindamycin is an acceptable choice for less severe infections. TMP-SMX and tetracyclines may have slightly better activity against CA-MRSA than clindamycin.

Smego RA, Nagar S, Maloba B, et al. A meta-analysis of salvage therapy for *Pneumocystis carinii* pneumonia. *Arch Intern Med*, 2001; 161: 1529–33.
Comments: Meta-analysis suggests clindamycin + primaquine is most effective alternative in patients unresponsive to conventional PCP treatment.

Safrin S, Finkelstein DM, Feinberg J, et al. Comparison of three regimens for treatment of mild to moderate *Pneumocystis carinii* pneumonia in patients with AIDS. A double-blind, randomized, trial of oral trimethoprim-sulfamethoxazole, dapsone-trimethoprim, and clindamycin-primaquine. ACTG 108 Study Group. *Ann Intern Med*, 1996; 124: 792–802.
Comments: Clindamycin-primaquine is acceptable alternative to TMP-SMX or dapsone-trimethoprim in management of mild or moderately severe PCP.

Katlama C, De Wit S, O'Doherty E, et al. Pyrimethamine-clindamycin vs. pyrimethamine-sulfadiazine as acute and long-term therapy for toxoplasmic encephalitis in patients with AIDS. *Clin Infect Dis*, 1996; 22: 268–75.
Comments: Pyrimethamine-clindamycin less effective than sulfadiazine-pyrimethamine but can be used as an alternative treatment regimen in sulfa-allergic patients.

CLOTRIMAZOLE

Paul A. Pham, PharmD and John G. Bartlett, MD

INDICATIONS

FDA
- Oral candidiasis (thrush).
- Vaginal candidiasis.
- Dermatomycoses.

FORMS TABLE

Brand name (mfr)	Forms†	Cost*
Mycelex (generic manufacturers)	Oral troche 10 mg	$1.60
Ivax (non-US brands) (generic manufacturers)	Vaginal cream 1% (45 g)	$12.00
	Vaginal tablet 200 mg (3)	$9.00
	Vaginal tablet 500 mg (1)	$13.88
	Topical cream (1%) 15 g and 30 g tube	$8.29/15 g; $12.57/30 g
	Topical soln/lotion (1%) 10 mL and 30 mL	$7.40/10 mL; $19.50/30 mL

*Prices represent cost per unit specified, are representative of Average Wholesale Price (AWP).
†Dosage is indicated in mg unless otherwise noted.

USUAL ADULT DOSING
- Oropharyngeal candidiasis (thrush): 10-mg troche 5 ×/day (dissolved in mouth).
- *Candida* vaginitis: 100-mg intravaginal tab twice daily × 3 days (preferred) or 100 mg once daily × 7 days or 500 mg × 1.
- Cutaneous candidiasis: apply cream, soln, or lotion to affected areas twice daily × 2–8 wks.

ADVERSE DRUG REACTIONS
Occasional
- Burning; itching; erythema (intravaginal and topical administration).
- Nausea and vomiting (lozenge).
- Elevated transaminases.

DRUG INTERACTIONS
- No known drug interactions.

PHARMACOLOGY
Mechanism
- Alteration of cell membrane permeability by binding with phospholipids resulting in cellular destruction.

Pharmacokinetic Parameters
- **Absorption:** very small amount absorbed systemically after intravaginal administration. Systemic absorption after lozenge administration has not been determined.
- **Distribution:** attains therapeutic concentration in saliva for up to 3 hrs after lozenge dissolution.

Pregnancy Risk
- Category C: teratogenic in animal studies at high doses. No human data available with lozenge. No adverse effect seen with intravaginal administration during the 2nd and 3rd trimester.

Breastfeeding Compatibility
- No data.

DOSING
Dosing for Decreased Hepatic Function
- Usual dose, monitor LFTs.

Renal Dosing
- No dose adjustment for renal impairment, dialysis, or hemofiltration.

Comments
- Slightly less effective (measured as disease-free period posttherapy) than fluconazole but preferred as 1st line due to the concern over azole-resistant candidiasis with long-term use of fluconazole.

SELECTED REFERENCES
Pons V, Greenspan D, Debruin M. Therapy for oropharyngeal candidiasis in HIV-infected patients: a randomized, prospective multicenter study of oral fluconazole versus clotrimazole troches. The Multicenter Study Group. *J Acquir Immune Defic Syndr*, 1993; 6: 1311–16.
Comments: Prospective randomized trial involving 334 HIV-infected patients. 98% and 94% of evaluable fluconazole and clotrimazole-treated patients, respectively, were cured or showed improvement (P = NS). Fluconazole-treated patients more likely to remain asymptomatic through 2nd wk of follow-up (82% vs 50%) (P <0.001). However, difference no longer evident by wk 4.

DAPSONE

Paul A. Pham, PharmD and John G. Bartlett, MD

DRUGS

INDICATIONS

FDA

- Leprosy.
- Dermatitis herpetiformis.
- Acne vulgaris (dapsone 5% gel).

Non-FDA Approved Uses

- PCP prophylaxis.
- Treatment of mild-to-moderately severe PCP (with trimethoprim).
- Toxoplasmosis prophylaxis (with pyrimethamine and leucovorin).

FORMS TABLE

Brand name (mfr)	Forms†	Cost*
Dapsone (generic manufacturers)	Oral tablet 25 mg; 100 mg	$0.20; $0.21
Aczone (QLT)	Topical gel 5% (30 g)	$166.50

*Prices represent cost per unit specified, are representative of Average Wholesale Price (AWP).
†Dosage is indicated in mg unless otherwise noted.

USUAL ADULT DOSING

- PCP prophylaxis: 100 mg PO once daily.
- Treatment of mild-to-moderately severe PCP: dapsone 100 mg PO once daily + trimethoprim 5 mg/kg q8h × 21 days.
- PCP and toxoplasmosis prophylaxis: dapsone 50 mg PO once daily + pyrimethamine 50 mg PO qwk + leucovorin 25 mg PO qwk OR dapsone 200 mg PO weekly + pyrimethamine 75 mg PO qwk + leucovorin 25 mg qwk.

ADVERSE DRUG REACTIONS

Common

- Nausea and anorexia.
- Hemolytic anemia with G6PD deficiency.

Occasional

- Blood dyscrasias (methemoglobinemia and sulfhemoglobinemia with or without G6PD deficiency).
- Hepatitis.
- Rash.
- Pruritus.
- Dose-dependent hemolytic anemia without G6PD deficiency.

Rare

- Sulfone syndrome: fever, malaise, exfoliative dermatitis, hepatic necrosis, lymphadenopathy, and hemolytic anemia w/ methemoglobinemia.
- Nephrotic syndrome; blurred vision, photosensitivity, tinnitus, insomnia, irritability, and headache.
- Neutropenia.

DRUG-DRUG INTERACTIONS—See Appendix I, p. 495, for table of drug-drug interactions.

PHARMACOLOGY

Mechanism

- Mechanism of action has not been fully elucidated, but most likely involves inhibition of dihydropteroate synthase, to disrupt folate synthesis.

Pharmacokinetic Parameters

- **Absorption:** complete absorption (except with achlorydria).
- **Metabolism and Excretion:** enterohepatic circulation. Hepatic metabolism to monoacetyl and diacetyl metabolite. Both unchanged drug (20%) and metabolite (70%–85%) are excreted in urine.
- **Protein Binding:** 50%–90%.
- **Cmax, Cmin, and AUC:** 3.1–3.3 mcg/mL after 100 mg PO dose administration.
- **T$_{\frac{1}{2}}$:** 30 hrs.
- **Distribution:** widely distributed in body tissue including skin, muscle, kidneys, liver, and sputum.

Pregnancy Risk

- Category C: no adverse effect reported with the use of dapsone in patients with Hansen's disease.

Breastfeeding Compatibility

- Excreted in breast milk. The American Academy of Pediatrics considers dapsone compatible with breastfeeding.

DOSING

Renal Dosing

- Dosing for GFR of <80: usual dose.
- Dosing for GFR of <10: no data; metabolite excreted renally, may need adjustment.
- Dosing in hemodialysis, peritoneal dialysis, and hemofiltration: no data.

COMMENTS

- Oral agent used for treatment and prevention of PCP and leprosy. Strong oxidizing agent; G6PD deficiency screening recommended (especially in high-risk patients including black men and males of Mediterranean descendent).
- Contraindicated use with Mediterranean but not African variant of G6PD deficiency. In addition to hemolytic anemia, may cause methemoglobinemia and bone marrow suppression.

SELECTED REFERENCES

Kaplan JE, Benson C, Holmes KH, et al. Guidelines for prevention and treatment of opportunistic infections in HIV-infected adults and adolescents: recommendations from CDC, the National Institutes of Health, and the HIV Medicine Association of the Infectious Diseases Society of America. *MMWR Recomm Rep*, 2009; 58: 1–207.
Comments: Current opportunistic infection guidelines.

Safrin S, Finkelstein DM, Feinberg J, et al. Comparison of three regimens for treatment of mild to moderate *Pneumocystis carinii* pneumonia in patients with AIDS. A double-blind, randomized, trial of oral trimethoprim-sulfamethoxazole, dapsone-trimethoprim, and clindamycin-primaquine. ACTG 108 Study Group. *Ann Intern Med*, 1996; 124: 792–802.
Comments: Trimethoprim + dapsone is acceptable alternative to TMP-SMX in management of mild or moderately severe PCP.

DOXYCYCLINE

Paul A. Pham, PharmD and John G. Bartlett, MD

INDICATIONS

FDA

- Anthrax due to *Bacillus anthracis*, including inhalation anthrax (postexposure). CDC recommends as 1st-line agent + 1–2 additional agents with *in vitro* activity.
- Granuloma inguinale caused by *Calymmatobacterium granulomatis*.

- If PCN-allergic: uncomplicated gonorrhea caused by *N. gonorrhoeae*; syphilis caused by *Treponema pallidum*; yaws caused by *T. pertenue*; listeriosis due to *L. monocytogenes*; Vincent's infection caused by *Fusobacterium fusiforme*; actinomycosis caused by *A. israelli*; infections caused by *Clostridium* spp.
- Psittacosis caused by *Chlamydia psitta*.
- Relapsing fever caused by *Borrelia recurrentis*.
- Pneumonia caused by *Mycoplasma pneumoniae*.
- Rocky mountain spotted fever, typhus, Q fever, rickettsial pox, and tick fevers caused by *Rickettsiae*.
- Uncomplicated urethral, endocervical, or rectal infections caused by *Chlamydia trachomatis*; nongonococcal urethritis caused by *Ureaplasma urealyticum*; lymphogranuloma venereum caused by *Chlamydia* spp.
- Trachoma; inclusion conjunctivitis caused by *C. trachomatis*.
- Gram-negative infections caused by: *H. ducreyi, Y. pestis, F. tularensis, V. cholerae, C. fetus, Brucella* spp., *B. bacilliformis, C. granulomatis*.

FORMS TABLE

Brand name (mfr)	Forms†	Cost*
Vibramycin (Pfizer)	Oral suspension 25 mg/5 mL Oral capsule 100 mg	$308.89 per 16 oz $6.56
Doxycycline; *Monodox*; *Adoxa* (Generic manufacturers [Imiren Pharmaceuticals, Watson/Schein Pharmaceuticals, and others])	Oral capsule 50 mg; 100 mg IV vial 100 mg Oral tablet 50 mg; 75 mg; 100 mg	50 mg: $0.73; 100 mg: $1.94 $18.55 50 mg: $0.40; 75 mg: $0.75; 100 mg: $1.15
Periostat (Collagenex Pharmaceuticals and generic manufacturer [Mutual Pharmaceutical])	Oral tablet 20 mg	$3.48

*Prices represent cost per unit specified, are representative of Average Wholesale Price (AWP).
†Dosage is indicated in mg unless otherwise noted.

USUAL ADULT DOSING

- Respiratory tract infections (community-acquired pneumonia, otitis, sinusitis): 100 mg PO twice daily w/ food × 7–14 days.
- *C. trachomatis* (alternative to azithromycin): 100 mg PO twice daily w/ food × 7 days.
- Uncomplicated non-GC (urethral, endocervical, or rectal): 100 mg PO twice daily × 7 days.
- Bacillary angiomatosis: 100 mg PO twice daily w/ food × >3 mos; consider lifelong Rx to prevent relapse.

ADVERSE DRUG REACTIONS

Occasional
- GI intolerance (dose related).
- Teeth stains and deformity in children up to 8 yrs old.
- Photosensitivity.

Rare
- *Candida* overgrowth (vaginitis and esophagitis).
- Worsening azotemia in patients with renal failure.
- Rash.
- "Black tongue" syndrome; benign fungus infection that is generally reversible upon drug discontinuation.
- Esophageal ulceration.
- Elevated liver function tests.

DRUGS

- Jarisch-Herxheimer reaction.
- *C. difficile* colitis (less likely compared to cephalosporins, carbapenems, and fluoroquinolones).
- Pseudotumor cerebri.
- Pancreatitis.

DRUG-DRUG INTERACTIONS—See Appendix I, p. 512, for table of drug-drug interactions.

RESISTANCE

- *S. pneumoniae:* 12% and 27% resistance in bloodstream infection and pneumonia, respectively. Cross-resistance with PCN-resistant *S. pneumoniae* with only 60% susceptible.
- Some strains of CA-MRSA are sensitive to doxycycline, but minocycline should be used due to better *in vitro* activity and demonstrated efficacy *in vivo*.

PHARMACOLOGY

Mechanism

- Inhibit protein synthesis by mainly binding to 30S ribosomal subunit and blocking binding of aminoacyl transfer-RNA.

Pharmacokinetic Parameters

- **Absorption:** 90% absorbed.
- **Metabolism and Excretion:** excreted mainly by nonrenal routes. Possible liver metabolism and intestinal inactivation. 20%–26% excreted in the urine, 20%–40% excreted in the feces.
- **Protein Binding:** 25%–91%.
- **Cmax, Cmin, and AUC:** Cmax: 1.5–2.1 mcg/mL.
- **$T_{\frac{1}{2}}$:** 18 hrs.
- **Distribution:** widely distributed into body tissues and fluids including pleural fluid, bronchial secretions, sputum, ascitic fluid, synovial fluid, aqueous and vitreous humor, and prostatic fluid. Better CSF penetration compared to tetracycline (26% of serum levels).

Pregnancy Risk

- Category D: contraindicated in pregnancy due to retardation of skeletal development and bone growth, enamel hypoplasia, and discoloration of teeth of fetus. Maternal liver toxicity has also been reported.

Breastfeeding Compatibility

- Excreted in breast milk at very low concentrations. There is theoretical possibility of dental staining and inhibition of bone growth, but infants exposed to tetracyclines have serum levels less than 0.05 mcg/mL.

DOSING

Dosing for Decreased Hepatic Function

- No data.

Renal Dosing

- No dose adjustment for renal impairment, dialysis, or hemofiltration.

COMMENTS

- Preferred tetracycline derivative due to more convenient twice daily dosing regimen and no food-drug interaction. Recommended tetracycline derivative in patients with renal failure.
- Agents of choice for *Rickettsia* and *Vibrio* infections. Minocycline preferred for mild-to-moderate soft tissue infections caused by CA-MRSA.

SELECTED REFERENCES

Cunha BA. Methicillin-resistant *Staphylococcus aureus*: clinical manifestations and antimicrobial therapy. *Clin Microbiol Infect*, 2005; 11 Suppl 4: 33–42.

Comments: This article underscores that clinicians should select a MRSA drug with proven *in vivo* effectiveness (i.e., daptomycin, linezolid, quinupristin/dalfopristin, minocycline, or vancomycin) and not rely on *in vitro* susceptibility data. For MRSA, doxycycline cannot be substituted for minocycline.

Jones RN, Sader HS, Fritsche TR. Doxycycline use for community-acquired pneumonia: contemporary *in vitro* spectrum of activity against *Streptococcus pneumoniae* (1999–2002). *Diagn Microbiol Infect Dis*, 2004; 49: 147–9.

Comments: Resistance to tetracyclines, in contrast to penicillin and the macrolides, seems more stable over the 1999–2002 monitored interval with 12% and 27% *S. pneumoniae* resistance in bloodstream infection and pneumonia, respectively.

Foucault C, Raoult D, Brouqui P. Randomized open trial of gentamicin and doxycycline for eradication of *Bartonella quintana* from blood in patients with chronic bacteremia. *Antimicrob Agents Chemother*, 2003; 47: 2204–7.
Comments: In an open-label study, gentamicin (3 mg/kg × 14 days) + doxycycline (200 mg/day × 28 days) is effective in the clearance of *B. quintana* bacteremia.

ENTECAVIR

Paul A. Pham, PharmD and John G. Bartlett, MD

INDICATIONS

FDA

- Treatment of chronic hepatitis B (HBV) infection in adult patients with evidence of active disease (active viral replication, elevated ALT or AST, or histologic evidence of active disease).

FORMS TABLE

Brand name (mfr)	Forms†	Cost*
Baraclude (Bristol-Myers Squibb)	Oral tablets 0.5 mg, 1 mg Oral soln 0.05 mg/mL (210 mL)	$27.11 $85.11

*Prices represent cost per unit specified, are representative of Average Wholesale Price (AWP).
†Dosage is indicated in mg unless otherwise noted.

USUAL ADULT DOSING

- For lamivudine (3TC) (see p. 294)-naïve patients: 0.5 mg PO daily on empty stomach (2 hrs before or after food).
- For 3TC-refractory patients: 1 mg PO daily on empty stomach (2 hrs before or after food).
- Avoid high-fat meals.

ADVERSE DRUG REACTIONS

General

- Generally well tolerated with side effect profile comparable to 3TC and placebo in clinical trials.

Rare

- Headache.
- Fatigue.
- Nausea, diarrhea.
- Insomnia.
- Low likelihood of lactic acidosis.
- Rash.
- Alopecia.

DRUG INTERACTIONS

- No drug interactions observed with the coadministration of entecavir and adefovir, TDF, or 3TC. *In vitro*, entecavir not antagonistic with ABC, ddI, 3TC, d4T, TDF, or ZDV.

PHARMACOLOGY

Mechanism

- Guanosine nucleoside analog that specifically inhibits HBV polymerase. A 150- to 1300-fold higher entecavir concentration would be needed to inhibit human cellular DNA polymerase.

Pharmacokinetic Parameters

- **Absorption:** food decreases absorption by 18%–20%.
- **Metabolism and Excretion:** renal excretion via glomerular filtration and tubular secretion accounts for 63%–73%.
- **Protein Binding:** 13% (*in vitro*).

DRUGS

- **Cmax, Cmin, and AUC:** Cmax = 4.2 ng/mL (with 0.5 mg) and 8.2 ng/mL (with 1 mg); AUC decreased by 18%–20% and Cmax decreased by 44%–46% when taken with food.
- **T$_\frac{1}{2}$:** serum: 128–149 hrs; intracellular: 15 hrs.
- **Distribution:** PK studies suggest it is widely distributed in tissues.

Pregnancy Risk
- Category C: negative embryotoxicity and maternal toxicity in rat and rabbit studies at 28 and 212 times levels achieved with highest daily dose (1 mg/day). Rat and rabbit embryo and fetal toxicities seen at 3100 times human drug levels. No studies in humans. Pregnancy registry for entecavir: 1-800-258-4263.

Breastfeeding Compatibility
- No human data, breast milk excretion in animal studies. Breastfeeding not recommended.

DOSING

Dosing for Decreased Hepatic Function
- Usual dose.

Renal Dosing
- Dosing for GFR of 50–80: usual dosing.
- Dosing for GFR of 30–49, 3TC-naïve: 0.25 mg daily; 3TC-resistant: 0.5 mg daily.
- Dosing for GFR of 10–29, 3TC-naïve: 0.15 mg daily; 3TC-resistant: 0.30 mg daily.
- Dosing for GFR of <10: nucleoside naïve: 0.05 mg daily; lamivudine (3TC)-refractory: 0.1 mg daily.
- Dosing in hemodialysis: 3TC-naïve: 0.05 mg daily (dose post-HD on days of dialysis); 3TC-refractory: 0.1 mg daily (dose post-HD on days of dialysis).
- Dosing in peritoneal dialysis: 3TC-naïve: 0.05 mg daily; 3TC-refractory: 0.1 mg daily.
- Dosing in hemofiltration: no data. Consider 0.5–1.0 mg daily.

COMMENTS
- Well tolerated and superior to 3TC for treatment of HBV-infected patients who are treatment naïve or 3TC-resistant. Ha activity against HIV, with ability to select for M184V; therefore HIV cross-resistance possible when entecavir used as monotherapy in coinfected patients. HIV/ HBV coinfected patients should not be treated with entecavir unless used in combination with fully suppressive ART regimen.

SELECTED REFERENCES

McMahon MA, Jilek BL, Brennan TP, et al. The HBV drug entecavir—effects on HIV-1 replication and resistance. *N Engl J Med*, 2007; 356(25): 2614–21.

Comments: A report showing that entecavir monotherapy led to a consistent 1-log(10) decrease in HIV-1 RNA in three HIV-1/HBV coinfection patients. Of these, one patient developed M184V mutation. Based on these reports, entecavir should not be used as monotherapy for treatment of HBV in HIV-coinfected patients who are not also receiving combination ART for treatment of their HIV infection due to the risk of developing HIV-associated resistance mutations.

Sherman M, Yurdaydin C, Sollano J, et al. Entecavir for treatment of lamivudine-refractory, HBeAg-positive chronic hepatitis B. *Gastroenterology*, 2006; 130: 2039–49.

Comments: A prospective, randomized, double-blind study compared entecavir (1 mg once daily) vs continued 3TC (100 mg once daily) × 52 wks in 286 patients with chronic HBV (HBeAg-positive) who failed 3TC treatment. Histologic improvement occurred in 55% (68/124) of entecavir-treated vs 28% (32/116) of 3TC-treated patients (P <.0001). Mean change from baseline in HBV DNA was −5.11 log for entecavir-treated patients and −0.48 log for 3TC-treated patients (P <0.0001).

Lai CL, Shouval D, Lok AS, et al. Entecavir versus lamivudine for patients with HBeAg-negative chronic hepatitis B. *N Engl J Med*, 2006; 354: 1011–20.

Comments: Prospective, randomized, double-blind study compared entecavir (0.5 mg once daily) vs 3TC (100 mg once daily) × 52 wks in 648 patients with chronic HBV (HBeAg-negative) who were NRTI-naïve. Histologic improvement after 48 weeks of treatment occurred in 208/296 (70%) patients in entecavir group vs 174/287 (61%) in 3TC group (P = 0.01). More patients in entecavir group than in 3TC group had undetectable serum HBV DNA levels (90% vs 72%, P <0.001) and normalization of ALT l (78% vs 71%, P = 0.045).

Wilkin Pessoa, B Gazzard, A Huang, et al. Entecavir in HIV/HBV Co-Infected Patients: Safety and Efficacy in a Phase II Study (ETV 038). presented at: 12th Conference on Retroviruses and Opportunistic Infections (CROI 2005); Boston, MA; Boston, MA.

Comments: Placebo-controlled study compared addition of entecavir or placebo to 3TC-containing ART regimen in HIV/HBV coinfected patients who experienced recurrent HBV viremia. At baseline, mean HBV DNA was 9.13 log, 99% of all patients were HBeAg+, and 88% had at least one 3TC resistance mutation. At 24 wks, entecavir-treated patients experienced significantly higher HBV DNA decrease of 3.66 log compared to 0.11 log increase in placebo Rx patients (P <0.0001). Proportion of patients with HBV DNA <400 or a >2 log reduction from baseline was also superior with entecavir (84% vs 0% for placebo, P <0.0001)

ETHAMBUTOL

Paul A. Pham, PharmD and John G. Bartlett, MD

INDICATIONS
FDA
- Treatment of all forms of TB in combination with other antituberculous drugs.

Non-FDA Approved Uses
- Treatment of *M. avium* complex (MAC) infection (in combination with a macrolide).
- Treatment of *M. kansasii* infection (in combination with INH and rifampin).

FORMS TABLE

Brand name (mfr)	Forms†	Cost*
Myambutol (Elan Pharmaceuticals)	Oral tablet 100 mg; 400 mg	$0.62; $1.80

*Prices represent cost per unit specified, are representative of Average Wholesale Price (AWP).
†Dosage is indicated in mg unless otherwise noted.

USUAL ADULT DOSING
- TB: 15–20 mg/kg (max 2 g) once daily (+ INH, PZA, rifamycin).
- Intermittent directly-observed treatment regimens: 50 mg/kg 2 ×/wk (max 4 g) or 25–30 mg/kg 3 ×/wk (max 2.4 g).
- MAC: 15 mg/kg/day (+ macrolide).
- *M. kansasii*: 25 mg/kg/day × 2 mos then 15 mg/kg/day (max 2.5 g/day) (+ INH and rifamycin).

ADVERSE DRUG REACTIONS
Occasional
- Optic neuritis: decreased acuity, reduced color discrimination, constricted fields, and scotomata (infrequent with 15 mg/kg/day; including risk w/ 25 mg/kg/day). Patients receiving 25 mg/kg/day should have baseline visual and color perception screening; repeated visual screening monthly. Ocular manifestation reversible with discontinuation, but irreversible blindness has been described.
- GI intolerance: anorexia, nausea, vomiting, and abdominal pain.

RARE
- Peripheral neuropathy.
- Hypersensitivity reaction.
- Confusion and dizziness.
- Acute gout.
- Hematologic: leukopenia, thrombocytopenia, eosinophilia, neutropenia, and lymphadenopathy.
- Dermatologic: rash, pruritus, dermatitis, and exfoliative dermatitis.
- Interstitial nephritis.

DRUG INTERACTIONS
- Ethionamide: may increase adverse effects of EMB.

PHARMACOLOGY
Mechanism
- Mechanism of action not fully elucidated, but it appears to suppress multiplication by interfering with RNA synthesis.

Pharmacokinetic Parameters
- **Absorption:** 75%–80% absorbed.
- **Metabolism and Excretion:** partially metabolized in the liver. Both unchanged drug and metabolite are excreted in the urine. Unabsorbed drug excreted unchanged in the feces.
- **Protein Binding:** 22%.
- **Cmax, Cmin, and AUC:** Cmax: 2–5 mcg/mL after 25 mg/kg PO.
- **T$\frac{1}{2}$:** 3–4 hrs.
- **Distribution:** widely distributed to most tissues and fluids, attaining high concentrations in kidneys, lungs, saliva, and erythrocyte. Poor CSF concentration (therapeutic levels usually not attained). Penetrates CSF with inflammation and is indicated as part of a four-drug regimen, but the added benefit of ethambutol has not been fully evaluated in TB meningitis.

Pregnancy Risk
- Category B: no congenital defects have been reported. CDC considers EMB safe in pregnancy.

Breastfeeding Compatibility
- Excreted in breast milk. American Academy of Pediatrics considers EMB compatible with breastfeeding.

DOSING

Dosing for Decreased Hepatic Function
- No data.

Renal Dosing
- Dosing for GFR of 50–80: 15 mg/kg/day (consider dose reduction with clearance <70).
- Dosing for GFR of 10–50: 15 mg/kg q24–36h.
- Dosing for GFR of <10: 15 mg/kg q48h.
- Dosing in hemodialysis: 15–20 mg/kg post-HD 3 × /wk.
- Dosing in peritoneal dialysis: 15 mg/kg q48 hrs.
- Dosing in hemofiltration: no data. Consider dose reduction.

COMMENTS
- 1st-line agent in combination for TB and MAC. Monitor visual acuity in patients receiving higher doses (25 mg/kg/day).

SELECTED REFERENCES

American Thoracic Society, CDC, Infectious Diseases Society of America. Treatment of tuberculosis. *MMWR Recomm Rep*, 2003; 52: 1–77.
Comments: Guidelines for the management of TB.

Ward TT, Rimland D, Kauffman C, et al. Randomized, open-label trial of azithromycin plus ethambutol vs. clarithromycin plus ethambutol as therapy for Mycobacterium avium complex bacteremia in patients with human immunodeficiency virus infection. Veterans Affairs HIV Research Consortium. *Clin Infect Dis*, 1998; 27: 1278–85.
Comments: Prospective randomized trial demonstrating the efficacy of a macrolide + EMB for treatment of disseminated MAC infection.

FAMCICLOVIR

Paul A. Pham, PharmD and John G. Bartlett, MD

INDICATIONS

FDA
- Recurrent genital herpes (suppression and treatment) in immunocompetent and HIV+ patients.
- Treatment of herpes zoster.

FORMS TABLE

Brand name (mfr)	Forms†	Cost*
Famvir (Novartis Pharmaceuticals)	Oral tablet 125 mg; 250 mg; 500 mg	$6.46; $7.02; $14.11
Famciclovir (Teva Pharmaceuticals [generic manufacturer])	Oral tablet 125 mg; 250 mg; 500 mg	$6.46; $7.02; $14.11

*Prices represent cost per unit specified, are representative of Average Wholesale Price (AWP).
†Dosage is indicated in mg unless otherwise noted.

USUAL ADULT DOSING
- Herpes zoster: 500 mg PO q8h × 7–10 days.
- HSV (initial): 250 mg PO q8h or 500 mg PO twice daily × 7 days.
- Recurrent HSV (oralabial or genital herpes infection): 125 mg PO q8h or 250–500 mg PO twice daily × 7 days.
- Suppression of recurrent genital HSV: 250 mg twice daily (up to 1 yr).
- Famciclovir is a prodrug of antiviral agent penciclovir.

ADVERSE DRUG REACTIONS
General
- Generally very well tolerated.
Occasional
- Headache and dizziness.
- GI intolerance: nausea and diarrhea.

DRUG INTERACTIONS
- Probenecid: may increase penciclovir concentrations.

PHARMACOLOGY
Mechanism
- Converted to penciclovir, a guanosine analog transformed in HSV and VZV infected cells into triphosphate form which inhibits viral DNA polymerase.
Pharmacokinetic Parameters
- **Absorption:** 77%.
- **Metabolism and Excretion:** Deacetylated and then oxidized to penciclovir (active), less than 1.5% of total dose is metabolized to inactive metabolite. 60%–65% of dose is excreted as penciclovir in the urine; 27% of dose excreted in feces.
- **Protein Binding:** 20%.
- **Cmax, Cmin, and AUC:** Cmax 3.3–4.2 mcg/mL after a single dose of 500 mg.
- **$T_{\frac{1}{2}}$:** 2–3 hrs.
- **Distribution:** good tissue penetration with blood/plasma ratio of 1.
Pregnancy Risk
- Category B: carcinogenic, but not embryotoxic or teratogenic in animal studies. No human data.
Breastfeeding Compatibility
- No data, but due to the probable excretion into breast milk and the carcinogenicity potential in animal studies, not recommended when breastfeeding.

DOSING
Dosing for Decreased Hepatic Function
- No data. Usual dose likely.
Renal Dosing
- Dosing for GFR of 50–80: usual dose.
- Dosing for GFR of 10–50: 125–500 mg q12–q24h.
- Dosing for GFR of <10: 125–250 mg q48h.
- Dosing in hemodialysis: 125–250 mg q48h, on days of dialysis dose after HD.
- Dosing in peritoneal dialysis: no data.
- Dosing in hemofiltration: no data.

DRUGS

COMMENTS
- An effective alternative to acyclovir or valacyclovir for treatment of HSV and VZV infections. Easier dosing than acyclovir; no clear advantage over valacyclovir.

SELECTED REFERENCES
Romanowski B, Aoki FY, Martel AY, et al. Efficacy and safety of famciclovir for treating mucocutaneous herpes simplex infection in HIV-infected individuals. Collaborative Famciclovir HIV Study Group. *AIDS*, 2000; 14: 1211–7.
Comments: Prospective, randomized trial comparing efficacy and safety of 7 days treatment with famciclovir 500 mg twice daily vs acyclovir 400 mg 5 ×/day for recurrent mucocutaneous HSV infection in HIV+ patients. Famciclovir equivalent to acyclovir in preventing new lesion formation.

CDC. 2010 STD treatment guidelines. *www.cdc.gov/std/treatment/2010*. Accessed May 15, 2011.
Comments: CDC STD treatment guidelines.

FLUCONAZOLE

Paul A. Pham, PharmD and John G. Bartlett, MD

INDICATIONS
FDA
- Candidiasis prophylaxis (patients undergoing bone marrow transplant who receive cytotoxic chemotherapy and/or radiation therapy).
- Treatment of oropharyngeal and esophageal candidiasis.
- Disseminated candidiasis (including peritonitis, pneumonia, and UTIs).
- Chronic mucocutaneous candidiasis.
- Vulvovaginal candidiasis.
- Disseminated cryptococcosis.
- Treatment and suppression of cryptococcal meningitis.

Non-FDA Approved Uses
- Coccidioidomycosis (treatment); itraconazole preferred (for nonmeningeal).
- Pityriasis versicolor.
- Histoplasmosis (treatment of mild disease); itraconazole preferred.

FORMS TABLE

Brand name (mfr)	Forms†	Cost*
Diflucan and generic fluconazole (Pfizer and generic manufacturers)	PO tablet 50 mg; 100 mg; 150 mg; 200 mg	$8.01; $12.58; $20.03; $20.59
	IV piggyback 200 mg; 400 mg PO suspension 10 mg/mL; 40 mg/mL	$128.00; $187.75 $35.80 (10 mg/mL; 35 mL); $132.45 (40 mg/mL; 35 mL)

*Prices represent cost per unit specified, are representative of Average Wholesale Price (AWP).
†Dosage is indicated in mg unless otherwise noted.

USUAL ADULT DOSING
- Cryptococcal meningitis induction phase: 1200 mg PO once daily + flucytosine (5-FC) 100 mg/kg/day × 6 wks (alternative regimen; amphotericin B or lipid amphotericin B + 5-FC a minimum of 2 wks preferred).
- Cryptococcal meningitis, consolidation phase after ≥2 wks of amphotericin + 5-FC: 400 mg PO once daily × 8 wks.
- Cryptococcal meningitis, maintenance phase: 200 mg PO once daily (until CD4 >100–200 × > 6 mos and after >1 yr of antifungal therapy).
- Vaginal candidiasis: 150 mg PO × 1. Multiple recurrences: fluconazole 150 mg PO qwk (topical azoles preferred).

- Esophageal candidiasis: 200 mg PO once daily × 14–21 days (or IV up to 800 mg/day). Use chronic maintenance therapy (same dose) for recurrent esophagitis.
- Oropharyngeal candidiasis (thrush): 100–200 mg PO once daily × 7–14 days (topical therapy with clotrimazole preferred to avoid azole resistance).
- Coccidioidomycosis, meningitis: 400–800 mg IV or PO. Nonmeningeal (diffuse pulmonary or disseminated): fluconazole 400–800 mg PO once daily (amphotericin B preferred); maintenance: 400 mg PO once daily (itraconazole equally effective).
- Histoplamosis: 800 mg daily (itraconazole preferred).
- For obese patients: 6 mg/kg/day up to 1200 mg/day.
- Cryptococcemia or cryptococcal pneumonia: 6 mg/kg (400 mg) once daily × 6–12 mos.

ADVERSE DRUG REACTIONS

General
- Generally well tolerated.

Occasional
- GI intolerance w/ bloating, nausea, vomiting, pain, anorexia.
- Reversible alopecia (with >400 mg/day).
- Transaminase elevation.

Rare
- Hepatitis (fatal hepatotoxicity in patients with serious underlying medical conditions; monitor LFTs).
- Dizziness.
- Headache.
- Hypokalemia.

DRUG INTERACTIONS
- CYP2C8/9/19 and CYP3A4 inhibitor resulting in an increase in CYP2C8/9/19 and CYP3A4 substrate. No clinically significant drug-drug interactions with PIs.

DRUG-DRUG INTERACTIONS—See Appendix I, p. 524, for table of drug-drug interactions.

PHARMACOLOGY

Mechanism
- Triazoles alter fungal cell membrane function by inhibiting C-14 alpha anosterol demethylase, thereby interfering with ergosterol synthesis, which results in increased cell permeability and leakage of essential elements.

Pharmacokinetic Parameters
- **Absorption:** >90% absorbed independent of gastric acidity.
- **Metabolism and Excretion:** partial metabolism. Both metabolite (11%) and unchanged drug (60%–80%) excreted in urine.
- **Protein Binding:** 11%–12%.
- **Cmax, Cmin, and AUC:** 6.72 mcg/mL after 400 mg PO dose administration. 3.9–5 mcg/mL after 6 days of 100 mg IV administration.
- **$T_{\frac{1}{2}}$:** 30 hrs.
- **Distribution:** widely distributed throughout body tissues and fluids such as kidney, skin, saliva, sputum, nail, blister fluid, prostate. Good CSF penetration (50%–94% of plasma serum concentration attained in the CSF).

Pregnancy Risk
- Category C: teratogenic in animal studies. Case reports of craniofacial, limb, and cardiac defects have been reported in 3 infants with 1st-trimester exposure to high-dose fluconazole. The risk of low-dose intermittent use has not been fully evaluated but appears to be low.

Breastfeeding Compatibility
- Fluconazole excreted into breast milk at high concentration (up to 83% of plasma concentration). Since no drug-induced toxicity encountered in infants during therapy with fluconazole, likelihood of toxicity during breastfeeding is low.

DOSING

Renal Dosing
- Dosing for GFR of 50–80: usual.
- Dosing for GFR of <50: 50% of dose.
- Dosing in hemodialysis: 100% of dose post-HD.

- Dosing in peritoneal dialysis: 50% of dose daily.
- Dosing in hemofiltration: CVVH: 200–400 mg once daily; CVVHD: 400–800 mg once daily.

COMMENTS
- Oral and parenteral azole with best oral bioavailability, independent of gastric pH. Use of fluconazole for treatment or suppression of thrush not recommended due to risk of azole-resistance; topical therapy (e.g., clotrimazole) preferred. However, if recurrences are frequent or mucocutaneous candidiasis is severe, oral fluconazole maintenance can be considered.
- Preferred drug for esophageal candidiasis. Fatal hepatotoxicity has been described.
- Fluconazole preferred over itraconazole for consolidation phase and maintenance of cryptococcal meningitis. Itraconazole has better *in vitro* activity against *Coccidioides immitis*; however due to better CNS penetration, fluconazole is recommended for meningitis.

SELECTED REFERENCES

Nussbaum JC, Jackson A, Namarika D, et al. Combination flucytosine and high-dose fluconazole compared with fluconazole monotherapy for the treatment of cryptococcal meningitis: a randomized trial in Malawi. *Clin Infect Dis*, 2010; 50: 338–44.
Comments: Randomized trial compared high-dose fluconazole (1200 mg/day) alone or in combination with 5-FC (25 mg/kg q6h) followed by fluconazole (800 mg/day) × 8 wks for treatment of cryptococcal meningitis in a resource-limited country. Improved survival rate with fluconazole + 5F-C observed at 2 wks (10% vs 37%).

Perfect JR, Dismukes WE, Dromer F, et al. Clinical practice guidelines for the management of cryptococcal disease: 2010 update by the Infectious Diseases Society of America. *Clin Infect Dis*, 2010; 50: 291–322.
Comments: Fluconazole 1200 mg/day + 5-FC × 6 wks OR fluconazole 1200 mg/day monotherapy (up to 2000 mg/day) × 10–12 wks can be considered during induction/consolidation phase as an alternative regimen in patients unable to tolerate amphotericin.

Kaplan JE, Benson C, Holmes KH, et al. Guidelines for prevention and treatment of opportunistic infections in HIV-infected adults and adolescents: recommendations from CDC, the National Institutes of Health, and the HIV Medicine Association of the Infectious Diseases Society of America. *MMWR Recomm Rep*, 2009; 58: 1–207.
Comments: Treatment guidelines recommend topical clotrimazole troches or nystatin suspension for the treatment of initial episodes of oropharyngeal candidiasis. Secondary prophylaxis for recurrent oropharyngeal or vulvovaginal candidiasis is generally not recommended because of the potential for resistant candidiasis. However, if recurrences are frequent or mucocutaneous candidiasis is severe, oral fluconazole can be used for either oropharyngeal or vulvovaginal. In addition, it is prudent to institute secondary prophylaxis in patients with fluconazole-refractory oropharyngeal or esophageal candidiasis who have responded to echinocandins, voriconazole, or posaconazole therapy because of high relapse rate until ART produces immune reconstitution.

Pappas PG, Rex JH, Sobel JD, et al. Practice guidelines for the management of candidiasis: 2009 update by the Infectious Diseases Society of America. *Clin Infect Dis*, 2009; 48: 35.
Comments: IDSA guidelines for treatment of candidiasis. For disseminated candidiasis, fluconazole may be given after AmB or caspofungin therapy if pt is clinically stable.

van der Horst CM, Saag MS, Cloud GA, et al. Treatment of cryptococcal meningitis associated with the acquired immunodeficiency syndrome. National Institute of Allergy and Infectious Diseases Mycoses Study Group and AIDS Clinical Trials Group. *N Engl J Med*, 1997; 337: 15–21.
Comments: Consolidation therapy with fluconazole associated with a higher rate of CSF sterilization compared to itraconazole.

Tumbarello M, Caldarola G, Tacconelli E, et al. Analysis of the risk factors associated with the emergence of azole resistant oral candidosis in the course of HIV infection. *J Antimicrob Chemother*, 1996; 38: 691–9.
Comments: Low CD4 and previous fluconazole therapy associated with development of fluconazole-resistant *Candida*. When possible, fluconazole use should be reserved for thrush refractory to topical treatment or *Candida* esophagitis.

FLUCYTOSINE

Paul A. Pham, PharmD and John G. Bartlett, MD

INDICATIONS
FDA
- Cryptococcal and *Candida* endocarditis (in addition to amphotericin B).
- Cryptococcal meningitis (in addition to amphotericin B or liposomal amphotericin).
- Cryptococcal and *Candida* pneumonia (in addition to amphotericin B).
- Cryptococcal and *Candida* septicemia (in addition to amphotericin B).
- Cryptococcal and *Candida* urinary tract infections (in addition to amphotericin B).

Brand name (mfr)	Forms†	Cost*
Ancobon (ICN Pharmaceuticals)	Oral capsule 250 mg; 500 mg	$22.64 per 100 caps; $43.81 per 100 caps

*Prices represent cost per unit specified, are representative of Average Wholesale Price (AWP).
†Dosage is indicated in mg unless otherwise noted.

USUAL ADULT DOSING
- 25 mg/kg q6h. Therapeutic monitoring recommended with renal insufficiency; goal peak of 30–80 mcg/mL 2 hrs postdose after 3–5 days.

ADVERSE DRUG REACTIONS

Occasional
- GI intolerance: diarrhea, dyspepsia, and abdominal pain.
- Marrow suppression w/ leukopenia or thrombocytopenia (with levels >100 mcg/mL).
- Headache.
- Taste perversion.
- Pruritis.

Rare
- Confusion.
- Rash.
- Hepatitis.
- Peripheral neuropathy.
- Enterocolitis.
- Photosensitivity.
- Fatal bone marrow aplasia.

DRUG INTERACTIONS
- Cytarabine: antagonism (avoid coadministration).
- Drugs that cause bone marrow suppression (i.e., AZT, ganciclovir, and interferon): increased bone marrow suppression.

PHARMACOLOGY

Mechanism
- Flucytosine interferes with protein synthesis by incorporation into fungal RNA after being converted to 5-FU intracellularly.

Pharmacokinetic Parameters
- **Absorption:** 75%–90%.
- **Metabolism and Excretion:** minimal metabolism; principally excreted unchanged in the urine. Unabsorbed drug excreted in feces.
- **Protein Binding:** 2%–4%.
- **Cmax, Cmin, and AUC:** 30–40 mcg/mL after 2 g PO.
- **$T_{\frac{1}{2}}$:** 2.5–6 hrs.
- **Distribution:** widely distributed into body tissues and fluids such as liver, kidney, spleen, heart, aqueous humor, and bronchial secretion. Good CNS penetration (60%–100% of serum concentration attained in the CSF).

Pregnancy Risk
- Category C: crosses placental barrier. Teratogenicity reported in animal studies. 3 case reports of 2nd and 3rd exposure found no defects in infants.

Breastfeeding Compatibility
- No data. Breastfeeding during flucytosine therapy not recommended.

DOSING

Dosing for Decreased Hepatic Function
- No data. Usual dose likely.

DRUGS

Renal Dosing

- Dosing for GFR of 50–80: 25 mg/kg q6h.
- Dosing for GFR of 10–50: 25 mg/kg q12–24h (monitor CBC and serum levels with appropriate dose adjustments).
- Dosing for GFR of <10: 25 mg/kg q24–48h (monitor CBC serum levels closely with appropriate dose adjustments).
- Dosing in hemodialysis: 25 mg/kg q24–48h. Dose postdialysis on days of dialysis (monitor CBC and serum levels w/ appropriate dose adjustment).
- Dosing in peritoneal dialysis: 0.5–1.0 g q24h (monitor CBC and serum levels w/ appropriate dose adjustments).
- Dosing in hemofiltration: CVVH and CVVHD: no data. Consider 25 mg/kg q12h for dialysis rate ≥ 1.5 L/hr or 25 mg/kg q24h for dialysis rate of 1 L/hr (monitor CBC and serum levels with appropriate dose adjustments).

COMMENTS

- Recommended in combination with amphotericin B or liposomal amphotericin for treatment of cryptococcal meningitis. Resulting in more rapid CSF sterilization, but clinical outcome similar with or without 5-FC. Should be used if tolerated, but can treat with amphotericin B alone if toxicity develops. Goal: peak of 30–80 mcg/mL 2 hrs postdose after 3–5 days.
- Close monitoring of renal function and serum level critical to prevent bone marrow suppression.

SELECTED REFERENCES

Perfect JR, Dismukes WE, Dromer F, et al. Clinical practice guidelines for the management of cryptococcal disease: 2010 update by the Infectious Diseases Society of America. *Clin Infect Dis*, 2010; 50: 291–322.
Comments: 5-FC + amphotericin B, liposomal amphotericin, or amphotericin lipid complex (for ≥2 wks) is recommended for treatment of cryptococcal meningitis. Without 5-FC, recommended amphotericin B treatment duration is 4–6 wks. Fluconazole 1200 mg/day + 5-FC × 6 wks is alternative in patients unable to tolerate amphotericin.

Saag MS, Cloud GA, Graybill JR, et al. A comparison of itraconazole versus fluconazole as maintenance therapy for AIDS-associated cryptococcal meningitis. National Institute of Allergy and Infectious Diseases Mycoses Study Group. *Clin Infect Dis*, 1999; 28: 291–6.
Comments: Fluconazole superior to itraconazole for maintenance therapy of cryptococcal meningitis. Factor best associated with relapse was having not received 5-FC during the initial 2 wks of primary treatment for cryptococcal disease (relative risk = 5.88; 95% CI, 1.27–27.14; P = 0.04).

van der Horst CM, Saag MS, Cloud GA, et al. Treatment of cryptococcal meningitis associated with the acquired immunodeficiency syndrome. National Institute of Allergy and Infectious Diseases Mycoses Study Group and AIDS Clinical Trials Group. *N Engl J Med*, 1997; 337: 15–21.
Comments: Addition of 5-FC to amphotericin resulted in faster CSF sterilization but did not improve clinical outcome.

FOSCARNET

Paul A. Pham, PharmD and John G. Bartlett, MD

INDICATIONS

FDA

- CMV retinitis in immunocompromised patients.
- Acyclovir-resistant mucocutaneous herpes simplex virus (HSV-1 and HSV-2) infections in immunocompromised patients.

Non-FDA Approved Uses

- Ganciclovir-resistant CMV retinitis.
- Extraocular CMV infection.

FORMS TABLE

Brand name (mfr)	Forms†	Cost*
Foscavir and generic (Astra Zeneca and generic manufacturers)	IV vial 24 mg/mL (250 mL; 500 mL)	$91.26 per 250-mL vial; $180.90 per 500-mL vial

*Prices represent cost per unit specified, are representative of Average Wholesale Price (AWP).
†Dosage is indicated in mg unless otherwise noted.

USUAL ADULT DOSING

- CMV retinitis: induction 90 mg/kg IV q12h × 14 days over 1 hr via infusion pump; maintenance 90–120 mg/kg IV once daily over 2 hrs via infusion pump (120 mg/kg IV daily after reinduction for a relapse).
- Extraocular CMV disease (e.g. GI, neuro): 90 mg/kg q12 × 14–21 days. Role of maintenance dose unclear but most recommend maintenance dose with reoccurrences.
- Acyclovir-resistant HSV and VZV: 60 mg/kg q12h × 3 wks.
- Infuse foscarnet over 2 hrs with 500 cc NS pre- and posthydration.
- Dose adjustment in renal failure: >1.4 mL/min/kg: 90 mg/kg q12h (induction); 90 mg/kg once daily (maintenance).
- Administer by controlled IV infusion (24 mg/mL via central venous line or 12 mg/mL via peripheral vein). Solns (with NL saline or 5% dextrose) should be used within 24 hrs of 1st entry into sealed foscarnet bottle. Do not coadminister with other drugs or supplements concurrently via the same catheter.
- Not recommended with CrCl <0.4 mL/min/kg (unless irreversible renal failure on HD).

ADVERSE DRUG REACTIONS

Common

- Renal failure (Cr 2 mg/dL in up to 37% of patients); often reversible if discontinued early. Hydrate adequately and monitor Cr 2–3 ×/wk during induction and weekly during maintenance. Discontinue if Cr >2.9 mg/dL.
- Electrolyte imbalance (hypocalcemia, hypophosphatemia, hypomagnesemia, and hypokalemia (8%–15%); monitor chem 2 ×/wk during induction and weekly during maintenance.

Occasional

- Paresthesias and seizures secondary to electrolyte imbalance.
- Penile ulcers.
- Nausea and vomiting.

Rare

- Fever.
- Rash.
- Bone marrow suppression.
- LFTs elevation.
- Headache.

DRUG INTERACTIONS

- Amphotericin B, aminoglycoside, cidofovir and other nephrotoxic agents: additive nephrotoxicity with foscarnet coadministration.
- Imipenem: possible increase in risk of seizure.
- Nephrotoxic agents: increased risk of nephrotoxicity.
- Pentamidine (IV): additive hypocalcemia and nephrotoxicity with coadministration.

RESISTANCE

- Foscarnet resistance mutations in DNA polymerase gene include V787L and E756Q and are associated with retinitis progression (OR 14; P = 0.016) (*J Infect Dis* 2003; 187: 77–84.)
- Foscarnet cross-resistance among ganciclovir-resistant strains is rare.

DRUGS

PHARMACOLOGY
Mechanism

- Pyrophosphate analog of phosphonoacetic acid that directly blocks pyrophosphate binding site of viral DNA polymerase, preventing cleavage of pyrophosphate from deoxynucleoside triphosphate and elongation of viral DNA chains. Unlike acyclovir and ganciclovir, foscarnet does not require thymidine kinase for activation.

Pharmacokinetic Parameters

- **Absorption:** poor absorption; 12%–22% (only given IV).
- **Metabolism and Excretion:** not metabolized; approximately 80%–87% of drug excreted unchanged in the urine via glomerular filtration and tubular secretion.
- **Protein Binding:** 14%–17%.
- **Cmax, Cmin, and AUC:** 575 mcg/L after 57 mg/kg administration.
- **T$_{\frac{1}{2}}$:** 3 hrs.
- **Distribution:** 43% CNS penetration; sequestered in bone and cartilage.

Pregnancy Risk

- Category C: skeletal malformation or variation in animal studies. No human data available; however, some experts feel that foscarnet should be used as 1st-line agent for sight-threatening CMV retinitis in pregnant women (due to high incidence of nephrotoxicity, antepartum testing of fetus and close monitoring of the amniotic fluid to observe for fetal nephrotoxicity recommended).

Breastfeeding Compatibility

- No data, most likely excreted in human milk; excreted in breast milk in animal studies. Due to potential for severe adverse reaction to foscarnet, mother should avoid foscarnet when breastfeeding.

DOSING
Dosing for Decreased Hepatic Function

- No data. Usual dose likely.

Renal Dosing

- CrCl of 1.0–1.4 mL/min/kg 70 mg/kg q12h (induction); 70 mg/kg once daily (maintenance).
- CrCl of 0.8–1.0 mL/min/kg 50 mg/kg q12h (induction); 50 mg/kg once daily (maintenance).
- CrCl of 0.6–0.8 mL/min/kg 80 mg/kg q24h (induction); 80 mg/kg every other day (maintenance).
- CrCl of 0.5–0.6 mL/min/kg 60 mg/kg q24h (induction); 60 mg/kg every other day (maintenance).
- CrCl of 0.4–0.5 mL/min/kg 50 mg/kg q24h (induction); 50 mg/kg every other day (maintenance).
- Dosing for GFR of <20: contraindicated (unless irreversible renal failure on HD).
- Dosing in hemodialysis: 38% removal, 60 mg/kg post-HD (consider monitoring serum levels: goal of 500–800 mcg).
- Dosing in peritoneal dialysis: dose for GFR <10 mL/min.

COMMENTS

- Parenteral antiviral agent with activity against HSV, VZV, and CMV.
- Generally considered 2nd line to valganciclovir or ganciclovir for CMV infections due to unfavorable side effect profile (nephrotoxicity and electrolyte imbalance). Close monitoring of electrolytes and renal function needed.
- Active against ganciclovir-resistant CMV and acyclovir-resistant HSV and VZV.

SELECTED REFERENCES

Kaplan JE, Benson C, Holmes KH, et al. Guidelines for prevention and treatment of opportunistic infections in HIV-infected adults and adolescents: recommendations from CDC, the National Institutes of Health, and the HIV Medicine Association of the Infectious Diseases Society of America. *MMWR Recomm Rep*, 2009; 58: 1–207.

Comments: Foscarnet is recommended treatment option in patients with CMV retinitis. Frequently used as an alternative to valganciclovir or ganciclovir due to high rates of nephrotoxicity and electrolyte imbalance. Should be considered if ganciclovir resistance suspected.

Jacobson MA, Wulfsohn M, Feinberg JE, et al. Phase II dose-ranging trial of foscarnet salvage therapy for cytomegalovirus retinitis in AIDS patients intolerant of or resistant to ganciclovir (ACTG protocol 093). AIDS Clinical Trials Group of the National Institute of Allergy and Infectious Diseases. *AIDS*, 1994; 8: 451–9.

Comments: Trial examined different doses of foscarnet in patients intolerant to or resistant to ganciclovir. Foscarnet effective in ganciclovir-resistant CMV retinitis, but time to CMV retinitis progression (pre-HAART) on therapy was disappointing (median 8 wks at all doses studied). 30% reduction in the risk of visual acuity loss with ART (*Ophthalmol*, 2003; 121(1): 99–107.)

GANCICLOVIR

Paul A. Pham, PharmD and John G. Bartlett, MD

INDICATIONS

FDA

- Treatment of CMV retinitis (IV) in immunocompromised patients.
- Prophylaxis and prevention of CMV disease reoccurrence in patients with AIDS and solid organ transplant recipients (use for primary prophylaxis in HIV is FDA approved but not currently recommended).
- Herpes keratitis (ophthalmic gel).

Non-FDA Approved Uses

- Castleman disease (limited data).

FORMS TABLE

Brand name (mfr)	Forms†	Cost*
Cytovene (Roche Pharmaceuticals)	IV vial 500 mg	$81.06
Gancicovir (generic) (Ranbaxy Pharmaceuticals)	Oral capsule 250 mg; 500 mg	$4.72; $9.44
Vitrasert ocular implant (Bausch and Lomb)	Ocular implant 4.5 mg	$19,200.00/per implant
Zirgan (Sirion Therapeutics)	Ocular ophthalmic gel 0.15%	$169

*Prices represent cost per unit specified, are representative of Average Wholesale Price (AWP).
†Dosage is indicated in mg unless otherwise noted.

USUAL ADULT DOSING

- CMV retinitis induction: 5 mg/kg IV q12h × 2 wks (alternative is valganciclovir 900 mg PO twice daily × 3 wks) + implant then maintenance valganciclovir.
- CMV retinitis maintenance: 5 mg/kg IV daily until immune reconstitution (CD4 >150 for 3–6 mos with inactive disease and follow-up by ophthalmologist). Decision to stop ganciclovir maintenance should take into account anatomic location of the retinal lesions, vision in contralateral eye, and feasibility of regular opthalmologic monitoring.
- Preferred maintenance regimen is valganciclovir (900 mg PO once daily). Provides serum concentrations comparable to those achieved with IV ganciclovir. IV reserved for patients unable to take PO or for seriously ill patients. For patients with small peripheral lesions oral valganciclovir alone may be adequate.
- IV foscarnet, IV cidofovir, valganciclovir, and ganciclovir (IV, implant) are all effective, but longest time to relapse with ocular implant.
- Implant: 4.5 mg ocular implant q6–9 mos (+ valganciclovir). Many opthalmologists recommend initial intravitreous injection of ganciclovir ASAP, until the ganciclovir implant can be placed.
- CMV encephalitis and CMV polyradiculitis: 5 mg/kg IV q12h (consider combination therapy with foscarnet), then 5 mg/kg q24h until immune reconstitution.
- CMV (GI): 5 mg/kg q12h × 3–6 wks. The role of maintenance ganciclovir is unclear. In an open label study, after an initial response, time to progression not significantly different between recipients (16 wks) and nonrecipients (13 wks) of maintenance therapy (*J Infect Dis*, 1995; 172(3): 622–8.)

DRUGS

- Herpes keratitis: ganciclovir ophthalmic gel 1 drop 5 × daily, until corneal ulcer heals, then 1 drop 3 × daily × 7 days.

ADVERSE DRUG REACTIONS

Common

- Neutropenia (reversible and responds to G-CSF).
- Reversible thrombocytopenia.
- Monitor CBC 2–3/wk and discontinue or add G-CSF if ANC <500; discontinue for PLT <25,000.

Occasional

- Anemia.
- Fever.
- Rash.
- Headache, seizures, confusion, change in mental status.
- Hepatoxicity.
- GI intolerance.

Rare

- Coma.

DRUG INTERACTIONS

- AZT: additive risk of neutropenia with coadministration.
- ddI: ddI AUC increased 111% with oral ganciclovir and 50%–70% with IV ganciclovir. Avoid or use with close monitoring for ddI-induced toxicity.
- Imipenem-cilastatin: potential for generalized seizures.
- Pyrimethamine, 5-FC, interferon: potential for additive bone marrow suppression.

PHARMACOLOGY

Mechanism

- Guanosine that requires TK (HSV/VZV) or protein kinase (CMV) as 1st step to convert to triphosphate, which inhibits viral DNA polymerase.

Pharmacokinetic Parameters

- **Absorption:** 5% (fasting); 6%–9% (with food).
- **Metabolism and Excretion:** not metabolized; 90%–99% excreted unchanged in the urine.
- **Protein Binding:** 1%–2%; low protein binding.
- **Cmax, Cmin, and AUC:** 9.5–11.6 mcg/mL after 5 mg/kg IV.
- **T$_{\frac{1}{2}}$:** 2.5–4 hrs.
- **Distribution:** 7%–67% CNS penetration. Good intraocular penetration.

Pregnancy Risk

- Category C: teratogenic, carcinogenic, and embryogenic; growth retardation; aplastic organ and aspermatogenesis in animal studies. No human data; use only for life-threatening CMV infection and warn patient of possible teratogenic effect.

Breastfeeding Compatibility

- No data; due to the potential for serious toxicity, mother should avoid breastfeeding.

DOSING

Dosing for Decreased Hepatic Function

- No data; usual dose likely.

Renal Dosing

- Dosing for GFR of 50–69: 2.5 mg/kg q12h or 500 mg PO 3 × daily.
- Dosing for GFR of 25–49: 2.5 mg/kg IV q24h or 1000 mg PO once daily.
- Dosing for GFR of 10–24: 1.25 mg/kg IV q24h or 500 mg PO once daily.
- Dosing for GFR of <10: induction dose: 1.25 mg/kg IV 3 ×/wk or 500 mg PO 3 ×/wk.
- Dosing in hemodialysis: 50% of dose removed after 4 hrs of HD. Induction dose: 1.25 mg/kg IV 3 ×/wk or 500 mg PO 3 ×/wk given post-HD.
- Dosing in peritoneal dialysis: no data, likely to be removed.
- Dosing in hemofiltration: removed in CVVHD. Limited data, consider 5 mg/kg q48h (induction) or 2.5 mg/kg q48h (maintenance).

COMMENTS
- An agent of choice for CMV infection due to better side effect profile vs foscarnet and cidofovir. Acyclovir-resistant HSV usually cross-resistant to ganciclovir.
- Oral ganciclovir replaced by valganciclovir for maintenance therapy of CMV retinitis due to poor absorption, high pill burden.
- Neutropenia (ANC <500) or thrombocytopenia (<25,000) are contraindications to initial use.

SELECTED REFERENCES

Kaplan JE, Benson C, Holmes KH, et al. Guidelines for prevention and treatment of opportunistic infections in HIV-infected adults and adolescents: recommendations from CDC, the National Institutes of Health, and the HIV Medicine Association of the Infectious Diseases Society of America. *MMWR Recomm Rep*, 2009; 58: 1–207.
Comments: Valganciclovir, IV ganciclovir, IV ganciclovir followed by valganciclovir, IV foscarnet, IV cidofovir, and ganciclovir intraocular implant + valganciclovir are all effective treatments for CMV retinitis.

Martin DF, Sierra-Madero J, Walmsley S, et al. A controlled trial of valganciclovir as induction therapy for cytomegalovirus retinitis. *N Engl J Med*, 2002; 346: 1119–26.
Comments: Valganciclovir 900 mg twice daily is bioequivalent to IV ganciclovir 5 mg/kg twice daily. Response rate comparable in the 2 groups; 47 of 61 patients (77%) assigned to IV ganciclovir and 46 of 64 (72%) assigned to valganciclovir had a satisfactory response (5.2% points; 95% CI, -20.4–10.1).

Martin DF, Parks DJ, Mellow SD, et al. Treatment of cytomegalovirus retinitis with an intraocular sustained-release ganciclovir implant. A randomized controlled clinical trial. *Arch Ophthalmol*, 1994; 112: 1531–9.
Comments: Ganciclovir implants were highly effective for treatment of CMV retinitis (median time to relapse 226 days). Systemic CMV disease and retinitis in contralateral eye observed in 31% and 50% of patients, respectively. Current recommendation is to administer oral valganciclovir in conjunction with ganciclovir implant to protect contralateral eye and prevent systemic CMV disease.

ISONIAZID

Paul A. Pham, PharmD and John G. Bartlett, MD

INDICATIONS
FDA
- Treatment and prevention of TB.

FORMS TABLE

Brand name (mfr)	Forms†	Cost*
Isoniazid (generic manufacturers [Barr Pharmaceuticals, Eon Pharmaceuticals, and others])	Oral tablet 100 mg; 300 mg Oral syrup 50 mg/5 mL (16 oz)	$0.09; $0.34 $58.00
Nydrazid (Geneva Pharmaceuticals)	IM vial 100 mg/mL (10 mL)	$24.90
Rifamate (Aventis Pharmaceuticals)	Oral capsule INH 150 mg/ RIF 300 mg	$3.71
Rifater (Aventis Pharmaceuticals)	Oral capsule INH 50 mg/RIF 120 mg/PZA 300 mg	$2.32

*Prices represent cost per unit specified, are representative of Average Wholesale Price (AWP).
†Dosage is indicated in mg unless otherwise noted.

USUAL ADULT DOSING
- Treatment of latent TB (prophylaxis): INH 5 mg/kg (max 300 mg) PO once daily × 9 mos or directly observed therapy (DOT): 15 mg/kg (max 900 mg) 2 ×/wk × 9 mos.
- Active TB treatment (with other anti-TB agents): 5 mg/kg (max 300 mg) PO once daily × 6–9 mos or DOT: 15 mg/kg (max 900 mg) 2–3 ×/wk × 6–9 mos.
- Active TB treatment continuation phase (with other anti-TB agents): 3 ×/wk for CD4 <100.

DRUGS

- Active TB treatment duration: 6 mos for most forms except severe cavitary pulmonary (9 mos), bone/joint (9 mos), miliary (9 mos), CNS (9–12 mos).
- Coadminister with pyridoxine 50 mg/day or 100 mg 2 ×/wk to prevent neuropathy.
- DOT preferred for active TB in all patients.
- Obtain CBC and LFTs at baseline and periodically throughout course of therapy. Monitor monthly for hepatitis Sx; consider monthly LFTs in patients with other risks for hepatotoxicity.
- Administer 1 hr before or 2 hrs after meals.

ADVERSE DRUG REACTIONS
Common
- Increased transaminases: increased ALT in 10%–20% (d/c if LFTs >5 × ULN).

Occasional
- GI intolerance (diarrhea with liquid INH; crushed tabs typically better tolerated in infants/children).

Rare
- Clinical hepatitis in 0.6% and fatal hepatitis in 0.02% (risk increased with age, alcohol use, prior liver disease, concurrent RIF, and pregnancy). May occur even after mos on treatment. In most cases, enzyme levels return to normal with discontinuation of therapy. Recommend monthly clinical and lab monitoring. Instruct patients to report Sxs of hepatitis. D/C if Sxs or signs of hepatic damage. Consider non-/less hepatotoxic alternatives. Reinstitute only after Sxs and lab abnormalities resolved. Restart with gradual dose escalation. Withdraw with any indication of recurrent liver damage.
- Peripheral neuropathy and optic neuropathy (dose-related and prevented by pyridoxine coadministration).
- Hypersensitivity reaction (rash, exfoliative dermatitis, urticaria, and edema).
- Fever.
- CNS toxicity: psychosis.
- Arthralgia.
- Bone marrow suppression.

DRUG INTERACTIONS
- Antacids: may decrease INH absorption (avoid coadministration).
- Benzodiazepines (i.e., diazepam, triazolam, midazolam): may increase benzodiazepine serum levels. Consider using oxazepam or lorazepam with INH coadministration.
- Carbamazepine: may increase carbamazepine levels. Monitor closely.
- Cycloserine: may increase central nervous system adverse effects. Monitor closely and discontinue if severe.
- Enflurane: in rapid acetylators of INH, high output renal failure may occur. Monitor closely.
- Ethanol: avoid.
- Ethionamide: may increase INH serum level. Monitor for toxicity (peripheral neuritis and hepatotoxicity) with coadministration.
- Ketoconazole: may decrease ketoconazole levels (based on case reports, clinical significance unknown).
- Phenytoin: may increase phenytoin levels. Monitor closely.
- Prednisone and prednisolone: may decrease INH serum levels. Monitor INH for therapeutic efficacy.
- Rifampin: possible additive hepatotoxicity due to production of secondary pathway metabolite of INH (hydrazine and isonicotinic acid). Consider rifabutin.
- Theophylline: serum level may be increased. Dose may need to be decreased.
- Tyramine rich foods (wine, cheese, etc.): may develop monoamine poisoning (avoid tyramine rich foods).
- Warfarin: may increase INR, monitor closely.

PHARMACOLOGY
Mechanism
- Inhibits mycolic acid synthesis which results in loss of acid-fastness and disruption of bacterial cell wall. May interfere with metabolism of bacterial proteins, nucleic acid, lipids, and carbohydrates.

Pharmacokinetic Parameters
- **Absorption:** 90% readily absorbed.
- **Metabolism and Excretion:** hepatic acetylation via N-acetyl transferase (rate of acetylation is genetically determined). 75%–95% excreted by the kidney mainly as inactive metabolite (90% as metabolite in fast acetylator, 63% as metabolite in slow acetylator). Approximately 50% of whites and blacks are slow acetylators. Rate of acetylation does not affect efficacy of standard once–daily or DOT regimens.
- **Protein Binding:** 0%–10%.
- **Cmax, Cmin, and AUC:** Cmax: 3–7 mcg/mL after 300 mg PO.
- **T$_{\frac{1}{2}}$:** 0.5–4 hrs.
- **Distribution:** 0.57–0.76 L/kg; widely distributed in all fluid and tissue, pleural and ascitic fluid, skin, sputum, saliva, lungs, muscle, and caseous tissue. Good CSF penetration (20%–90% of serum levels attained in the CSF); therapeutic level attained in CSF.

Pregnancy Risk
- Category C: animal studies show embryocidal effect, but not teratogenic. Retrospective analysis of more than 4900 exposures to INH did not result in increased rate of fetal malformation. Pregnant women with active TB should be treated immediately. American Academy of Pediatrics recommends that pregnant women with + PPD should receive INH if HIV +, have recent contact or X-ray showing old TB; begin after 1st trimester if possible. Treatment of latent TB should be deferred in patients with acute hepatic diseases.

Breastfeeding Compatibility
- Excreted in breast milk at levels insufficient for Rx of active or latent TB. American Academy of Pediatrics considers INH safe with breastfeeding.

DOSING

Dosing for Decreased Hepatic Function
- Use with caution in hepatic impairment; use is contraindicated if acute liver disease or history of INH-associated hepatitis.

Renal Dosing
- Dosing for GFR of 10–80: usual dose.
- Dosing for GFR of <10: if slow acetylator use 150 mg PO once daily; HD: 5 mg/kg postdialysis.
- Dosing in hemodialysis: 5 mg/kg postdialysis.
- Dosing in peritoneal dialysis: once daily dose postdialysis (50% of dose if slow acetylator).
- Dosing in hemofiltration: no data.

COMMENTS
- 1st-line agent for treatment and prophylaxis of TB. Because of high prevalence of INH resistance, treatment with RIF-containing regimen should be strongly considered in the treatment of latent TB for immigrants from Vietnam, Haiti, and Philippines (NEJM 2002; 347: 1850).

SELECTED REFERENCES

Blumberg HM, Burman WJ, Chaisson RE, et al. Treatment of tuberculosis: American Thoracic Society/Centers for Disease Control and Prevention/Infectious Diseases Society of America. *Am J Respir Crit Care Med*, 2003; 167: 603–62.
Comments: Current guidelines for treatment of active TB in the US.

American Thoracic Society. Targeted tuberculin testing and treatment of latent tuberculosis infection. *Am J Respir Crit Care Med*, 2000; 161: S221–47.
Comments: Current guidelines for tuberculin (PPD) testing and treatment of latent TB in the US.

ITRACONAZOLE

Paul A. Pham, PharmD and John G. Bartlett, MD

INDICATIONS

FDA
- Histoplasmosis, including chronic cavitary pulmonary disease and disseminated nonmeningeal histoplasmosis (oral capsule). Pulmonary and extrapulmonary blastomycosis in immunocompromised and nonimmunocompromised patients (oral capsule).

DRUGS

ANTIMICROBIAL AGENTS

- Onychomycosis (oral capsule).
- Oropharyngeal and esophageal candidiasis (oral liquid).
- Neutropenic fever in patients with a suspected fungal infection (oral liquid).
- Aspergillosis treatment in patients intolerant of or refractory to amphotericin B therapy (oral capsule no longer preferred; see Voriconazole p. 260).

Non-FDA Approved Uses
- Coccidioidomycosis.
- Cryptococcosis.
- Penicilliosis.
- Sporotrichosis.
- *Candida* vaginitis.
- Fluconazole-resistant esophageal candidiasis.
- Prophylaxis of invasive fungal infections, susceptible hosts (prolonged neutropenia, GVH).

FORMS TABLE

Brand name (mfr)	Forms†	Cost*
Sporanox (JOM Pharmaceutical)	Oral capsule 100 mg Oral soln 10 mg/mL (150 mL) IV vial 10 mg/mL (250 mg)	$14.48 $202.94 n/a (no longer available in the US)
Itraconazole (Sandoz generic manufacturer)	100 mg capsule	$9.28

*Prices represent cost per unit specified, are representative of Average Wholesale Price (AWP).
†Dosage is indicated in mg unless otherwise noted.

USUAL ADULT DOSING
- Aspergillosis: 200 mg twice daily (caps). Voriconazole is preferred azole.
- Blastomycosis: 200 mg once or twice daily (caps). Preferred azole for nonmeningeal cases (fluconazole preferred for meningeal cases). Initial therapy with amphotericin B recommended.
- *Candida* esophagitis: 200 mg liquid swish and swallow once daily × 14 days (fluconazole preferred).
- *Candida* vaginitis: 200 mg once daily (caps) × 3 days or 200 mg PO twice daily × 1 day (fluconazole preferred).
- Coccidioidomycosis: 200–400 mg (caps) PO twice daily (acute treatment of nonmeningeal coccidioidomycosis) then maintenance with 200 mg (caps) PO twice daily. Preferred azole for nonmeningeal coccidioidomycosis (fluconazole preferred for meningeal cases).
- Cryptococcal meningitis: 200 mg PO once-daily (caps) maintenance (after 2 wks of amphotericin B in patients who can not tolerate fluconazole).
- Nonmeningeal cryptococcosis: 200 mg PO twice daily (caps) × 8 wks then 200 mg PO once-daily maintenance (fluconazole preferred).
- Histoplasmosis: 200 mg PO 3 × daily × 3 days (loading dose) then 200 mg PO twice daily. Preferred azole but amphotericin B indicated for initial treatment of severe disseminated disease.
- Onychomycosis: pulse therapy with 200 mg twice daily (caps) × 1 wk per mo × 2 mos (fingernails). For toenails treat with 200 mg once daily (caps) × 3 mos. Not recommended in patients with CHF.
- Penicilliosis: 200 mg PO twice daily (caps) + amphotericin B 0.7 mg/kg × 1–2 wks then 200 mg PO twice-daily (caps) maintenance (preferred azole).
- Sporotrichosis: 200 mg PO twice daily (caps) × 3–6 mos. Preferred azole for lymphocutaneous cases. Amphotericin B preferred for disseminated cases.
- Neutropenic fever: no longer generally used for acute treatment of suspected invasive fungal infections, but still employed by some institutions for prophylaxis, 200 mg (oral soln preferred) PO twice daily.
- Take caps with food and acidic beverage (e.g., colas), since absorption dependent on acidity. Avoid PPIs and H2 blockers that reduce gastric acidity.

- Liquid preparation has superior bioavailability; take on empty stomach (food decreases absorption of liquid by 30%).
- Most studies have been performed with capsule formulation, but liquid should be considered if desired serum concentrations are not achieved.
- Target serum concentrations (Cmax at steady state) for invasive fungal diseases: >1 mcg/mL 2 hrs postdose after 5 days of therapy. Send 2–4 mL in frozen state to Dr. Rinaldi's lab (210–567–4131).
- Loading doses: 200 mg caps 3 × daily (caps) × 3 days. Monitoring of serum level recommended for all serious systemic infections.
- Dose conversion from capsule to liquid: 200-mg capsule = 100-mg liquid (variable serum concentrations; therefore, TDM recommended for invasive fungal diseases).

ADVERSE DRUG REACTIONS
Common
- GI intolerance (nausea and vomiting).
Occasional
- Headache.
- Rash.
- Increased transaminases.
Rare
- Hypokalemia; adrenal insufficiency (generally with long-term use of high dose), impotence; gynecomastia; and leg edema associated with high dose (>600 mg/day).
- Cardiotoxicity with negative inotropic effect.
- Severe hepatitis.
- Neuropathy.
- Hearing loss.

DRUG INTERACTIONS
- CYP3A4 substrates may be significantly increased. Avoid or use with close monitoring.
- Itraconazole is substrate and inhibitor of CYP3A4.

DRUG-DRUG INTERACTIONS—See Appendix I, p. 545, for table of drug-drug interactions.
PHARMACOLOGY
Mechanism
- Triazoles alter fungal cell membrane function by inhibiting C-14 alpha anosterol demethylase, thereby interfering with ergosterol synthesis, which results in increased cell permeability and leakage of essential elements.
Pharmacokinetic Parameters
- **Absorption:** variable and dependent on gastric acidity (decreased absorption with achlorhydria; common in AIDS); increased absorption with soln (administer on empty stomach); capsule (administer with food).
- **Metabolism and Excretion:** extensive liver metabolism to active (hydroxyitraconazole) and inactive metabolite. 55% biliary excretion and 35% renal excretion of both active and inactive metabolites.
- **Protein Binding:** 90%–99%.
- **Cmax, Cmin, and AUC:** Cmax: 2 mcg/mL steady-state concentration after 200 mg PO twice-daily dose administration. Range of 0.5–1.1 mcg/mL after single-dose 100-mg dose administration.
- $T_{\frac{1}{2}}$: 56–64 hrs.
- **Distribution:** good tissue penetration including skin, liver, bone, adipose tissue, endometrium cervical mucus. Good nail and bronchial fluid distribution. Negligible CSF penetration; however treatment has been successfully reported for cryptococcal and coccidioidal meningitis.
Pregnancy Risk
- Category C: teratogenic in animal studies. Generally not recommended in pregnancy but some studies have found it to be safe (*Am J Obstet Gynecol. 2000; 183: 617–20*).
Breastfeeding Compatibility
- High breast milk excretion (up to 177% of plasma concentration). Because safety of itraconazole has not been evaluated, use of itraconazole during breastfeeding should be avoided.

DOSING

Dosing for Decreased Hepatic Function
- Use with caution. Usual dose likely based on a small study. Consider monitoring serum level.

Renal Dosing
- Dosing for GFR of 10–80: usual dose.
- Dosing for GFR of <10: usual dose; some recommend decreasing dose by 50%; HD: 100 mg q12–24h.
- Dosing in hemodialysis: no significant itraconazole removal during HD. 100 mg q12–24h.
- Dosing in peritoneal dialysis: no significant itraconazole removal during HD. 100 mg q12–24h.
- Dosing in hemofiltration: no data.

COMMENTS

- Absorption of capsules is pH dependent; therefore H2 blockers, PPIs, and antacid coadministration should be avoided. Improved absorption is achieved with acidic gastric environment (cola).
- Liquid formulation may be preferred due to better absorption but most studies have been performed with capsule formulation.
- Itraconazole is CYP3A4 substrate and inhibitor with potential for many drug-drug interactions. IV formulation no longer available in US.

SELECTED REFERENCES

Pappas PG, Rex JH, Sobel JD, et al. Guidelines for treatment of candidiasis. *Clin Infect Dis*, 2004; 38: 161–89.
Comments: Fluconazole, itraconazole soln, or voriconazole are recommended agents for esophagitis. Fluconazole preferred due to more reliable absorption and less drug-drug interactions.

Patterson TF, Kirkpatrick WR, White M, et al. Invasive aspergillosis. Disease spectrum, treatment practices, and outcomes. I3 Aspergillus Study Group. *Medicine* (Baltimore), 2000; 79: 250–60.
Comments: This is a report of 595 patients with proven or probable invasive aspergillosis. Only 25% of patients treated with amphotericin B responded, and mortality rate was 65%. Results were better with itraconazole, but these patients were less seriously immunosuppressed so that conclusions regarding relative merits were limited. Voriconazole is preferred agent for aspergillosis (*NEJM* 2002; 347: 408–15.)

Galgiani JN, Catanzaro A, Cloud GA, et al. Comparison of oral fluconazole and itraconazole for progressive, nonmeningeal coccidioidomycosis. A randomized, double-blind trial. Mycoses Study Group. *Ann Intern Med*, 2000; 133: 676–86.
Comments: Randomized, double-blind, placebo-controlled trial of oral fluconazole, 400 mg/day vs itraconazole, 200-mg tabs twice daily for 198 patients with chronic pulmonary, soft tissue or skeletal infections due to *C. immitis*. Response rate was 50% (47/94) for those treated with fluconazole and 63% (61/97) for those treated with itraconazole (P = 0.08). Authors concluded that these 2 azoles are comparably effective in nonmeningeal coccidioidomycosis, although there is a trend toward greater efficacy with itraconazole.

van der Horst CM, Saag MS, Cloud GA, et al. Treatment of cryptococcal meningitis associated with the acquired immunodeficiency syndrome. National Institute of Allergy and Infectious Diseases Mycoses Study Group and AIDS Clinical Trials Group. *N Engl J Med*, 1997; 337: 15–21.
Comments: Consolidation therapy with fluconazole associated with a higher rate of CSF sterilization compared to itraconazole.

KETOCONAZOLE

Paul A. Pham, PharmD and John G. Bartlett, MD

INDICATIONS

FDA
- Treatment of severe recalcitrant cutaneous dermatophyte infections (*Tinea corporis* and *Tinea cruris*) unresponsive to topical therapy or oral griseofulvin.
- Treatment of mucocutaneous candidiasis (esophagitis, oral thrush) and candiduria.
- Treatment of blastomycosis, coccidioidomycosis, histoplasmosis, chromomycosis, and paracoccidioidomycosis.

FORMS TABLE

Brand name (mfr)	Forms†	Cost*
Nizoral and generic (Janssen Pharmaceuticals and generic manufacturers)	Oral tablet 200 mg	$4.74 (brand); $3.16 (generic)
Nizoral and generic shampoo and generic (McNeil Pharmaceutical and generic manufacturers)	Topical shampoo 2% (4 oz)	$27.75
Nizoral cream and generic (generic manufacturers)	Topical cream 2% (15 g)	$16.46

*Prices represent cost per unit specified, are representative of Average Wholesale Price (AWP).
†Dosage is indicated in mg unless otherwise noted.

USUAL ADULT DOSING
- Thrush: 200 mg PO once daily to twice daily × 7–10 days (topical therapy with clotrimazole preferred).
- *Candida* esophagitis: 200–400 mg PO twice daily (fluconazole preferred) × 2–3 wks.
- *Candida* vaginitis: 200–400 mg/day × 7 days or 400 mg/day × 3 days.
- Nonmeningeal blastomycosis: 400–800 mg/day >6 mos (itraconazole preferred).
- Nonmeningeal coccidioidomycosis: 400 mg/day >1 y (itraconazole or fluconazole preferred).
- Histoplasmosis: not generally recommended (itraconazole preferred).
- Chromomycosis: not generally recommended (itraconazole preferred).
- Tinea: 200 mg PO once daily × 2–4 wks.
- Absorption dependent on gastric acidity, which decreases with advanced HIV disease. Administer with acidic drinks (orange juice, colas, etc).

ADVERSE DRUG REACTIONS
Common
- GI upset and abdominal pain.
- Transient transaminitis.

Occasional
- Decreased steroid and testosterone synthesis generally seen with prolonged use of doses >600 mg/day. Impotence, gynecomastia, oligospermia, reduced libido, and menstrual abnormalities secondary to decreased steroid synthesis.
- CNS: headache, somnolence, dizziness, photophobia.
- Hepatitis (more common compared to other azoles).
- Asthenia.

Rare
- Hepatic necrosis.
- Bone marrow suppression.
- Hallucination.
- Hypothyroidism.
- Adrenal crisis reported with prolonged use of high doses.

DRUG-DRUG INTERACTIONS—See Appendix I, p. 549, for table of drug-drug interactions.
PHARMACOLOGY
Mechanism
- Imidazoles alter fungal cell membrane function by interfering with ergosterol synthesis, which results in increased cell permeability and leakage of essential elements.

Pharmacokinetic Parameters
- **Absorption:** variable absorption. Dependent on gastric acidity; decreased absorption with achlorhydria (common in AIDS).
- **Metabolism and Excretion:** partially metabolized. Primarily excreted as unchanged drug and metabolite in feces via biliary excretion. Only a small amount excreted in urine.
- **Protein Binding:** 84%–99%.
- **Cmax, Cmin, and AUC:** Cmax: 4.2 mcg/mL after 200 mg PO dose administration.

DRUGS

- $T_{\frac{1}{2}}$: 8 hrs.
- **Distribution:** high concentration attained in liver, pituitary, adrenals. Lung, kidney, bladder, bone marrow, myocardium, and various glandular tissue distribution also noted. Low and unpredictable CSF concentration.

Pregnancy Risk

- Category C: teratogenic in animal studies. In surveillance study of Michigan Medicaid recipients, no birth defects found in 20 newborns exposed to oral ketoconazole during the 1st trimester. Since this study, FDA has received 6 reports of limb defects.

Breastfeeding Compatibility

- Breast milk excretion likely. Effect on the fetus unknown.

DOSING

Dosing for Decreased Hepatic Function

- Use with caution.

Renal Dosing

- No dose adjustment for renal impairment or dialysis.
- Dosing in hemofiltration: no data; usual dose likely.

COMMENTS

- Oral azole with pH-dependent absorption. Improved absorption achieved with an acidic gastric environment; avoid proton-pump inhibitor, H2 blocker, and antacid coadministration.
- Cheaper than fluconazole, but fluconazole preferred for treatment of *Candida* esophagitis due to more predictable absorption, better efficacy, and fewer drug-drug interactions.

SELECTED REFERENCES

Kaplan JE, Benson C, Holmes KH, et al. Guidelines for prevention and treatment of opportunistic infections in HIV-infected adults and adolescents: recommendations from CDC, the National Institutes of Health, and the HIV Medicine Association of the Infectious Diseases Society of America. *MMWR Recomm Rep*, 2009; 58: 1–207.
Comments: Due to variable absorption, ketoconazole less effective than fluconazole in treatment of oropharyngeal and esophageal candidiasis. Updated OI guidelines do not recommend ketoconazole for treatment of invasive or mucosal candidiasis.

de Repentigny L, Ratelle J. Comparison of itraconazole and ketoconazole in HIV-positive patients with oropharyngeal or esophageal candidiasis. Human Immunodeficiency Virus Itraconazole Ketoconazole Project Group. *Chemotherapy*, 1997; 42: 374–83.
Comments: Ketoconazole 200 mg/day compared to itraconazole 200 mg/day for treatment of oropharyngeal and esophageal candidiasis. Esophageal candidiasis cleared at 41 days in 100% and 91% of patients receiving itraconazole and ketoconazole, respectively (P = 0.08). Mean rates of infection relapse not statistically different in the 2 treatment groups. Comparable efficacy also demonstrated in other trials.

De Wit S, Weerts D, Goossens H, et al. Comparison of fluconazole and ketoconazole for oropharyngeal candidiasis in AIDS. *Lancet*, 1989; 1: 746–8.
Comments: Fluconazole 50 mg/day superior to ketoconazole 200 mg/day in treatment of oropharyngeal candidiasis (100% vs 75% clinical response, respectively).

LEVOFLOXACIN

Paul A. Pham, PharmD and John G. Bartlett, MD

INDICATIONS

FDA

- Acute bacterial exacerbations of chronic bronchitis (ABECB); acute bacterial sinusitis.
- Community-acquired pneumonia (CAP) (including those due to PCN-resistant *S. pneumoniae*) and nosocomial pneumonia (750 mg once daily).
- Inhalational anthrax (postexposure).
- Uncomplicated and complicated skin and soft tissue infections (750 mg once daily).
- Uncomplicated and complicated UTIs.
- Bacterial conjunctivitis (*Quixin* 0.5% opthalmic drops); treatment of corneal ulcer (1.5% ophthalmic soln).
- Chronic bacterial prostatitis.

FORMS TABLE

Brand name (mfr)	Forms†	Cost*
Levaquin (JOM Pharmaceutical)	Oral tablet 250 mg; 500 mg IV vial 500 mg/20 mL; 750 mg/30 mL Oral tablet 750 mg	$15.48; $17.74 $43.82; $58.16 $33.23
Levofloxacin (various generic manufacturers)	250 mg and 500 mg tabs	$16.81; $19.26
Quixin (JOM Pharmaceutical)	Topical ophthalmic soln (5 mL) 0.5%	$78.54
Iquix (JOM Pharmaceutical)	Topical ophthalmic soln (5 mL) 1.5%	$78.54

*Prices represent cost per unit specified, are representative of Average Wholesale Price (AWP).
†Dosage is indicated in mg unless otherwise noted.

USUAL ADULT DOSING
- CAP: 500 mg IV or PO once daily × 7–14 days.
- CAP: 750 mg IV or PO once daily × 5 days.
- Complicated skin and skin structure infections: 750 mg IV/PO once daily × 7–14 days.
- Nosocomial pneumonia: 750 mg IV/PO once daily × 7–14 days.
- UTI (uncomplicated): 250 mg PO once daily × 3 days.
- UTI (complicated): 250 mg PO once daily × 10 days.
- Chronic prostatitis: 500 mg PO once daily × 28 days.
- Acute sinusitis: 500 mg PO once daily × 7–14 days (r/o viral etiology 1st).
- ABECB: 500 mg PO once daily × 7 days (r/o viral etiology 1st).
- Bacterial conjunctivitis: 0.5% ophth. soln: 1–2 gtts in affected eye q2 hrs (up to 8 ×/day) × 2 days, then q4 hrs while awake (up to 4 ×/day) × 5 days.
- Corneal ulceration: 1–2 gtt (1.5%) in affected eye(s) q 30 min–2 hrs while awake and 4 and 6 hrs at night × 3 days, then 1–2 gtts in affected eye(s) q1–4 hrs while awake until completion.

ADVERSE DRUG REACTIONS
General
- Generally well tolerated.

Occasional
- GI intolerance: diarrhea.
- CNS: headache, malaise, insomnia, restlessness, dizziness.
- Allergic reactions.
- Photosensitivity/phototoxicity (can be severe).
- *C. difficile* colitis.

Rare
- Peripheral neuropathy.
- Increased hepatic enzymes.
- QTc prolongation (elderly patients may be more susceptible).
- Tendon rupture (increased incidence especially seen in patients >60, concurrent use of corticosteroids, kidney, heart, and lung transplant recipients).
- Seizure.
- Severe allergic reactions (TEN, Stevens-Johnsons syndrome, allergic pneumonitis, hepatitis, and bone marrow suppression).
- Interstitial nephritis.
- Hepatitis (generally occurred within 14 days of initiation and most cases occurred within 6 days).

DRUG INTERACTIONS
- Avoid concurrent use with other drugs that prolong the QT interval including Class Ia or Class III antiarrhythmic agents, in patients with hypokalemia, significant bradycardia, or cardiomyopathy.

DRUGS

- Divalent or trivalent cations (i.e., antacids, sucralfate, buffered ddI, vitamins, and minerals): interferes with levofloxacin absorption. Do not coadminister or administer levofloxacin 2 hrs before cation.
- NSAIDS: may increase risk of CNS side effects (clinical significance unknown).
- NFV: no drug interactions with levofloxacin. No data with other PIs but interaction unlikely.
- NVP: no drug interactions with levofloxacin. No data with other NNRTIs but interaction unlikely.
- Warfarin: may increase INR with coadministration. Monitor closely.

RESISTANCE
- PCN-resistant *S. pneumoniae* to levofloxacin is low but with increased use resistance is a concern.

PHARMACOLOGY
Mechanism
- Fluoroquinolones inhibits DNA topoisomerases (DNA gyrase and topoisomerase 4) by binding to DNA-enzyme complexes, thereby interfering with bacterial DNA replication and some aspects of transcription, repair, recombination, and transposition.

Pharmacokinetic Parameters
- **Absorption:** 98% absorbed. Can be administered without regard to food.
- **Metabolism and Excretion:** minimal hepatic metabolism. 87% of dose excreted unchanged in the urine within 48 hrs via glomerular filtration and tubular secretion.
- **Protein Binding:** 24%–38%.
- **Cmax, Cmin, AUC:** Cmax: 6.2 mcg/mL after 500 mg IV dose administration and 5.7 mcg/mL after 500 mg PO dose administration.
- **$T_{\frac{1}{2}}$:** 7 hrs.
- **Distribution:** mean Vd = 74–112 L. Widely distributed in kidneys, gallbladder, GYN tissues, liver, lung, prostatic tissue, phagocytic cells, urine, sputum, blister fluid, lungs, and bile. 30%–50% of serum attained in CSF with inflamed meninges.

Pregnancy Risk
- Category C: in a prospective follow-up study conducted by European Network of Teratology Information Services (ENTIS), 666 cases of fluoroquinolone exposure (majority of exposures were during 1st trimester) showed congenital malformation rate of 4.8%. From previous epidemiologic data, 4.8% did not exceed background rate. Animal data demonstrated arthropathy in immature animals with erosions in joint cartilage. Because of animal data and availability of alternative agents, use of fluoroquinolones during pregnancy is contraindicated.

Breastfeeding Compatibility
- Fluoroquinolones not recommended during breastfeeding due to potential for arthropathy (based on animal data).

DOSING
Dosing for Decreased Hepatic Function
- Usual dose likely.

Renal Dosing
- Dosing for GFR of 50–80: 500–750 mg once daily.
- Dosing for GFR of 20–49: 500–750 mg × 1, then 500 mg once daily or 750 mg every other day.
- Dosing for GFR of 10–19: 500–750 mg × 1, then 250–500 mg every other day.
- Dosing for GFR of <10: 500–750 mg, then 250–500 mg every other day.
- Dosing in hemodialysis: 500–750 mg, then 250–500 mg every other day.
- Dosing in peritoneal dialysis: 500–750 mg, then 250–500 mg every other day.
- Dosing in hemofiltration: 500–750 mg, then 250 mg once daily.

COMMENTS
- Levofloxacin is L-isomer of ofloxacin with good *in vitro* and clinical experience against *S. pneumoniae* and atypical agents of pneumonia. Used primarily for lower respiratory tract infections and FDA approved for PCN-resistant *S. pneumoniae* and nosocomial pneumonia. Comparable to moxifloxacin for treatment of community-acquired pneumonia. May result in false-positive opiate urine screen (*JAMA* 2001; 286: 3115–9).

SELECTED REFERENCES
Jacobson KR, Tierney DB, Jeon CY, et al. Treatment outcomes among patients with extensively drug-resistant tuberculosis: systematic review and meta-analysis. *Clin Infect Dis*, 2010; 51: 6–14.

Comments: A meta-analysis of 13 observational studies involving 560 patients found that younger patients and the use of later generation fluoroquinolone (e.g., moxifloxacin, levofloxacin) were associated with favorable treatment outcomes (OR 3.7; P = 0.012).

Mandell LA, Wunderink RG, Anzueto A, et al. Infectious Diseases Society of America/American Thoracic Society consensus guidelines on the management of community-acquired pneumonia in adults. *Clin Infect Dis*, 2007; 44 (suppl 2): S27–72.

Comments: IDSA guidelines recommend respiratory fluoroquinolone (i.e., levofloxacin, moxifloxacin, or gemifloxacin) for outpatient treatment of CAP in patients with comorbidities or in patients requiring hospital admissions (non-ICU). In ICU patients with CAP, cefotaxime or ceftriaxone should be used in combination with a respiratory fluoroquinolone.

Ho PL, Que TL, Chiu SS, et al. Fluoroquinolone and other antimicrobial resistance in invasive pneumococci, Hong Kong, 1995–2001. *Emerg Infect Dis*, 2004; 10: 1250–7.

Comments: In 265 invasive isolates of pneumococci obtained during 1995–2001, prevalence of levofloxacin resistance (MIC >8 μg/mL) was 3.8% but increased to 15.2% among PNC-resistant isolates. Resistance to levofloxacin remains low in the US but is a concern with widespread use.

Villani P, Viale P, Signorini L, et al. Pharmacokinetic evaluation of oral levofloxacin in human immunodeficiency virus-infected subjects receiving concomitant antiretroviral therapy. *Antimicrob Agents Chemother*, 2001; 45: 2160–2.
Comments: No drug interactions between levofloxacin, NVP, and NFV.

Frothingham R. Rates of torsades de pointes associated with ciprofloxacin, ofloxacin, levofloxacin, gatifloxacin, and moxifloxacin. *Pharmacotherapy*, 2001; 21: 1468–72.
Comments: True rates of torsades de pointes associated with fluoroquinolones remains to be determined. Clinicians should use ALL fluoroquinolones with caution in patients with risk factors for QT prolongation.

File TM, Segreti J, Dunbar L, et al. A multicenter, randomized study comparing the efficacy and safety of intravenous and/or oral levofloxacin versus ceftriaxone and/or cefuroxime axetil in treatment of adults with community-acquired pneumonia. *Antimicrob Agents Chemother*, 1997; 41: 1965–72.
Comments: Patients treated with levofloxacin had a higher clinical success (96% vs 90%) and bacterial eradication rates (98% vs 85%) compared to the ceftriaxone/cefuroxime + erythromycin group. *S. pneumoniae* was isolated in 15% of clinically evaluable patients whereas atypical bacterial pathogens were implicated in 38% (150/456). Possible explanation for these results is that cultures for *S. pneumoniae* were insensitive and serology for atypicals was nonspecific.

METRONIDAZOLE

Paul A. Pham, PharmD and John G. Bartlett, MD

INDICATIONS
FDA
- Anaerobic infections: intraabdominal infections; skin and skin structure infections; bone and joint infections.
- Bacterial septicemia; endocarditis (caused by *Bacteroides* spp.).
- Gynecologic infections (endometritis, endomyometritis, tubo-ovarian abscess, and postsurgical vaginal cuff infection) caused by anaerobes.
- Lower respiratory tract infections (in combination with another agent with activity against microaerophilic *Streptococcus*).
- Adjunct treatment for gastritis and duodenal ulcer associated with *Helicobacter pylori*.
- CNS infections (meningitis and brain abscess).
- Treatment of acute intestinal amebiasis and amebic liver abscess.
- Treatment of symptomatic and asymptomatic periodontal disease and trichomoniasis.
- Bacterial vaginosis (vaginal gel).
- Rosacea (topical gel).
Non-FDA Approved Uses
- Colitis, antibiotic-associated (treatment).
- Periodontal disease.
- Elective colorectal surgery prophylaxis (classified as contaminated or potentially contaminated).
- Treatment of giardiasis and dracunculiasis.

DRUGS

FORMS TABLE

Brand name (mfr)	Forms†	Cost*
Flagyl and generic (Pfizer and generic manufacturers)	Oral tablet 250 mg Oral cap 375 mg Oral tablet 500 mg IV vial 500 mg	$0.48 $5.24 $0.72 $2.58
Metrocream; Metrolotion (Galderma)	Topical cream 0.75% (45 g) Topical lotion 0.75% (70 g)	$249.40 $281.40 (2 oz)
MetroGel (vaginal) (Prasco)	Topical gel 0.75% (70 g)	$36.00
MetroGel and generic (Galderma; Taro)	Topical gel 0.75% (1.5 oz) Topical gel 1.0% (60 g)	$71.15 $193.20
Flagyl ER (Pfizer)	Oral extended release tab 750 mg	$12.70

*Prices represent cost per unit specified, are representative of Average Wholesale Price (AWP).
†Dosage is indicated in mg unless otherwise noted.

USUAL ADULT DOSING
- Susceptible anaerobic infections: 250–500 mg PO 3 × daily or 500 mg IV q6h (manufacturer's recommendation) or consider 0.5–1 g PO or IV q12h (based on PK data).
- *C. difficile* colitis: 500 mg PO 3 × daily or 250 mg PO 4 ×/day × 10–14 days.
- Bacterial vaginosis: 500 mg twice daily PO × 7 days or *Flagyl ER* 750 mg PO once daily × 7 days.
- Trichomoniasis: single 2 g × 1 dose or 500 mg PO twice daily × 7 days (alternative).
- Amebiasis: 750 mg PO 3 × daily × 5–10 days.
- Giardiasis: 250 mg PO 3 × daily × 5–10 days.

ADVERSE DRUG REACTIONS
Common
- GI intolerance.
- Metallic taste.
- Headache.
- Dark urine (harmless).

Occasional
- Peripheral neuropathy (with prolonged use—usually reversible).
- Phlebitis at injection sites.
- Disulfiram-like reaction with alcohol.
- Insomnia.
- Stomatitis.

Rare
- Seizures.
- Encephalopathy, aseptic meningitis, optic neuropathy, dysarthria.
- Stevens-Johnson syndrome.

DRUG INTERACTIONS
- Alcohol (including drugs coformulated with alcohol) should be avoided, and disulfiram should be discontinued 2 wks prior to use of metronidazole. Nausea, vomiting, headache, abdominal cramps, and flushing can occur. Acute of psychosis or confusional state have been reported.

DRUG-DRUG INTERACTIONS—See Appendix I, p. 568, for table of drug-drug interactions.
RESISTANCE
- *H. pylori* resistance rate up to 20%–30%. High metronidazole doses (1.5 g/day) may overcome resistance.

PHARMACOLOGY
Mechanism
- Exact mechanism not fully elucidated, but reduction of metronidazole may lead to a polar metabolite that disrupts DNA and inhibits nucleic acid synthesis.

Pharmacokinetic Parameters

- **Absorption:** 90% absorbed with oral administration (IV only if oral administration is contraindicated).
- **Metabolism and Excretion:** hepatic hydroxylation, oxidation, and glucuronide conjugation to an active metabolite (2-hydroxy metronidazole) accounts for 30%–60% of administered dose. 77% of the dose excreted in urine and 14% in feces as unchanged drug and metabolites within 5 days.
- **Protein Binding:** 20%.
- **Cmax, Cmin, and AUC:** 20–25 mcg/mL after 500 mg PO or IV dose administration.
- **$T_{\frac{1}{2}}$:** 6–14 hrs.
- **Distribution:** distributed to saliva, bile, seminal fluid, bone, liver, and liver abscesses, lungs, vaginal secretions. Good CSF penetration (30%–100% of serum levels attained in the CSF).

Pregnancy Risk

- Category B: animal (rodents) data show risk of carcinogenicity. Use of metronidazole in pregnancy is controversial; reports in humans have arrived at conflicting data (but most studies show no risk). Manufacturer and CDC consider metronidazole to be contraindicated in 1st trimester.

Breastfeeding Compatibility

- Excreted in breast milk. American Academy of Pediatrics recommends using metronidazole with caution; discontinuation of breastfeeding for 12–24 hrs recommended to allow excretion of drug.

DOSING

Dosing for Decreased Hepatic Function

- Decreased dose in severe hepatic impairment.

Renal Dosing

- No dose adjustment for renal impairment, or dialysis.
- Dosing in hemofiltration: no data. Usual dose likely.

COMMENTS

- Metronidazole is gold standard anti-anaerobic agent.
- Active against virtually all anaerobes with exception of *Actinomyces*, *Propionibacterium acnes*, and *Lactobacillus* spp. Additional antibiotic coverage needed for combined aerobes/anaerobes infections (metronidazole only active against anaerobes).
- 1st-line agent for giardiasis, trichomoniasis, and amebiasis. Oral vancomycin and metronidazole are equivalent in the treatment of mild colitis with comparable rates of response and relapse, but most experts recommend oral vancomycin in moderate to severe disease.

SELECTED REFERENCES

Zar FA, Bakkanagari SR, Moorthi KM, et al. A comparison of vancomycin and metronidazole for the treatment of *Clostridium difficile*-associated diarrhea, stratified by disease severity. *Clin Infect Dis*, 2007; 45: 302–7.

Comments: Prospective, randomized, double-blind, placebo-controlled trial compared oral vancomycin to oral metronidazole in 172 patients with *C. difficile*-associated diarrhea (CDAD). Patients stratified based on disease severity. Severe CDAD defined as pseudomembranous colitis or 2 of following: (1) age >60; (2) albumin <2.5; (3) WBC >15K; (4) temp >38.3. Treatment with metronidazole or vancomycin resulted in clinical cure in 90% and 98% of patients with mild disease, respectively (P = 0.36). However, among patients with severe CDAD, vancomycin superior to metronidazole with clinical cure in 97% and 76%, respectively (P = 0.02). CDAD relapse rates similar between metronidazole and vancomycin treated groups.

Bartlett JG. Narrative review: the new epidemic of *Clostridium difficile*-associated enteric disease. *Ann Intern Med*, 2006; 145: 758–64.

Comments: *C. difficile* has been more frequent, more severe, more refractory to standard therapy, and more likely to relapse. This pattern is wildly distributed in US, Canada, and Europe and is now attributed to a new strain of *C. difficile* designated BI, NAP1, or ribotype 027 (synonymous terms). This strain appears more virulent, possibly because of production of large amounts of toxins, and fluoroquinolones are now major inducing agents along with cephalosporins, which presumably reflects newly acquired *in vitro* resistance and escalating rates of use. Recent experience does not change principles of management of individual patient, but it emphasizes need for better diagnostics, early recognition, improved methods to manage severe disease and relapsing disease, and greater attention to infection control and antibiotic restraint.

Joesoef MR, Schmid GP. Bacterial vaginosis: review of treatment options and potential clinical Indications for therapy. Clin Infect Dis, 1995; 20 (suppl 1): S72–9.

Comments: Sexually transmitted guidelines 2010 / Vol. 59 / No. RR-12 Recommended treatment for BV: metronidazole 500 mg bid x 7 days, metronidazole 0.75% (5 gm applicator) once daily x 5 days, or clindamycin 2% (5 gm applicator) x 7 days.

MOXIFLOXACIN

Paul A. Pham, PharmD and John G. Bartlett, MD

INDICATIONS

FDA

- Acute bacterial exacerbation of chronic bronchitis (ABECB). Acute bacterial sinusitis.
- Community-acquired pneumonia (CAP), including those caused by multidrug resistant (MDR) *Streptococcus pneumoniae*.
- Uncomplicated skin and skin structure infections (oral and IV). Complicated skin and skin structure infections, including diabetic foot infections (oral and IV).
- Complicated intraabdominal infections, including polymicrobial infections such as abscesses. Author's opinion: due to potential resistance of *B. fragilis*, use in mild-to-moderate intraabdominal infections only. Consider addition of metronidazole for severe infections.
- Bacterial conjunctivitis (ophthalmic drops).

Non-FDA Approved Uses

- Treatment of tuberculosis, including MDR and extremely drug resistant (XDR) TB (in combination w/ other agents).
- Treatment of MAC (in combination w/ other agents).

FORMS TABLE

Brand name (mfr)	Forms†	Cost*
Avelox (Merck/Schering-Plough [Bayer])	Oral tablet 400 mg IV piggyback 400 mg	$16.35 $42.00
Vigamox (Alcon Laboratories)	Ophthalmic soln 0.5% (3 mL)	$81.66

*Prices represent cost per unit specified, are representative of Average Wholesale Price (AWP).
†Dosage is indicated in mg unless otherwise noted.

USUAL ADULT DOSING

- CAP: 400 mg IV or PO once daily × 7–14 days.
- Uncomplicated skin and skin structure infections: 400 mg IV or PO once daily × 7 days. Complicated skin and skin structure infections: 400 mg IV once daily × 7–21 days.
- Acute sinusitis: 400 mg PO once daily × 5–10 days.
- ABECB: 400 mg PO once daily × 5 days.
- Mild-to-moderate intraabdominal infections, including polymicrobial infections: 400 mg IV or PO once daily × 5–21 days. Consider addition of metronidazole for severe intraabdominal infections.
- Bacterial conjunctivitis: 1 drop (0.5% ophthalmic soln) to affected eye q8h × 7 days.

ADVERSE DRUG REACTIONS

General

- Generally well tolerated.

Occasional

- GI intolerance: diarrhea.
- CNS: headache, malaise, insomnia, restlessness, dizziness. Use with caution in patients with CNS disorders, especially elderly.
- Increased transaminases.
- Photosensitivity/phototoxicity reactions (can be severe).
- *C. difficile* colitis.

Rare

- Allergic reactions.
- QTc prolongation.
- Tendon rupture. Can occur during or after therapy with moxifloxacin. Increased incidence especially seen in older patients over age 60, concurrent use of corticosteroids, kidney, heart, and lung transplant recipients. D/c if patient experiences pain or tendon rupture.
- Peripheral neuropathy.
- Seizure.

- Severe allergic reactions (TEN, Stevens-Johnsons syndrome, allergic pneumonitis, hepatitis, and bone marrow suppression).
- Interstitial nephritis.
- Exacerabation of myasthenia gravis Sx.

DRUG INTERACTIONS
- Any divalent and trivalent cations (i.e., antacid, multivitamin, zinc, calcium, iron, sucralfate, buffered ddI, etc.): significant decrease in moxifloxacin serum levels. Avoid coadministration or moxifloxacin should be taken 4 hrs before or 8 hrs after divalent/trivalent cations administration.
- Class IA (e.g., quinidine, procainamide) or Class III (e.g., amiodarone, sotalol) antiarrhythmic agents: avoid in patients with known prolongation of QT interval and patients with uncorrected hypokalemia due to the potential for additive QTc prolongation. Other drugs that have potential for causing QTc prolongation should be used with caution.
- Sevelamer may decrease moxifloxacin absorption. Avoid coadministration or give moxifloxacin 2 hrs before sevelamer.

RESISTANCE
- *S. pneumoniae* resistance to newer fluoroquinolones remains very low (*Clin Microbiol Infect* 2004;10:645–51) but drug resistant *S. pneumoniae* (DRSP) can be a concern.

PHARMACOLOGY
Mechanism
- Inhibits DNA topoisomerases (DNA gyrase and topoisomerase 4) by binding to DNA-enzyme complexes, thereby interfering with bacterial DNA replication and some aspects of transcription, repair, recombination, and transposition.

Pharmacokinetic Parameters
- **Absorption:** 90%; may be taken with or without meals.
- **Metabolism and Excretion:** metabolized in the liver to an inactive metabolite. CYP450 enzymes are not involved in moxifloxacin metabolism, and not affected by moxifloxacin.
- **Protein Binding:** 48%.
- **Cmax, Cmin, and AUC:** Cmax: 4.5 mcg/mL; AUC 48 mcg/mL hr with 400 mg q day at steady state.
- **T$_{1/2}$:** 13 hrs.
- **Distribution:** Vd 2.7–3.5 L/kg; widely distributed. Good CNS penetration with and without inflamed meninges (*JAC* 2008; 61: 1328). Can be considered in combination for TB meningitis.

Pregnancy Risk
- Category C: no data for moxifloxacin. In prospective follow-up study conducted by European Network of Teratology Information Services (ENTIS), 666 cases of fluoroquinolone exposure (majority of exposures were during 1st trimester) showed congenital malformation rate of 4.8%. From previous epidemiologic data, 4.8% did not exceed background rate. Animal data demonstrated arthropathy in immature animals with erosions in joint cartilage. Because of animal data and availability of alternative antimicrobial agents, use of fluoroquinolones during pregnancy is contraindicated.

Breastfeeding Compatibility
- No data. Fluoroquinolones not recommended during breastfeeding due to potential for arthropathy.

DOSING
Renal Dosing
- No dose adjustment for renal impairment or dialysis.
- Dosing in hemofiltration: no data.

COMMENTS
- Oral and parenteral fluoroquinolone with spectrum of activity similar to levofloxacin (including enhanced activity against *S. pneumoniae*). Best anaerobic and mycobacterial activity among quinolones. Activity against *Pseudomonas* poor compared to ciprofloxacin and levofloxacin.
- Lower urinary drug concentrations means moxifloxacin should not be used for complicated UTIs. May result in false positive opiate screening test (*JAMA*. 2001; 286: 3115–3119).

DRUGS

SELECTED REFERENCES

Jacobson KR, Tierney DB, Jeon CY, et al. Treatment outcomes among patients with extensively drug-resistant tuberculosis: systematic review and meta-analysis. *Clin Infect Dis*, 2010; 51: 6–14.

Comments: A meta-analysis of 13 observational studies involving 560 patients found that younger patients and use of later generation fluoroquinolone (e.g., moxifloxacin, levofloxacin) associated with favorable treatment outcomes (OR 3.7; P = 0.012).

Mandell LA, Wunderink RG, Anzueto A, et al. Infectious Diseases Society of America/American Thoracic Society consensus guidelines on the management of community-acquired pneumonia in adults. *Clin Infect Dis*, 2007; 44 (suppl 2): S27–72.

Comments: The IDSA guidelines recommend a respiratory fluoroquinolone (i.e., levofloxacin, moxifloxacin, or gemifloxacin) for outpatient treatment of CAP in patients with comorbidities or in patients requiring hospital admissions (non-ICU). In ICU patients with CAP, cefotaxime or ceftriaxone should be used in combination with a respiratory fluoroquinolone.

Ho PL, Que TL, Chiu SS, et al. Fluoroquinolone and other antimicrobial resistance in invasive pneumococci, Hong Kong, 1995–2001. *Emerg Infect Dis*, 2004; 10: 1250–7.

Comments: In 265 invasive isolates of pneumococci obtained during 1995–2001, prevalence of levofloxacin resistance (MIC ≥8 µg/mL) was 3.8% but increased to 15.2% among the PNC-resistant isolates. Resistance to levofloxacin remains low in US but is a concern with widespread use.

Pletz MW, De Roux A, Roth A, et al. Early bactericidal activity of moxifloxacin in treatment of pulmonary tuberculosis: a prospective, randomized study. *Antimicrob Agents Chemother*, 2004; 48: 780–2.

Comments: This preliminary study found that moxifloxacin exhibits early bactericidal activity comparable to that of isoniazid. Ongoing studies are evaluating role of moxifloxacin in combination with currently available agents in the treatment of M. TB.

Valerio G, Bracciale P, Manisco V, et al. Long-term tolerance and effectiveness of moxifloxacin therapy for tuberculosis: preliminary results. *J Chemother*, 2003; 15: 66–70.

Comments: *In vitro* and in a mouse model, moxifloxacin is most active fluoroquinolone against M. TB. These preliminary results found good tolerance and efficacy for treatment of tuberculosis.

NYSTATIN

Paul A. Pham, PharmD and John G. Bartlett, MD

INDICATIONS

FDA

- Oropharyngeal candidiasis.
- Vulvovaginal candidiasis.
- Cutaneous candidiasis.

FORMS TABLE

Brand name (mfr)	Forms†	Cost*
Nystatin (generic manufacturers [Paddock Laboratories, Teva Pharmaceuticals, and others])	Oral tablet 500,000 U Vaginal tablet 100,000 U	$0.68 $0.47
Mycostatin (Generic manufacturers [Apothecon Pharmaceuticals, Bristol-Myers Squibb, and others])	Oral suspension 100,000 U/mL (60 mL or 480 mL)	$1.67 per 5 mL
	Topical powder 100,000 U/g (50-mm unit)	$35.45
	Topical cream or ointment 100,000 U/g (15 g; 30 g)	$4.25 (15 g); $6.50 (30 g)

*Prices represent cost per unit specified, are representative of Average Wholesale Price (AWP).
†Dosage is indicated in mg unless otherwise noted.

USUAL ADULT DOSING

- Oropharungeal candidiasis (thrush): 500,000–1,000,000 U (1–2 tabs or 5–10 mL) 3–5 × days.
- Vaginitis: 1 vaginal tablet (100,000 U) daily for 2 wks.
- Topical candidiases: apply cream or ointment to affected areas twice daily.

ADVERSE DRUG REACTIONS
Common
- Oral preparations: bad taste.
Occasional
- Oral preparations: GI distress: nausea, vomiting, and diarrhea.
- Topical preparations: skin irritation.
DRUG INTERACTIONS
- None.
PHARMACOLOGY
Mechanism
- Binds to sterols in the fungal cell membrane resulting in loss of function.
Pharmacokinetic Parameters
- **Absorption:** no systemic absorption.
- **Metabolism and Excretion:** not metabolized.
- **Protein Binding:** n/a.
- **Cmax, Cmin, and AUC:** minimal absorption; salivary concentration 1000 U/mL 1 hr post-dose.
- $T_{\frac{1}{2}}$: 4 hrs.
- **Distribution:** concentrated in saliva.
Pregnancy Risk
- Category B: no fetal harm has been reported.
Breastfeeding Compatibility
- Compatible with breastfeeding.
DOSING
Dosing for Decreased Hepatic Function
- Usual dose.
Renal Dosing
- No dose adjustment for renal impairment, dialysis, or hemofiltration.
COMMENTS
- Causes GI side effects and may not be as effective as clotrimazole since the bitter taste prevents patients from keeping it in their mouths for prolonged periods of time. Poor adherence due to 4 ×/day administration (suspension). Efficacy dependent on contact time with mucosa. Clotrimazole lozenges preferred by most patients.
- In contrast to topical clotrimazole, topical nystatin not effective for *Tinea corporis*.

SELECTED REFERENCES
Kaplan JE, Benson C, Holmes KH, et al. Guidelines for prevention and treatment of opportunistic infections in HIV-infected adults and adolescents: recommendations from CDC, the National Institutes of Health, and the HIV Medicine Association of the Infectious Diseases Society of America. *MMWR Recomm Rep*, 2009; 58: 1–207.
Comments: Initial episodes of oropharyngeal candidiasis can be treated with topical therapy, such as clotrimazole troches or nystatin suspension.

Pappas PG, Rex JH, Sobel JD, et al. Guidelines for treatment of candidiasis. *Clin Infect Dis*, 2004; 38: 161–89.
Comments: Guidelines for the management of different forms of candidiasis.

Pons V, Greenspan D, Lozada-Nur F, et al. Oropharyngeal candidiasis in patients with AIDS: randomized comparison of fluconazole versus nystatin oral suspensions. *Clin Infect Dis*, 1997; 24: 1204–7.
Comments: Systemic fluconazole therapy more effective than topical nystatin with response seen in 87% of the fluconazole-treated patients compared to 52% in the nystatin-treated group (P <0.001). Obvious concern is development of azole-resistance with chronic fluconazole treatment.

PAROMOMYCIN

Paul A. Pham, PharmD and John G. Bartlett, MD

INDICATIONS
FDA
- Intestinal amebiasis.
- Hepatic coma.

DRUGS

Non-FDA Approved Uses
• Cryptosporidiosis.

FORMS TABLE

Brand name (mfr)	Forms†	Cost*
Humatin (Monarch Pharmaceuticals and generic manufacturers)	Oral capsule 250 mg	$2.73

*Prices represent cost per unit specified, are representative of Average Wholesale Price (AWP).
†Dosage is indicated in mg unless otherwise noted.

USUAL ADULT DOSING
• Cryptosporidiosis: 500 mg PO q6h or 1 g PO q12h (no cures with marginal benefit in clinical trials; ART is treatment of choice).
• Intestinal amebiasis: 500–1000 mg PO q6h.

ADVERSE DRUG REACTIONS
Common
• Anorexia, nausea, vomiting, cramps, epigastric burning pain.
Rare
• Rash, headaches, vertigo, nephrotoxicity, and ototoxicity (paromomycin is an aminoglycoside with minimal absorption, but monitor closely in patients with renal failure).

DRUG INTERACTIONS
• Digoxin: decreased digoxin serum concentrations by 30%–82%.

PHARMACOLOGY
Mechanism
• Inhibition of protein synthesis by binding to 30S segment of the ribosome.
Pharmacokinetic Parameters
• **Absorption:** minimal absorption.
• **Metabolism and Excretion:** excreted unchanged in feces.
Pregnancy Risk
• Category C: limited human data, due to poor systemic absorption risk of teratogenicity is low.
Breastfeeding Compatibility
• No data; not likely to be excreted in breast milk.

DOSING
Dosing for Decreased Hepatic Function
• Usual dose.
Renal Dosing
• Dosing for GFR of 50–80: usual dose.
• Dosing for GFR of 10–50: usual dose. Monitor closely for ototoxicity and worsening nephrotoxicity.
• Dosing for GFR of <10: usual dose; HD: usual dose. Monitor closely for ototoxicity and worsening nephrotoxicity.
• Dosing in hemodialysis: usual dose.
• Dosing in peritoneal dialysis: usual dose.
• Dosing in hemofiltration: no data. Usual dose likely.

COMMENTS
• In HIV-infected patients, used primarily to treat cryptosporidiosis, but with marginal efficacy in clinical trials (ART is treatment of choice).

SELECTED REFERENCES
Hewitt RG, Yiannoutsos CT, Higgs ES, et al. Paromomycin: no more effective than placebo for treatment of cryptosporidiosis in patients with advanced human immunodeficiency virus infection. AIDS Clinical Trial Group. *Clin Infect Dis*, 2000; 31: 1084–92.
Comments: Contrary to the findings of an earlier trial showing a slight benefit with paromomycin (*J Infect Dis.* 1994;170:419–24), this prospective, randomized, double-blind, placebo-controlled (pre-HAART) trial found no significant difference between paromomycin and placebo.

PENTAMIDINE

Paul A. Pham, PharmD and John G. Bartlett, MD

INDICATIONS

FDA

- Treatment (IV pentamidine) and prophylaxis (aerosolized pentamidine) of PCP.

FORMS TABLE

Brand name (mfr)	Forms†	Cost*
Pentam 300 (Generic manufacturers [American Pharmaceutical Partners])	IV vial 300 mg	$98.75
NebuPent (Generic manufacturers [American Pharmaceutical Partners])	Inhalation powder 300 mg	$98.75
Pentamidine (APP Pharmaceuticals)	IV vial 300 mg	$94.80

*Prices represent cost per unit specified, are representative of Average Wholesale Price (AWP).
†Dosage is indicated in mg unless otherwise noted.

USUAL ADULT DOSING

- PCP treatment: 4 mg/kg IV once daily over 1 hr × 21 days (TMP-SMX or clindamycin/primaquin preferred).
- PCP prophylaxis: 300 mg aerosolized pentamidine (AP) monthly (TMP-SMX or dapsone preferred). 300 mg diluted in 6 mL of sterile water delivered at 6L/min by a *Respigard II* nebulizer.
- AP should not be used for PCP treatment.

ADVERSE DRUG REACTIONS

Common

- Nephrotoxicity (25%–50%): usually reversible with discontinuation but may progress to ARF.
- Hypoglycemia: most commonly seen after 5–7 days but can occur at anytime, including after therapy have been stopped (treat with IV glucose and/or diazoxide).
- Hyperglycemia and IDDM.
- GI intolerance: anorexia, abdominal pain, dysgeusia, nausea, and vomiting.
- Phlebitis at IV infusion site.
- Cough and wheezing with AP: consider pretreatment with inhaled beta-2 agonist.

Occasional

- Hypotension: give IV over 60 min in supine position with hydration to reduce risk.
- Marrow suppression: leukopenia and thrombocytopenia.
- Hypocalcemia, hypomagnesemia, and hypokalemia: laboratory monitoring recommended.

Rare

- Pancreatitis.
- Torsade de pointes.
- Fever.
- Rash, including TEN.
- Dizziness and confusion.
- Hepatitis.
- Laryngitis, chest pain, and dyspnea with aerosolized pentamidine.

DRUG INTERACTIONS

- Amphotericin B and foscarnet: may increase risk of severe hypocalcemia.
- ddI: may increase risk of pancreatitis.
- Nephrotoxic agents (aminoglycoside, foscarnet, cidofovir, amphotericin B): may increase risk of nephrotoxicity.

DRUGS

PHARMACOLOGY
Mechanism
- Exact mechanism of action of pentamidine not fully elucidated, but may involve interference with incorporation of nucleotides into RNA and DNA and inhibition of oxidative phosphorylation and biosynthesis of DNA, RNA, protein, and phospholipid.

Pharmacokinetic Parameters
- **Metabolism and Excretion:** unknown metabolism. 4%–17% excreted in the urine, due to the long terminal half-life excretion that can last up to 8 wks following last dose.
- **Protein Binding:** 69%.
- **Cmax, Cmin, and AUC:** 0.5–3.4 mcg/mL after 4 mg/kg IV dose administration.
- **$T_{\frac{1}{2}}$:** 7 hrs (terminal half-life up to 4 wks).
- **Distribution:** high concentration attained in liver, kidney, adrenal glands, and spleen. Slow CNS penetration, only detected 30 days after the start of therapy. Lung concentration also attained.

Pregnancy Risk
- Category C: both manufacturer and CDC advise against the use of pentamidine in pregnancy. Spontaneous abortion reported; however causal relationship has not been established.

Breastfeeding Compatibility
- No data.

DOSING
Renal Dosing
- Dosing for GFR of 50–80: usual.
- Dosing for GFR of 10–50: 4 mg/kg q24–36h.
- Dosing for GFR of <10: consider dose adjustment to 4 mg/kg q48h; HD: nonsignificant increase in elimination half-life during HD. No dosage adjustment needed.
- Dosing in hemodialysis: nonsignificant increase in elimination half-life during hemodialysis. No dosage adjustment needed.
- Dosing in peritoneal dialysis: no data, no supplemental dose needed.
- Dosing in hemofiltration: no data.

COMMENTS
- Parenteral agent used for treatment of severe PCP in patients intolerant to TMP/SMX or clindamycin/primaquine. AP used for PCP prophylaxis in patients intolerant of TMP/SMX or dapsone.
- Parenteral: toxicities such as hypotension, hypoglycemia, and renal failure limit its use. Close monitoring of vital signs and blood sugar with infusion recommended. Avoid concurrent administration of nephrotoxic drugs due to additive nephrotoxicity. Unclear whether AP may increase risk of extrapulmonary infection and pneumothorax.
- Risk of TB transmission to healthcare workers during AP administration; do not use if suspicion of active TB.

SELECTED REFERENCES
Bozzette SA, Finkelstein DM, Spector SA, et al. A randomized trial of three antipneumocystis agents in patients with advanced human immunodeficiency virus infection. NIAID AIDS Clinical Trials Group. *N Engl J Med*, 1995; 332: 693–9. **Comments:** Open-label study comparing TMP/SMX vs dapsone vs AP. 36-mo cumulative risks of PCP were 18%, 17%, and 21% in the TMP/SMX, dapsone, and AP groups, respectively (P = 0.22). In patients with CD4 <100 risk was 33% with AP vs 19% with TMP/SMX and 22% with dapsone (P = 0.04). AP may be an alternative in patients who cannot tolerate TMP/SMX or dapsone.

Klein NC, Duncanson FP, Lenox TH, et al. Trimethoprim-sulfamethoxazole versus pentamidine for *Pneumocystis carinii* pneumonia in AIDS patients: results of a large prospective randomized treatment trial. *AIDS*, 1992; 6: 301–5. **Comments:** Survival rate was 67% in patients initially administered TMP-SMX vs 74% in patients initially administered pentamidine (P = 0.402). This study indicates that patients who switch from TMP/SMX to pentamidine due to "clinical failure" do not have improved clinical outcomes. However, if switch due to drug toxicity, survival rate higher. TMP/SMX is drug of choice due to its better safety profile.

POSACONAZOLE

Paul A. Pham, PharmD and John G. Bartlett, MD

INDICATIONS
FDA

- Prophylaxis of invasive aspergillosis and disseminated candidiasis in severely immunocompromised hosts, such as hemapoietic stem cell transplant recipients with graft versus host disease (GVHD) or those with hematologic malignancies with prolonged neutropenia from chemotherapy.
- Treatment of oropharyngeal candidiasis, including itraconazole and/or fluconazole-refractory cases.

Non-FDA Approved Uses

- Treatment of invasive fungal infections due to *Aspergillus* spp., *Candida* spp., and zygomycoses (e.g., *Rhizomucor*, *Cunninghamella*, *Absidia*) spp.

FORMS TABLE

Brand name (mfr)	Forms†	Cost*
Noxafil (Schering Corporation)	Oral suspension 40 mg/mL (105 mL)	$743.84 per 105-mL bottle

*Prices represent cost per unit specified, are representative of Average Wholesale Price (AWP).
†Dosage is indicated in mg unless otherwise noted.

USUAL ADULT DOSING

- Administration of oral drug with full meal or liquid nutritional supplement significantly increases drug levels. Food critical for absorption.
- Prophylaxis of invasive fungal infections: 200 mg (5 mL) PO q8h.
- Treatment of invasive fungal infections: 200 mg PO 4 × daily or 400 mg PO twice daily. Some experts recommend increasing to 400 mg q8h for severe infection, lack of clinical response, and/or low poscanazole serum concentrations.
- Oropharyngeal candidiasis (thrush): 100 mg twice daily × 2 (loading dose on d 1), then 100 mg once daily × 13 days. Generally not recommended due to high cost and availability of generic or topical alternatives.
- Oropharyngeal and esophageal candidiasis refractory to itraconazole and/or fluconazole: 400 mg twice daily (duration of therapy based on clinical response).
- Consider therapeutic drug monitoring. Target: >1.25 mcg/mL for invasive fungal disease.

ADVERSE DRUG REACTIONS
General

- Generally well tolerated with comparable side effect profile to fluconazole.

Occasional

- Nausea, vomiting, diarrhea, abdominal pain.
- Increased liver enzymes.
- Hyperbilirubinemia.

Rare

- Adrenal insufficiency.
- Hypersensitivity reaction.
- QTc prolongation.

DRUG INTERACTIONS

- Metabolized via UDP glucuronidation (phase II enzymes). It is a substrate of Pgp efflux and inhibitor of CYP3A4. As a result, CYP3A4 substrate may be increased. Posaconazole serum concentrations may be decreased with coadministration of UDP glucuronidation or Pgp inducers.
- Contraindicated drugs: terfenadine, astemizole, cisapride, pimozide, halofantrine, quinidine, ergotamine, and dihydroergotamine serum concentrations may be significantly increased.
- Avoid coadministration: rifabutin, phenytoin, and cimetidine decreased posaconazole AUC by 49%, 50%, and 39%, respectively. Rifabutin AUC increased by 72%.
- Use with dose adjustment and close monitoring—cyclosporine: decrease cyclosporine dose by 25% with TDM. Tacrolimus: decrease tacrolimus dose by 2/3 with TDM. Sirolimus dose should

DRUGS

also be reduced and monitored. Midazolam AUC increased by 83%, consider alternative: lorazepam.

- Posaconazole may increase the serum concentrations of other benzodiazepines (triazolam, alprazolam, diazepam), carbamazepine, sirolimus, irinotecan, dofetilide, amiodarone, vincristine, vinblastine, calcium channel blockers, corticosteroid, drugs used for the treatment of ED (sildenafil, tadalafil, and vardenafil), simvastatin, lovastatin, and other CYP3A4 substrates.
- Posaconazole serum concentration may be significantly decreased with rifampin, tipranavir, nelfinavir, and lopinavir coadministration. Avoid coadministration with rifampin. Use TPV, NFV, and LPV/r with close monitoring of posaconazole serum concentrations.
- No significant interaction observed with RTV (600 mg twice daily), antacids, glipizide, H2 blockers (other than cimetidine), and proton pump inhibitors (per FDA labeling).
- In a recent study, esomeprazole decreases posaconazole AUC 33% (AAC 2009; 53: 958). Avoid coadministration.

DRUG-DRUG INTERACTIONS—See Appendix I, p. 583, for table of drug-drug interactions.

PHARMACOLOGY

Mechanism

- Mechanism of action: posaconazole is a triazole antifungal that inhibits fungal ergosterol synthesis.

Pharmacokinetic Parameters

- **Absorption:** well absorbed when administered with food or a nutritional supplement (e.g., Boost Plus). The mean AUC and Cmax of posaconazole were approximately 3–4 × higher with food.
- **Metabolism and Excretion:** primarily metabolized in the liver, where it undergoes glucuronidation and is transformed into biologically inactive metabolites. Posaconazole is predominantly eliminated in the feces (71%). Renal clearance is a minor elimination pathway (13%).
- **Protein Binding:** >98%.
- **Cmax, Cmin, and AUC:** mean average concentration after 200 mg PO 3 ×/day with food at steady state: 583–1103 g/mL with a relative large CV% of 65%–67%.
- **$T_{\frac{1}{2}}$:** 35 hrs (steady state attained at 7–10 days). Although the half-life would suggest less frequent dosing, more frequent dosing results in better bioavailability.
- **Distribution:** widely distributed with a Vd of 1774 L.

Pregnancy Risk

- Category C: no human data. Shown to cause skeletal malformations in rats, but not in rabbits, given 3–5 × human exposure.

Breastfeeding Compatibility

- No human data. Posaconazole is excreted in milk of lactating rats.

DOSING

Dosing for Decreased Hepatic Function

- Limited data, consider standard dose. Use with caution.

Renal Dosing

- Dosing for GFR of 20–80: standard dose.
- Dosing for GFR of <20: Due to a large pharmacokinetic variability (CV = 96%), closer monitoring for breakthrough infection recommended with CrCl <20 mL/min.
- Dosing in hemodialysis: no data. Standard dose likely. Dose post-HD on days of HD.
- Dosing in peritoneal dialysis: no data. Standard dose likely.
- Dosing in hemofiltration: no data. Standard dose likely.

COMMENTS

- Active against all *Candida* spp. (including many azole-resistant *Candida* spp.) and *Aspergillus* spp. (including *A. terreus*). Although *Fusarium* spp. are generally resistant *in vitro*, clinical successes have been reported. The high PK variability (dependent on food administration), the lack of IV formulation, and the 1-wk lag time to reach steady state may limit the use of posaconazole in severe invasive fungal infections. Nevertheless, activities against certain *Zygomycetes* spp. and good efficacy in preliminary open-label observational studies are encouraging. Prospective, randomized studies are needed to better define role of posaconazole in invasive fungal infections.

SELECTED REFERENCES

Noxafil (poscanazole) [package insert]. Kenilworth, NJ: Schering Corporation.

Comments: FDA approval of posaconazole was based on 2 prophylaxis studies comparing posaconazole to fluconazole (or itraconazole) in hematopoietic stem cell transplant recipients with graft versus host disease (study 1) and hematologic malignancies with prolonged neutropenia from chemotherapy (study 2). In stem cell recipient, clinical failure rate of posaconazole (33%) similar to fluconazole (37%). In hematologic malignancies with prolonged neutropenia patients, clinical failure rate (27% vs 42%) and mortality (14% vs 21%) were lower in posaconazole-treated patients vs fluconazole or itraconazole treated patients. Difference attributed to fewer breakthrough infections caused by *Aspergillus* spp. in posaconazole-treated patients.

Vazquez JA, Skiest DJ, Tissot-Dupont H, et al. Safety and efficacy of posaconazole in the long-term treatment of azole-refractory oropharyngeal and esophageal candidiasis in patients with HIV infection. *HIV Clin Trials*, 2007; 8: 86–97.

Comments: In this nonrandomized, open-label study, posaconazole was effective in treatment of azole-refractory oropharyngeal and esophageal candidiasis in HIV+ patients. Clinical response (cure or improvement) occurred in 85.6% (77/90) at end of 3 mos. It should be noted that only 1/3 to 1/2 of isolates had MIC >32 mcg/mL and cost of posaconazole for 3 mos is $11,700.

Vazquez JA, Skiest DJ, Nieto L, et al. A multicenter randomized trial evaluating posaconazole versus fluconazole for the treatment of oropharyngeal candidiasis in subjects with HIV/AIDS. *Clin Infect Dis*, 2006; 42: 1179–86.

Comments: This prospective, randomized trial demonstrated that posaconazole (200 mg on day 1, then 100 mg once daily for 13 days) was noninferior to fluconazole in treatment of oropharyngeal candidiasis. Clinical success observed in 91.7% and 92.5% of fluconazole and posaconazole groups (95% CI, −6.61–5.04%). High clinical response rate consistent with prior studies; however, in order to limit development of azole resistance, topical treatment with clotrimazole or nystatin preferred in treatment of oropharyngeal candidiasis. Systemic antifungal therapy should be reserved for esophageal candidiasis.

DRUGS

PRIMAQUINE

Paul A. Pham, PharmD and John G. Bartlett, MD

INDICATIONS

FDA

- Malaria prevention of relapses (radical cure) caused by *Plasmodium vivax*. Also effective against gametocytes of *P. falciparum*.

Non-FDA Approved Uses

- Treatment of PCP (in combination with clindamycin).

FORMS TABLE

Brand name (mfr)	Forms†	Cost*
Primaquine (Sanofi-Aventis US)	Oral tablet 26.3 mg (15-mg base)	$1.51

*Prices represent cost per unit specified, are representative of Average Wholesale Price (AWP).
†Dosage is indicated in mg unless otherwise noted.

USUAL ADULT DOSING

- Treatment of PCP: 15–30 mg (base) once daily with food (in combination with clindamycin).

ADVERSE DRUG REACTIONS

Occasional

- Hemolytic anemia (in patients with G6PD deficiency). Screen for G6PD deficiency (African and Mediterranean descent).
- Methemoglobinemia.
- Neutropenia and leukopenia (incidence may be higher with primaquine 30 mg).
- GI intolerance (abdominal pain, nausea, and vomiting).

Rare

- Blurred vision.
- Headache.
- Pruritis.

DRUG INTERACTIONS
- Bone marrow suppressive drugs (i.e., AZT, ganciclovir, pyrimethamine, 5-FC, interferon): potential for additive bone marrow suppression with coadministration.

PHARMACOLOGY
Mechanism
- Exact mechanism of action not fully elucidated, but appears to interfere with pyrimidine synthesis and mitochondrial electron transport chain.

Pharmacokinetic Parameters
- **Absorption:** well absorbed.
- **Metabolism and Excretion:** hepatic metabolism to carboxy metabolite. Both metabolite and a small amount of unchanged drug are excreted unchanged in urine.
- **Protein Binding:** no data.
- **Cmax, Cmin, and AUC:** 104 ng/mL steady-state concentration after 30 mg PO.
- **$T_{\frac{1}{2}}$:** 5.8 hrs.
- **Distribution:** lack of data, however appears to be widely distributed.

Pregnancy Risk
- Category C: no studies available. Theoretical concern is hemolytic anemia in G6PD deficient fetus.

Breastfeeding Compatibility
- No data available.

DOSING
Renal Dosing
- No dose adjustment for renal impairment.
- Dosing in hemodialysis: no data, dose post-HD.
- Dosing in peritoneal dialysis: no data.
- Dosing in hemofiltration: no data.

COMMENTS
- Primaquine in combination with clindamycin is good 2nd-line treatment for mild, moderate, and severe PCP in patients intolerant of TMP/SMX. Prior screening for G6PD deficiency recommended to prevent hemolytic anemia.

SELECTED REFERENCES
Kaplan JE, Benson C, Holmes KH, et al. Guidelines for prevention and treatment of opportunistic infections in HIV-infected adults and adolescents: recommendations from CDC, the National Institutes of Health, and the HIV Medicine Association of the Infectious Diseases Society of America. *MMWR Recomm Rep*, 2009; 58: 1–207.
Comments: Although primaquine/clindamycin efficacy data not as robust as data supporting IV pentamidine for treatment of severe PCP, OI treatment guidelines recommend that primaquine/clindamycin OR IV pentamidine be considered as alternatives to TMP/SMX for patients with moderate-to-severe PCP.

Safrin S, Finkelstein DM, Feinberg J, et al. Comparison of three regimens for treatment of mild to moderate *Pneumocystis carinii* pneumonia in patients with AIDS. A double-blind, randomized, trial of oral trimethoprim-sulfamethoxazole, dapsone-trimethoprim, and clindamycin-primaquine. ACTG 108 Study Group. *Ann Intern Med*, 1996; 124: 792–802.
Comments: Clindamycin-primaquine efficacy comparable to TMP-SMX and TMP-dapsone for PCP. Hematologic toxicities (neutropenia, anemia, thrombocytopenia, or methemoglobinemia) occurred more frequently in clindamycin-primaquine group.

PYRAZINAMIDE

Paul A. Pham, PharmD and John G. Bartlett, MD

INDICATIONS
FDA
- TB (active, latent) treatment (in combination with other antituberculous drugs).

FORMS TABLE

Brand name (mfr)	Forms†	Cost*
Pyrazinamide (Several generic manufacturers [Stada Pharmaceuticals, UDL Laboratories, and others])	Oral tablet 500 mg	$1.26
Rifater (Aventis Pharmaceuticals)	Oral capsule PZA 300 mg/ INH 50 mg/RIF 120 mg	$3.10

*Prices represent cost per unit specified, are representative of Average Wholesale Price (AWP).
†Dosage is indicated in mg unless otherwise noted.

USUAL ADULT DOSING

- Active TB (induction phase): 20–25 mg/kg (max 2 g) once daily in combination with RIF, ethambutol (EMB), and INH × 8 wks.
- DOT active TB treatment (in combination with RIF + EMB + INH): 40–55 kg: 1500 mg 3 ×/wk or 2000 mg 2 ×/wk; 56–75 kg: 2500 mg 3 ×/wk or 3000 mg 2 ×/wk; 76–90 kg: 3000 mg 3 ×/wk or 4000 mg 2 ×/wk. MAX DOSE: 2000 mg/day; 3000 mg 3 ×/wk; 4000 mg 2 ×/wk.
- Patients with CD4 <100 should receive once-daily or 3 ×/wk therapy for active TB.
- PZA + RIF × 2 mos for treatment of latent TB no longer recommended by the CDC due to hepatotoxicity; however, a subsequent analysis showed no deaths or serious reactions among the 792 HIV+ infected patients who took RIF/PZA; the rate of AST >250 U/l at 2 mos was 2.1% (*CID* 2004; 39: 561).
- Treatment with *Rifater*: wt <65 kg: 1 tab/10 kg/day; >65 kg: 6 tabs/day.

ADVERSE DRUG REACTIONS

General
- For *Rifater* ADRs: see also INH (p. 206) and RIF (p. 241).

Common
- Nongouty polyarthralgia (up to 40%, Rx with ASA).
- Asymptomatic hyperuricemia.

Occasional
- Dose-related hepatitis (1% at 25 mg/kg, but up to 15% with >3 g/day). Monitor for Sx suggestive of hepatitis at baseline and 2, 4, 6, and 8 wks. Bilirubin, AST, and ALT at baseline and 2, 4, and 6 wks. D/c if LFTs >5 × ULN in asymptomatic patient or at any level above normal range in symptomatic patient. Risk increased with alcohol consumption.
- GI intolerance.

Rare
- Gout (Rx w/ allopurinol and probenecid). D/c and do not restart if hyperuricemia accompanied by acute gouty arthritis.

DRUG INTERACTIONS
- For *Rifater* drug interactions: see also INH (p. 206) and RIF (p. 241).
- Ethionamide: may increase risk of hepatotoxicity.

RESISTANCE
- *M. kansasii* intrinsically resistant to PZA.

PHARMACOLOGY

Mechanism
- Converted to pyrazinoic acid (in susceptible strains). Pyrazinoic acid may lower pH of local environment below that necessary for growth of *M. tuberculosis*; also may have direct antimycobacterial activity though unknown mechanism.

Pharmacokinetic Parameters
- **Absorption:** near complete absorption.
- **Metabolism and Excretion:** metabolized in liver to pyrazoic acid (active metabolite). Both metabolite and small amount of unchanged drug are excreted in urine.
- **Protein Binding:** 17%.
- **Cmax, Cmin, and AUC:** Cmax: 30–50 mcg/ml after 20–25 mg/kg PO.

DRUGS

- $T_{\frac{1}{2}}$: 9.5 hrs.
- **Distribution:** widely distributed into body tissues and fluids. Good levels in liver and lungs. Good CNS penetration, with therapeutic levels attained (85%–100% of serum levels).

Pregnancy Risk

- Category C: no animal data available. No human data available. For active TB Rx during pregnancy, CDC guidelines for US are INH + RIF+ EMB (without PZA, due to insufficient safety data) for 2 mos then INH + RIF for additional 7 mos (9 mos total). Worldwide, WHO recommends PZA for routine use in pregnant women with active TB.

Breastfeeding Compatibility

- Excreted in breast milk.

DOSING

Dosing for Decreased Hepatic Function

- Consider withholding. Consult with a TB expert.

Renal Dosing

- Dosing for GFR of 10–80: usual dose.
- Dosing for GFR of <10: 12–20 mg/kg/day. Risk of hyperuricemia may be increased; HD: usual dose post-HD on days of HD.
- Dosing in hemodialysis: HD: usual dose post-HD on days of HD. Risk of hyperuricemia may be increased.
- Dosing in peritoneal dialysis: no data; avoid.
- Dosing in hemofiltration: no data.

COMMENTS

- 1st-line agent in combination with other antituberculous drugs for TB treatment. Monitor LFTs closely with RIF coadministration; use with caution in patients with gout due to potential for PZA-induced hyperuricemia.

SELECTED REFERENCES

Kaplan JE, Benson C, Holmes KH, et al. Guidelines for prevention and treatment of opportunistic infections in HIV-infected adults and adolescents: recommendations from CDC, the National Institutes of Health, and the HIV Medicine Association of the Infectious Diseases Society of America. *MMWR Recomm Rep*, 2009; 58: 1–207.
Comments: Current OI treatment guidelines.

Blumberg HM, Burman WJ, Chaisson RE, et al. American Thoracic Society/Centers for Disease Control and Prevention/Infectious Diseases Society of America: treatment of tuberculosis. *Am J Respir Crit Care Med*, 2003; 167: 603–62.
Comments: Treatment guidelines for TB.

Centers for Disease Control and Prevention (CDC). Fatal and severe hepatitis associated with rifampin and pyrazinamide for the treatment of latent tuberculosis infection—New York and Georgia, 2000. *MMWR*, 2001; 50: 289–91.
Comments: To date, 40 cases of severe liver injury in patients on 2-mo regimen of RIF + PZA for treatment of latent TB; 8 deaths. Risk of death unclear, but retrospective data suggest 1/1000. Risk may be same whether given once daily or twice weekly. PZA and RFA for 2 mos for latent TB treatment no longer recommended.

PYRIMETHAMINE

Paul A. Pham, PharmD and John G. Bartlett, MD

INDICATIONS

FDA

- Malaria (acute) in combination with sulfadoxine and quinine in treatment of chloroquine-resistant *Plasmodium falciparum* malaria. Resistance prevalent worldwide; not recommended as prophylactic agent for travelers to most areas.
- Toxoplasmosis (in combination with sulfadiazine or clindamycin + leucovorin).

FORMS TABLE

Brand name (mfr)	Forms†	Cost*
Daraprim (GlaxoSmithKline)	Oral tablet 25 mg	$0.58
Fansidar (Roche Pharmaceuticals)	Oral tablet pyrimethamine 25 mg + sulfadoxine 500 mg	$4.14

*Prices represent cost per unit specified, are representative of Average Wholesale Price (AWP).
†Dosage is indicated in mg unless otherwise noted.

USUAL ADULT DOSING

- CNS toxoplasmosis, induction therapy: 200 mg × 1, then 50–75 mg once daily (+ folinic acid 10–20 mg/day + sulfadiazine 1.5 g q6h or clindamycin 600 mg IV q6h) × >6 wks.
- CNS toxoplasmosis, maintenance therapy: 25–50 mg (+ folinic acid 15 mg + sulfadiazine 0.5–1 g q6h or clindamycin 300–450 mg q6h) until immune reconstitution (CD4 >200 × 6 mos, induction therapy completed, and asymptomatic). Reintroduce maintenance therapy if CD4 count decreases to <200.
- Toxoplasmosis prophylaxis: 50 mg/wk (+ folinic acid 25 mg/wk + dapsone 50–100 mg once daily + leucovorin 25 mg/wk OR atovaquone 1500 mg/day ± pyrimethamine 25 mg/day + leucovorin 10 mg/day). Note: TMP/SMX 1 DS daily preferred.
- Toxoplasmosis primary prophylaxis can be discontinued in patients who have responded to ART with increase in CD4 count to >200 for >3 mos, but should be reintroduced if CD4 decreases to <100–200.
- Malaria prophylaxis: *Fansidar* 1 tab (pyrimethamine 25 mg/sulfadoxine 500 mg) wkly or OR 2 tabs qow; start 1–2 days before arrival in endemic area and continue during stay and for 4–6 wks after leaving endemic area. Generally not recommended due to high incidence of rash.
- Acute malaria, acute: *Fansidar* 2–3 tabs (pyrimethamine 50–75 mg/sufadoxine 1000–1500 mg) as single dose.

ADVERSE DRUG REACTIONS

Occasional

- Reversible pancytopenia (megaloblastic anemia, leucopenia, agranulocytosis, and thrombocytopenia) secondary to depletion of folic acid stores. Generally prevented with coadministration of leucovorin. Consider increasing leucovorin dose to 50–100 mg/day if hematologic toxicity observed.
- GI intolerance: abdominal pain and vomiting (improved by administration with meals).
- Headache, dizziness, and insomnia.
- With sulfonamide coadministration: rash, hepatitis.

Rare

- Neurologic: tremors, ataxia, and seizure.
- With sulfonamide coadministration: Stevens-Johnson syndrome, TEN, erythema multiforme, and anaphylaxis can occur.

DRUG INTERACTIONS

- Lorazepam: may increase risk of hepatotoxicity.
- TMP/SMX, dapsone, ganciclovir, AZT, and interferon: potential for additive bone marrow suppression.

PHARMACOLOGY

Mechanism

- Binds to dihydrofolate reductase inhibiting the reduction of dihydrofolic to tetrahydrofolic acid (folinic acid).

Pharmacokinetic Parameters

- **Absorption:** well absorbed.
- **Metabolism and Excretion:** hepatic metabolism. Both metabolite and 20%–30% of unchanged drug excreted in the urine.
- **Protein Binding:** 80%–87%.
- **Cmax, Cmin, and AUC:** Cmax: 0.13–0.31 mcg/mL after 25 mg PO.

DRUGS

- $T_{\frac{1}{2}}$: 80–123 hrs (139 ± 34 hrs in patients with AIDS) (*Antimicrob Agents Chemother* 1996; 40: 1360–5).
- **Distribution:** distributed into kidneys, lungs, liver, and spleen. 13%–26% of serum concentration penetrates the CSF.

Pregnancy Risk
- Category C: teratogenic in animal studies. No adverse fetal effects reported in 2 reviews of treatment of toxoplasmosis in pregnancy. If pyrimethamine used during pregnancy, folinic acid 5 mg/day supplementation recommended, especially during 1st trimester, to prevent folate deficiency.

Breastfeeding Compatibility
- Excreted in breast milk. The American Academy of Pediatrics considers pyrimethamine compatible with breastfeeding.

Dosing
Renal Dosing
- No dose adjustment for renal impairment.
- Dosing in hemodialysis: no data, usual dose likely (dose post-HD on days of HD).
- Dosing in peritoneal dialysis: 47% removed after PD.
- Dosing in hemofiltration: no data. Usual dose likely.

Comments
- Treatment of choice (with sulfadiazine and leucovorin) for CNS toxoplasmosis. *Fansidar* (pyrimethamine/sulfadoxine) is not 1st-line agent for malaria prophylaxis due to high incidence of rash and availability of better-tolerated alternatives (e.g., atovaquone/proguanil, mefloquine, and doxycycline).

Selected References
Kaplan JE, Benson C, Holmes KH, et al. Guidelines for prevention and treatment of opportunistic infections in HIV-infected adults and adolescents: recommendations from CDC, the National Institutes of Health, and the HIV Medicine Association of the Infectious Diseases Society of America. *MMWR Recomm Rep*, 2009; 58: 1–207.
Comments: Initial therapy of choice for CNS toxoplasmosis is pyrimethamine + sulfadiazine + leucovorin.

Katlama C, De Wit S, O'Doherty E, et al. Pyrimethamine-clindamycin vs. pyrimethamine-sulfadiazine as acute and long-term therapy for toxoplasmic encephalitis in patients with AIDS. *Clin Infect Dis*, 1996; 22: 268–75.
Comments: Randomized trial comparing pyrimethamine + sulfadiazine (P/S) vs pyrimethamine + clindamycin (P/C) for CNS *Toxoplasma encephalitis* (TE). P/C less effective than PIs; overall risk of TE progression was 1.84 × higher for patients on P/C. No statistically significant difference in efficacy during acute therapy, however rate of crossover motivated by lack of response higher among P/C recipients.

RIBAVIRIN

Paul A. Pham, PharmD and John G. Bartlett, MD

Indications
FDA
- Respiratory syncytial virus (RSV) infection (including bronchiolitis and pneumonia).
- Hepatitis C (in combination with interferon alfa or peginterferon alfa).

Forms Table

Brand name (mfr)	Forms†	Cost*
Rebetol (Schering-Plough)	Oral capsule 200 mg Oral soln 40 mg/mL	$10.60 $232.80 (4 oz)
Virazole (Valeant Pharmaceuticals)	Inhalation vial 6 g	$4512.21 (per vial)
Riba-Pak (Three River Pharmaceuticals)	Oral tab pack 800 mg; 1000 mg; 1200 mg	$19.14; $24.00; $28.80

FORMS TABLE *(Continued)*

Brand name (mfr)	Forms†	Cost*
Copegus (Roche Pharmaceuticals)	Oral tablet 200 mg	$15.19
Ribasphere (Three River Pharmaceuticals and generic manufacturers)	Oral capsule 200 mg	$9.93

*Prices represent cost per unit specified, are representative of Average Wholesale Price (AWP).
†Dosage is indicated in mg unless otherwise noted.

USUAL ADULT DOSING

- HCV (genotype I): ribavirin 1000 mg/day (<75 kg) or 1200 mg/day (>75 kg) × 48 wks + peginterferon in combination with telapravir for the 1st 12 wks. HCV (genotype II and III): RBV 800 mg/day × 24 wks + peginterferon in patients who are <40 kg (88 lbs).
- In patients without CV history: consider dose reduction to 600 mg/day with Hgb <10 g/dL or d/c with Hgb <8.5 g/dL. Consider erythropoietin.
- In patients with CV history: consider dose reduction to 600 mg/day with a Hgb drop >2 g/dL. If Hgb remains <12 g/dL over next 4 wks after reduction to 600 mg, d/c ribavavirin. Consider erythropoietin.

ADVERSE DRUG REACTIONS

Common

- Hemolytic anemia (dose-related and reversible. Develops in 2–4 wks; avg. drop 2.5–3 g Hgb). Consider erythropoietin coadministration.
- Dry cough.
- Dyspnea.

Occasional

- Fatigue.
- Dyspepsia (may respond to antacid).
- Headache.
- Insomnia.
- Bronchospasm (aerosolized ribavirin).
- Anorexia.
- Nausea.
- Gout.

Rare

- Lactic acidosis (especially when combined with ddI).
- Decrease or loss of vision (case reports when used in combination with interferon).
- Pure red cell aplasia.
- Interstitial pneumonitis with acute respiratory distress syndrome (ARDS).

DRUG INTERACTIONS

- ABC: potential antagonism. Consider alternative agent (e.g., TDF).
- AZT: additive anemia. Monitor for anemia with coadministration; consider alternative NRTI or use with erythropoietin.
- AZT, d4T, 3TC: *in vitro* antagonism but not clinically significant.
- ddI: increases intracellular concentrations of ddI; may increase risk of lactic acidosis and/or pancreatitis. Avoid coadministration.

PHARMACOLOGY

Mechanism

- Synthetic guanosine nucleoside analog that interferes with synthesis of guanosine triphosphate thereby inhibiting nucleic acid synthesis. May also inhibit some viral RNA polymerases.

Pharmacokinetic Parameters

- **Absorption:** 64% (increased with high-fat meal).

DRUGS

- **Metabolism and Excretion:** metabolized by phosphorylation and deribosylation. Metabolites excreted in urine.
- **Protein Binding:** no significant protein binding.
- **Cmax, Cmin, and AUC:** Cmax: 5.1 μmol/L (600-mg dose).
- **T$\frac{1}{2}$:** inhalation: 9.5 hrs; IV and oral: 0.5–2 hrs; erythrocyte intracellular half-life 40 days.
- **Distribution:** large volume of distribution (Vd: 802 L). Concentrated in plasma, respiratory tract secretion, and RBCs. CNS concentration found (up to 67%) after prolonged administration.

Pregnancy Risk

- Category X: embryotoxic and teratogenic in all animal species. **Note:** contraindicated in pregnant women and in male partners of pregnant women per manufacturer and CDC. Women of childbearing age must use effective form of contraception during treatment and 6-mo after completion of treatment.

Breastfeeding Compatibility

- No data.

DOSING

Dosing for Decreased Hepatic Function

- Usual dose.

Renal Dosing

- Dosing for GFR of 50–80: usual dose.
- Dosing for GFR 30–50: 200 mg alternate with 400 mg every other day.
- Dosing of GFR <30: 200 mg daily.
- HD: 200 mg daily.
- Dosing in hemodialysis: Small amount removed in dialysis; dose: 200 mg/d, dose postdialysis on days of dialysis.
- Dosing in peritoneal dialysis: no data. Not recommended.
- Dosing in hemofiltration: no data. Not recommended.

COMMENTS

- Preferred agent for hepatitis C infection when combined with pegylated alfa interferon. Monitor closely for hemolytic anemia in 1st few wks of therapy. In management of hemolytic anemia, addition of erythropoietin preferred over decreasing ribavirin dose since sustained virologic response rate is higher with standard dose (1000–1200 mg).
- Contraindicated in pregnancy and coadministration with ddI. Warn patients of teratogenic effect of ribavirin and need for adequate forms of contraception.
- Additive anemia with AZT and potential antagonism with ABC; consider alternative agent (e.g., TDF). Avoid use with renal failure and/or hemoglobinopathies.

SELECTED REFERENCES

Payan C, Pivert A, Morand P, et al. Rapid and early virologic response to chronic Hep C treatment with IFN alpha-2b or PEG-IFN alpha-2b plus ribavirin in HIV/HCV co-infected patients. *Gut*, 2007; 56: 1111–1116.
Comments: Rapid virologic response (RVR) studied in 323 patients from the ANRS HC02 RIBAVIC trial, comparing IFN alfa-2b 3 MU 63/wk with pegylated IFN alfa-2b 1.5 mg/kg/wk, each combined with ribavirin 800 mg/day over 48 wks. RVR at wk 4 of therapy was predictor of sustained virologic response (PPV 97%).

Hadziyannis SJ, Sette H, Morgan TR, et al. Peginterferon-alpha2a and ribavirin combination therapy in chronic hepatitis C: a randomized study of treatment duration and ribavirin dose. *Ann Intern Med*, 2004; 140: 346–55.
Comments: HCV (genotype I) infected patients treated with ribavirin 1000–1200 mg/day (+ peginterferon) had 11.2% better sustained virologic response rate compared to low-dose ribavirin (800 mg/day). No significant difference between standard-dose and low-dose ribavirin for HCV (genotype 2 and 3).

Chung RT, Andersen J, Volberding P, et al. Peginterferon alfa-2a plus ribavirin versus interferon alfa-2a plus ribavirin for chronic hepatitis C in HIV-coinfected persons. *N Engl J Med*, 2004; 351: 451–9.
Comments: Randomized trial with 133 patients with chronic HCV/HIV-coinfection. Peginterferon alfa-2a (Pegasys 180 mcg) weekly for 48 wks compared to IFN alfa-2a (6 million IU) 3 × wkly for 12 wks followed by 3 million IU 3 × wkly for 36 wks. Both groups received ribavirin. Treatment with peg-IFN and ribavirin associated with significantly higher SVR than treatment with IFN and ribavirin (27% vs 12%, P = 0.03). In group given peginterferon and ribavirin, only 14% of subjects with HCV genotype 1 infection had a sustained virologic response compared with 73% of subjects with HCV genotype other than 1 (11 of 15, P<0.001). Histologic response observed in 35% of patients with no virologic response who underwent liver Bx. SVR rate disappointing and significantly lower than those observed in previous trials involving HIV-negative patients.

Cummings KJ, Lee SM, West ES, et al. Interferon and ribavirin vs interferon alone in the re-treatment of chronic hepatitis C previously nonresponsive to interferon: a meta-analysis of randomized trials. *JAMA*, 2001; 285: 193–9.

Comments: Meta-analysis of 12 trials with 941 patients compared interferon + ribavirin vs interferon alone in patients who failed initial treatment with interferon. Pooled virologic response rate for the combination treatment with ribavirin (1000–1200 mg/day) was 16% (better than interferon alone). No difference when comparing interferon alone and interferon + ribavirin at 600–800 mg/day.

RIFABUTIN

Paul A. Pham, PharmD and John G. Bartlett, MD

INDICATIONS
FDA
- Prophylaxis of MAC in patients with AIDS.

Non-FDA Approved Uses
- Treatment of disseminated MAC in patients with AIDS (in combination with macrolide + EMB).
- Treatment of TB in patients with AIDS who are taking PIs or NNRTIs.
- Treatment of latent TB in patients intolerant to INH. Rifabutin × 4 mos can be considered.

FORMS TABLE

Brand name (mfr)	Forms†	Cost*
Mycobutin (Pfizer)	Oral capsule 150 mg	$12.75

*Prices represent cost per unit specified, are representative of Average Wholesale Price (AWP).
†Dosage is indicated in mg unless otherwise noted.

USUAL ADULT DOSING
- MAC prophylaxis: 300 mg PO once daily (azithromycin preferred).
- MAC treatment: 5 mg/kg (300 mg) PO once daily combined with EMB + either clarithromycin or azithromycin.
- With unboosted PIs (IDV, NFV, FPV): rifabutin 150 mg once daily (OR 300 mg 3 times weekly).
- With boosted PIs (IDV/r, FPV/r, DRV/r, LPV/r, TPV/r, ATV/r) and unboosted ATV: rifabutin 150 mg qod (OR 150 mg 3 × wk). For the treatment of TB, most experts recommend rifabutin 150 mg/d with PI/r (TDM should be considered).
- With NVP: rifabutin 300 mg once daily.
- With EFV: rifabutin 450 mg once daily (OR 600 mg 3 times weekly).
- With ETR: rifabutin 300 mg once daily + ETR 200 mg twice daily.
- With MVC: no data, MVC 300 mg twice daily.
- With RAL: no data, consider standard doses.

ADVERSE DRUG REACTIONS
Common
- Orange discoloration of urine, tears, and sweat.

Occasional
- Uveitis seen with high doses; dose-related (600 mg/day or concurrent use with CYP3A4 inhibitors such as fluconazole, clarithromycin or most PIs); D/C immediately and consult an ophthalmologist.
- Myalgia and arthralgia.

Rare
- Neutropenia.
- Hepatotoxicity (<1%) and pseudojaundice (w/ normal bilirubin).
- Loss of taste.

DRUG INTERACTIONS
- Rifabutin is a substrate and mild inducer of CYP3A4.

DRUG-DRUG INTERACTIONS — See Appendix I, p. 588, for table of drug-drug interactions.

PHARMACOLOGY

Mechanism

- Inhibits initiation of chain formation for RNA synthesis by inhibiting DNA-dependent RNA polymerase.

Pharmacokinetic Parameters

- **Absorption:** 20%.
- **Metabolism and Excretion:** extensive hepatic metabolism via CYP3A4 (25-O-desacetyl and 31-hydroxy most predominant metabolite; activity equivalent to rifabutin). CYP3A4 inducer, although effect less pronounced than rifampin. Metabolites excreted in urine. 30% of drug also excreted in feces. Small amount of drug excreted unchanged in urine and bile.
- **Protein Binding:** 85%.
- **Cmax, Cmin, and AUC:** Cmax: 375 ng/mL after 300 mg. Proposed target peak for mycobacterial infections: 0.3–0.9 mcg/mL 3–4 hrs post-dose (fasted state) or 4–5 hrs post-dose (if given with food).
- $T_{\frac{1}{2}}$: 2–4 hrs.
- **Distribution:** widely distributed with high intracellular uptake due to high lipophilicity. 50% of serum concentration penetrates into CSF; penetrates inflamed meninges.

Pregnancy Risk

- Category B: animal data show skeletal abnormalities. No human data available.

Breastfeeding Compatibility

- No data available.

DOSING

Dosing for Decreased Hepatic Function

- Dose reduction may be necessary with severe liver dysfunction.

Renal Dosing

- Dosing for GFR of 50–80: usual dose.
- Dosing for GFR of 10–50: 50% of dose once daily with CrCl <30 mL/min.
- Dosing for GFR of <10: 50% of dose once daily.
- Dosing in hemodialysis: no data, no supplementation needed.
- Dosing in peritoneal dialysis: no data.
- Dosing in hemofiltration: no data.

COMMENTS

- Benefit of addition of rifabutin to clarithromycin + EMB in treatment of disseminated MAC has been debated. Fear of drug interactions should not deter clinicians, since rifabutin may have survival benefit in addition to protecting against macrolide resistance.
- Addition of rifabutin should be considered in patients with advanced immuno-suppression, high mycobacterial burden, or in absence of effective ART. Good alternative to rifampin for treatment of active and latent TB when needed for concurrent use with PIs or NNRTIs.

SELECTED REFERENCES

Department of Health and Human Services Centers for Disease Control and Prevention; 2007. Managing drug interactions in the treatment of HIV-related tuberculosis. *www.cdc.gov/tb/publications/guidelines/TB_HIV_Drugs/default.htm*. Accessed June 22, 2011.
Comments: Recommendations on the management of drug interactions between rifamycin and ARVs.

Benson CA, Williams PL, Currier JS, et al. A prospective, randomized trial examining the efficacy and safety of clarithromycin in combination with ethambutol, rifabutin, or both for the treatment of disseminated Mycobacterium avium complex disease in persons with acquired immunodeficiency syndrome. *Clin Infect Dis*, 2003; 37: 1234–43.
Comments: Microbiologic response rates were similar between all 3 groups. Clarithromycin + EMB + rifabutin group had improved survival compared to clarithromycin + EMB group (HR 0.44; 95% CI, 0.23–0.83).

Gordin FM, Sullam PM, Shafran SD, et al. A randomized, placebo-controlled study of rifabutin added to a regimen of clarithromycin and ethambutol for treatment of disseminated infection with Mycobacterium avium complex. *Clin Infect Dis*, 1999; 28: 1080–5.
Comments: Addition of rifabutin did not improve bacteriologic response or survival, but may have protected against development of clarithromycin resistance in patients who responded to therapy. 1/44 (2%) receiving rifabutin vs 6/42 (14%) in the placebo group developed clarithromycin resistance (P = 0.055).

RIFAMPIN

Paul A. Pham, PharmD and John G. Bartlett, MD

INDICATIONS
FDA
- Treatment of active TB.
- Treatment of asymptomatic carriers of *Neisseria meningitidis* to eliminate meningococci from the nasopharynx.

Non-FDA Approved Uses
- Treatment of latent TB.
- Treatment of orthopedic implant-related staphylococcal infections (in combination).
- Treatment of prosthetic valve endocarditis (in combination with vancomycin + aminoglycoside).

FORMS TABLE

Brand name (mfr)	Forms†	Cost*
Rifadin (Eon Pharmaceuticals)	Oral capsule 150 mg; 300 mg	$2.57; $3.64
Rifamate (Aventis Pharmaceuticals)	Oral capsule RIF 300 mg/INH 150 mg	$4.19
Rifampin (various generic manufacturers)	150 mg and 300 mg capsules	$2.27; $2.57
Rifater (Aventis Pharmaceuticals)	Oral capsule RIF 120 mg/INH 50 mg/PZA 300 mg	$3.10

*Prices represent cost per unit specified, are representative of Average Wholesale Price (AWP).
†Dosage is indicated in mg unless otherwise noted.

USUAL ADULT DOSING
- TB treatment (in combination with other anti-TB drugs): 10 mg/kg/day (max 600 mg PO or IV once daily). DOT: 600 mg 2–3 ×/wk. HIV+ patients with CD4 <100 should receive DOT 3 ×/wk (not 2 ×/wk, since they are more prone to rifamycin resistance).
- *Rifamate*: 2 caps (RIF/INH 600/300 mg) once daily, 1 hr before or 2 hrs after meals.
- *Rifater*: <44 kg: 4 tabs once daily; 45–54 kg: 5 tabs once daily; >55 kg: 6 tabs once daily, administered 1 hr before or 2 hrs after meals.
- Treatment of latent TB: 10 mg/kg (max 600 mg) once daily for 4 mos (alternative to INH in patients intolerant of INH or exposed to INH-resistant TB).
- Meningococcal prophylaxis: 600 mg twice daily × 2 days. Due to reports of fluoroquinolone resistance, rifampin recommended in selected counties in North Dakota and Minnesota (*MMWR* 2008;57:173).
- Contraindicated with all PIs except with LPV/r + RTV (see below).
- With LPV/r: consider LPV/r 400/100 mg (2 tabs) + RTV 300 mg twice daily (monitor LFTs, GI intolerance, and lipids) or consider switching to rifabutin.
- With RTV+ SQV: not recommended due to high incidence of hepatitis.
- With EFV: EFV 800 mg once daily + RIF 600 mg once daily (monitor CNS side effects). Consider TDM.
- With NVP: coadministration not recommended by manufacturer. Consider EFV.
- With ETR: avoid coadministration.
- With MVC: MVC 600 mg twice daily.
- With RAL: avoid coadministration due to lack of clinical data. If co-administration needed, use RAL 800 mg bid and standard dose rifampin.

ADVERSE DRUG REACTIONS
Common
- Orange discoloration of urine, tears, sweat.

Occasional
- Hepatitis (2.7% w/ other TB Rx) with cholestatic changes in 1st month; jaundice.
- GI intolerance.
- Flu-like syndrome (0.4%–0.7% when taking RIF 2 ×/wk): Sx include fever and chills, headache, dizziness, bone pain, abdominal pain, and generalized pruritus.

Rare
- Hypersensitivity (0.07%–0.3%).
- Thrombocytopenia and hemolytic anemia.
- Headache and dizziness.
- Drug fever.

DRUG INTERACTIONS
- Substrate and potent inducer of CYP3A4. Also an inducer of CYP2B6, 2C8, 2C9, 2C19, 2D6, and glucuronosyl transferase.
- NVP: NVP Cmin decreased by 37%–68% and AUC decreased 37%–58%. RIF AUC increased by 11%. Due to higher risk of hypersensitivity reaction with NVP 300 mg twice daily, CDC recommends standard dose NVP with rifampin coadministration but this was found to be virologically inferior vs HIV. Consider rifabutin with coadministration.

DRUG-DRUG INTERACTIONS—See Appendix I, p. 591, for table of drug-drug interactions.

PHARMACOLOGY
Mechanism
- Inhibits initiation of chain formation for RNA synthesis by inhibiting DNA-dependent RNA polymerase.

Pharmacokinetic Parameters
- **Absorption:** well absorbed with a mean peak concentration is 7.0 mcg/mL, but can vary significantly (4 to 32 mcg/mL). Absorption reduced by ~30% with food.
- **Metabolism and Excretion:** hepatic metabolism to active deacetylated metabolite. Potent CYP3A4 inducer prone to multiple drug interactions. Both unchanged drug and active metabolite primarily excreted via biliary excretion. Unchanged drug undergoes enterohepatic circulation. 3%–30% excreted in urine as metabolite and unchanged drug.
- **Protein Binding:** 75%.
- **Cmax, Cmin, and AUC:** Cmax: 7–9 mcg/mL after 600 mg PO. 17.5 mcg/mL after 600 mg IV.
- **T$_{\frac{1}{2}}$:** 2–5 hrs.
- **Distribution:** widely distributed into most tissue and fluids including liver, lungs, bile, pleural fluid, prostate, seminal fluid, bone, and saliva. With inflamed meninges (approximately 20%) therapeutic CSF concentration attained (consider using high dose 600 mg q12h).

Pregnancy Risk
- Category C: considered safe in pregnancy. Animal data show congenital malformations: cleft palate, spina bifida, embryotoxicity. Administration in last wks of pregnancy may cause postnatal hemorrhage. Several reviews concluded that RIF is not proven teratogen and recommended use of RIF with INH and EMB if necessary.

Breastfeeding Compatibility
- Excreted in breast milk. American Academy of Pediatrics considers RIF compatible with breastfeeding.

DOSING
Dosing for Decreased Hepatic Function
- Clearance may be impaired. Should be given with close monitoring.

Renal Dosing
- Dosing for GFR of 10–80: usual dose.
- Dosing for GFR of <10: usual dose. Some recommend a 50% decrease in dose.
- Dosing in hemodialysis: 300–600 mg once daily.
- Dosing in peritoneal dialysis: 300–600 mg once daily.
- Dosing in hemofiltration: no data.

COMMENTS
- Oral and parenteral rifamycin used for treatment of active and latent TB, treatment and prophylaxis of MOTT, meningococcal prophylaxis, and occasional adjunctive therapy for infections involving *S. aureus*.

- Significant reduction of CYP3A4 substrates serum level (i.e., PIs and NNRTIs) and therefore RIF should be substituted with rifabutin in patients receiving most ART regimens.
- Although data are limited, rifampin's biofilm penetration may make this agent an ideal candidate (in combination with other antibiotics) for treating infections associated with prosthetic devices.

SELECTED REFERENCES

Centers for Disease Control and Prevention (CDC), American Thoracic Society. Update: adverse event data and revised American Thoracic Society/CDC recommendations against the use of rifampin and pyrazinamide for treatment of latent tuberculosis infection—United States, 2003. *MMWR*, 2003; 52: 735–9.
Comments: Two mos RIF and PZA for treatment of latent tuberculosis infection is no longer recommended.

Sterling TR, Pham PA, Chaisson RE. HIV infection-related tuberculosis: clinical manifestations and treatment. *Clin Infect Dos*, 2010; 50 (suppl): S223–30.
Comments: Review on drug-drug interaction involving PIs, NNRTIs, and rifamycins. Updated guidelines are also available online (*www.cdc.gov/nchstp/tb/TB_HIV_Drugs/PDF/tbhiv.pdf*. Accessed July 22, 2011).

SULFADIAZINE

Paul A. Pham, PharmD and John G. Bartlett, MD

DRUGS

INDICATIONS
FDA
- CNS and ocular toxoplasmosis (in combination with pyrimethamine); nocardiosis.
- Malaria due to chloroquine-resistant *P. falciparum* malaria (in combination with quinine and pyrimethamine).
- UTI (also FDA indicated for pyelonephritis, but generally reserved for uncomplicated UTI). Sulfamethoxazole preferred.
- FDA indicated, but not generally recommended: chancroid; trachoma; inclusion conjunctivitis.
- FDA indicated, but not generally recommended: prophylaxis of meningococcal meningitis when sulfonamide-sensitive group A strains known to prevail; meningococcal meningitis; acute otitis media due to *H. influenzae* (in combination with PCN); prophylaxis against recurrences of rheumatic fever (alternative to penicillin); *H. influenzae* meningitis (in combination with streptomycin).

FORMS TABLE

Brand name (mfr)	Forms†	Cost*
Sulfadiazine (Sandoz)	Oral tab 500 mg	$2.50 per 500 mg tab

*Prices represent cost per unit specified, are representative of Average Wholesale Price (AWP).
†Dosage is indicated in mg unless otherwise noted.

USUAL ADULT DOSING
- CNS and ocular toxoplasmosis (induction phase): sulfadiazine 1–1.5 g PO q6h (+ leucovorin 10–20 mg PO once daily and pyrimethamine 100–200 mg PO loading dose, then 50–100 mg PO once daily × 6 wks).
- CNS and ocular toxoplasmosis (maintenance phase): sulfadiazine 500 mg PO q6h (+ leucovorin 10–20 mg PO once daily and pyrimethamine 25–50 mg PO once daily) until immune reconstition (CD4 >200 × 6 mos and on stable ART).
- Treatment of norcardiosis: 1.5 g PO q6h × >6 mos; SMX/TMP preferred (*CID* 1996; 22: 891–903). Target serum level: 100–150 g/mL (2 hrs after dose).
- Ocular toxoplasmosis: sulfadiazine 1 g q6h (+ leucovorin 15 mg PO once daily and pyrimethamine 100 mg PO × 1, then 50 mg PO once daily × 4 wks). Additional treatment if patient has dense vitreous floaters, active retinal inflammation, or both (*Am J Ophthalmol* 2002; 134: 34–40).

ADVERSE DRUG REACTIONS

Common
- GI intolerance with nausea and vomiting.
- Rash and pruritus.

Occasional
- Bone marrow suppression (anemia, thrombocytopenia, leukopenia).
- Serum sickness and drug fever.
- Crystalluria with azotemia, urolithiasis, oliguria. May be prevented by adequate hydration (daily urinary output >1500 mL) and alkalinizing urine to pH >7.15.
- Photosensitivity.
- Hepatitis.

Rare
- TEN and Stevens-Johnson syndrome.
- Encephalopathy.
- Pancreatitis.

DRUG INTERACTIONS
- Cyclosporine: may decrease cyclosporine serum levels. Monitor levels closely; may require dose increase.
- Para-aminobenzoic acid (PABA) and derivatives (such as benzocaine, procaine, tetracaine): theoretical antagonism. Avoid coadministration.
- Phenytoin: may increase phenytoin serum levels. Monitor free phenytoin levels with coadministration.
- Porfimer: may increase the risk of photosensitivity reaction. Avoid coadministration.
- Sulfonylurea: may increase hypoglycemia. Monitor closely with coadministration.
- Warfarin: may increase INR. Monitor closely.

PHARMACOLOGY

Mechanism
- Structural analog of para-aminobenzoic acid (PABA); competitively inhibits dihydrofolic acid synthesis, which is necessary for conversion of PABA to folic acid.

Pharmacokinetic Parameters
- **Absorption:** well absorbed.
- **Metabolism and Excretion:** metabolized extensively in liver to acetylated metabolite. 30%–44% excretion of unchanged drug in urine, while 15%–40% excreted as acetylated metabolite. Renal excretion dependent on urinary pH.
- **Protein Binding:** 38%–48%.
- **Cmax, Cmin, and AUC:** Cmax: 100–150 mcg/mL. Consider therapeutic drug monitoring for serious infections. Target 120–150 mcg/mL. >200 mcg/mL associated with ADR.
- **T$_\frac{1}{2}$:** 7–17 hrs of parent compound.
- **Distribution:** 0.29 L/kg, 40%–60% CNS penetration.

Pregnancy Risk
- Category C: contraindicated near term due to potential for kernicterus in newborn.

Breastfeeding Compatibility
- Excreted in breast milk. Breastfeeding generally not recommended with sulfonamide administration.

DOSING

DOSING FOR DECREASED HEPATIC FUNCTION
- No data. Consider 0.5–1.0 g q6h.

Renal Dosing
- Dosing for GFR of 50–80: 0.5–1.5 gm q6h.
- Dosing for GFR of 10–50: 0.5–1.5 g q8–12h (approximately half dose).
- Dosing for GFR of <10: 0.5–1.5 g q12–24h (approximately 1/3 dose); HD: no data, dose post-HD.
- Dosing in hemodialysis: no data; consider 0.5–1.5 g q12–24h.
- Dosing in peritoneal dialysis: no data; consider 0.5–1.5 g q12–24h.
- Dosing in hemofiltration: no data; consider 0.5–1.5 g q8h–12h.

COMMENTS
- Agent of choice for toxoplasmosis (with pyrimethamine) due to superior CNS penetration and extensive clinical data. Higher incidence of crystaluria compared to other sulfonamides. This regimen also provides PCP prophylaxis.

SELECTED REFERENCES
Katlama C, De Wit S, O'Doherty E, et al. Pyrimethamine-clindamycin vs. pyrimethamine-sulfadiazine as acute and long-term therapy for toxoplasmic encephalitis in patients with AIDS. *Clin Infect Dis*, 1996; 22: 268–75.
Comments: Prospective randomized trial involving 299 patients. Overall risk of progression of toxoplasmosis encephalitis 1.84 × higher for patients receiving pyrimethamine + clindamycin compared to pyrimethamine + sulfadiazine. No significant difference in efficacy during acute therapy, but rate of crossover due to lack of response during induction phase is higher among pyrimethamine + clindamycin recipients.

Dannemann B, McCutchan JA, Israelski D, et al. Treatment of toxoplasmic encephalitis in patients with AIDS. A randomized trial comparing pyrimethamine plus clindamycin to pyrimethamine plus sulfadiazine. The California Collaborative Treatment Group. *Ann Intern Med*, 1992; 116: 33–43.
Comments: Clindamycin + pyrimethamine equivalent to sulfadiazine + pyrimethamine for treatment of toxoplamosis encephalitis in this small prospective clinical trial.

TELBIVUDINE

Paul A. Pham, PharmD and Chloe Lynne Thio, MD

INDICATIONS
FDA
- Treatment of chronic hepatitis B (HBeAg-negative or HBeAg+) with ongoing viral replication and evidence of transferase elevation or histologically active disease.

FORMS TABLE

Brand name (mfr)	Forms†	Cost*
Tyzeka (Novartis Pharmaceuticals)	Oral tablet 600 mg	$26.72 per tablet

*Prices represent cost per unit specified, are representative of Average Wholesale Price (AWP).
†Dosage is indicated in mg unless otherwise noted.

USUAL ADULT DOSING
- 600 mg PO once daily with or without food.

ADVERSE DRUG REACTIONS
General
- Generally well tolerated with adverse reactions comparable to lamivudine and adefovir.
Occasional
- Compared to lamivudine, CK elevation more common in telbivudine-treated patients (9% vs 3%).
- Potential for acute exacerbations of hepatitis B with discontinuation.
Rare
- Although lactic acidosis and severe hepatomegaly with steatosis not reported with telbivudine, nucleoside analogs have potential for causing these potentially fatal adverse reactions.
- Peripheral neuropathy.

DRUG INTERACTIONS
- Not a substrate, inducer, or inhibitor of CYP450 isoenzymes.
- Interactions with PIs and NNRTI unlikely.
- No antagonism observed with other NRTIs *in vitro*. No significant interactions observed with lamivudine, adefovir, cyclosporine, and pegylated IFN-alfa.

RESISTANCE
- M204I genotypic substitution accounts for 74%–94% of observed mutations associated with resistance (*Gastro* 2006;130:A765; Standring, et al. EASL 2006). Additional reported mutations include L80I/V, A181T, L180M, L229W/V.

- In 2-yr follow-up, resistance developed in 8.6% and 21.6% of telbivudine-treated who were HBeAg- and HBeAg+, respectively. Although overall resistance rates were high, in subset of who successfully suppressed to undetectable at 24 wks, resistance rates were only 2%–4%. Clinical implication of this finding unclear, but some experts advocate using monotherapy for 24 wks with "intensification" only if VL remains detectable. Efficacy of telbivudine against HBV harboring lamivudine and adefovir resistance remains to be determined. *In vitro*, telbivudine active against lamivudine-resistant virus with M204V mutation alone, but not against lamivudine-treated virus with L180M/M204V double mutation or M204I mutation. However, clinical relevance of these *in vitro* observations unclear.
- Adefovir-resistant HBV with A181V mutation associated with 3–5-fold reduction in susceptibility.

PHARMACOLOGY
Mechanism
- Telbivudine, a synthetic thymidine analog, inhibits HBV DNA polymerase reverse transcriptase by competing with natural substrate thymidine 5′–triphosphate.

Pharmacokinetic Parameters
- **Absorption:** well absorbed.
- **Metabolism and Excretion:** not metabolized, and is primarily excreted via glomerular filtration.
- **Protein Binding:** low (3.3%).
- **Cmax, Cmin, and AUC:** Cmax 3.69, AUC 26.1 mcg hr/mL, and Cmin 0.2–0.3 mcg/mL after 600 mg once daily at steady state.
- **T$_{\frac{1}{2}}$:** terminal half-life of 40–49 hrs.
- **Distribution:** Widely distributed.

Pregnancy Risk
- Category B: not teratogenic in animal studies. No human data.

Breastfeeding Compatibility
- Excreted in breast milk (animal data).

DOSING
Dosing for Decreased Hepatic Function
- 600 mg once daily.

Renal Dosing
- Dosing for GFR of 50–80: GFR >50: 600 mg once daily.
- Dosing for GFR of 10–50: GFR 30–49: 600 mg qod; GFR <30 (no HD): 600 mg q72h.
- Dosing for GFR of <10: GFR <30 (no HD): 600 mg q72h.
- Dosing in hemodialysis: ESRD (HD): 600 mg q96h (on days of HD, dose post-HD).
- Dosing in peritoneal dialysis: no data.
- Dosing in hemofiltration: no data.

COMMENTS
- In treatment of chronic hepatitis B, telbivudine is more potent than lamivudine and adefovir. Active *in vitro* against lamivudine-resistant strains with M204V mutation, but due to similar resistance mutation, some experts do not recommend telbivudine for treatment of lamivudine-resistant HBV. Compared to lamivudine, resistance less likely and slower to develop. In addition, a unique mutation (M204I), may allow sequencing. *In vitro* telbivudine is not active against HIV-1; however, a case report suggest activity against HIV-1 (Low E, et al. *AIDS* 2009; 23: 546). Head-to-head comparison with more potent agents (e.g., entecavir), combination studies, and studies evaluating sequencing strategies needed to establish role of telbivudine.

SELECTED REFERENCES
Lai CL, Gane E, Liaw YF, et al. Telbivudine versus lamivudine in patients with chronic hepatitis B. *N Engl J Med*, 2007; 357: 2576–88.
Comments: The GLOBE study was randomized, blinded phase III trial comparing telbivudine (600 mg/day) vs lamivudine (100 mg/day) in 1370 naïve-patients with chronic HBV. Patients had HBV VL >6 log c/mL, an ALT 1.3–10 × ULN, and compensated liver disease. Therapeutic response, defined as HBV VL <5 log with HBeAg loss or ALT normalization. At wk 52, significantly higher proportion of HBeAg+ patients receiving telbivudine than had therapeutic response (75.3% vs 67.0%,

P = 0.005) or histologic response (64.7% vs 56.3%, P = 0.01). Tolerability comparable between treatment groups, but elevated CK more common in patients treated with telbivudine (3 cases of reversible myositis).

Chan HL, Heathcote EJ, Marcellin P, et al. Treatment of hepatitis B e antigen positive chronic hepatitis with telbivudine or adefovir: a randomized trial. *Ann Intern Med*, 2007; 147: 745–54.

Comments: Multicenter, randomized study involving 135 treatment-naïve patients with compensated liver disease compared telbivudine, adefovir, and adefovir-telbivudine (adefovir for 1st 24 wks followed by switch to telbivudine for 28 wks). Patients were HBeAg+ with HBV VL >6 log and ALT 1.3–10 × ULN. Compared to adefovir, telbivudine-treated patients had >1.4 log VL decline (P <0.001) at 24 wks. More patients in telbivudine-treated group were HBV PCR negative (39% vs 12%; OR 4.46 [CI, 1.86–10.72]; P = 0.001); however, HBeAg loss and ALT normalization comparable between 2 groups. In patients who switched from adefovir to telbivudine at 24 wks, an additional 1 log drop in HBV VL was observed; HBV viral suppression in these patients was comparable to those patients who received adefovir for 52 wks.

Gane E, Safadi R, Xie Q, et al. A randomized trial of telbivudine (LdT) versus lamivudine in lamivudine-experienced patients—week 24 primary analysis. Poster 1007 presented at: 57th Conference of the American Association for the Study of Liver Diseases (AASLD); October 27–31, 2006: Boston, MA.

Comments: 256 lamivudine-experienced patients with persistent viremia (HBV VL >3 log) despite 3–12 mos of lamivudine treatment randomized to switch to telbivudine or continue therapy with lamivudine. At preliminary 24 wks evaluation, serum HBV VL suppressed to below 5 log in 80% of patients switched to telbivudine vs 56% in lamivudine group, and undetectable HBV VL achieved in 41% and 31%, respectively.

TRIMETHOPRIM + SULFAMETHOXAZOLE

Paul A. Pham, PharmD and John G. Bartlett, MD

DRUGS

INDICATIONS
FDA
- Acute exacerbation of chronic bronchitis (AECB).
- Otitis media (in *S. pneumoniae*-sensitive cases only).
- PCP prophylaxis.
- PCP treatment.
- Traveler's diarrhea, shigellosis.
- Urinary tract infections.

Non-FDA Approved Uses
- *Nocardia* infection.
- Toxoplasmosis treatment and prophylaxis.
- Bacterial cystitis prophylaxis.
- *Isospora* infections.
- *Salmonella* infections.
- MSSA and community-acquired MRSA soft tissue infections.
- Legionellosis treatment (2nd line).
- Listeriosis treatment (2nd line for PCN-allergic patients).

FORMS TABLE

Brand name (mfr)	Forms†	Cost*
Bactrim or Septra (brand and generic manufacturers)	Oral tablet 400 mg/80 mg (SS); 800 mg/160 mg (DS)	$0.66; $2.89
	IV vial 80 mg/16 mg per mL (30 mL)	$10.98 (30 mL)
	Oral suspension 400/80 mg/5 mL (16-oz bottle)	$57.95 (16 oz)

*Prices represent cost per unit specified, are representative of Average Wholesale Price (AWP).
†Dosage is indicated in mg unless otherwise noted.

USUAL ADULT DOSING
- PCP treatment: 5 mg/kg (TMP component) IV or PO q8h × 21 days (usually 5–6 DS/day but must dose based on weight using TMP component).
- PCP prophylaxis: 1 DS or 1 SS PO once daily or 1 DS 3 ×/wk (alternative).

- Toxoplasmosis prophylaxis: 1 DS PO once daily.
- Toxoplasmosis treatment: 5 mg/kg (TMP component) PO or IV q12h × 6 wks, then 1/2 dose for maintenance (sulfadiazine + pyrimethamine preferred).
- UTI: 1 DS PO twice daily × 3–14 days (3 days recommended for uncomplicated cystitis in women).
- Traveler's diarrhea, *Salmonella, Shigella, E. coli*, and *Cyclospora*: 1 DS PO twice daily × 5–7 days.
- Skin and soft tissue infections (including CA-MRSA): 1–2 DS PO q12h.
- *Nocardia*: 2–3 DS PO twice daily × >6 mos.
- *Isospora*: 1 DS PO twice daily × 7–10 days, then 1 DS 3 ×/wk.
- Gradual dose escalation over 6 days may improve long-term tolerability of TMP/SMX compared to direct rechallenge, but dosing may be impractical for some patients. Start with 12.5% of SS TMP/SMX (10-mg TMP component), then increase by 12.5%/day until target dose of 1 SS TMP/SMX on day 6 (*J Infect Dis.* 2001;184:992–7).
- Acute exacerbations of chronic bronchitis (bacterial): 1 DS twice daily × 14 days.

ADVERSE DRUG REACTIONS
General
- Generally well tolerated in the immunocompetent host. HIV+ patients at increased risk for developing SMX-TMP-associated ADRs.

Common
- GI intolerance with nausea and vomiting (in 20%–50% receiving high dose >15 mg/kg).
- Rash and pruritus (usually 7–14 days after starting SMX/TMP).
- Continue treatment if Sx not disabling.
- Pseudoelevation in serum creatinine (an average increase of 18%) (*Chemotherapy*. 1981; 27: 229–32).

Occasional
- Reversible hyperkalemia (with higher TMP doses ± chronic renal insufficiency).
- Bone marrow suppression (anemia with folate deficiency, thrombocytopenia, and leukopenia; more common with higher doses).
- Serum sickness and drug fever.
- Hepatitis (may be cholestatic).
- Photosensitivity.
- Methemoglobinemia (with severe G6PD deficiency). Black patients with mild-to-moderate G6PD deficiency can tolerate TMP-SMX.

Rare
- Crystalluria with azotemia, urolithiasis, and oliguria (more common with sulfadiazine).
- Stevens-Johnson syndrome or toxic epidermal necrolysis (TEN).
- Aseptic meningitis.
- Pancreatitis.
- Neurologic toxicity (tremor, ataxia, apathy, and ankle clonus).
- Interstitial nephritis.
- Sweet's syndrome (fever; leukocytosis; and tender, erythematous, dense neutrophilic infiltrative papules).

DRUG INTERACTIONS
- Cyclosporine: may decrease cyclosporine serum levels. Monitor cyclosporine serum levels.
- Folinic acid: possible antagonism. Avoid coadministration.
- Para-aminobenzoic acid (PABA) and derivatives (such as benzocaine, procaine, tetracaine): theoretical antagonism.
- Phenytoin: may increase phenytoin serum levels. Monitor free phenytoin levels with coadministration.
- Porfimer: may increase the risk of photosensitivity reaction. Avoid coadministration.
- Sulfonylurea: may increase hypoglycemia. Monitor closely with coadministration.
- Warfarin: may increase INR. Monitor closely.

RESISTANCE
- *E. coli* (urine isolates): certain regions in US and worldwide >20% resistance.
- *S. pneumoniae:* 15%–30% resistance.

- *P. jiroveci:* increasing rates of mutations in the dihydropteroate synthase (DHPS) gene of *P. jiroveci* associated with resistance to sulfonamide and dapsone but not clinically significant since clinical outcome was not worse with DHPS mutation in a prospective trial (*Lancet* 2001; 358: 545–9).
- CA-MRSA: low resistance rates to TMP-SMX.

PHARMACOLOGY

Mechanism

- TMP acts synergistically with SMX by interfering with folic acid production. TMP binds to dihydrofolate reductase inhibiting the reduction of dihydrofolic acid to tetrahydrofolic acid (folinic acid). Sulfonamides are structural analog of para-aminobenzoic acid (PABA); it competitively inhibits dihydrofolic acid synthesis, which is necessary for the conversion of PABA to folic acid.

Pharmacokinetic Parameters

- **Absorption:** 90%–100% absorption.
- **Metabolism and Excretion:** extensive liver metabolism of SMX to n-acetyl and n-glucuronidate metabolite. 10%–30% of SMX and 50%–70% of TMP excreted in urine.
- **Protein Binding:** SMX (70%); TMP (44%–62%).
- **Cmax, Cmin, and AUC:** steady-state peak concentration is 9 mcg/mL and 105 mcg/mL for TMP and SMX, respectively, with 160/800 mg IV q8h administration. For nocardiosis, peak (2 hrs post-dose) of 100–150 mcg/mL is recommended.
- **$T_{\frac{1}{2}}$:** 11 hrs (TMP); 9 hrs (SMX).
- **Distribution:** TMP: 2.0 L/kg; SMX: 360 mL/kg. Good CSF penetration with high doses (15–20 mg/kg/day).

Pregnancy Risk

- Category C: in surveillance study of Michigan Medicaid recipients, 2296 exposures to TMP-SMX in 1st trimester resulted in 5.5% birth defects. This incidence is suggestive of association between drug and congenital defects (cardiovascular); however, other factors such as mother's disease, concurrent drug used, and chance may be involved. Although manufacturers do not recommend use near term/late 3rd trimester due to theoretical risk of kernicterus, adult OI guidelines recommend TMP/SMX for treatment and prophylaxis of PCP in pregnant women.

Breastfeeding Compatibility

- Excreted in breast milk at low concentrations. The American Academy of Pediatrics considers TMP-SMX to be compatible with breastfeeding.

DOSING

Dosing for Decreased Hepatic Function

- No data. Consider usual dose with close monitoring.

Renal Dosing

- Dosing for GFR of 30–80: usual dose.
- Dosing for GFR of 10–30: 5 mg/kg IV q12h; oral 50% of dose.
- Dosing for GFR of <10: manufacturer recommends avoiding. For severe PCP or serious infections, authors recommend 5–7.5 mg/kg/day in 2–3 divided doses (1/2–1/3 standard dose) for GFR <10. HD: 5–7.5 mg/kg/day (1/2–1/3 standard dose). PCP prophylaxis: consider 1 SS PO once daily.
- Dosing in hemodialysis: dialyzed out, consider 5–7.5 mg/kg/day in 2–3 divided doses (dose post-HD on days of dialysis). PCP prophylaxis: consider 1 SS PO once daily.
- Dosing in peritoneal dialysis: not dialyzed out. PCP prophylaxis: consider 1 DS PO every other day. PCP treatment: consider 5 mg/kg/day.
- Dosing in hemofiltration: CVVH and CVVHD: limited data. Consider 5 mg/kg IV q8–12h.

COMMENTS

- 1st-line agent for PCP prophylaxis and treatment. Active against other pathogens (*T. gondii*, *Listeria*, *Legionella*, 70% of *S. pneumoniae*, many *S. aureus* including CA-MRSA, and *H. influenzae*), which may protect patients against CAP and soft tissue infections. Although generally well tolerated in immunocompetent host, there is higher incidence of intolerance requiring discontinuation in HIV+ patients.

DRUGS

SELECTED REFERENCES

Kaplan JE, Benson C, Holmes KH, et al. Guidelines for prevention and treatment of opportunistic infections in HIV-infected adults and adolescents: recommendations from CDC, the National Institutes of Health, and the HIV Medicine Association of the Infectious Diseases Society of America. *MMWR Recomm Rep*, 2009; 58: 1–207.
Comments: TMP-SMX usage recommendations in HIV patients. TMP-SMX is the preferred agent for PCP prophylaxis and treatment.

Lin D, Li WK, Rieder MJ. Cotrimoxazole for prophylaxis or treatment of opportunistic infections of HIV/AIDS in patients with previous history of hypersensitivity to cotrimoxazole. *Cochrane Database Syst Rev*, 2007; 2: CD005646.
Comments: Meta-analysis of 3 randomized trials comparing treating-through, rechallenge, or desensitization of cotrimoxazole treatment or prophylaxis in HIV+ patients found beneficial effect of desensitization protocol over rechallenge protocol at 6 mos of follow-up for preventing discontinuation of cotrimoxazole (number needed to treat (NNT) 7.14, 95% CI 4.0–33.0), and for lower incidence of overall hypersensitivity (NNT 4.55, 95% CI 3.03–9.09). No severe hypersensitivity reactions occurred in these protocols. Desensitization did not change outcome compared with rechallenge in other studies (Biomed Pharmacother 2000; 54: 45).

Safrin S, Finkelstein DM, Feinberg J, et al. Comparison of three regimens for treatment of mild to moderate *Pneumocystis carinii* pneumonia in patients with AIDS. A double-blind, randomized, trial of oral trimethoprim-sulfamethoxazole, dapsone-trimethoprim, and clindamycin-primaquine. ACTG 108 Study Group. *Ann Intern Med*, 1996; 124: 792–802.
Comments: TMP/SMX, TMP/dapsone, and primaquine/clindamycin equivalent in management of mild or moderately severe PCP. Patients treated with TMP-SMX experienced more rash and hepatitis compared to the other 2 groups.

Bozzette SA, Finkelstein DM, Spector SA, et al. A randomized trial of three antipneumocystis agents in patients with advanced human immunodeficiency virus infection. NIAID AIDS Clinical Trials Group. *N Engl J Med*, 1995; 332: 693–9.
Comments: Open-label study comparing TMP/SMX vs dapsone vs aerosolized pentamidine (AP). 36-mos cumulative risks of PCP were 18%, 17%, and 21% in TMP/SMX, dapsone, and AP groups, respectively (P = 0.22). In patients with CD4 <100, risk was 33% with AP vs 19% with TMP/SMX and 22% with dapsone (P = 0.04). AP may be an alternative in patients who can not tolerate TMP/SMX or dapsone.

Klein NC, Duncanson FP, Lenox TH, et al. Trimethoprim-sulfamethoxazole versus pentamidine for *Pneumocystis carinii* pneumonia in AIDS patients: results of a large prospective randomized treatment trial. *AIDS*, 1992; 6: 301–5.
Comments: Survival was 67% in patients initially administered TMP/SMX vs 74% in patients initially administered AP (P = 0.402). This study indicates that patients who switch from TMP/SMX to IV pentamidine due to "clinical failure" do not have improved clinical outcomes. However, higher survival rate if switch due to drug toxicity. TMP/SMX is drug of choice due to better safety profile.

VALACYCLOVIR

Paul A. Pham, PharmD and John G. Bartlett, MD

INDICATIONS

FDA

- Treatment of initial episode of genital herpes in immunocompetent adults.
- Suppression of recurrent episodes of genital herpes in immunocompetent and HIV+ adults.
- Treatment of recurrent episodes of genital herpes in immunocompetent adults.
- Treatment of herpes zoster in immunocompetent adults.
- Treatment of herpes labialis.

Non-FDA Approved Uses

- Treatment of initial episode and recurrent episodes of genital herpes in HIV+ patients.
- Treatment of herpes zoster in HIV+ patients.
- Treatment of perianal herpes and disseminated HSV.

FORMS TABLE

Brand name (mfr)	Forms†	Cost*
Valtrex (GlaxoSmithKline)	Oral tablet 500 mg; 1000 mg	$8.21; $14.06
Valacyclovir (various generic manufactures)	500 mg and 1000 mg tablets	$7.22; $12.64

*Prices represent cost per unit specified, are representative of Average Wholesale Price (AWP).
†Dosage is indicated in mg unless otherwise noted.

USUAL ADULT DOSING

- Dermatomal herpes zoster: 1 g PO q8h × 7–10 days.
- Treatment of 1st episode of genital HSV: 1 g PO twice daily × 7–10 days.
- Treatment of recurrent genital HSV: 500 mg PO twice daily (1 g PO twice daily if severe).
- Suppressive therapy for genital HSV: 500 mg PO twice daily.
- Herpes labialis: 2 g PO q12h × 1 day.
- Treatment of adult varicella: consider 1 g PO q8h within 24 hrs of rash onset (no data with valacyclovir but efficacy demonstrated with ACV [*Ann Intern Med* 1992; 117: 358–63]).

ADVERSE DRUG REACTIONS

General
- Generally well tolerated.

Occasional
- Nausea and vomiting.
- Rash.

Rare
- Agitation, dizziness, headache, confusion, hallucination, seizure (more common in elderly patients).
- Transaminase elevation.
- Anemia, neutropenia.
- Hypotension.
- Thrombotic thrombocytopenic purpura/hemolytic uremic syndrome (TTP/HUS) reported in immunocompromised patients receiving valacyclovir 8 g/day.

DRUG INTERACTIONS
- Probenecid: may increase ACV levels. No dose adjustment needed.

PHARMACOLOGY

Mechanism
- Cleaved by valine hydrolase into ACV. ACV converted by viral thymidine kinase (TK) to active ACV monophosphate; cellular enzyme catalase converts ACV monophosphate to ACV triphosphate, which competitively inhibits viral DNA polymerase.

Pharmacokinetic Parameters
- **Absorption:** 54% (3–5-fold increase in bioavailability compared to oral ACV).
- **Metabolism and Excretion:** rapidly converted to ACV via intestinal and hepatic 1st-pass metabolism. ACV converted to inactive metabolites by alcohol and aldehyde dehydrogenase. 80%–89% of ACV recovered in the urine unchanged.
- **Protein Binding:** 14%–18%.
- **Cmax, Cmin, and AUC:** Cmax: 3.3–3.7 mcg/mL after 500 mg administration; AUC: 18–20 hr/mcg/mL. Cmax: 4.6–5.5 mcg/mL after 1 g oral administration.
- **$T_{\frac{1}{2}}$:** 2.5–3.3 hrs.
- **Distribution:** high concentration found in kidneys, liver, and intestines. CNS penetration 50% of serum. Also distributed to lung, aqueous humor, tears, muscle, spleen, breast milk, uterine, vaginal mucosa, semen, and amniotic fluid.

Pregnancy Risk
- Category B: not teratogenic in animal studies. No human data available but likely to be similar to ACV. Prophylaxis not recommended in pregnancy.

DRUGS

Breastfeeding Compatibility

• No data: most likely distributed into breast milk as ACV. Not associated with any problems in the newborn.

Dosing

Dosing for Decreased Hepatic Function

• No data. Dose reduction unlikely.

Renal Dosing

• Dosing for GFR of 50–80: usual dose.
• Dosing for GFR of 30–49: 1000 mg PO twice daily.
• Dosing for GFR of 10–29: 1000 mg once daily.
• Dosing for GFR of <10: 500 mg PO once daily.
• Dosing in hemodialysis: 500 mg once daily, 33% removed with HD. On days of dialysis dose post-dialysis.
• Dosing in peritoneal dialysis: 500 mg PO q24–48h;, no supplemental dose needed (*Nephron* 2002; 91: 164).
• Dosing in hemofiltration: not effectively removed. Consider 500 mg PO once daily.

COMMENTS

• Prodrug of ACV with better absorption, higher blood levels, and more convenient dosing vs oral ACV. Alternatives are ACV and famciclovir (see Herpes simplex, p. 71, and Herpes zoster, p. 72).
• More effective at decreasing postherpetic neuralgia than ACV in immunocompetent host.

SELECTED REFERENCES

MacDougall C, Guglielmo BJ. Pharmacokinetics of valaciclovir. *J Antimicrob Chemother*, 2004; 53: 899–901.

Comments: Review of valacyclovir PKs. When switching from IV ACV to PO valacyclovir, remember that valacyclovir 1 g PO q8h does not provide equivalent PK to ACV 10 mg/kg IV q8h. Valacyclovir 2000 mg 4 ×/day provides AUC similar to IV ACV (10 mg/kg q8h).

Conant MA, Schacker TW, Murphy RL, et al. Valaciclovir versus aciclovir for herpes simplex virus infection in HIV-infected individuals: two randomized trials. *Int J STD AIDS*, 2002; 13: 12–21.

Comments: ACV as effective as valacyclovir for suppression and episodic treatment of herpes. Most experts now recommend valacyclovir over ACV due to better absorption and more convenient dosing schedule.

Sexually transmitted guidelines 2010 / Vol. 59 / No. RR-12.

Comments: CDC recommendation for the use of ACV, famciclovir, and valacyclovir in the treatment of HSV infections.

Beutner KR, Friedman DJ, Forszpaniak C, et al. Valaciclovir compared with acyclovir for improved therapy for herpes zoster in immunocompetent adults. *Antimicrob Agents Chemother*, 1995; 39: 1546–53.

Comments: In immunocompetent host, valacyclovir significantly accelerated the resolution of herpes zoster-associated pain 44 days vs 51 days (P = 0.001, respectively) compared to ACV. Treatment with valacyclovir also significantly reduced the duration of postherpetic neuralgia and decreased the proportion of patients with pain persisting for 6 mos (19.3% vs 25.7%). The use of valacyclovir for the treatment of zoster has not been evaluated in patients with AIDS. Use with close monitoring in patients with disseminated zoster since treatment failure has been reported (*AIDS Patient Care* STDS 2004; 18: 255–7).

VALGANCICLOVIR

Paul A. Pham, PharmD and John G. Bartlett, MD

INDICATIONS

FDA

• Treatment of CMV retinitis in patients with AIDS.
• Prevention of CMV disease in kidney, heart, and kidney-pancreas transplant patients at high risk for CMV disease (e.g., donor positive, recipient negative). Not indicated in liver transplant patients.

Non-FDA Approved Uses

• Prevention of CMV retinitis of the contralateral eye in patients treated with intraocular ganciclovir implant.
• Treatment of GI CMV disease (in patients tolerating PO intake).

FORMS TABLE

Brand name (mfr)	Forms†	Cost*
Valcyte (Roche)	Oral tablet 450 mg	$46.99

*Prices represent cost per unit specified, are representative of Average Wholesale Price (AWP).
†Dosage is indicated in mg unless otherwise noted.

USUAL ADULT DOSING

- CMV retinitis (induction): 900 mg PO twice daily with food × 3 wks (+ ganciclovir implant).
- CMV retinitis (maintenance): 900 mg PO once daily with food until immune reconstitution (CD4 >150 × 3–6 mos w/ ophthalmology consultation confirming quiescence).
- Gastrointestinal CMV disease: 900 mg twice daily with food × 3–6 wks (consider maintenance therapy with severe disease and/or with relapse).
- Prevention of CMV disease in kidney, heart, and kidney-pancreas transplant patients at high risk for CMV disease (e.g., donor [+] CMV/recipient negative): 900 mg daily with food beginning within 10 days of transplantation and continuing through day 100 post-transplantation.
- Monitor CBC 2–3 ×/wk. Discontinue drug or add G-CSF if ANC <500. Discontinue if platelet count <25,000 or consider d/c if Hgb <8 g/dL.

ADVERSE DRUG REACTIONS

Common
- Neutropenia (reversible and responds to G-CSF). Reversible within 3–7 days of discontinuation or dose reduction.
- Reversible thrombocytopenia.
- Diarrhea and nausea.

Occasional
- Anemia.
- Fever.
- Rash.
- Headache.
- Seizures.
- Confusion.
- Mental status changes.

Rare
- Hepatoxicity.

DRUG INTERACTIONS

- ddI (buffered or EC): not studied with valganciclovir but ddI levels may be increased. PK study with ddI (buffered) and ganciclovir (GCV) resulted in a 111% increase in ddI AUC. GCV AUC decreased by 21%. Monitor closely for ddI toxicity. Consider ddI dose reduction or alternative NRTI.
- Drug interactions with PIs, NNRTIs, RAL, MVC, and ENF unlikely.
- Myelosuppressive drugs (e.g., AZT, interferon, 5-FC, pyrimethamine, etc.): may increase risk of hematologic toxicity. Monitor closely with coadministration. Consider alternative agents or support with GCSF.
- Probenecid: may increase GCV serum levels. Monitor for GCV toxicity.
- Trimethoprim: may increase GCV serum levels. Monitor for GCV toxicity.

PHARMACOLOGY

Mechanism
- Prodrug of GCV with improved bioavailability. GCV is a synthetic analogue of 2-deoxyguanosine. Once phosphorylated, GCV triphosphate inhibits viral DNA synthesis.

Pharmacokinetic Parameters
- **Absorption:** 60% (well absorbed, should be administered with food).
- **Metabolism and Excretion:** rapidly hydrolyzed to GCV, which is renally excreted via glomerular filtration and active tubular secretion.
- **Protein Binding:** 1%–2%.

DRUGS

- **Cmax, Cmin, and AUC:** Cmax: 5.61 mcg/mL after 900-mg dose (with food). AUC: 29 mcg hr/mL after 900-mg dose (comparable to 5 mg/kg GCV IV).
- **T$_\frac{1}{2}$:** 4 hrs (serum), 18 hrs (intracellular).
- **Distribution:** Vd = 0.7 L/kg.

Pregnancy Risk
- Category C: teratogenic, carcinogenic, embryogenic and causes aspermatogenesis; growth retardation; aplastic organ in animal studies. No human data, use only for life-threatening CMV infection and warn patient of possible teratogenic effect. Effective form of contraception is recommended.

Breastfeeding Compatibility
- No data. Due to potential for serious toxicity, mother should avoid breastfeeding.

DOSING

Dosing for Decreased Hepatic Function
- No data. Usual dose likely.

Renal Dosing
- Dosing for GFR of 40–59: 450 mg twice daily (induction) then 450 mg once daily (maintenance).
- Dosing for GFR of 25–39: 450 mg once daily (induction) then 450 mg every other day (maintenance).
- Dosing for GFR of 10–24: 450 mg every other day (induction) then 450 mg twice weekly (maintenance).
- Dosing for GFR of <10: not recommended by manufacturer.
- Dosing in hemodialysis: not recommended by manufacturer (HD removes approximately 50% of GCV). Consider using 1.25 mg/kg IV ganciclovir post-HD (induction).
- Dosing in peritoneal dialysis: no data.
- Dosing in hemofiltration: no data.

COMMENTS
- Oral valganciclovir has 10-fold better absorption than oral GCV. AUC of oral valganciclovir 900 mg comparable to GCV 5 mg/kg IV. Oral valganciclovir equivalent to IV GCV for treatment of CMV retinitis in HIV+ patients and is preferred due to oral administration.
- Contraindicated by manufacturer in patients with severe neutropenia (ANC <500/dL), thrombocytopenia (<25,000/dL), severe anemia (Hgb <8 g/dL) and renal failure. Neutropenia and anemia generally responsive to G-CSF and erythropoietin.

SELECTED REFERENCES

Kaplan JE, Benson C, Holmes KH, et al. Guidelines for prevention and treatment of opportunistic infections in HIV-infected adults and adolescents: recommendations from CDC, the National Institutes of Health, and the HIV Medicine Association of the Infectious Diseases Society of America. MMWR Recomm Rep, 2009; 58: 1–207.
Comments: In patients tolerating PO intake, oral valganciclovir + ganciclovir implant is recommended for the treatment of CMV retinitis.

Khoury JA, Storch GA, Bohl DL, et al. Prophylactic versus preemptive oral valganciclovir for the management of cytomegalovirus infection in adult renal transplant recipients. *Am J Transplant*, 2006; 6: 2134–43.
Comments: Both prophylactic and preemptive treatment strategies were effective in preventing symptomatic CMV in kidney transplant recipients at risk for CMV (D+/R–, D+/R+, D–/R+) disease. As expected, more patients in the preemptive group (59%) than in the prophylaxis group (29%) developed CMV DNAemia, but symptomatic infection did not significantly differ between the 2 groups.

Lalezari J, Lindley J, Walmsley S, et al. A safety study of oral valganciclovir maintenance treatment of cytomegalovirus retinitis. *J Acquir Immune Defic Syndr*, 2002; 30: 392–400.
Comments: With exception of GI intolerance seen with valganciclovir and line infections seen with IV GCV, ADRs are comparable between IV GCV and valganciclovir.

Martin DF, Sierra-Madero J, Walmsley S, et al. A controlled trial of valganciclovir as induction therapy for cytomegalovirus retinitis. *N Engl J Med*, 2002; 346: 1119–26.
Comments: Valganciclovir 900 mg twice daily bioequivalent to IV GCV 5 mg/kg twice daily. Response rate comparable in the 2 groups; 47/61 patients (77%) assigned to IV GCV and 46/64 (72%) assigned to valganciclovir had a satisfactory response (5.2 percentage points; 95% CI, -20.4–10.1).

VANCOMYCIN

Paul A. Pham, PharmD and John G. Bartlett, MD

INDICATIONS

FDA

- Bone and joint infections.
- Pneumonia.
- Septicemia.
- Endocarditis treatment and prophylaxis (in PCN-allergic patients).
- Oral vancomycin: antibiotic-associated pseudomembranous colitis caused by *C. difficile* and enterocolitis caused by *S. aureus* (including MRSA).

Non-FDA Approved Uses

- Hardware-associated infections.

FORMS TABLE

Brand name (mfr)	Forms†	Cost*
Vancomycin (generic manufacturer)	IV vial 500 mg; 1000 mg	$4.56; $7.78
Vancocin pulvule (ViroPharma)	Oral pulvule 125 mg; 250 mg	$26.60; $49.03

*Prices represent cost per unit specified, are representative of Average Wholesale Price (AWP).
†Dosage is indicated in mg unless otherwise noted.

USUAL ADULT DOSING

- **Systemic infections caused by MRSA and other resistant Gram-positive organisms:** 15 mg/kg IV q12h (dose based on actual body weight). Typical dose 1 g IV q12h for 70-kg patient with normal renal function. Higher dose (15 mg/kg IV q8h or 22.5 mg/kg IV q12h) recommended for CNS infections. Loading dose 25–30 mg/kg ×1 in critically ill patients (20–25 mg/kg can be considered in critically ill patients with baseline renal insufficiency).
- Target trough: 15–20 mcg/mL (endocarditis and pneumonia); 20 mcg/mL (CNS infections); 10–15 mcg/mL (bacteremia with MRSA MIC <2). Consider alternative to vancomycin with MIC ≥2.
- *C. difficile colitis:* 125 mg PO q6h × 7–10 days. Higher doses 250–500 mg PO q6h (± IV metrondiazole) may be given with ileus or severe disease.
- Oral preparation not systemically absorbed and ineffective for any infections other than *C. difficile* colitis and *S. aureus* enterocolitis. Parenteral formulation not effective for treatment of staphylococcal enterocolitis and pseudomembranous colitis caused by *C. difficile*.
- **Staphylococcal enterocolitis:** 500–2000 mg PO/day in 3–4 divided doses × 7–10 days.
- IV vancomycin can be given orally for *C. difficile* colitis to decrease cost ($5 vs $80/day).
- Intraventricular or intrathecal dose: vancomycin 20 mg/day (up to 30 mg). Use preservative-free vancomycin 1-g vial for reconstitution.

ADVERSE DRUG REACTIONS

General

- Generally well tolerated.

Occasional

- "Red man syndrome": flushing over chest/face ± hypotension and pruritis (infusion over >60 min may reverse or prevent; pretreatment w/ antihistamine may alleviate symptoms). Red man syndrome should not be construed as a true allergy.
- Phlebitis.
- Renal function impairment (most often in combination with aminoglycosides). Uncommon with modern formulations of drug but controversial.

Rare

- Neutropenia.
- Eosinophilia.

DRUGS

- Drug fever.
- Allergic reactions: IgA bullous dermatitis; drug rash with eosinophilia and systemic syndrome (DRESS).
- Tissue irritation.
- Ototoxicity (controversial).
- Thrombocytopenia.

DRUG INTERACTIONS

- Aminoglycoside: controversial but higher incidence of nephrotoxicity associated with vancomycin and aminoglycoside coadministration.
- Cholestyramine: binds to oral vancomycin. Do not coadminister; consider oral metronidazole with cholestyramineco-administration.
- Linezolid: in a rabbit MRSA aortic valve endocarditis model, addition of linezolid to vancomycin was antagonistic (*AAC* 2003; 47: 3002). Clinical significance unknown but avoid coadministration.
- Nondepolarizing muscle relaxants (succinylcholine, atracurium, vecuronium, pancuronium, tubocurarine): case reports of enhanced neuromuscular blockade. Monitor closely with coadministration.

RESISTANCE

- Vancomycin-resistant *S. aureus* (VRSA): MIC = 16 mcg/mL (7 isolates reported to date).
- Vancomycin-intermediate *S. aureus* (VISA): MIC range 4–8 mcg/mL.
- Heteroresistant *S. aureus* (hetero VISA): MIC = 4 mcg/mL (but contain subpopulation of organisms that have MICs of 4–8 mcg/mL).
- Vancomycin-sensitive *S. aureus*: MIC = 2 mcg/mL or lower (former breakpoint was 4 mcg/mL).
- *Enterococci:* MIC breakpoint of 4 mcg/mL.

PHARMACOLOGY

Mechanism

- Inhibits bacterial cell wall biosynthesis by binding to D-alanyl-D-alanine precursor thereby blocking peptidoglycan polymerization.

ABSORPTION

- **Absorption**: oral vancomycin is not absorbed in the GI tract (therefore should not be given for systemic infections).
- **Metabolism and Excretion**: excreted unchanged in the urine primarily glomerular filtration.
- **Protein Binding**: 50%–60%.
- **Cmax, Cmin, and AUC**: Cmax: 20–50 mcg/mL and Cmin 10 mcg/mL after 1-g IV dose administration.
- $T_{\frac{1}{2}}$: 4–6 hrs.
- **Distribution**: following parenteral administration, widely distributed in body tissue and fluids. Lower tissue concentrations in diabetic patients (3.7 mcg/mL vs 11.9 mcg/mL; P = 0.002). Good level attained in pericardial, pleural, ascitic, and synovial fluid. Low concentration attained in CSF with inflamed meninges (1%–53% of serum concentration attained with high dose with inflamed meninges).

Pregnancy Risk

- Category C: manufacturer has received reports on use of vancomycin in pregnancy without adverse fetal effects.

Breastfeeding Compatibility

- Excreted in breast milk.

DOSING

Dosing for Decreased Hepatic Function

- Usual dose.

Renal Dosing

- Dosing for GFR of >60: 15 mg/kg IV q12 (monitor serum concentrations). Target Cmin: 10–20 mcg/mL.
- Dosing for GFR of 30–59: 15 mg/kg q24h.
- Dosing for GFR of 15–29: 15 mg/kg IV q48h (monitor serum concentrations). Target Cmin: 10–20 mcg/mL.

- Dosing for GFR of <10: 15 mg/kg IV, then redose based on serum concentrations; redose when Cmin <10–20 mcg/mL).
- Dosing in hemodialysis: 15 mg/kg, then redose based on serum concentrations; redose when Cmin <10–20 mcg/mL) IV. Generally twice a wk administration required.
- Dosing in peritoneal dialysis: intraperitoneal 1 g loading dose followed by 30 mg/L dialysate OR intraperitoneal 30 mg/kg once weekly [*Am J Kidney Dis* 1988]. 15 mg/kg IV once to twice per wk (monitor serum concentrations; redose when Cmin <10–20 mcg/mL).
- Dosing in hemofiltration: CVVH: 15 mg/kg q48h; CVVHD: 15 mg/kg IV q24h (monitor serum concentrations; redose when Cmin <10–20 mcg/mL).

COMMENTS

- Vancomycin appropriate in following conditions: (1) treatment of serious infections caused by beta-lactam resistant Gram-positive microorganisms; (2) treatment of infections caused by Gram-positive microorganisms in patients who have serious allergies to beta-lactam antimicrobials; (3) when antibiotic-associated colitis fails to respond to metronidazole therapy or is moderate to severe and potentially life-threatening; (4) prophylaxis, as recommended by American Heart Association, for endocarditis following certain procedures in patients at high risk for endocarditis; (5) prophylaxis for major surgical procedures involving implantation of prosthetic materials or devices (e.g., cardiac and vascular procedures and total hip replacement) at institutions that have high rate of infections caused by MRSA or methicillin-resistant *S. epidermidis*.
- Single dose of vancomycin administered immediately before surgery is sufficient unless procedure lasts >6 hrs, in which case dose should be repeated. Prophylaxis should be discontinued after maximum of 2 doses.

SELECTED REFERENCES

Zar FA, Bakkanagari SR, Moorthi KM, et al. A comparison of vancomycin and metronidazole for the treatment of *Clostridium difficile*-associated diarrhea, stratified by disease severity. *Clin Infect Dis*, 2007; 45: 302.
Comments: Prospective, randomized, double-blind, placebo-controlled trial compared oral vancomycin to oral metronidazole in 172 patients with *C. difficile*-associated diarrhea (CDAD). Patients stratified based on disease severity. Severe CDAD was defined as pseudomembranous colitis or 2 of following: (1) age >60; (2) alb <2.5; (3) WBC> 15K, Temp >38.3. Treatment with metronidazole or vancomycin resulted in clinical cure in 90% and 98% of patients with mild disease, respectively (P = 0.36). However, among patients with severe CDAD, vancomycin was superior to metronidazole with clinical cure in 97% and 76%, respectively (P = 0.02). CDAD relapse rates were similar between metronidazole and vancomycin-treated groups.

Hidayat LK, Hsu DI, Quist R, et al. High-dose vancomycin therapy for methicillin-resistant *Staphylococcus aureus* infections: efficacy and toxicity. *Arch Intern Med*, 2006; 166: 2138–44.
Comments: Use of TDM to guide vancomycin dosing remains controversial. This prospective cohort study of 95 adult patients infected with MRSA was performed to determine if treatment outcomes with vancomycin doses targeting an unbound trough of at least 4 × the MIC (i.e., trough >15 mcg/mL for MRSA with MIC of >2 mcg/mL) results in better outcome. 54% of patients were infected with high-MIC strains (>2 mcg/mL) and 77% had pneumonia and/or bacteremia. Although initial (within 72h) clinical response was significantly better if target trough was achieved, the patients infected with MRSA with a high MIC had lower end-of-treatment responses (24/39 [62%] vs 34/40 [85%]; P = 0.02) and higher infection-related mortality (11/51 [24%] vs 4/44 [10%]; P = 0.16).

Lu SS, Schwartz JM, Simon DM, et al. *Clostridium difficile*-associated diarrhea in patients with HIV positivity and AIDS: a prospective controlled study. *Am J Gastroenterol*, 1994; 89: 1226–9.
Comments: *C. difficile* infection behaves no differently in HIV+ patients compared to control subjects.

Levine DP, Fromm BS, Reddy BR. Slow response to vancomycin or vancomycin plus rifampin in methicillin-resistant *Staphylococcus aureus* endocarditis. *Ann Intern Med*, 1991; 115: 674–80.
Comments: *In vitro* data demonstrated that vancomycin is less bactericidal than nafcillin *in vitro*. This study confirmed this finding with slow clinical response (median duration of bacteremia is 7–9 days) for MRSA endocarditis who are treated with vancomycin or vancomycin + rifampin.

Teasley DG, Gerding DN, Olson MM, et al. Prospective randomised trial of metronidazole versus vancomycin for *Clostridium difficile*-associated diarrhoea and colitis. *Lancet*, 1983; 2: 1043–6.
Comments: Prospectively randomized trial involving 101 patients with *C. difficile* colitis. Metronidazole and vancomycin had equivalent efficacy and relapse rates after 10-day course. This study has been criticized as inconclusive because most patients had mild disease that may have responded to withdrawal of inducing agent. Subsequent comparisons included more seriously ill patients. Oral metronidazole should be 1st-line treatment for mild CDAD. Lack of response should prompt evaluation of adherence and search for alternative Dx or complications such as ileus or toxic megacolon.

DRUGS

VORICONAZOLE

Paul A. Pham, PharmD and John G. Bartlett, MD

INDICATIONS

FDA

- *P. boydii* (*S. apiospermum*) and *Fusarium* spp. (including *F. solani*) infections in persons intolerant of, or refractory to, other therapy.
- Esophageal candidiasis.
- Invasive aspergillosis.
- Treatment of candidemia in nonneutropenic patients.

FORMS TABLE

Brand name (mfr)	Forms†	Cost*
VFEND (Pfizer)	Oral tablet 50 mg; 200 mg IV vial 200 mg/20mL Oral suspension 45 g per bottle (40 mg/mL)	$12.19; $48.76 $143.50 $837.23/45-g bottle

*Prices represent cost per unit specified, are representative of Average Wholesale Price (AWP).
†Dosage is indicated in mg unless otherwise noted.

USUAL ADULT DOSING

- **Invasive aspergillosis:** 6 mg/kg IV q12h × 2 doses (load), then 4 mg/kg IV q12h infused over 1–2 hrs. >40 kg: 200 mg PO twice daily (but should consider 300 mg PO twice daily for severe disease); may be increased to 300 mg PO twice daily. <40 kg: 100 mg PO twice daily; may be increased to 150 mg PO twice daily. Treatment indefinite or until immune reconstitution.
- *Candida* esophagitis (may be active against fluconazole-resistant esophagitis): 200 mg PO twice daily (>40 kg) or 100 mg PO twice daily (<40 kg) × 14 days or 7 days after Sx resolution.
- **Candidemia in nonneutropenic patients:** 6 mg/kg IV q12h × 2 then 3 mg/kg q12h.
- Administer oral doses on empty stomach, avoid high-fat food.
- Monitor serum concentrations (target trough >2.05 mcg/mL) with invasive disease.

ADVERSE DRUG REACTIONS

Common

- Visual disturbances ("abnormal" vision described as blurriness, color changes, and enhanced vision) seen in 21% of patients but less than <1% required discontinuation. Duration of abnormality usually <30 min, typically starting 30 min after dosing.

Occasional

- Increased transaminases (13%) and alkaline phosphatase; d/c required in 4%–8%. Elevation associated with duration of therapy >400 days.
- Rash (6%).
- Hallucination (4.3%).
- Nausea and vomiting.
- Increase in total bilirubin.
- Encephalopathy (associated with trough >5.5 mcg/mL).

DRUG INTERACTIONS

- *In vitro* a substrate of CYP2C19>>CYP2C9 >CYP3A4, and inhibitor of CYP2C19, CYP2C9, and CYP3A4.
- Contraindicated: sirolimus, terfenadine, astemizole, cisapride, pimozide, quinidine, rifabutin, rifampin, carbamazepine, long-acting barbiturates, and ergot alkaloids.

DRUG-DRUG INTERACTIONS—See Appendix I, p. 631, for table of drug-drug interactions.

RESISTANCE

- Isolates with low-level resistance to fluconazole and/or itraconazole exhibit 15% cross-resistance to voriconazole. However, high-level resistance to fluconazole results in 50% cross-resistance to voriconazole.

- No reliable activity against members of the zygomycetes family (e.g., mucor, *Rhizopus*). Not active against zygomycetes. 83% and 60% *in vitro* resistance seen with *Fusaria* and *Rhizopus*, respectively (*J Clin Microbiol* 2003; 41: 3623), but case reports of success reported with *Fusarium* spp.

PHARMACOLOGY

Mechanism

- Voriconazole is a triazole antifungal that inhibits fungal ergosterol biosynthesis.

Pharmacokinetic Parameters

- **Absorption:** 96% (CV 13%) absorbed on an empty stomach (1 hr before or 2 hrs after meals). Absorption independent of gastric pH but reduced by 24% with high-fat meals.
- **Metabolism and Excretion:** metabolized by CYP2C19>>CYP2C9 >CYP3A4 (based on *in vitro* data) to inactive metabolite (N-oxide voriconazole) that is excreted in urine. Less than 2% of unchanged drug excreted in urine.
- **Protein Binding:** 58% (low).
- **Cmax, Cmin, and AUC:** Cmax: 2.51–4.6 mcg/mL.
- **T$_\frac{1}{2}$:** dose dependent terminal half-life.
- **Distribution:** widely distributed with a Vd of 4.6 L/kg. CSF: serum ratio of 0.5:1 (animal data). CNS tissue:serum ratio of 2:1 (animal data).

Pregnancy Risk

- Category D: avoid in pregnancy. No human data, but teratogenic in animal studies.

Breastfeeding Compatibility

- No data. Not recommended.

DOSING

Dosing for Decreased Hepatic Function

- Mild-to-moderate hepatic insufficiency (Child-Pugh Class A and B): 6 mg/kg q12h × 2 doses (load), then 2 mg/kg IV q12h.

Renal Dosing

- Dosing for GFR of 50–80: standard dose.
- Dosing for GFR of 10–50: standard dosing of PO voriconazole. IV voriconazole not recommended due to potential for toxicity of the sulfobutylether-cyclodextrin (SBECD) vehicle.
- Dosing for GFR of <10: standard dosing of oral voriconazole. IV voriconazole not recommended due to potential for toxicity of the sulfobutylether-cyclodextrin (SBECD) vehicle.
- Dosing in hemodialysis: voriconazole is dialyzed. Standard dosing of PO voriconazole (dose after HD). IV voriconazole not recommended.
- Dosing in peritoneal dialysis: no data. Standard PO dose likely. IV voriconazole not recommended.
- Dosing in hemofiltration: CVVHDF: usual dose recommended (*JAC* 2007; 60: 1085–90.)

COMMENTS

- Active against *P. boydii*, *Fusarium* spp., *Candida* spp. (including *C. glabrata* and *C. krusei*) and *Aspergillus* spp. In treatment of aspergillosis, voriconazole resulted in better clinical response at 12 wks compared to amphotericin.
- Generally well tolerated with reversible visual disturbances (blurriness, color changes, and enhanced vision) reported in 20.6% of patients.
- May be considered for the treatment of fluconazole-resistant esophagitis but similar to itraconazole, up to 50% cross-resistance to other azoles has been reported.

SELECTED REFERENCES

Kaplan JE, Benson C, Holmes KH, et al. Guidelines for prevention and treatment of opportunistic infections in HIV-infected adults and adolescents: recommendations from CDC, the National Institutes of Health, and the HIV Medicine Association of the Infectious Diseases Society of America. *MMWR Recomm Rep*, 2009; 58: 1–207.

Comments: Voriconazole, posaconazole, amphotericin, anidulafungin, caspofungin, and micafungin can be considered in flucononazole- and itraconazole-refractory esophageal candidiasis.

Pascual A, Calandra T, Bolay S, et al. Voriconazole therapeutic drug monitoring in patients with invasive mycoses improves efficacy and safety outcomes. *Clin Infect Dis*, 2008; 46: 201–211.

DRUGS

Comments: Retrospective analysis found that lack of response to therapy more frequent in patients with voriconazole concentrations >1 mg/L compared to concentrations <1 mg/L (6 [46%] of 13 patients vs (15 [12%] of 39 patients; P = 0.02). After increasing dose, concentrations of >1 mg/L were reached, with complete resolution of infection in all 6 patients. Voriconazole troughs >5.5 mg/L associated with development of encephalopathy (P = 0.002). Due to high variability of voriconazole serum concentrations, careful assessment of patient's clinical status is critical before voriconazole dose adjustments are made. Prospective trials needed to validate "therapeutic serum concentrations" for voriconazole.

Herbrecht R, Denning DW, Patterson TF, et al. Voriconazole versus amphotericin B for primary therapy of invasive aspergillosis. *N Engl J Med*, 2002; 347: 408–15.

Comments: Satisfactory global response at 12 wks (complete or partial resolution of all attributable signs, symptoms, and radiographic/bronchoscopic abnormalities present at baseline assessed by an independent Data Review Committee) was seen in 53% of voriconazole-treated patients compared to 32% of amphotericin B-treated patients (P <0.0001). Improved survival rate at 12 wks with voriconazole (71%) compared to amphotericin (58%) (HR 0.59; 95% CI, 0.4–0.88).

Ally R, Schürmann D, Kreisel W, et al. A randomized, double-blind, double-dummy, multicenter trial of voriconazole and fluconazole in the treatment of esophageal candidiasis in immunocompromised patients. *Clin Infect Dis*, 2001; 33: 1447–54.

Comments: Randomized, double-blind, multicenter trial showed equivalency between voriconazole and fluconazole for the treatment of esophageal candidiasis. Success rates of 98.3% were seen in the voriconazole group compared to 95.1% seen in the fluconazole group (95% CI -1%, 7.5%). Comments: *in vitro* data suggest that the majority of fluconazole-resistant candida (MIC >8mcg/mL) retains susceptibility to voriconazole (*J Med Microbiol* 2002; 51: 479-83). However, with high level resistance (MIC >32), cross-resistance is reported to be up to 50%.

Antiretrovirals

ABACAVIR

Paul A. Pham, PharmD and John G. Bartlett, MD

INDICATIONS

FDA
- Treatment of HIV infection in combination with other ARVs.

FORMS TABLE

Brand name (mfr)	Forms†	Cost*
Ziagen (ViiV Healthcare by GlaxoSmithKline)	Oral tablet 300 mg Oral suspension 10 mg/mL (240-mL bottle)	$10.26 per tab $161.78 (per 240 mL)
Trizivir (ViiV Healthcare by GlaxoSmithKline)	Oral tablet ABC 300 mg/ AZT 300 mg/3TC 150 mg	$26.81 per tab
Epzicom (ViiV Healthcare by GlaxoSmithKline)	Oral tablet ABC 600 mg + 3TC 300 mg	$35.78 per tab
Kivexa (available in Europe) (Viiv Healthcare by GlaxoSmithKline)	Oral tablet ABC 600 mg + 3TC 300 mg	Variable (not available in US)

*Prices represent cost per unit specified, are representative of Average Wholesale Price (AWP).
†Dosage is indicated in mg unless otherwise noted.

USUAL ADULT DOSING
- Pill burden: 2 pills/day (*Ziagen, Trizivir*) or 1 pill/day (*Epzicom, Kivexa*).
- ABC 300 mg PO twice daily with or without food (as *Ziagen* or *Trizivir*).
- ABC 600 mg PO once daily with or without food (as *Ziagen, Epzicom,* or *Kivexa*).

ADVERSE DRUG REACTIONS

Common
- Nausea, abdominal pain, malaise, and headache reported in approximately 7% of patients in clinical trials (8%–11% when given with AZT).

Occasional
- Hypersensitivity reaction (HSR) noted in ~4% of patients: fever, rash, fatigue, malaise, GI Sx, myalgias, and arthralgias. Over 93% occur within 1st 6 wks of therapy, with median time on onset of 11 days. Requires discontinuation, but can continue ABC with close monitoring until Dx certain or likely (Sx generally worsen with each dose). Do not rechallenge, since anaphylactic-like reaction and death reported. HSR more common in Caucasians and associated with HLA-DR7, HLA-DQ3, and HLA-B*5701 haplotypes. Genetic testing for HLA-B*5701 (cost $70–$80) virtually eliminates risk of HSR, though patients should still be counseled about HSR before initiation. ABC should not be given to patients with positive test.

Rare
- Mitochondrial toxicity: lipoatrophy and lactic acidosis with hepatic steatosis described with NRTI class, although most common with ddI, d4T, ddC, and AZT; unclear whether it occurs at all with ABC, since ABC is one of the least likely NRTIs to cause mitochondrial toxicity *in vitro.*
- Possible increased risk of myocardial infarction (D:A:D Study Group; SMART/INSIGHT Study Group).

DRUGS

DRUG INTERACTIONS
- Not a substrate, inducer, or inhibitor of CYP3A4. No interaction likely with PIs, NNRTIs, MVC, and RAL. ABC metabolized by alcohol dehydrogenase and glucoronyl transferase.

DRUG-DRUG INTERACTIONS — See Appendix I, p. 480, for table of drug-drug interactions.

RESISTANCE
- 74V: intermediate resistance to ABC and ddI. Most common mutation to be selected by ABC/3TC-containing regimens without thymidine analog. M184V further decreases susceptibility.
- 65R: low-level resistance, and intermediate resistance to ddI, TDF, 3TC, FTC. Can be selected by ABC/3TC-containing regimens without thymidine analog, though 74V more common. Intermediate ABC and ddI resistance with 65R + 184V. M184V partially restores TDF susceptibility.
- 184V + >3 TAMs: intermediate-to high-level resistance. Greater ABC resistance with 41L/210W/215Y TAM pathway than with 67N/70R/219 pathway. High-level resistance with >4 TAMs.
- 115F: can be selected by ABC, and causes low-level resistance. Intermediate resistance with 115F + 184V.
- 184V: can cause low-level loss of susceptibility to ABC, but by itself is not associated with clinically relevant resistance.

PHARMACOLOGY
Mechanism
- Intracellular phosphorylation to active carbovir triphosphate, which competitively inhibits HIV DNA polymerase.

Pharmacokinetic Parameters
- **Absorption:** well absorbed with 83% oral bioavailability.
- **Metabolism and Excretion:** 81% metabolized by alcohol dehydrogenase and glucuronyl transferase with renal excretion of metabolites; 16% recovered in stool and 1% unchanged in urine.
- **Protein Binding:** 50%.
- **Cmax, Cmin, and AUC:** mean steady-state Cmax = 3 mcg/mL; AUC = 6 mcg hr/mL. Intracellular levels of carbovir triphosphate 100 FM/million cells.
- **T$_{\frac{1}{2}}$:** serum: 1.5 hrs; intercellular (carbovir triphosphate): 12–20 hrs.

Pregnancy Risk
- Category C: rodent studies demonstrated placental passage. Teratogenic in rodent studies resulting in anasarca, skeletal malformation at 1000 mg/kg dose (35× human therapeutic levels) during organogenesis. However, rabbit studies using 8.5× human therapeutic levels did not result in fetal malformation. No adequate human data, placental passage was 32%–66%.

Breastfeeding Compatibility
- No human data. Breastfeeding is not recommended in the US in order to avoid postnatal transmission of HIV to the child, who may not yet be infected.

DOSING
Dosing for Decreased Hepatic Function
- Usual dose or 200 mg twice daily (limited clinical data).

Renal Dosing
- No dose adjustment for renal impairment.
- Dosing in hemodialysis: usual dose.
- Dosing in peritoneal dialysis: no data. usual dose likely.
- Dosing in hemofiltration: no data. usual dose likely.

COMMENTS
- *Trizivir* (AZT/3TC/ABC) equivalent to unboosted IDV-based ART regimen in patients with baseline VL <100,000, but inferior to EFV-based ART regimens. Since *Trizivir* (without a PI or NNRTI) is inferior to EFV-based regimen, it is recommended by the DHHS Guidelines only as alternative regimen when PI- or NNRTI-based regimens cannot be used (ACTG 5095). Addition of ABC to AZT/3TC/EFV did not improve virologic response in ART-naïve patients. HLA-B*5701 should be ordered in all patients before starting ABC, and ABC should not be given to those who test positive. Recent data suggest decreased virologic response compared to TDF/FTC in patients with baseline VL >100,000, and possible increased risk of MI.

- **Pros:** one of most potent Nrtis, with VL reduction of 1.5–2.0 logs in monotherapy; good data on ABC/3TC as a well-tolerated and effective once-daily dual-NRTI backbone; development of 74V mutation with failure may allow sequencing to TDF, though clinical data lacking; coformulated with 3TC (*Epzicom, Kivexa*) and with AZT/3TC (*Trizivir*); HLA B*5701 prescreening essentially eliminates HSR risks discussed below.
- **Cons:** hypersensitivity reaction; requires pretreatment screening and counseling/education; can be fatal with rechallenge; shorter intracellular half-life than TDF, and no susceptibility benefit with M184V. Less long-term data than with TDF. Inferior compared to TDF in patients with baseline VL >100,000 c/mL (ACTG 5202). Increased risk of cardiovascular disease in some observational studies (D:A:D and SMART Study Groups) but not on others or in clinical trials.

REFERENCES

Sax PE, Tierney C, Collier AC, et al. Abacavir-lamivudine versus tenofovir-emtricitabine for initial HIV-1 therapy. *N Engl J Med*, 2009; 361: 2230.

Comments: Randomized controlled trial compared TDF/FTC and ABC/3TC in combination with EFV or boosted ATV. At a median follow-up of 60 wks, among patients with VL >100,000 c/mL, the time to virologic failure was significantly shorter in the ABC/3TC group than in the TDF/FTC group (HR, 2.33; 95% CI, 1.46–3.72; P <0.001), 57 virologic failures (14%) were observed in the ABC/3TC group vs 26 (7%) in the TDF/FTC group. In patients with VL <100,000 c/mL, there was no significant difference in time to virological failure between groups.

D:A:D Study Group, Sabin CA, Worm SW, et al. Use of nucleoside reverse transcriptase inhibitors and risk of myocardial infarction in HIV-infected patients enrolled in the D:A:D study: a multi-cohort collaboration. *Lancet*, 2008; 371: 1417–26.

Comments: A retrospective review of D:A:D observational cohort for cardiovascular disease risks associated with NRTI use included 33,347 patients (157,912 patient of follow-up). There were 517 MIs, including 192 in patients receiving ABC-containing regimens. After adjusting for confounding risk factors, relative risk for ABC use within last 6 mos was 1.9 (95% CI 1.5–2.5). There was also increased risk associated with ddI treatment, but not d4T or AZT. Greatest risk (and greatest increased risk) in patients with risk factors for cardiovascular disease. Pathophysiologic mechanism of this effect, if real, has not been identified. Other studies have not shown this risk, but they may have been underpowered to show a risk of an infrequent toxicity. However, the usual caveats with observational studies apply.

SMART/INSIGHT and D:A:D Study Groups. Use of nucleoside reverse transcriptase inhibitors and risk of myocardial infarction in HIV-infected patients. *AIDS*, 2008; 22: F17–24.

Comments: Retrospective review of 2752 patients enrolled in continuous treatment arm of SMART evaluated cardiovascular (CV) disease risks associated with NRTI components of ARV regimens. CV risk factors comparable between groups: median age of 40, 73% males, 39% smokers, 7% with diabetes, and 4% with prior CV disease. Use of ABC associated with increased risk of MI (AHR = 4.3), CV-related death (AHR = 1.8), with signficantly increased risk seen in those with 5 or more CV risk factors.

Gulick RM, Ribaudo HJ, Shikuma CM, et al. Three- vs four-drug antiretroviral regimens for the initial treatment of HIV-1 infection: a randomized controlled trial. *JAMA*, 2006; 296: 769–81.

Comments: Continuation of ACTG 5095 compared AZT/3TC/EFV to AZT/ABC/3TC/EFV in ART-naïve patients. No significant differences between 3- vs 4-drug regimens; approximately 80% of patients had VL <50 through 3 yrs. 10% treated with AZT/3TC/ABC/EFV had ABC HSR, vs 7% on AZT/3TC/EFV.

Gallant JE, Rodriguez AE, Weinberg WG, et al. Early virologic nonresponse to tenofovir, abacavir, and lamivudine in HIV-infected antiretroviral-naive subjects. *J Infect Dis*, 2005; 192: 1921–30.

Comments: High rate of virologic failure in the TDF + ABC + 3TC arm, with 49% experiencing virologic failure compared to 5.4% of patients taking EFV. Among TDF-treated patients for whom virologic data are available, 64% had both the K65R and M184V mutations and 36% had M184V alone. TDF/ABC/3TC is not recommended as a triple-NRTI regimen, and data minimal for use with a 4th agent.

Moyle GJ, DeJesus E, Cahn P, et al. Abacavir once or twice daily combined with once-daily lamivudine and efavirenz for the treatment of antiretroviral-naive HIV-infected adults: results of the Ziagen Once Daily in Antiretroviral Combination Study. *J Acquir Immune Defic Syndr*, 2005; 38: 417–25.

Comments: EFV + once- or twice-daily ABC as part of an ABC/3TC backbone were equivalent, with 66% and 68% of patients achieving VL <50, respectively.

Gulick RM, Ribaudo HJ, Shikuma CM, et al. Triple-nucleoside regimens versus efavirenz-containing regimens for the initial treatment of HIV-1 infection. *N Engl J Med*, 2004; 350: 1850–61.

Comments: Compared triple-NRTI regimen of AZT/3TC/ABC with 2 EFV-containing regimens, AZT/3TC + EFV and AZT/3TC/ABC + EFV. Triple-NRTI arm was stopped early because of higher rate of virologic failure vs EFV-based regimens (21% vs 10%, P <0.001). Triple NRTI regimens should only be used as alternative in patients who cannot take PI or NNRTI-based regimens.

DeJesus E, Herrera G, Teofilo E, et al. Abacavir versus zidovudine combined with lamivudine and efavirenz, for the treatment of antiretroviral-naive HIV-infected adults. *Clin Infect Dis*, 2004; 39: 1038–46.

Comments: ABC/3TC + EFV was noninferior to AZT/3TC + EFV in a randomized, double-blind study involving 649 naïve patients. Response rate (<50) through wk 48 was 70% and 69% in ABC and AZT group, respectively. Patients on ABC/3TC had less nausea, vomiting, fatigue, and anemia than patients taking AZT, but more HSR. ABC/3TC associated with greater increase in CD4 (209 vs 155) and CD4%.

Mallal S, Nolan D, Witt C, et al. Association between presence of HLA-B*5701, HLA-DR7, and HLA-DQ3 and hypersensitivity to HIV-1 reverse-transcriptase inhibitor abacavir. *Lancet*, 2002; 359: 727–32.

Comments: This study found an extraordinary association between presence of HLA-B*5701, HLA-DR7, and HLA-DQ3 alleles and HSR to ABC (OR 822 [43–15675], P <0.0001). Authors concluded that if ABC was withheld in presence of these alleles, prevalence of HSR would decrease from 9.5% to 2.5%. Positive predictive value for HSR 100%, negative predictive value 97%.

Staszewski S, Keiser P, Montaner J, et al. Abacavir-lamivudine-zidovudine vs indinavir-lamivudine-zidovudine in antiretroviral-naive HIV-infected adults: a randomized equivalence trial. *JAMA*, 2001; 285: 1155–63.

Comments: AZT/3TC + ABC was equivalent to AZT/3TC + unboosted IDV, with 51% in both group achieving VL <400 at 48 wks. Trend favoring IDV-based regimen in patients with baseline VL >100,000, with 45% vs 31% achieving <50 (a treatment difference −14% [95% CI, −27%–0%]). Although this trial demonstrated equivalency at <400 endpoint, the decreased potency at high VL suggests lower potency overall.

Mallal S, Phillips E, Carosi G, et al. HLA-B*5701 screening for hypersensitivity to abacavir. *N Engl J Med*, 2008: 358: 568–79.

Comments: Study randomized 1956 ABC-naïve patients to standard of care or screening with HLA-B*5701 test before starting ABC. Incidence of both clinically diagnosed and immunologically confirmed HSR significantly lower in screening arm vs control arm. No cases of immunologically confirmed HSR observed in prospective screening arm. HLA-B*5701 had a 100% sensitivity.

ATAZANAVIR

Paul A. Pham, PharmD and John G. Bartlett, MD

INDICATIONS
FDA
• Treatment of HIV infection in combination with other ARVs.

FORMS TABLE

Brand name (mfr)	Forms†	Cost*
Reyataz (Bristol-Myers Squibb)	Oral capsule 100 mg; 150 mg; 200 mg; 300 mg	$18.12 per 100 mg, 150 mg, or 200 mg cap; $35.91 per 300 mg

*Prices represent cost per unit specified, are representative of Average Wholesale Price (AWP).
†Dosage is indicated in mg unless otherwise noted.

USUAL ADULT DOSING
• Pill burden: 2/day (ATV 400 mg once daily or ATV 300 mg + RTV 100 mg once daily).
• ATV 400 mg once daily w/ food (FDA approved dose for treatment-naïve patients; consider ATV/r 300/100 mg daily due to superior PK). ATV 400 mg daily (without RTV) not recommended with TDF, EFV, ddI, NVP, and ETR coadministration.
• ATV 300 mg + RTV 100 mg once daily w/ food (FDA approved dose for treatment-experienced patients, but preferred dose for treatment-naïve patients also).
• With EFV: ATV 400 mg + RTV 100 mg once daily + EFV 600 mg at bedtime (consider TDM; coadministration not recommended in patients w/ PI resistance).
• With TDF: ATV 300 mg + RTV 100 mg once daily + TDF 300 mg daily.
• With SQV: ATV 400 mg + SQV 1200 mg once daily (did not perform well in trials) or consider ATV 300 mg + RTV 100 mg + SQV 1500–2000 mg daily (limited data).
• With LPV/r: ATV 300 mg once daily + LPV/r 400/100 mg twice daily.

- With FPV: insufficient data; avoid or consider TDM (studied regimen FPV 1400 mg once daily + ATV 400 mg once daily).
- No dosing recommendation with coadministration of other PIs (IDV, NFV) or DLV.
- With NVP: avoid coadministration.
- With TPV: ATV may be significantly decreased. Avoid coadministration.
- With ETR: coadministration not recommended by manufacturer, but clinical significance unclear. Consider ATV/r 300/100 mg once daily + ETR 200 mg twice daily with TDM.
- With RAL: ATV 300 mg + RTV 100 mg once daily + RAL 400 mg twice daily.
- With MVC: ATV 300 mg + RTV 100 mg once daily + MVC 150 mg twice daily In PI-naïve patients, unboosted ATV can also be considered with MVC.
- With DRV: ATV 300 mg once daily + DRV/r 600/100 mg twice daily.
- With ddI + either FTC or 3TC: avoid with unboosted ATV (poor clinical response).
- Dose in pregnancy: ATV 300 mg + RTV 100 mg once daily (resulted in comparable PK parameters in 3rd trimester).

ADVERSE DRUG REACTIONS
Common
- Reversible indirect hyperbilirubinemia, with Grade 3–4 ($>2.6 \times$ UNL) occurring in 35%–47% of patients. Clinically benign: does not indicate liver disease and does not require discontinuation. Trough >0.85 mcg/mL associated higher incidence of hyperbilirubinemia.

Occasional
- Jaundice with scleral icterus in up to 7%–8% of patients. In comparison of ATV vs ATV/r, Grade 2–4 jaundice seen in $<1\%$ on ATV, 3% on ATV/r. Reversible with discontinuation.
- Nausea, vomiting, abdominal pain less common than with LPV/r.
- Rash, headache, mild transaminase elevation (unrelated to phase II conjugation UGT1A1 inhibition).
- Diabetes, hyperlipidemia: minimal or no effect on lipid profile or insulin resistance. Lipids slightly higher with RTV boosting.
- Lipodystrophy listed, but unboosted ATV may unlikely to cause fat accumulation.

Rare
- Dose-dependent QTc and PR interval prolongation. Use with caution in patients with baseline altered cardiac conduction and with drugs that can alter cardiac conduction (i.e., diltiazem and clarithromycin; see Drug-Drug Interactions in Appendix I on p. 480 for dosing recommendation).
- Studies with ATV/r 300/100 mg once daily showed slight but not significant increases in PR interval averaging 3 msec and no change at 1 mo. 2nd- and 3rd-degree AV block and left bundle branch block have been reported.
- Nephrolithiasis secondary to precipitation of ATV (30 cases reported to FDA from Dec 2002–Jan 2007).
- Interstitial nephritis (1 case report).
- Cholestasis, cholelithiasis, and cholecystitis.
- Hepatitis.
- Severe rash (Stevens-Johnson syndrome, erythema multiforme, and toxic skin eruptions have been reported).

DRUG INTERACTIONS
- Substrate and inhibitor of CYP3A4. Weak inhibitor of CYP1A2 and CYP2C9 *in vitro* but clinical significance unknown. Inhibitor of phase II conjugation (UGT1A1). CYP3A4 inhibitors may increase ATV levels. CYP3A4 inducers may decrease ATV levels. ATV may increase levels of CYP3A4 substrates. NRTI levels generally not affected by ATV.

DRUG-DRUG INTERACTIONS—See Appendix I, p. 480, for table of drug-drug interactions.
RESISTANCE
- I50L: unique primary ATV mutation, selected by unboosted ATV. Results in intermediate resistance to ATV but susceptibility (or hypersusceptibility) to other PIs. Typically followed by A71V (in 40% of patients). Limited data suggest that PI resistance less common with failure of ATV/r as initial PI.
- L10Y/F, I50L, L63P, A71V, N88S, V32I, M46I, I84V, and L89M: 4-5 of the following mutations resulted in >90-fold resistance to ATV *in vitro*.

DRUGS

- PI mutations (L33F, 82A/F/T/S, 84V/A/C, 90M, 46I/L) and (L10I/F/V, K20R/M/I, L24I, V32I, M36I/L/V, I50L, I54V, L63P, A71V, G73C/S/T/A) >4 mutations: decreased potency of ATV (post-hoc analysis of 045 study).
- ATV mutation score: 10F/I/V, 16E, 33F/I/V, 46I/L, 60E, I84V, 85V, and 90M. Response: 0–1 mutation = 100%; 2 mutation = 80%; 3 mutations = 42%; 4 mutations = 0%.

PHARMACOLOGY

Mechanism

- Inhibition of HIV protease, which results in nonfunctional, immature and noninfectious virions.

Pharmacokinetic Parameters

- **Absorption:** well absorbed with food.
- **Metabolism and Excretion:** CYP3A4 substrate and inhibitor. Metabolized to 2 inactive metabolites and excreted primarily via biliary excretion. 13% of ATV and/or its metabolites are excreted in the urine.
- **Protein Binding:** 86%.
- **Cmax, Cmin, and AUC:** mean Cmax = 3.152 mcg/mL; Cmin = 0.273 mcg/mL; AUC = 22.3 mcg hr/mL (ATV 400 mg once daily at steady state). Cmin 0.15–0.85 mcg/mL associated with good response.
- **$T_{\frac{1}{2}}$:** 6.5 hrs.
- **Distribution:** highly variable and poor CNS penetration. Poor seminal fluid penetration.

Pregnancy Risk

- Category B: no human data. In animal studies, ATV did not result in embryonic or fetal toxicity when given maternally toxic doses. AUC reduced but trough levels adequate in 3rd trimester of pregnancy with ATV/r 300/100 mg once daily, but inadequate data to recommend routine use of ATV in pregnancy.

Breastfeeding Compatibility

- No data.

DOSING

Dosing for Decreased Hepatic Function

- ATV AUC increased by 45% with mild-to-moderate hepatic insufficiency. Consider decreasing dose to ATV to 300 mg daily, but no clinical data.

Renal dosing

- Dosing for GFR of <80: no data. Usual dose likely.
- Dosing in hemodialysis: serum concentrations may be lower in HD patients. Unboosted ATV should be avoided; use ATV/r 300/100 mg once daily. Consider TDM.
- Dosing in peritoneal dialysis: no data. Unboosted ATV should be avoided; use ATV/r 300/100 mg once daily. Consider TDM.
- Dosing in hemofiltration: no data. Unboosted ATV should be avoided; use ATV/r 300/100 mg once daily. Consider TDM.

COMMENTS

- **Pros:** excellent potency, especially when boosted with RTV; lowest pill burden among PIs; once-daily regimen; minimal effect on lipids; good GI tolerability; less likely to cause insulin resistance and possibly fat accumulation than some other PIs (especially those using 200 mg/day of RTV); resistance profile favorable with failure of unboosted ATV in PI-naïve patients, and PI resistance uncommon with failure of ATV/r. ATV/r comparable to LPV/r in PI-experienced patients at 96 wks. Noninferior to LPV/r in treatment-naïve patients with less GI side effects and less triglyceride elevation. The only boosted PI to show noninferiority to EFV (ACTG 5202), with less resistance with failure and more favorable lipid effects. Best PI option when RTV boosting not possible (combined with ABC/3TC or AZT/3TC but not TDF/FTC).
- **Cons:** jaundice or scleral icterus may be problematic for some patients; drug interactions with PPIs, H2 blocker, and antacids (not recommended with PPIs); food requirement. RTV-boosting improves potency, but with slight increase in lipids and jaundice vs unboosted ATV. Not recommended for use in combination with NVP.

SELECTED REFERENCES

Daar ES, Tierney C, Fischl MA, et al. Atazanavir plus ritonavir or efavirenz as part of a 3-drug regimen for initial treatment of HIV-1. *Ann Intern Med*, 2011; 154: 445–56.

Comments: ACTG 5202 randomized ARV-naïve patients to ATV/r (N = 463) or EFV (N = 465), both with ABC/3TC or TDF/FTC. At 96 wks, virologic response rates were similar between ATV/r and EFV treated patients.

Malan N, Krantz E, David N, et al. 96-week efficacy and safety of atazanavir, with and without ritonavir, in a ART regimen in treatment-naive patients. *J Int Assoc Physicians AIDS Care*, 2010; 9: 34–42.

Comments: 200 ARV-naïve patients randomized to ATV/r 300/100 mg (N = 95) or ATV 400 mg (N = 105), both in combination with 3TC and d4T XR, all daily. At 96 wks, response rates comparable between ATV/r and ATV (75% and 70% had VL <50 by ITT analysis, respectively). However, study not powered to determine noninferiority of ATV vs ATV/r, and there were numerically more virologic failures in ATV arm, with more apparent PI and NRTI resistance. Jaundice more common in ATV/r arm, and lipids somewhat higher, though few patients required lipid-lowering therapy.

Squires K, Young B, DeJesus E, et al. Similar efficacy and tolerability of atazanavir compared to atazanavir/ritonavir, each in combination with abacavir/lamivudine (ABC/3TC), after initial suppression with ABC/3TC + ATV/r in HIV-1 infected patients: 84 week results of the ARIES trial. Abstract WELBB103. Presented at: 5th International Aids Society (IAS) Conference on HIV Pathogenesis, Treatment, and Prevention; July 19–22, 2009: Cape Town.

Comments: ARIES randomized 419 treatment-naïve patients whose VL <50 after 36 wks of ATV/r + ABC/3TC to either continue ATV/r or switch to unboosted ATV + ABC/3TC. At 84 wks, 86% taking ATV had VL <50 vs 81% of of those on ATV/r (ITT, P = 0.14). Virologic suppression also comparable between ATV/r and ATV in patients with baseline VL >100,000. Hyperbilirubinemia, cholesterol, and TG elevation lower in patients who switched to ATV.

Molina J, Andrade-Villanueva J, Echevarria J et al. Once-daily atazanavir/ritonavir compared with twice-daily lopinavir/ritonavir, each in combination with tenofovir and emtricitabine, for management of antiretroviral-naive HIV-1-infected patients: 96-week efficacy and safety results of the CASTLE study. *J Acquir Immune Defic Syndr*, 2010; 53(3): 323–32.

Comments: CASTLE compared ATV/r 300/100 mg daily vs LPV/r 400/100 mg (caps) twice daily, both combined with TDF/FTC in 883 treatment-naïve patients. 96-wk results showed comparable rates of VL suppression (74% for ATV/r vs 68% for LPV/r <50 c/mL). On both regimens, 7% were virologic failures by 96 wks. Response rates comparable with VL >100K; however, lower rate of virologic suppression in LPV/r-treated patients with lower baseline CD4 count (80% with CD4 >200 vs 63% with CD4 <50; P = 0.0085). Fasting cholesterol, triglycerides, and GI intolerance higher in LPV/r-treated group (P <0.0001).

Johnson M, Grinsztejn B, Rodriguez C, et al. Atazanavir plus ritonavir or saquinavir, and lopinavir/ritonavir in patients experiencing multiple virological failures. *AIDS*, 2005; 19: 685–94.

Comments: 358 patients who had failed at least 2 ART regimens containing at least 1 PI, NNRTI, and NRTI randomized to ATV/RTV 300/100 mg once daily, ATV/SQV 400/1200 mg once daily, or LPV/r 400/100 mg twice daily each combined with TDF + 1 NRTI. At 48 wks, 58% vs 56% achieved VL <400 in LPV/r and ATV/RTV arm, respectively. Trend favoring LPV/r, with 46% vs 38% achieving VL endpoint of <50, but not statistically significant. ATV/SQV arm did not perform as well as other 2 groups. Note that not all patients in this trial were heavily PI-experienced. Only 33% of the ATV/RTV arm and 37% of the LPV/r arm had >4 PI mutations (10, 20, 24, 32, 33, 36, 46, 50, 54, 63, 71, 73, 82, 84, 90). In a post-hoc analysis of these patients with >4 PI mutations at baseline, LPV/r regimen demonstrated greater decline in VL compared to the ATV/RTV arm (1.47 log and 1.38, respectively). The limitation of this genotypic analysis is that the percent of critical PI mutation (i.e., 32, 33, 54, 82, 84, and 90) in each group is not known. In addition, only 1/3 of patients were on a PI-containing regimen at the time of the genotype analysis. The post-hoc analysis of the more heavily PI-experienced patients was under powered to show difference between 2 groups. For the mean time it is safe to say that boosted-ATV is noninferior to LPV/r in moderately PI-experienced patients, and these data can probably be extrapolated to PI-naïve patients as well.

Cohen C, Nieto-Cisneros L, Zala C, et al. Comparison of atazanavir with lopinavir/ritonavir in patients with prior protease inhibitor failure: a randomized multinational trial. *Curr Med Res Opin*, 2005; 21: 1683–92.

Comments: Phase III trial that compared ATV (400 mg once daily) with LPV/r (400/100 mg twice daily), each in combination with 2 NRTIs, in 300 treatment-experienced patients with virologic failure following a single PI-based regimen. At 24 wks LPV/r showed a better virologic response: 75% vs 54% with VL <400 and 50% vs 34% with VL <50. Unboosted ATV is inferior to LPV/r and should not be used in PI-experienced patients.

DARUNAVIR

Paul A. Pham, PharmD and John G. Bartlett, MD

INDICATIONS
FDA
- Treatment of HIV-infected patients who are treatment-experienced and have virus resistant to >1 PI, in combination with other antiretrovirals (DRV/r 600/100 mg twice daily).

- Treatment of HIV-infected patients who are treatment-naïve or treatment experienced without DRV resistance (DRV/r 800/100 mg once daily).
- Treatment of HIV-1 infection in pediatric patient ≥3 yrs.

FORMS TABLE

Brand name (mfr)	Forms†	Cost*
Prezista (Janssen Therapeutics)	Oral tablet 75 mg; 150 mg; 400 mg; 600 mg	$2.30; $4.59; $18.37; $18.37

*Prices represent cost per unit specified, are representative of Average Wholesale Price (AWP).
†Dosage is indicated in mg unless otherwise noted.

USUAL ADULT DOSING

- Pill burden: 3/day (two 400-mg tabs + 1 RTV 100-mg tab) or 4/day (two 600-mg tabs + 2 RTV 100-mg tabs).
- In ART-naïve patients or ART-experienced patients with no DRV mutations (V11I, V32I, L33F, I47V, I50V, I54L, I54M, T74P, L76V, I84V, and L89V): DRV 800 mg (two 400-mg tabs or 8 ml suspension) + RTV 100 mg once daily with food.
- In treatment-experienced patients with >1 DRV mutation (V11I, V32I, L33F, I47V, I50V, I54L, I54M, T74P, L76V, I84V, and L89V): DRV 600 mg (one 600-mg tab) + RTV 100 mg twice daily with food.
- With ATV: standard dose DRV/r + ATV 300 mg once daily.
- With NVP: standard dose of both drugs (limited data).
- Not recommended with LPV/r and SQV.
- With IDV: dose not established.
- No data with FPV, TPV, and NFV; avoid coadministration.
- With ENF: standard dose of both drugs.
- With ETR: standard dose ETR + DRV/r 600/100 mg twice daily.
- With MVC: standard dose DRV/r + MVC 150 mg twice daily.
- With RAL: standard dose of both drugs.
- With EFV: dose not established; consider DRV/r 800–900 mg/100 mg once daily (PI-naïve patients) or DRV/r 600/100 mg twice daily in (PI-experienced patients).

ADVERSE DRUG REACTIONS

General

- Adverse reactions comparable to comparator PIs in POWER studies. Discontinuation due to AEs: 9% and 5% in the DRV/r and comparator PI arms, respectively.

Common

- GI intolerance (nausea, vomiting, and/or diarrhea) in 20%. Moderate-to-severe diarrhea less common than with LPV/r.
- Headache in 15%.

Occasional

- Contains sulfonamide moiety and should be used with caution in patients with severe sulfa allergy.
- Rash observed in 7% of patients with 0.3% discontinuation rate.
- Lipodystrophy.
- Insulin resistance and hyperglycemia.
- Hyperlipidemia.
- Transaminase elevation.

Rare

- Severe rash.
- Severe hepatitis (reported in 0.5%).

DRUG INTERACTIONS

- Substrate and inhibitor of CYP3A4. With RTV coadministration, net effect of DRV/r on CYP3A4 is generally inhibitory. CYP3A4 inhibitors and inducers may increase or decrease DRV serum concentrations, respectively.

RESISTANCE
- Baseline phenotypic DRV fold-change (FC) was strongest predictor of virologic response in POWER studies. At wk 24, 50%, 25%, and 13% of patients with FC <10, 10–40, and >40 achieved VL <50, respectively. FCs of <10, 10–40, and >40 were associated with <10, 10 or 11, and >12 IAS PI mutations. The following mutations were more predictive of virologic outcome than IAS PI mutations: 11I, 32I, 33F, 47V, 50V, 54L/M, 73S, 76V, 84V, and 89V (XV International HIV Drug Resistance Workshop, 2006, Abstract 73). With 0–2, 3, or >4 of these mutations at baseline, the virologic response (VL <50 c/mL at wk 24) was 50%, 22%, and 10% respectively.
- In vitro, pathway to DRV resistance is different from other PIs. Among mutations emerging during virologic failure (patients with virologic rebound or never suppressed) in POWER studies, most common substitutions occurred at position V32 (30% of isolates), I54 (20% isolates), and I15, L33, I47, G73, and L89 (10–20% of isolates). In these isolates, median DRV phenotypic FC increased from 21-fold at baseline to 94-fold at failure.
- In vitro, 77% and 70% of clinical isolates (n = 2682) that have decreased susceptibility to LPV and TPV, respectively, were susceptible (FC<10) to DRV (XV International HIV Drug Resistance Workshop, 2006, Abstract 73). Using Virco's lower DRV FC cutoff of 3.4, other investigators reported higher cross-resistance rates. Analyses of >50,000 isolates found that only 42% and 28% of isolates with resistance to LPV and TPV will have predicted response to DRV (XV International HIV Drug Resistance Workshop, 2006, Abstract 28). However, clinical isolates (n = 586) with decreased susceptibility to DRV retained susceptibility to LPV and TPVin only 0.5% and 53% of cases, respectively (XV International HIV Drug Resistance Workshop, 2006, Abstract 73).
- Current fold-change cut offs for DRV susceptibility: Monogram PhenoSense lower clinical cut off (LCCO) 10, upper CCO 90; Virco Antivirogram LCCO 10, UCCO 40; Virco VircoTYPE LCCO 10, UCCO 106.9.

PHARMACOLOGY
Mechanism
- HIV-protease inhibitor.

Pharmacokinetic Parameters
- **Absorption:** with RTV coadministration, DRV is well absorbed with an absolute bioavailability of 82%. Food (a light snack or a full meal) increases DRV AUC by 30%.
- **Metabolism and Excretion:** DRV undergoes extensive oxidative metabolism via CYP3A4 to weakly active oxidative.
- **Protein Binding:** 95%.
- **Cmax, Cmin, and AUC:** at steady state, the geometric mean DRV AUC and Cmin was 62.35 mcg/mL/hr and 3.54 mcg/mL, respectively. DRV trough was 6-fold higher than the EC50 for resistant virus and 18-fold higher than the EC90 for wild type virus.
- **T$\frac{1}{2}$:** 15 hours.
- **Distribution:** CNS penetration: 13%. Free DRV concentration of 542 ng/mL is ~20-fold above IC of wild-type virus.

Pregnancy Risk
- Category C: no human data. DRV has shown no embryotoxicity or teratogenicity in mice, rats, and rabbits. Based on animal studies, serum concentrations may be significantly decreased in pregnancy. Inadequate data to recommend in pregnancy.

Breastfeeding Compatibility
- No data. Not recommended.

DOSING
Dosing for Decreased Hepatic Function
- Avoid or use with caution. Severe hepatitis reported in 0.5% of patients treated with DRV/r.
Renal Dosing
- Dosing for GFR of 10–80: usual dose.
- Dosing for GFR of <10: consider usual dose (limited data).
- Dosing in hemodialysis: consider usual dose (limited data).

DRUGS

- Dosing in peritoneal dialysis: consider usual dose (limited data).
- Dosing in hemofiltration: consider usual dose (no data).

COMMENTS

- **Pros:** effective in highly treatment-experienced patients with better safety profile than TPV/r. Superior to LPV/r in LPV/r-naïve, treatment-experienced patients (noninferior in those with baseline LPV susceptibility, but trend toward better outcome with DRV/r, and less virologic failure and emergence of new mutations). Once-daily DRV/r superior to LPV/r in treatment-naïve patients with baseline VL >100,000, with more favorable GI tolerability and lipid effects.
- **Cons:** PI-class adverse effects. Greater potential for rash than with most other PIs. Severe hepatitis reported; as with other PIs, greatest risk in patients with chronic HBV or HCV infection.

SELECTED REFERENCES

Mills AM, Nelson M, Jayaweera D, et al. Once-daily darunavir/ritonavir vs. lopinavir/ritonavir in treatment-naive, HIV-1-infected patients: 96-week analysis. *AIDS*, 2009; 23: 1679–88.

Comments: ARTEMIS evaluated DRV/r (800/100 mg once daily) vs LPV/r (once or twice daily, but majority received twice-daily dosing) both combined with TDF/FTC in treatment-naïve patients. Characteristics of patients (N = 689) comparable at baseline with a median VL of approximately 70,000 and CD4 220. At wk 96 (per protocol), 79% of DRV/r-treated patients and 71% of LPV/r-treated patients achieved VL <50, difference was 8.4% (P <0.001). DRV/r met noninferiority (per protocol) and superiority (P = 0.012; ITT). In patients with baseline VL >100,000, DRV/r was superior (79% vs 67%; P <0.05), which was subsequently attributed to use of once-daily LPV/r. Median CD4 increase comparable between 2 groups (171 for DRV/r and 188 for LPV/r). Grade 2–4 GI intolerance significantly higher in the LPV/r-treated patients (11% vs 4%) whereas Grade 2–4 treatment-related rash occurred in 3% in DRV/r vs 1% in LPV/r-treated patients.

Madruga JV, Berger D, McMurchie M, et al. Efficacy and safety of darunavir-ritonavir compared with that of lopinavir-ritonavir at 48 weeks in treatment-experienced, HIV-infected patients in TITAN: a randomised controlled phase III trial. *Lancet*, 2007; 370: 49–58.

Comments: TITAN trial evaluated DRV/r (600/100 mg twice daily) vs LPV/r (400/100 mg twice daily) both with OBT in patients who had failed prior therapy and were naïve to LPV/r. Baseline patients characteristic (N = 595) comparable between 2 groups: median VL 4.31 log, CD4 232, 31% were PI-naïve; 82% were susceptible to 4 or more PIs. At wk 48, significantly more DRV/r- than LPV/r-treated patients had VL <400 (77% vs 68%; estimated difference 9%, 95% CI 2–16) and within 12% margin of noninferiority.

Clotet B, Bellos N, Molina JM, et al. Efficacy and safety of darunavir-ritonavir at week 48 in treatment-experienced patients with HIV-1 infection in POWER 1 and 2: a pooled subgroup analysis of data from two randomised trials. *Lancet*, 2007; 369: 1169–78.

Comments: POWER 1 and 2 demonstrated high rates of virologic suppression in highly treatment-experienced patients treated with DRV/r. All were 3-class (NRTI, NNRTI, PI) experienced and had >1 primary PI mutation at screening. Baseline characteristics (N = 131) of patients on DRV/r + OBR were: VL = 4.52 log, CD4 153, 8 IAS PI mutations associated with resistance (>3 primary mutations in 54%), and phenotypic resistance to all approved PIs (with exception of TPV/r due to availability) in 64% of patients. After initial dose-finding phase, patients randomized to receive an OBR (>2 NRTIs ± ENF with DRV/r 600/100 mg twice daily OR investigator choice of PIs, including boosted or dual-boosted PIs (control group). Primary efficacy endpoint defined as decrease in VL >1 log vs baseline. By ITT analysis, 61% of DRV/r-treated patients and 15% of control patients achieved >1 log reduction in VL though wk 48. VL<50 achieved in 45% and 10% of DRV/r and control patients, respectively (P <0.0001). Mean CD4 increase was 102 and 19 in DRV/r-treated patients and control patients, respectively. Adverse drug reactions were comparable between the two groups.

DELAVIRDINE

Paul A. Pham, PharmD and John G. Bartlett, MD

INDICATIONS

FDA

- Treatment of HIV infection in combination with other antiretroviral agents.

Brand name (mfr)	Forms†	Cost*
Rescriptor (ViiV Healthcare)	Oral tablet 100 mg; 200 mg	$0.88; $1.75

*Prices represent cost per unit specified, are representative of Average Wholesale Price (AWP).
†Dosage is indicated in mg unless otherwise noted.

USUAL ADULT DOSING
- Pill burden: 6 tabs/day (200-mg tabs).
- 400 mg PO 3 ×/day with or without food (100-mg tab should be dispersed in at least 3 oz of water before administration; 200-mg tab is taken intact).
- With IDV: DLV 400 mg 3 ×/day + IDV 600 mg q8h (GI intolerance and high pill burden).
- With SQV: high rates of GI intolerance and high pill burden. No data with SQV hgc *Invirase*; avoid use.
- Not recommended with NFV, APV, and FPV.
- No data with DRV/r, TPV/r, LPV/r, and ATV. Avoid use.
- With MVC: DLV 400 mg 3 ×/day + MVC 150 mg twice daily. (No clinical data; avoid use.).
- With EFV, NVP, and ETR: avoid coadministration.

ADVERSE DRUG REACTIONS
Common
- Rash in 18%; usually lasts 2 wks and does not require discontinuation unless desquamation or mucous membrane involvement; approximately 4% discontinue due to rash. High rates (70%) of cross-allergy between DLV and NVP (*Ann Pharmacother* 2000; 34: 940).
- Headache and fatigue (11%–17%).
Occasional
- Transaminase elevation in 2%–5% of patients (less common and severe than with NVP).
- Nausea, vomiting, diarrhea, dyspepsia, and abdominal pain.
Rare
- Erythema multiforme or Stevens-Johnson syndrome.
- Proteinuria.

DRUG INTERACTIONS
- CYP3A4 substrate and inhibitor. DLV may increase serum levels of other CYP3A4 substrates.

DRUG-DRUG INTERACTIONS — See Appendix I, p. 501, for table of drug-drug interactions
RESISTANCE
- K103N; Y181C, V106M; 188L, P236L: high-level resistance.
- G190A, G190S, P225H, F227L: sensitive or even hypersusceptible (but no clinical data).

PHARMACOLOGY
Mechanism
- Noncompetitive inhibition of HIV DNA polymerase resulting in disruption of catalytic site of the enzyme.
Pharmacokinetic Parameters
- **Absorption:** bioavailability 85%. Absorption highly dependent on gastric acidity.
- **Metabolism and Excretion:** metabolized by CYP3A4 to several hydroxylated metabolites, which undergo subsequent glucuronidation. Both unchanged drug and metabolites are excreted in the feces.
- **Protein Binding:** 98%–99%.
- **Cmax, Cmin, and AUC:** steady-state mean AUC = 83 mcg hr/mL; Cmax = 16 mcg/mL; Cmin = 7 mcg/mL (400 mg 3×/day).
- $T_{\frac{1}{2}}$: 5.8 hrs.
Pregnancy Risk
- Category C: placental passage of 4%–15% in late-term rodent studies. Teratogenicity in rodent studies resulting in ventricular septal defects. Maternal toxicity, embryotoxicity, and decreased pup survival seen with doses 5× the human dose. No data on carcinogenicity.

DRUGS

Breastfeeding Compatibility
- Unknown breast milk excretion. Breastfeeding is not recommended in the US in order to avoid postnatal transmission of HIV to the child, who may not yet be infected.

DOSING

Dosing for Decreased Hepatic Function
- No data. Consider dose reduction in ESLD.

Renal Dosing
- Dosing for GFR of 50–80: 400 mg 3×/day.
- Dosing for GFR of 10–50: usual dose.
- Dosing for GFR of <10: usual dose.
- Dosing in hemodialysis: no data. Usual dose likely; unlikely to be removed in dialysis due to high protein binding.
- Dosing in peritoneal dialysis: no data. Usual dose likely.
- Dosing in hemofiltration: no data. Usual dose likely.

COMMENTS

- **Pros:** may still have activity in patients with resistance to EFV and NVP due to G190A, and G190S, P225H, F227L mutations, but little clinical data; increases drug levels of some PIs.
- **Cons:** low potency; less clinical data than for other NNRTIs; 3×/day dosing.

SELECTED REFERENCES

Friedland GH, Pollard R, Griffith B, et al. Efficacy and safety of delavirdine mesylate with zidovudine and didanosine compared with two-drug combinations of these agents in persons with HIV disease with CD4 counts of 100 to 500 cells/mm³ (ACTG 261). ACTG 261 Team. *J Acquir Immune Defic Syndr*, 1999; 21: 281–92.

Comments: Prospective randomized study comparing the following regimens: DLV + AZT + ddI, DLV + AZT, DLV + ddI, and AZT + ddI in naïve patients (<6 mos of therapy). Therapy with DLV + AZT + ddI showed only modest antiviral activity and CD4 benefit compared with 2-drug regimens. VL reduction was not significantly different between AZT + ddI compared to DLV + AZT or DLV + ddI. This study is consistent with other studies showing only modest antiviral potency with DLV-containing regimens.

Para MF, Meehan P, Holden-Wiltse J, et al. ACTG 260: a randomized, phase I-II, dose-ranging trial of the anti-human immunodeficiency virus activity of delavirdine monotherapy. The AIDS Clinical Trials Group Protocol 260 Team. *Antimicrob Agents Chemother*, 1999; 43: 1373–8.

Comments: Phase I-II dose-finding study. DLV monotherapy decreased VL by only 0.87–1.08 log by wk 2 (less potent than EFV or NVP). Subjects developed rapid DLV resistance.

DIDANOSINE

Paul A. Pham, PharmD and John G. Bartlett, MD

INDICATIONS

FDA
- Treatment of HIV infection in combination with other antiretrovirals.

FORMS TABLE

Brand name (mfr)	Forms†	Cost*
Videx (Bristol-Myers Squibb)	Oral pediatric powder 2 g (4 oz); 4 g (8 oz)	$57.04; $124.51
Videx EC (Bristol-Myers Squibb)	Oral enteric coated caps 400 mg	$14.18
Didanosine EC (generic) (Barr Laboratories, Inc.)	Oral capsule 200 mg; 250 mg; 400 mg	$6.16; $7.87; $12.27

*Prices represent cost per unit specified, are representative of Average Wholesale Price (AWP).
†Dosage is indicated in mg unless otherwise noted.

USUAL ADULT DOSING
- Pill burden: 1/day (ddI EC).
- Wt >60 kg dose: 400 mg PO once daily. EC cap on an empty stomach (>1 hr before or >2 hrs after meals).
- Wt <60 kg dose: 250 mg PO once daily. EC cap on an empty stomach (>1 hr before or >2 hrs after meals).
- Total daily dose may also be taken in 2 divided doses if GI tolerance is an issue.
- Dose adjustment with tenofovir coadministration: <60 kg, 200 mg once daily; >60 kg, 250 mg once daily (see Drug-Drug Interactions in Appendix 1 on p. 509 for additional warnings).

ADVERSE DRUG REACTIONS
General
- Fewer GI side effects with EC formulation than with buffered, powder, or pediatric soln formulations.

Common
- Time- and dose-dependent peripheral neuropathy (5%–12% of patients after 2–6 mos of therapy). Relative risk of neuropathy is 135% higher when combined with hydroxyurea (HU), 250% higher with d4T, and 680% higher with d4T + HU. Irreversible and debilitating neuropathy with continued use despite early Sxs.
- GI intolerance (nausea, vomiting, and diarrhea) especially with buffered tablets.

Occasional
- Dose-dependent pancreatitis (in 1%–9% of patients, with 6% cases fatal). Risk factors associated with ddI-induced pancreatitis: alcohol use, renal failure, obesity, and concurrent use of d4T, HU, allopurinol, or pentamidine.
- Reversible transaminase elevation. Noncirrhotic portal hypertension resulting in esophageal variceal bleed, liver failure, and death have been reported.
- Lipoatrophy. Best characterized with ddI + d4T; may occur when ddI used without d4T.

Rare
- Lactic acidosis and severe hepatomegaly with steatosis (can be fatal in severe cases).
- Rash and optic neuritis.
- Increased risk of MI.

DRUG INTERACTIONS
- ddI does not interact with CYP3A4. Majority of drug interactions with buffered formulation, as buffer can decrease the absorption of some coadministered drugs.

DRUG-DRUG INTERACTIONS—See Appendix I, p. 509, for table of drug-drug interactions.
RESISTANCE
- K65R: selected by ddI, resulting in intermediate resistance to ddI, TDF, 3TC, FTC, and low-level resistance to ABC and possibly d4T. When present with 184V, susceptibility to TDF improves, susceptibility to ABC and ddI further decreased.
- L74V: selected by ddI, resulting in intermediate resistance to ddI and low-level resistance to ABC. When present with 184V, causes further loss of susceptibility to ABC and ddI. May increase susceptibility to AZT, d4T, and TDF.
- Q151M complex: high-level resistance.
- T69S insertion: high-level resistance.
- TAMs (41L, 210W, 215Y/F, 219Q/E, 44D, 67N, 70R, 118I): intermediate- or high-level resistance with 3 or more TAMs, especially with 41L/210W/215Y pathway.
- 184V: slight decrease in sensitivity to ddI but not clinically significant.

PHARMACOLOGY
Mechanism
- Metabolized intracellularly to ddATP (active metabolite), which competitively inhibits HIV DNA polymerase.

Pharmacokinetic Parameters
- **Absorption:** 30% absorption with powder.
- **Metabolism and Excretion:** 50% excreted unchanged in the urine via glomerular filtration and tubular secretion.
- **Protein Binding:** <5%.

DRUGS

- **Cmax, Cmin, and AUC:** Cmax = 1.6 mcg/mL after a single dose of 375 mg.
- **$T_{\frac{1}{2}}$:** serum: 1.6 hrs; intracellular: 25–40 hrs.

Pregnancy Risk

- Category B: human studies demonstrated 35% (range 23%–59%) placental passage. In 8 patients studied, no toxicities were observed in mothers or infants. Due to the small number of patients no firm conclusion can be made. In a phase I study (PACTG 249) ddI was well tolerated by women and fetus when started at wk 26–36. Pregnant patients may be at increased risk of lactic acidosis (FDA warns against its use in combination with d4T in pregnant patients).

Breastfeeding Compatibility

- Unknown breast milk excretion. Breastfeeding not recommended in the US in order to avoid postnatal transmission of HIV to the child, who may not yet be infected.

Dosing

Dosing for Decreased Hepatic Function

- No data: usual dose likely.

Renal Dosing

- Dosing for GFR of 50–80: wt >60 kg dose: 400 mg PO once daily (tabs) or 500 mg PO once daily (powder). Wt <60 kg dose: 250 mg PO once daily (tabs) or 334 mg PO once daily (powder).
- Dosing for GFR of 10–50: 50% of usual dose once daily.
- Dosing for GFR of <10: 25% of usual dose once daily.
- Dosing in hemodialysis: 25% of usual dose once daily, on days of dialysis give post-dialysis.
- Dosing in peritoneal dialysis: 25% of usual dose (little effect on removal with PD) (*Clin Pharmacol Ther* 1996;60(5):535).
- Dosing in hemofiltration: no data.

Comments

- **Pros:** good clinical track record; once-daily administration; excellent results in uncontrolled trials when combined with 3TC or FTC + 3rd agent.
- **Cons:** GI intolerance with pediatric soln; needs to be taken on an empty stomach; pancreatitis, neuropathy, and mitochondrial toxicity; relative lack of controlled data in ART era for ddI + 3TC or ddI + FTC compared to other dual-NRTI backbones; lack of coformulation; cross-resistance with TDF, ABC; not preferred as a 1st-line NRTI in current DHHS treatment guidelines. May increase risk of MI, especially in patients with cardiovascular risk factors. Association with noncirrhotic portal hypertension in postmarketing reports.

Selected References

D:A:D Study Group, Sabin CA, Worm SW, et al. Use of nucleoside reverse transcriptase inhibitors and risk of myocardial infarction in HIV-infected patients enrolled in the study: a multi-cohort collaboration. *Lancet*, 2008; 371: 1417–26.
Comments: A retrospective review of the D:A:D observational cohort for cardiovascular disease risks associated with NRTI use included 33347 patients (157,912 patient yrs of follow-up). ddI-containing regimens were associated with an increased risk of MI (RR 1.49, 95% CI 1.14–1.95). There was also an increased risk associated with ABC treatment, but not d4T or AZT. Apparent pathophysiologic mechanism of this finding has not been identified.

Molina JM, Journot V, Furco A, et al. Five-year follow up of once-daily therapy with emtricitabine, didanosine and efavirenz (Montana ANRS 091 trial). *Antivir Ther*, 2007; 12: 417–22.
Comments: An observational study involving 40 ART-naïve HIV-1-infected patients treated with once-daily FTC/ddI/EFV demonstrated good long-term virologic efficacy. After 5 yrs, 73% and 68% of patients had plasma HIV RNA levels <400 and <50 c/mL, respectively (ITT analysis).

Saag MS, Cahn P, Raffi F, et al. Efficacy and safety of emtricitabine vs stavudine in combination therapy in antiretroviral-naive patients: a randomized trial. *JAMA*, 2004; 292: 180–9.
Comments: FTC 301 study: 48 wk double-blind study that compared once-daily FTC or twice-daily d4T, both given in combination with ddI and EFV. 571 naïve patients with mean baseline CD4 of 318 (range 5–1317) and median baseline VL of 4.9 log (range 2.6–7.0) randomized to receive FTC once daily or d4T twice daily, both in combination with ddI, and EFV once daily. Probability of persistent virological response (VL <50) through wk 60 was 76% for the FTC group vs 54% for the d4T group (P <.001).

Robbins GK, De Gruttola V, Shafer RW, et al. Comparison of sequential three-drug regimens as initial therapy for HIV-1 infection. *N Engl J Med*, 2003; 349: 2293–303.

Comments: ACTG 384: 620 patients randomized to compare sequential 3-drug regimens in four groups: EFV combined with AZT/3TC or d4T/ddI OR NFV + AZT/3TC or d4T/ddI. EFV outperformed NFV in all arms. With a median of 2.3 yrs of follow-up, EFV combined with AZT/3TC had virologic failure in 14% and 23% of patients with the 1st and 2nd regimen, respectively. There was a higher rate of virologic failure in the EFV/d4T/ddI arm, with 31% and 58% of patients with the 1st and 2nd regimen, respectively. Lipoatrophy also occurred more rapidly in the ddI/d4T arm. Consistent with the DHHS guidelines, the authors recommend EFV/AZT/3TC as a preferred initial regimen.

Jemsek J, Hutcherson P, Harper E. Poor virologic response and early emergence of resistance in treatment naive, HIV-infected patients receiving a once daily triple nucleoside regimen of ddI, 3TC, and TDF. Abstract 51. Presented at: 11th Conference on Retroviruses and Opportunistic Infections (CROI 2004); February 8–11, 2004; San Francisco, CA.
Comments: The triple-NRTI regimen of ddI + TDF + 3TC was associated with an unusually high rate of virologic failure (91%) and NRTI resistance in this small trial.

Molina J, Marcelin AG, Marcelin J et al. Didanosine in treatment-experienced HIV-infected patients: results from a ran-domised double-blind study (A1454-176 Jaguar). Abstract H-447. Presented at: 43rd Interscience Conference on Antimi-crobial Agents and Chemotherapy (ICAAC); September 13–17, 2003; Chicago, IL.
Comments: ddI intensification after virologic failure produced a median decrease in VL of 0.5 log c/mL at wk 4. The decrease in VL correlated with the number of TAMs, with no significant response with >3 TAMs. L74V also predicted no response.

US Food and Drug Administration. FDA drug safety communication: serious liver disorder associated with the use of Videx/Videx EC (didanosine). January 29, 2010. http://www.fda.gov/Drugs/DrugSafety/ucm199169.htm. Accessed August 13, 2011.
Comments: FDA reports 42 post-marketing cases of noncirrhotic portal hypertension in patients using didanosine.

DRUGS

EFAVIRENZ

Paul A. Pham, PharmD and John G. Bartlett, MD

INDICATIONS
FDA
• Treatment of HIV infection in combination with other ARV agents.

FORMS TABLE

Brand name (mfr)	Forms†	Cost*
Sustiva (available in US, Canada, and Europe) (Bristol-Myers Squibb)	Oral capsule 50 mg Oral tablet 600 mg Oral capsule 200 mg	$1.77 $21.25 $7.08
Stocrin (available in South Africa, Southeast Asia, and other parts of the world) (Merck)	Oral capsule 50 mg; 100 mg; 200 mg Oral tablet 600 mg Oral soln 30 mg/30 mL (180-mL bottle)	variable (not available in US) variable (not available in US) variable (not available in US)
Atripla (available in the US, Canada, and Europe) (Bristol-Myers Squibb and Gilead Sciences)	Oral tablet EFV 600 mg/ TDF 300 mg/FTC 200 mg	$61.09

*Prices represent cost per unit specified, are representative of Average Wholesale Price (AWP).
†Dosage is indicated in mg unless otherwise noted.

USUAL ADULT DOSING
• Pill burden: 1 tab/day.
• EFV 600 mg PO once daily. Evening dosing on an empty stomach recommended initially to decrease side effects.
• Can be administered as a coformulated product with TDF/FTC (Atripla) 1 tab PO once daily.
• Administration with food, especially with high-fat meal, may increase CNS side effects: EFV peak levels increased by 40% (caps) and 80% (tabs).

- For GI intolerance, consider taking with food after resolution of CNS side effects.
- Morning CNS side effects may be decreased if taken several hrs before bedtime. Some patients can tolerate morning dosing after resolution of initial CNS side effects.
- With LPV/r: LPV/r 500/125 mg twice daily + EFV 600 mg once daily, especially for PI-experienced patients. In PI-naïve patients, standard dose of 400/100 (2 tabs) twice daily may be adequate.
- With FPV: FPV 700 mg twice daily + RTV 100 mg twice daily OR FPV 1400 mg + RTV 300 mg once daily + EFV 600 mg once daily.
- With ATV: ATV 400 mg once daily + RTV 100 mg once daily + EFV 600 mg once daily. Consider TDM.
- With IDV: IDV 800 mg twice daily + RTV 200 mg twice daily + EFV 600 mg once daily.
- With SQV: SQV 1000 mg twice daily + RTV 100 mg twice daily with EFV 600 mg once daily.
- With NFV: NFV 1250 mg twice daily + EFV 600 mg once daily.
- With DRV: dose not established. Consider DRV/r 600/100 mg twice daily + EFV 600 mg once daily. With once-daily DRV/r, only 900/100 mg dose has been tested with EFV. Consider DRV/r 800/100 mg or 900/100 mg once daily + EFV 600 mg once daily in PI-naïve patients. Consider TDM.
- With TPV: TPV/r 500/200 mg twice daily + EFV 600 mg once daily.
- With RAL: RAL 400 mg twice daily + EFV 600 mg once daily.
- With MVC: MVC 600 mg twice daily + EFV 600 mg once daily. Note: if PIs (i.e., LPV/r or SQV/r) contained in regimen, MVC 150 mg twice daily recommended.
- With ETR or NVP: avoid coadministration.
- Planned EFV discontinuation: stop EFV and continue NRTIs for 1–2 wks, but may require up to 4 wks with CYP2B6 polymorphism ("staggered discontinuation") OR substitute PI-based ART for 1 mo ("substituted discontinuation"). Substitution associated with less NNRTI resistance than staggered discontinuation in SMART study.

ADVERSE DRUG REACTIONS

General

- Generally well tolerated after resolution of CNS side effects (2–4 wks).

Common

- CNS effects: vivid dreams including nightmares, nocturnal dizziness, morning confusion, depersonalization; usually seen during 1st 2–4 wks with gradual resolution in most patients. Dose escalation over 2 wks decreases CNS side effects by approximately 50%, but not recommended due potential risk of resistance.
- Patients experiencing early CNS toxicity should avoid tasks that require concentration, such as driving, especially in the morning.
- Patients should be advised of additive effects of alcohol and other psychoactive agents when coadministered with EFV.
- Morbilliform rash in up to 26% of patients requiring discontinuation in 1.7% (median onset 11 days, duration 16 days); incidence and severity lower than NVP. Generally resolves with continued use of EFV. A meta-analysis of 13 reports with 239 patients indicated 13% of patients developed recurrence of rash when switched from NVP to EFV.
- False-positive urine toxicology screening test for cannabinoids (w/ CEDIA DAU Multilevel THC assay only); confirmatory tests negative.
- False-positive benzodiazepine screening test (e.g., Triage 8, Drug Screen Multi 5).

Occasional

- Elevated triglycerides and cholesterol (incidence higher than with NVP).
- Elevated transaminases (2%–8%; incidence and severity lower than with NVP). Frequency increased with concurrent hepatoxic drugs and HCV coinfection.
- Possible reduction in vitamin D levels.

Rare

- Erythema multiforme and Stevens-Johnson syndrome (0.1%).
- Gynecomastia.
- Severe psychiatric disorders, primarily depression reported in 2.4%.

DRUG INTERACTIONS
- Substrate of CYP2B6 >CYP3A4; inducer of CYP3A4 and CYP2B6; weak inhibitor of CYP3A4, 2B6, 2C9, and 2C19. Inducers of CYP3A4 and CYP2B6 may decrease EFV serum levels. EFV generally decreases serum levels of CYP3A4 and CYP2B6 substrates.

DRUG-DRUG INTERACTIONS — See Appendix I, p. 514, for table of drug-drug interactions.

RESISTANCE
- K103N: most common mutation selected by EFV, resulting in high-level resistance to EFV, NVP, DLV.
- Y181 mutations: 181C/I: resistance to NPV, DLV, low-level resistance to EFV (minimal clinical data on use of EFV with 181C/I). 181C can partially reverse TAM-mediated AZT, TDF resistance to V108I.
- Y188 mutations: 188L high-level resistance to NVP, EFV, intermediate resistance to DLV; 188C: high-level resistance to NVP, low-level resistance to EFV, DLV; 188H: low-level resistance to NVP, EFV, DLV.
- G190 mutations: 190A: high-level resistance to NVP, intermediate resistance to EFV; 190S: high-level resistance to NPV, EFV; both cause hypersusceptibility to DLV (unknown clinical significance).
- L100I: intermediate resistance to EFV, DLV; low-level resistance to NVP; can partially reverse TAM-mediated AZT, TDF resistance.
- V106 mutations: 106A: low-level EFV resistance, high-level NPV resistance, intermediate DLV resistance; 106M: high-level resistance to EFV, NPV, intermediate resistance to DLV; 106I: not associated with resistance.
- P225H: increases EFV resistance when combined with other NNRTI mutations.
- V108I: low-level resistance to EFV and other NNRTIs. Clinically insignificant when present as sole mutation.

PHARMACOLOGY

Mechanism
- Noncompetitive inhibition of HIV DNA polymerase resulting in disruption of catalytic site of the enzyme.

Pharmacokinetic Parameters
- **Absorption:** 40%–45% absorption with or without food; high-fat meals increase absorption by 39% (caps) to 79% (tabs).
- **Metabolism and Excretion:** metabolized by CYP2B6 >CYP3A4 to several hydroxylated metabolites, which undergo subsequent glucuronidation. Both unchanged drug and metabolites are excreted in the feces.
- **Protein Binding:** 99.5%–99.75%.
- **Cmax, Cmin, and AUC:** steady-state (600 mg) mean Cmax = 13 μmol per mL; Cmin = 5.6 μmol/mL; AUC = 184 μmol/mL hr.
- **T$_\frac{1}{2}$:** 36–100 hrs. Recent study found that the 516T/T genotype (more frequently found in blacks) was associated with higher plasma EFV concentrations, slower clearance, and increased CNS toxicity.

Pregnancy Risk
- Category D: placental passage of 100% seen in cynomolgus monkeys, rats, and rabbits. Teratogenicity demonstrated in cynomolgus monkeys resulting in anencephaly. Women with childbearing potential should be counseled about adequate contraceptive protection. The Antiretroviral Pregnancy Registry showed birth defects in 7 of 281 live births with 1st trimester exposure. Safety in 2nd or 3rd trimester not established but may be safe since neural tube has closed.

Breastfeeding Compatibility
- No human data, breast milk excretion in animal studies. Breastfeeding is not recommended in the US in order to avoid postnatal transmission of HIV to the child, who may not yet be infected.

DOSING

Dosing for Decreased Hepatic Function
- 600 mg at bedtime (serum level may be increased with ESLD).

Renal Dosing
- Dosing for GFR of 50–80: usual dose.
- Dosing for GFR of <50: usual dose. Avoid EFV/TDF/FTC coformulation.

DRUGS

- Dosing in hemodialysis: 600 mg once daily (EFV PK not affected by HD). Avoid EFV/TDF/FTC coformulated tab with GFR <50 mL/min.
- Dosing in peritoneal dialysis: 600 mg once daily (limited data). Avoid EFV/TDF/FTC coformulated tab with GFR <50 mL/min.
- Dosing in hemofiltration: no data. Consider usual dose.

COMMENTS

- **Pros:** multiple studies demonstrating potency and durability, including inpatients with high VL and/or low CD4; convenient (1 pill once daily), including coformulation with TDF and FTC (Atripla); generally well tolerated; minimal long-term toxicity; less hepatotoxicity and less severe rash than with NVP; long half-life (forgiving of delayed or missed doses); a preferred agent in DHHS guidelines with more rapid 1st phase virologic decay and superior virologic efficacy compared to LPV/r containing regimen in ACTG 5142.
- **Cons:** early CNS side effects common and require patient education/counseling; more hyperlipidemia than with NVP (though less than with most PIs); low genetic barrier (single point mutation) to resistance; long half-life may increase risk of resistance inpatients who interrupt therapy. Lower CD4 increase and more lipoatrophy than with LPV/r in ACTG 5142. (Lipoatrophy difference probably applies only to d4T- or AZT-containing regimens.). More lipid effects than ATV/r in ACTG 5202.

SELECTED REFERENCES

Arribas JR, Pozniak AL, Gallant JE, et al. Tenofovir disoproxil fumarate, emtricitabine, and efavirenz compared with zid-ovudine/lamivudine and efavirenz in treatment-naive patients: 144-week analysis. *J Acquir Immune Defic Syndr*, 2008; 47: 74–8.
Comments: 144-wk multicenter, open-label trial comparing TDF + FTC vs coformulated AZT/3TC, both administered in combination with EFV, in 509 treatment-naïve patients. Mean baseline VL 5.0 log. At 144 wks, 71% in TDF + FTC arm had Vl <400 vs 58% in AZT/3TC arm (P = 0.002) by FDA-mandated TLOVR analysis. Suppression to <50 achieved in 64% and 56% of patients, respectively (P = 0.08). At 144 wks, more patients in ZDV/3TC arm (105 patients [41%]) discontinued study regimen than in TDF/FTC and EFV group (75 patients [29%]; P = 0.004). Discontinuation attributable to virologic failure, and ADR higher in AZT/3TC-treated group. Limb fat at wk 96 was significantly greater in the TDF + FTC + EFV group vs the ZDV/3TC + EFV group (7.9 vs 4.5 kg; P <0.001).

Riddler SA, Haubrich R, DiRienzo G, et al. Class-sparing regimens for initial treatment of HIV-1 infection (ACTG 5142). *N Engl J Med*, 2008; 358: 2095–2106.
Comments: 757 ARV-naïve patients randomized to 3 regimens: LPV/r + NRTIs, EFV + NRTIs, and LPV/r + EFV. At median follow-up of 112 wks, time to virologic failure longer in EFV-treated patients (P = 0.006). At 96 wks, 89% of patients in EFV + 2 NRTIs arm had VL <50 vs 77% in LPV/r + 2 NRTIs arm (P = 0.003). LPV/r + EFV arm had similar virologic efficacy compared to EFV + 2 NRTIs (83% vs 89%). No difference between 3 arms in time to 1st treatment-limiting toxicity, but significant triglyceride elevation more common in EFV + LPV/r-treated patients. Despite superior virologic response in EFV + 2 NRTIs regimen, LPV/r-containing regimen resulted in greater CD4 increase (241 vs 285, P = 0.01). In patients with virologic failure, development of resistance observed in 70%, 48%, and 21% in EFV + LPV/r arm, EFV + 2 NRTIS, and LPV/r + 2 NRTIs, respectively.

Bartlett JA, Johnson J, Herrera G, et al. Long-term results of initial therapy with abacavir and lamivudine combined with efavirenz, amprenavir/ritonavir, or stavudine. *J Acquir Immune Defic Syndr*, 2006; 43: 284–92.
Comments: 291 naïve patients with median baseline VL 63,000–79,000 and CD4 296–307 received ABC/3TC 300/150 mg twice daily combined with either an NNRTI once daily, PI once daily, or NRTI twice daily. Patients in EFV arm had longer duration of VL suppression compared to the NRTI arm (VL <400, P = 0.007). However, at wk 96, there were no differences between arms in the percentage of subjects with VL <400 and <50. Median CD4 increase and incidence of AEs were similar between arms.

Gulick RM, Ribaudo HJ, Shikuma CM, et al. Three- vs four-drug antiretroviral regimens for the initial treatment of HIV-1 infection: a randomized controlled trial. *JAMA*, 2006; 296: 769–81.
Comments: Continuation of ACTG 5095 compared AZT/3TC/EFV to AZT/ABC/3TC/EFV in ART-naïve patients. No signifi-cant differences between 3- vs 4-drug regimens; approximately 80% of patients had VL <50 through 3 yrs. 10% treated with AZT/3TC/ABC/EFV had ABC HSR, vs 7% on AZT/3TC/EFV.

van Leth F, Phanuphak P, Ruxrungtham K, et al. Comparison of first-line antiretroviral therapy with regimens including nevirapine, efavirenz, or both drugs, plus stavudine and lamivudine: a randomised open-label trial, the 2NN Study. *Lancet*, 2004; 363: 1253–63.
Comments: Large, prospective, randomized trial comparing NVP 400 mg once daily, NVP 200 mg twice daily, EFV 600 mg once daily, or NVP 400 mg + EFV 800 mg once daily, + d4T and 3TC, for 48 wks in 1216 naïve patients. EFV and NVP regimens comparable, with VL <50 in 65% vs 60%, respectively at 48 wks (P = 0.193), but did not meet study criteria for noninferiority (within the 10% limit). Hepatotoxicity more common in NVP arm (9.6% vs 3.5%).

Squires K, Lazzarin A, Gatell JM, et al. Comparison of once-daily atazanavir with efavirenz, each in combination with fixed-dose zidovudine and lamivudine, as initial therapy for patients infected with HIV. *J Acquir Immune Defic Syndr*, 2004; 36: 1011–9.
Comments: Randomized, double-blind study involving 810 naïve patients compared ATV 400 mg once daily to EFV 600 mg at bedtime in combination with open-label fixed-dose AZT/3TC twice daily. At wk 48, VL <400 in 70% of patients receiving ATV and 64% of patients receiving EFV (NS). Unboosted ATV was equivalent to EFV in ART-naïve patients.

Gallant JE, Staszewski S, Pozniak AL, et al. Efficacy and safety of tenofovir DF vs stavudine in combination therapy in antiretroviral-naive patients: a 3-year randomized trial. *JAMA*, 2004; 292: 191–201.
Comments: 602 ART-naïve patients randomized to receive either TDF (N = 299) or d4T (N = 303), with placebo, in combination with 3TC and EFV. The proportion of patients with VL <400 at wk 48 was 239/299 (80%) and 253/301 (84%) in patients receiving TDF and d4T, respectively. Virologic results equivalent but more lipoatrophy, neuropathy, and hyperlipidemia in d4T arm.

Gulick RM, Ribaudo HJ, Shikuma CM, et al. Triple-nucleoside regimens versus efavirenz-containing regimens for the initial treatment of HIV-1 infection. *N Engl J Med*, 2004; 350: 1850–61.
Comments: Randomized, double-blind study comparing 3 regimens (AZT/3TC/ABC, AZT/3TC + EFV, AZT/3TC/ABC + EFV) as initial treatment in ART-naïve patients. After median follow-up of 32 wks, 82/382 subjects in triple-NRTI arm (21%) and 85/765 in combined EFV groups (11%) had virologic failure; time to virologic failure significantly shorter in the triple-NRTI arm (P <0.001).

Haas D, Ribaudo H, Kim R, et al. Pharmacogenetics of efavirenz and central nervous system side effects: an Adult AIDS Clinical Trials Group study. *AIDS*, 2004; 18: 2391–400.
Comments: 516T/T genotype (more frequently found in blacks) was associated with higher plasma EFV concentrations, slower clearance, and increased CNS toxicity.

Robbins GK, De Gruttola V, Shafer RW, et al. Comparison of sequential three-drug regimens as initial therapy for HIV-1 infection. *N Engl J Med*, 2003; 349: 2293–303.
Comments: 620 patients randomized to compare sequential 3-drug regimens in 3 groups: EFV-based ART combined with AZT/3TC or d4T/ddI OR NFV + AZT/3TC or d4T/ddI. EFV out performed NFV in all arms. With a median of 2–3 yr follow-up virologic failure in 14% and 23% of EFV + AZT/3TC-treated patients with the 1st and 2nd regimen, respectively. Higher rate of virologic failure in EFV + d4T + ddI arm (31% and 58%).

Staszewski S, Morales-Ramirez J, Tashima KT, et al. Efavirenz plus zidovudine and lamivudine, efavirenz plus indinavir, and indinavir plus zidovudine and lamivudine in the treatment of HIV-1 infection in adults. Study 006 Team. *N Engl J Med*, 1999; 341: 1865–73.
Comments: Open-label study involving 450 patients naïve to 3TC, NNRTIs, and PIs: randomized to receive EFV + AZT/3TC, IDV + AZT/3TC, or EFV + IDV. At 48 wks, VL <50 was achieved in more patients in EFV + AZT/3TC group than in IDV + AZT/3TC group by ITT analysis (64% vs 43%, P <0.01). More patients discontinuing treatment because of ADRs in the IDV arm compared to EFV arm (43% vs 27%, P = 0.005).

Saag M, Ive P, Heera J, et al. A multicenter, randomized, double-blind, comparative trial of a novel CCR5 antagonist, maraviroc, versus efavirenz, both in combination with Combivir (zidovudine [ZDV]/lamivudine [3TC]), for the treatment of antiretroviral-naive patients infected with R5 HIV1: week 48 results of the MERIT study. Abstract WESS104. Presented at: 4th International Aids Society (IAS) Conference on HIV Pathogenesis, Treatment and Prevention; July 22–25, 2007; Sydney, Australia.
Comments: Over 700 patients with mean baseline VL 4.8 logs and median CD4 approximately 250 randomized to received AZT/3TC + either EFV or MVC for 48 wks. MVC (twice daily) noninferior to EFV in viral suppression to <400 (71% vs 73%, respectively), but did not meet noninferiority threshold using <50 assay (65% vs 69%). Post-hoc analysis found that difference accounted for by patients who had R5 virus at screen but D/M virus at baseline. Patients with baseline VL >100,000 less likely to achieve VL<50 with MVC than EFV (59.6% vs 66.6%), although suppression similar with VL <100,000. Mean CD4 increases 170 and 144 in MVC- and EFV-treated patients, respectively. Overall discontinuation rates similar between groups, but patients on MVC more likely to withdraw for lack of treatment effect, while those on EFV more likely to withdraw for AEs. CNS side effects more common in EFV-treated group.

EMTRICITABINE

Paul A. Pham, PharmD and John G. Bartlett, MD

INDICATIONS
FDA
- Treatment of HIV infection in combination with other antiretroviral agents.
Non-FDA Approved Uses
- Treatment of hepatitis B in HIV-HBV coinfected patients or in HBV monoinfected patients.

FORMS TABLE

Brand name (mfr)	Forms†	Cost*
Emtriva (Gilead Sciences)	Oral capsule 200 mg Oral soln 10 mg/mL (170 mL)	$15.58 per cap $110.38 (170-mL bottle)
Complera (Gilead Sciences)	TDF/FTC/RPV 300/200/25 mg tablet	$68.19/tablet
Truvada (Gilead Sciences)	Oral tablet FTC 200 mg/ TDF 300 mg	$39.84 per tab
Atripla (Bristol-Myers Squibb; Gilead Sciences)	Oral tablet FTC 200 mg/TDF 300 mg/EFV 600 mg	$61.09 per tab

*Prices represent cost per unit specified, are representative of Average Wholesale Price (AWP).
†Dosage is indicated in mg unless otherwise noted.

USUAL ADULT DOSING

- Pill burden: 1 cap or tab/day.
- FTC 200 mg: 1 tab once daily, with or without food.
- Adult dose: *Complera* 1 tablet once-daily with meals.
- Can be administered as a coformulated product with tenofovir DF (*Truvada*) 1 tab PO once daily with or without food and TDF/EFV (*Atripla*) 1 tab once daily. Evening dosing on an empty stomach recommended with initial *Atripla* therapy to decrease EFV-associated side effects.

ADVERSE DRUG REACTIONS
General

- Generally well tolerated. For *Atripla*, see EFV for EFV-associated side effects (p. 276) and TDF for TDF-associated side effects (p. 320).
- Adult dose: *Complera* 1 tablet once-daily with meals.

Occasional

- Mild asymptomatic skin hyperpigmentation on the palm and/or soles noted in 3% of patients, with increased frequency in dark-skinned individuals.
- Asymptomatic and transient CPK elevation.
- Headache, diarrhea, nausea, asthenia, and rash that required discontinuation in approximately 1% of patients.

Rare

- Lactic acidosis (categorized as NRTI class adverse effect, but not expected to occur frequently with FTC).

DRUG INTERACTION

- Not a substrate, inhibitor, or inducer of any CYP450 isoforms. No clinically significant drug interactions.

DRUG-DRUG INTERACTIONS—See Appendix I, p. 520, for table of drug-drug interactions.
RESISTANCE

- 184V: high-level resistance.
- T69ins: high-level resistance.
- Q151M complex: unknown data, but low-level resistance likely.
- TAMs (41L, 210W, 215Y/F, 219Q/E, 44D, 67N, 70R, 118I): high level resistance with multiple TAMs.

PHARMACOLOGY
Mechanism

- Intracellular phosphorylation to active triphosphate, which competitively inhibits HIV DNA polymerase.

Pharmacokinetic Parameters

- **Absorption:** FTC is well absorbed with an absolute bioavailability of 93%.

- **Metabolism and Excretion:** only 13% of administered dose is metabolized to sulfadoxide and glucuronide metabolites. Metabolites and unchanged drug are excreted primarily via glomerular filtration and tubular secretion.
- **Protein Binding:** <4%.
- **Cmax, Cmin, and AUC:** mean Cmax = 1.8 g/mL; Cmin = 0.09 g/mL; AUC 10 mcg hr/mL after 200 mg once daily at steady state.
- **T$_{\frac{1}{2}}$:** 10 hrs.

Pregnancy Risk
- Category B: no human data. In animal studies, FTC at 120-fold higher than human exposure did not result in fetal malformation.

Breastfeeding Compatibility
- No data. Breastfeeding is not recommended for HIV-infected patients in the US.

DOSING

Dosing for Decreased Hepatic Function
- No data: usual dose likely.

Renal Dosing
- Dosing for GFR of 30–49: FTC 200 mg every other day or TDF/FTC coformulation (*Truvada*) 1 tab every other day; TDF/FTC/EFV (*Atripla*) not recommended with GFR <50.
- Dosing for GFR of 15–29: FTC 200 mg q3 days. TDF/FTC (*Truvada*) not recommended with GFR <30. EFV/TDF/FTC (*Atripla*) not recommended with GFR <50.
- Dosing for GFR of <15: 200 mg q4 days; TDF/FTC (*Truvada*) and EFV/TDF/FTC (*Atripla*) not recommended.
- Dosing in hemodialysis: 200 mg q4 days post-HD (30% of dose removed with 3-hr HD). TDF/FTC (*Truvada*) not recommended with GFR <30. EFV/TDF/FTC (*Atripla*) not recommended with GFR <50.
- Dosing in peritoneal dialysis: no data. Consider dose reduction. TDF/FTC (*Truvada*) not recommended with GFR <30 and EFV/TDF/FTC (*Atripla*) not recommended with GFR <50.
- Dosing in hemofiltration: no data. Consider dose reduction.

COMMENTS
- **Pros:** activity against HBV; well tolerated; once-daily dosing; coformulation with TDF; similar to 3TC with respect to activity, tolerability, and resistance profile.
- **Cons:** hyperpigmentation in some patients.

SELECTED REFERENCES
Arribas JR, Pozniak AL, Gallant JE, et al. Tenofovir disoproxil fumarate, emtricitabine, and efavirenz compared with zidovudine/lamivudine and efavirenz in treatment-naive patients: 144-week analysis. *J Acquir Immune Defic Syndr*, 2008; 47: 74–8.
Comments: 144-wk multicenter, open-label trial comparing TDF + FTC vs coformulated AZT/3TC, both administered in combination with EFV, in 509 treatment-naïve patients. Mean baseline VL 5.0 log10 and no patients discontinued because of renal events. At 144 wks, 71% of evaluable patients in the TDF + FTC arm had a Vl <400 compared to 58% in the AZT/3TC arm (P = 0.004) by the FDA-mandated time to loss of viral response analysis. Suppression to <50 was achieved in 80 and 70% of patients, respectively (P = 0.02). Higher ITT success rate in the TDF/FTC arm was due to a higher rate of discontinuation caused by AEs in the AZT/3TC arm (11% vs 5%; P = 0.016); discontinuing due to anemia was higher in AZT/3TC arm. Patients in the ZDV/3TC arm had significantly less limb fat than patients in the TDF/FTC arm (5.4 vs 7.9 kg; P <0.001).

Molina JM, Journot V, Furco A, et al. Five-year follow up of once-daily therapy with emtricitabine, didanosine and efavirenz (Montana ANRS 091 trial). *Antivir Ther*, 2007; 12: 417–22.
Comments: This open-label trial enrolled 40 ARV-naïve patients who received a once-daily regimen of FTC/ddI/EFV. At 5 yrs, 73% and 68% of patients had plasma HIV RNA levels <400 and <50.

Molina JM, Journot V, Morand-Joubert L. Simplification therapy with once-daily emtricitabine, didanosine, and efavirenz in HIV-1-infected adults with viral suppression receiving a protease inhibitor-based regimen: a randomized trial. *J Infect Dis*, 2005; 191: 830–9.
Comments: ANRS 099 (Alize Study): open-label, noninferiority study involving 355 patients receiving a PI-based regimen with VL <400. Patients randomized to continue PI-based regimen or switch to once-daily regimen of FTC, ddI, and EFV. Noninferiority defined as a difference in proportion of success between the 2 groups of <15%. In an ITT analysis, 87% and 95% of patients randomized to PI-based regimen vs once-daily regimen maintained VL <50, respectively (P <0.05).

Saag MS, Cahn P, Raffi F, et al. Efficacy and safety of emtricitabine vs stavudine in combination therapy in antiretroviral-naive patients: a randomized trial. *JAMA*, 2004; 292: 180–9.

DRUGS

Comments: FTC 301 study: 48 wk double-blind study that compared once-daily FTC or twice-daily d4T, both given in combination with ddI and EFV. 571-naïve patients with a mean baseline CD4 of 318 (range 5–1317) and median baseline VL of 4.9 (range 2.6–7.0) randomized to receive FTC once daily or d4T twice daily, both in combination with ddI and EFV once daily. The probability of persistent virological response <50 through wk 60 was 76% for the FTC group vs 54% for the d4T group (P <0.001).

Benson CA, van der Horst C, Lamarca A, et al. A randomized study of emtricitabine and lamivudine in stably suppressed patients with HIV. *AIDS*, 2004; 18: 2269–76.

Comments: FTC 303/350 study: 440 patients on a 3TC-containing regimen with VL <400 randomized to switch to FTC or continue 3TC with maintenance of background regimen. 67% and 72% of patients randomized to FTC and 3TC achieved and maintained VL <50 through wk 48 (P = NS), respectively. Mean increase from baseline CD4 was 29 for FTC and 61 for 3TC. In patients who elected to continue FTC after wk 48, the probability of virologic failure was 11% after 4 yrs follow-up.

ENFUVIRTIDE

Paul A. Pham, PharmD and John G. Bartlett, MD

INDICATIONS
FDA
- Indicated for use in combination with other ARV agents for treatment of HIV-1 infection in treatment-experienced patients with evidence of HIV replication despite ongoing ART.

FORMS TABLE

Brand name (mfr)	Forms†	Cost*
Fuzeon (Roche)	SC vial 90 mg	$51.04

*Prices represent cost per unit specified, are representative of Average Wholesale Price (AWP).
†Dosage is indicated in mg unless otherwise noted.

USUAL ADULT DOSING
- 90 mg (1 mL) SC q12h into upper arm, anterior thigh, or abdomen with each injection given at a site different from preceding injection site. Do not inject where large nerves course close to skin, over blood vessels, into moles, scar tissue, tattoos, burn sites, or around umblicus.
- Prior to administration, reconstitute with 1.1 mL of sterile water, giving volume of 1.2 mL.
- Once reconstituted must be refrigerated and used within 24 hrs.

ADVERSE DRUG REACTIONS
Common
- Local injection site reaction including pain (9%), erythema (32%), pruritus (4%), induration (57%), and nodules or cysts (26%), leading to discontinuation in 3%.
Occasional
- Eosinophilia.
- Bacterial pneumonia (6.7 vs 0.60 events per 100 patients-yr in treatment and control arms, respectively). Mechanism unknown.
- With use of Biojector needle-free device: nerve pain (neuralgia and/or paresthesia) lasting up to 6 mos at anatomical sites where large nerves course close to the skin; bruising; hematomas.

DRUG INTERACTIONS
- Not inhibitor or inducer CYP3A4, CYP2D6, CYP1A2, CYP2C19, or CYP2E1 substrates as expected, does not interact with SQV, RTV, or rifampin.
- In observational study, TPV Cmin increased by approximately 50% with ENF coadministration.
- Critical factor such as food effect and adherence not objectively measured. Limitations of study design could also have affected results.
- No significant interaction with PIs, NNRTIs, NRTIs, RAL, and MVC.
Resistance
- No cross-resistance with RAL, MVC, NRTIs, NNRTIs, or PIs. *In vitro*, clinical isolates resistant to NRTI, NNRTI, or PIs retained susceptibility to ENF.

- A 21-fold (range, <1–422-fold) decrease in susceptibility to ENF has been correlated with genotypic changes in the 1st heptad repeat (HR1) region of gp41 amino acids 36D/S, 37V, 38A/M/E, 39R, 40H, 42T, and 43D.

PHARMACOLOGY

Mechanism

- ENF binds to HR1 site in gp41 subunit of the viral envelope glycoprotein and prevents conformational change required for viral fusion and entry into cells.

Pharmacokinetic Parameters

- **Absorption:** well absorbed from SC site with bioavailability of 84.3% (± 15.5%).
- **Metabolism and Excretion:** undergoes catabolism with 17% converted to an active deaminated form. *In vitro*, undergoes a non-NADPH dependent hydrolysis.
- **Protein Binding:** 92%.
- **Cmax, Cmin, and AUC:** following 90 mg SC, mean Cmax was 5.0 ± 1.7 mcg/mL, Cmin was 3.3 ± 1.6 mcg/mL, and AUC was 48.7 ± 19.1 mcg/mL hr. Cmin 2.2 mcg/mL was associated with virologic suppression.
- **T$_{\frac{1}{2}}$:** 3.8 ± 0.6 h.
- **Distribution:** Vd = 5.5 ± 1.1L. Limited CNS penetration.

Pregnancy Risk

- Category B: not teratogenic in animal studies. Does not cross placenta (limited data). Inadequate data for use in pregnant women.

Breastfeeding Compatibility

- No data. Breastfeeding not recommended in US.

DOSING

Dosing for Decreased Hepatic Function

- No data. Usual dose likely.

Renal Dosing

- Dosing for GFR of 50–80: 90 mg SC q12h.
- Dosing for GFR 35–50: no significant change in PK parameters. Usual dose likely.
- Dosing for GFR <35: no data, usual dose likely.
- Dosing in hemodialysis: no data, usual dose likely.
- Dosing in peritoneal dialysis: no data, usual dose likely.
- Dosing in hemofiltration: no data, usual dose likely.

COMMENTS

- **Pros:** active against PI-, NNRTI-, and NRTI-resistance virus; good response if background regimen includes >2 active ARTs; well studied in ART-experienced patients.
- **Cons:** SC administration; injection site reactions; time consuming reconstitution process; expensive; requires extensive patient education and training. Easier and more convenient alternatives now available for most treatment-experienced patients.

SELECTED REFERENCES

Clotet B, Bellos N, Molina JM, et al. Efficacy and safety of darunavir-ritonavir at week 48 in treatment-experienced patients with HIV-1 infection in POWER 1 and 2: a pooled subgroup analysis of data from two randomised trials. *Lancet*, 2007; 369: 1169–78.
Comments: 61% of DRV/r-treated patients and 15% of control patients achieved >1 log reduction in VL though wk 48. VL <50 achieved in 46% and 10% of DRV/r and control patients, respectively (P <0.003). Darunavir-treated patients who were naïve to ENF had a significantly greater VL if they included ENF in their background regimen. 21/36 achieved a VL reduction of at least 1 log, compared with only 4/35 ENF-naïve patients who did not receive DRV/r.

Hicks CB, Cahn P, Cooper DA, et al. Durable efficacy of tipranavir-ritonavir in combination with an optimised background regimen of antiretroviral drugs for treatment-experienced HIV-1-infected patients at 48 weeks in the Randomized Evaluation of Strategic Intervention in multi-drug reSistant patients with Tipranavir (RESIST) studies: an analysis of combined data from two randomised open-label trials. *Lancet*, 2006; 368: 466–75.
Comments: Similar to DRV studies, patients on TPV/r + an optimized background regimen (OBR) that included ENF had a better virologic response rate (VL reduction of 1.67 log vs 0.98 log).

Lalezari JP, Henry K, O'Hearn M, et al. Enfuvirtide, an HIV-1 fusion inhibitor, for drug-resistant HIV infection in North and South America. *N Engl J Med*, 2003; 348: 2175–85.
Comments: Pooled data presented to FDA from 2 randomized, controlled, open-label studies (TORO 1 and TORO 2) involving 995 treatment-experienced patients. ENF + an optimized background regimen (OBR) superior to OB regimen

DRUGS

alone. Patients had baseline VL of 5.2 logs, mean of 12 prior ART agents, and 80%–90% had >5 resistance mutations to NRTIs, NNRTIs, or PIs. VL change from baseline to wk 24 was −1.52 log for patients receiving ENF + OB regimen arm compared to −0.73 log in OB arm. As expected, patients with >2 active agents in their OB regimen were more likely to achieve undetectable VL.

ETRAVIRINE

Paul A. Pham, PharmD

INDICATIONS
FDA
- In combination with other ARV agents for the treatment of HIV-1 infection in treatment-experienced patients with PIs, NRTIs, and NNRTI-resistant variants.
Non-FDA Approved Uses
- Potential for use in 1st-line therapy for patients infected with NNRTI-resistant virus (untested).
FORMS TABLE

Brand name (mfr)	Forms†	Cost*
Intelence (Tibotec Pharmaceuticals)	Oral tablet 100 mg; 200 mg	$7.31 per tab; $15.32 for the 200 mg tab $7.67 for the 100 mg tab.

*Prices represent cost per unit specified, are representative of Average Wholesale Price (AWP).
†Dosage is indicated in mg unless otherwise noted.

USUAL ADULT DOSING
- Pill burden: 2 tablets/day (200-mg tab).
- ETR 200 mg PO twice daily with food. Tablets can also be dissolved in water.
- With MVC: MVC 600 mg twice daily + ETR 200 mg twice daily with food.
- With MVC + boosted PI: MVC 150 mg twice daily + ETR 200 mg twice daily with food.
- With RAL: RAL 400 mg twice daily + ETR 200 mg twice daily with food.
- With exception of DRV/r, LPV/r, and SQV/r, manufacturer recommends avoiding coadministration or use with caution with other PIs, but clinical significance unclear.
- With DRV/r: DRV/r 600/100mg twice daily + ETR 200 mg twice daily with food. Based on a PK study, DRV 800/100 mg once daily + ETR 400 mg once daily with food can be considered (clinical studies ongoing).
- With SQV/r: SQV/r 1000/100 mg twice daily + ETR 200 mg twice daily with food.
- With LPV/r: LPV/r 400/100 mg twice daily + ETR 200 mg twice daily with food.
- With TPV/r: avoid coadministration.
- With ATV/r: avoid coadministration, but clinical significance unclear. With coadministration consider ATV/r 400/100 mg once daily and TDM.
- With FPV/r: avoid coadministration, but clinical significance unclear. With coadministration consider TDM.
- With any unboosted PIs (IDV, NFV, ATV) and high-dose RTV: avoid coadministration.
ADVERSE DRUG REACTIONS
General
- Generally well tolerated.
Common
- In patients also treated with DRV/r, rash occurred in 17% of ETR-treated group vs 9% of placebo-treated patients.
- In general, rash was mild to moderate (but Grade 3 and 4 rashes reported in 1.3% of patients), occurred in 2nd wk and resolved within 1–2 wks on continued therapy. 2% required

ETR discontinuation. Rash more common in women. ETR should be discontinued for severe rash or if rash accompanied by fever, hepatitis, and other systemic Sx.

- Patients with history of NNRTI-related rash did not have higher risk of rash with ETR.

Occasional

- With DRV/r coadministration, moderate to severe (Grade 2–4) nausea, abdominal pain, diarrhea, and vomiting reported in approximately 15% of patients comparable to placebo.
- Grade of 2 or greater LFTs and bilirubin elevations more common in HBV and HCV coinfected patients.
- AST, ALT, and bilirubin elevation occurred in 22.8%, 21.4%, and 5.7%, respectively, vs 5.5%, 6.1%, and 1.2% of noncoinfected patients treated with ETR. Grade 3 hepatotoxicity (ALT or AST >5× ULN) in 2%–3%, but rates 4× higher with HBV or HCV coinfection.
- Fatigue (3.3%).
- Peripheral neuropathy (2.8%).
- Headache (2.7%).
- Hypertension (2.8%).
- Total cholesterol elevation (>240 mg/dL) reported in 24% of ETR-treated patients vs 17% of placebo-treated patients.
- Triglyceride elevation (>500 mg/dL) in 14% of ETR-treated patients vs 11% of placebo-treated patients.
- Hyperglycemia (>161 mg/dL) in 16% of ETR-treated patients compared to 13% of placebo-treated patients.
- GI intolerance (2%–5%), but not significantly different compared to placebo-treated patients.

Rare

- Severe rash including Stevens-Johnson syndrome, erythema multiforme, toxic epidermal necrolysis (resulting in one fatality).

DRUG INTERACTIONS

- *In vitro* ETR is CYP3A4, 2C19, and 2C9 substrate. Also undergoes glucuronidation. Not a Pgp substrate. Does not induce or inhibit its own metabolism.
- ETR inhibits 2C9 and 2C19.
- Mild inducer of CYP3A4, 2B6, and glucuronidation *in vitro*.

DRUG-DRUG INTERACTIONS—See Appendix I, p. 521, for table of drug-drug interactions.

RESISTANCE

- ETR maintained activity against multiple NNRTI resistance, including K103N and Y181C.
- 3 or more of following mutations at baseline associated with decreased response to ETR: V90I, A98G, L100I, K101E, K101P, V106I, V179D/F, Y181C/I, Y181V, G190A/s. Note: the FDA approved labeling also include other IAS-USA mutations to this list, but clinical significance unclear.
- Highest level of resistance observed with following combination of mutations: V179F + Y181C (187-fold change), V179F + Y181I (123-fold change), or V179F + Y181C + F227C (888-fold change).
- Mutations that emerged most commonly in subjects with virologic failure were V179F, V179I, Y181C, and Y181I.
- Weighted scoring system to predict phenotypic susceptibility:
  - 4 points: 100I, 101P, 181C/I.
  - 3 points: 138A/G, 179E, 190Q, 230L, 238N.
  - 2 points: 101E, 106A, 138K, 179L, 188L.
  - 1 point: 90I, 101H, 106M, 138Q, 179D/F/M, 181F, 189I, 190E/T, 221Y, 225H, 238T.
  - A score of 4+ points associated with reduced susceptibility.
- Weighted scoring system to predict response in DUET trials (6/08, Janssen Therapeutics):
  - 3 points: 181I/V.
  - 2.5 points: 101P, 100I, 181C, 230L.
  - 1.5 points: 138A, 106I, 190S, 179F.
  - 1 point: 90I, 179D, 101E, 101H, 98G, 179T, 190A.
  - 0–2 points: 74% response; 2.5–3.5 points: 52% response; 4+ points: 38% response.

DRUGS

PHARMACOLOGY

Pharmacokinetic Parameters

- **Absorption:** absolute bioavailability unknown.
- **Metabolism and Excretion:** ETR undergoes oxidative metabolism by CYP3A4, CYP2C9, and CYP2C19 *in vitro*. ETR's methylhydroxylated metabolites have 90% less activity against wild-type virus compared to ETR. Primarily excreted in the feces with only 1.2% recovered in the urine.
- **Protein Binding:** 99.9%.
- **Cmax, Cmin, and AUC:** with DRV/r coadministration: ETR AUC 12h (GM ± SD): 4531 ± 4543 ng h/m; ETR Cmin (GM ± SD): 296 ± 377 ng/mL.
- **T$_{\frac{1}{2}}$:** 41 (± 20) hrs.
- **Distribution:** unknown distribution into CSF and genital tract secretion, but presumed to be low.

Pregnancy Risk

- Category B: no human data. Not teratogenic in animal studies.

Breastfeeding Compatibility

- No data. Breastfeeding is not recommended in the US in order to avoid postnatal transmission of HIV to the child, who may not yet be infected.

DOSING

Dosing for Decreased Hepatic Function

- Child-Pugh Class A and B: 200 mg twice daily. Child-Pugh Class C: no data. Use with caution.

Renal Dosing

- Dosing for GFR of >50: 200 mg twice daily.
- Dosing for GFR of <50: no data. Usual dose likely since ETR and metabolites are not significantly excreted in urine.
- Dosing in hemodialysis: no data. Due to high protein binding, ETR is unlikely to be removed in dialysis. Usual dose likely.
- Dosing in peritoneal dialysis: no data. Due to high protein binding, ETR is unlikely to be removed in dialysis. Usual dose likely.
- Dosing in hemofiltration: no data. Due to high protein binding, ETR is unlikely to be removed in dialysis. Usual dose likely.

COMMENTS

- **Pros:** active against most of EFV- and NVP-resistant strains, generally well tolerated, with higher genetic barrier to resistance compared to EFV and NVP. Can be dissolved in water for liquid dosing.
- **Cons:** twice-daily dosing (though PK supports once-daily dosing), food requirement, rash (including TEN and SJS), and many drug interactions.

SELECTED REFERENCES

Katlama C, Haubrich R, Lalezari J, et al. Efficacy and safety of etravirine in treatment-experienced, HIV-1 patients: pooled 48 week analysis of two randomized, controlled trials. *AIDS*, 2009; 23: 2289–300.
Comments: Treatment-experienced patients (N = 1203) with at least 1 NNRTI mutation and at least 3 PI mutations randomized to placebo or ETR (+ DRV/r + OBR). Baseline characteristics (N = 599) of patients on ETR were: VL = 4.8 log, CD4 99. 2/3 had extensive ARV treatment history (10–15 ARVs), 69% had >2 detectable NNRTI mutations, 62% had >4 primary PI mutations, and only 4% had prior use of DRV/r. Virologic suppression (VL <50) at 48 wks achieved in 61% of patients in ETR arms compared with 40% in placebo arms (P <0.0001). Pooled DUET-1 and -2 data found mean −2.25 log reduction in ETR arm vs −1.49 in placebo arm (P <0.0001). Mean increase in CD4 from baseline was higher in ETR arm (98 vs 73, P = 0.0006). If ENF was used *de novo*, 71% of ETR-treated patients and 59% of placebo-treated patients achieved virologic suppression. ETR generally well tolerated with rash occurring in 22% and 17% (DUET-1 and -2, respectively) in ETR group vs only 11% in placebo group. However, rash led to discontinuation in 2% of ETR-treated patients.

FOSAMPRENAVIR

Paul A. Pham, PharmD and John G. Bartlett, MD

INDICATIONS
FDA
• Treatment of HIV-infected patients in combination with other ARVs.

FORMS TABLE

Brand name (mfr)	Forms†	Cost*
Lexiva (US); Telzir (Europe) (ViiV Healthcare)	Oral tablet 700 mg Oral suspension 50 mg/mL (225-mL bottle)	$14.49 $133.20

*Prices represent cost per unit specified, are representative of Average Wholesale Price (AWP).
†Dosage is indicated in mg unless otherwise noted.

USUAL ADULT DOSING
• Pill burden: 4 tabs/day (unboosted or boosted with RTV).
• FPV/r 700/100 mg twice daily with or w/o food or FPV/r 1400/100-200 mg once daily with or w/o food (PI-naïve patients only). Unboosted FPV (1400 mg twice daily) no longer recommended due to potential for DRV cross-resistance.
• With EFV: FPV 700 mg twice daily + RTV 100 mg twice daily + EFV 600 mg at bedtime OR FPV 1400 mg once daily + RTV 300 mg once daily + EFV 600 mg at bedtime.
• With LPV/r: generally not recommended. Consider FPV 1400 mg twice daily + LPV/r 600/150 mg twice daily with TDM.
• With NFV, IDV: inadequate data; avoid coadministration.
• With ATV: inadequate data; avoid or consider ATV 300 mg once daily + FPV/r 700/100 mg twice daily.
• With SQV: inadequate data; avoid or consider SQV/r 1000/100–200 mg twice daily + FPV 700 mg twice daily.
• With TPV: not recommended.
• With NVP: FPV/r 700/100 mg twice daily + NVP 200 mg twice daily.
• With RAL: avoid unboosted FPV. Consider FPV/r 700/100 mg twice daily + standard dose RAL with close monitoring or consider an alternative boosted PI.
• With ETR: avoid coadministration per manufacturer, but clinical significance unclear. Consider FPV/r 700/100 mg twice daily + standard dose etravirine.
• With MVC: no data. Consider FPV/r 700/100 mg twice daily + MVC 150 mg twice daily.
• With DRV/r: no data. Avoid coadministration.
• FPV tablets and liquid formulations interchangeable, but liquid formulation should be administered on empty stomach in adults (but with food in children).
• Dose in pregnancy: FPV 700 mg + RTV 100 mg twice daily resulted in 36% AUC decrease, but trough adequate in patients without PI-resistance.

ADVERSE DRUG REACTIONS
General
• ADRs similar to comparator PIs (NFV and LPV/r). GI intolerance and triglyceride elevation slightly higher compared to ATV/r.
Common
• Rash in 12%–33% of patients (<1% require discontinuation).
• GI intolerance in up to 40%–53% (severe in 5%–10%). Diarrhea less common than with NFV, but higher compared to ATV/r.
Occasional
• Triglyceride and LDL elevation (lower incidence compared to NFV); with RTV (200 mg/day) coadministration, incidence of hypertriglyceridemia (>750 mg/dL) was 11%. With FPV/r 1400/100 mg once daily, LDL elevation comparable to ATV/r; however, triglyceride elevation was slightly higher in the FPV/r-treated group (34 vs 7 g/dL increase from baseline).
• Insulin resistance.

DRUGS

- Elevated transaminases in 6%–8%.
- Fat accumulation.

Rare
- Stevens-Johnson syndrome reported. FPV has a sulfa moiety; incidence of cross-reaction with other sulfa drugs unknown. Use with caution in patients with severe skin reaction secondary to sulfonamides.
- Angioedema.
- Nephrolithiasis (unclear association).
- Myocardial infarction (OR: 1.52 per additional yr of exposure; 95% CI, 1.19–1.95) (CROI 2009, Abstract #43LB).

DRUG INTERACTIONS
- Substrate, inhibitor, and likely an inducer of CYP3A4. CYP3A4 inhibitors may increase APV levels. CYP3A4 inducers may decrease APV levels. FPV may increase or decrease levels of CYP3A4 substrates.

DRUG-DRUG INTERACTIONS—See Appendix I, p. 525, for table of drug-drug interactions.

RESISTANCE
- As with other boosted PIs, PI mutations uncommon with failure of FPV/r in previously PI-naive patients.
- I50V: primary mutation selected by APV and FPV that confers intermediate resistance to APV and low-level resistance to LPV.
- I54M/L: selected by APV and FPV, causes low-to-intermediate level APV resistance.
- I84V: primary PI mutations that causes intermediate APV resistance.
- Other PI mutations (10F/I/R/V, 32I, 46I/L, 47V, 54V, 73S, 76V, 82A/F/S/T, 90M): increasing APV resistance with multiple mutations.
- Predominant mutation observed in clinical trials: 32I, 33F, 46I, 47V, and 54L/V/M.
- Use of FPV (without RTV) may lead to cross-resistance with DRV due to selection of DRV mutations (I50V, I54M/L, I84V, 32I, 33F, 47V).

PHARMACOLOGY

Mechanism
- Rapidly hydrolyzed by cellular phosphatases to APV in the gut epithelium as it is absorbed. APV inhibits HIV protease, which results in nonfunctional, immature, and noninfectious virions.

Pharmacokinetic Parameters
- **Absorption:** independent of food.
- **Metabolism and Excretion:** metabolized by CYP3A4. The metabolite is excreted primarily in feces (75%) with 14% excreted in urine.
- **Protein Binding:** 90%.
- **Cmax, Cmin, and AUC:** Cmax = 4.85 mcg/mL, Cmin=0.35 mcg/mL after 1400-mg dose.
- **$T_\frac{1}{2}$:** 7.7 hrs.

Pregnancy Risk
- Category C: no human data. In animal studies FPV showed no embryo-fetal development abnormalities; however rate of abortion was increased.

Breastfeeding Compatibility
- No data: not recommended in the US in order to avoid postnatal transmission of HIV to the child, who may not yet be infected.

DOSING

Dosing for Decreased Hepatic Function
- No clinical data. Consider dose adjustment based on PK data: adjustment to 700 mg twice daily with Child Pugh score 5–9 (in PI-naïve patients); FPV/r 700/100 mg twice daily with Child Pugh score 5–6 (in PI-naïve or experienced); FPV/r 450/100 mg twice daily with Child Pugh score 7–9 (PI-naïve or experienced); FPV 350 mg twice daily with Child Pugh score 10–12 (PI-naïve). No data with RTV boosting in severe hepatic impairment.

Renal Dosing
- Dosing for GFR of >50: usual dose.
- Dosing for GFR of <50: no data. Usual dose likely.
- Dosing in hemodialysis: no data. Usual dose likely (on days of HD dose post-HD).

- Dosing in peritoneal dialysis: no data. Usual dose likely.
- Dosing in hemofiltration: no data.

COMMENTS

- **Pros:** noninferior to LPV/r in treatment-naïve patients; option for once-daily administration (with RTV in PI-naïve patients); can be taken with or without food; no significant PPI or H2 blocker drug-interactions when boosted with RTV; no PI resistance and reduced NRTI resistance with failure of FPV/r compared to FPV; FPV/r with lower dose RTV (1400/100 mg once daily) effective in treatment-naïve patients with similar tolerability and lipid effects as ATV/r.

- **Cons:** higher pill burden than ATV or ATV/r; FPV/r has comparable ADRs to LPV/r when used with 200 mg/day of RTV without advantage of coformuation; may not be as effective as LPV/r in PI-experienced patients. 1400/100 mg once-daily dose not as extensively studied as once-daily DRV or ATV/r; greater potential for rash than LPV/r or ATV/r. Failure of unboosted FPV can lead to DRV cross-resistance.

REFERENCES

Smith K, Weinberg W, DeJesus E, et al. Fosamprenavir or atazanavir once daily boosted with ritonavir 100 mg, plus tenofovir/emtricitabine, for the initial treatment of HIV infection: 48-week results of ALERT. *AIDS Res Ther*, 2008; 28: 5. **Comments:** Randomized clinical trial involving 106 ART-naïve, HIV+ patients. Patients received either FPV/r 1400/100 mg daily or ATV/r 300/100 mg daily, each with TDF/FTC. At wk 48, virologic suppression with daily FPV/r comparable to ATV/r-treated group, with 83% of patients in ATV/r group and 75% in the FPV/r group achieving VL <50 (P = 0.338). **Note:** This study was not powered to demonstrate noninferiority. No significant LDL elevation observed between two groups; however, TG elevation slightly higher in FPV/r-treated group (34 vs 7 g/dL increase from baseline). Diarrhea in 53% and 25% of FPV/r and ATV/r-treated patients, respectively.

Eron J, Yeni P, Gathe J, et al. The KLEAN study of fosamprenavir-ritonavir versus lopinavir-ritonavir, each in combination with abacavir-lamivudine, for initial treatment of HIV infection over 48 weeks: a randomised non-inferiority trial. *Lancet*, 2006; 368: 476–82. **Comments:** Open-label, randomized study involving 878 naïve patients who were randomized to receive FPV/r 700/100 mg twice daily or LPV/r 400/100 mg twice daily, each with ABC/3TC. At wk 48, FPV/r noninferior to LPV/r (95% CI 4.84–7.05), with 73% patients in FPV/r group and 71% in LPV/r group achieving VL <400. ADRs comparable between the two groups.

Gathe JC, Ive P, Wood R, et al. SOLO: 48-week efficacy and safety comparison of once-daily fosamprenavir/ritonavir versus twice-daily nelfinavir in naive HIV-1-infected patients. *AIDS*, 2004; 18: 1529–37. **Comments:** Open-label, randomized study involving 649 naïve patients with median CD4 170 and VL 4.81 log. Patients received FPV/r 1400/200 mg once daily + ABC/3TC or NFV 1250 mg twice daily + ABC/3TC. ITT analysis: VL <400 through wk 48 in 69% of FPV-treated patients and 68% of NFV-treated patients, difference of 1% (95% CI, -6%, 8%). VL <400 through wk 48 in 55% of FPV-treated patients vs 53% of NFV-treated patients. In a sub-analysis, patients with VL >100,000, both FPV and NFV (66% vs 64%, respectively) achieved VL <400. Daily FPV/r noninferior to NFV in PI-naïve patients. Unfortunately, this study compared FPV with NFV, a PI known to have inferior efficacy and PK profile compared to other agents in its class.

Rodriguez-French A, Boghossian J, Gray GE, et al. The NEAT study: a 48-week open-label study to compare the antiviral efficacy and safety of GW433908 versus nelfinavir in antiretroviral therapy-naive HIV-1-infected patients. *J Acquir Immune Defic Syndr*, 2004; 35: 22–32. **Comments:** Open-label, randomized study involving 249 naïve patients with median CD4 212 and VL 4.83 log. Patients received FPV 1400 mg twice daily + ABC/3TC OR NFV 1250 mg twice daily + ABC/3TC. ITT analysis: VL <400 through wk 48 in 66% of FPV-treated patients vs 51% of NFV-treated patients, difference of 15% (95% CI, 2%, 28%). VL <50 through wk 48 in 55% of FPV-treated patients vs 41% of NFV-treated patients, difference of 14% (95% CI 2%, 27%). FPV more effective in patients with VL >100,000 vs NFV (55% vs 24% VL <50, respectively). Mean VL comparable between groups at wk 48: −2.41 log for FPV group and −2.32 log for NFV group. Mean treatment difference in average change in viral load or average AUC minus baseline (AAUCMB) was −0.08 (95% CI: −0.333–0.169). Study showed that FPV (unboosted) is noninferior to NFV.

DeJesus E, LaMarca A, Sension M, et al. The context study: efficacy and safety of GW433908/RTV in PI-experienced subjects with virological failure (24-week results). Presented at: 10th Conference on Retroviruses and Opportunistic Infections (CROI 2003); February 10–14, 2003: Boston, MA. **Comments:** Open-label, randomized study involving 315 patients with virologic failure on 1 or 2 prior PI-containing regimens. Median CD4 263 and VL 4.14 log. Time-average change in VL from baseline at 48 wks were −1.53 log for twice-daily FPV and −1.76 log for LPV/r, difference of 0.244 (97.5% CI −0.017, 0.561). VL <50 through wk 48 observed in 37%, 46%, and 50% receiving once-daily FPV, twice-daily FPV, and LPV/r, respectively. Once-daily FPV performed poorly and should not be used in PI-experienced patients. Trend favoring LPV/r, although time-average change in VL from baseline not statistically different vs twice-daily FPV/r. In PI-experienced patients, FPV 700 mg twice daily + RTV 100 mg twice daily is not noninferior to LPV/r as defined by the time-average decline in VL from baseline. It should be noted that secondary endpoint of VL <50 at 48 wks was underpowered to detect difference between treatment groups.

INDINAVIR

Paul A. Pham, PharmD and John G. Bartlett, MD

INDICATIONS
FDA
• Treatment of HIV infection in combination with other ARVs.

FORMS TABLE

Brand name (mfr)	Forms†	Cost*
Crixivan (Merck Pharmaceuticals)	Oral capsule 400 mg	$3.05

*Prices represent cost per unit specified, are representative of Average Wholesale Price (AWP).
†Dosage is indicated in mg unless otherwise noted.

USUAL ADULT DOSING
• Pill burden: 6/day (based on IDV 800 mg + RTV 100 mg twice daily using 400-mg caps).
• IDV 800 mg q8h on an empty stomach or with a light snack (>1 hr ac and >2 hrs pc). Food restrictions apply to all unboosted IDV regimens below.
• With RTV (preferred): IDV 800 mg twice daily + RTV 100 mg twice daily with or w/o food (higher rate of nephrotoxicity) or IDV 400 mg twice daily + RTV 400 mg twice daily with or w/o food (higher rate of GI side effects).
• With EFV: IDV 1000 mg q8h + EFV 600 mg at bedtime or IDV 800 mg twice daily + RTV 200 mg twice daily with or w/o food + EFV 600 mg at bedtime.
• With NFV: IDV 1200 mg twice daily + NFV 1250 mg twice daily (rarely used; limited data).
• With LPV/r: IDV 600 mg or 666 mg twice daily + LPV/r 400/100 mg twice daily.
• With NVP: IDV 1000 mg q8h + NVP 200 mg twice daily or IDV 800 mg twice daily + RTV 200 mg twice daily + NVP standard dose.
• Not recommended with ATV (due to potential for additive hyperbilirubinemia) or SQV (due to *in vitro* antagonism).
• FPV: no data.
• TPV: no data. Avoid coadministration.
• DRV: dose not established. May increase risk of nephrolithiasis.
• ETR: avoid coadministration.
• RAL: no data. Usual dose likely.
• MVC: IDV standard dose + MVC 150 mg twice daily.

ADVERSE DRUG REACTIONS
Common
• GI intolerance: nausea, vomiting, and diarrhea.
• >2 retinoid-like side effects (alopecia, dry skin, mouth, and eyes) in up to 30%; paronychia in 4%–9%.
Occasional
• Nephrolithiasis ± hematuria: 5%–20% (highest risk with IDV 800 mg twice daily + RTV 100–200 mg twice daily, lowest risk with IDV 400 mg twice daily + RTV 400 mg twice daily). Encourage adequate oral hydration.
• Indirect hyperbilirubinemia (>2.5 mg/dL in 10%–15% of patients but clinically insignificant).
• Lipodystrophy, especially fat accumulation or gynecomastia.
• Insulin resistance ± hyperglycemia ± diabetes.
• Hyperlipidemia: increased triglycerides and/or cholesterol.

- Increased transaminases.
- Nephropathy: sterile leukocyturia, hematuria, IDV crystalluria, and albumin loss (35% with increased serum creatinine).
- Interstitial nephritis with pyuria and renal insufficiency reported in 2% (*Clin Infect Dis* 2002;34:1122).

Rare
- Pruritis and rash.

DRUG INTERACTIONS
- Substrate and inhibitor of CYP3A4 and weak inhibitor of CYP2D6. May increase levels of CYP3A4 (and possibly 2D6) substrates. CYP3A4 inhibitors and inducers may increase and decrease IDV levels, respectively.

DRUG-DRUG INTERACTIONS—See Appendix I, p. 535, for table of drug-drug interactions.

RESISTANCE
- V82A/T/F/S: most common mutations with IDV monotherapy, results in intermediate IDV resistance and cross-resistance to other PIs. 82I does not cause PI resistance. Primary mutation (82A/F/T/S, 84V, 46I/L): low to intermediate resistance with individual mutations, but significant IDV resistance with multiple mutations.
- Other PI mutations: (10I/R/V, 20M/R, 24I, 32I, 36I, 54V, 71V/T, 73S/A, 76V, 77I, 90M): >3 results in >4-fold decrease in susceptibility.
- RTV boosting increases activity against PI-resistant virus.

PHARMACOLOGY
Mechanism
- Inhibition of HIV protease, which results in nonfunctional, immature and noninfectious virions.

Pharmacokinetic Parameters
- **Absorption:** 65% absorption in fasting state (food decreases absorption by 77%).
- **Metabolism and Excretion:** metabolized by the CYP3A4 to several hydroxylated metabolite, which undergo subsequent glucuronidation. Both unchanged drug and metabolites are excreted in the feces.
- **Protein Binding:** 60% (variable).
- **Cmax, Cmin, and AUC:** mean steady-state AUC = 18.8 mcg hr/mL; Cmax = 7.7 mcg/mL; Cmin = 0.154 mcg/mL. Serum levels significantly decreased in pregnancy.
- **$T_{\frac{1}{2}}$:** 1.5–2 hrs.

Pregnancy Risk
- Category C: placental passage is significant in rats, but low in rabbits. Not teratogenic in rodent studies (but extra ribs have been reported). Incidence of hyperbilirubinemia in neonatal Rhesus monkeys approximately 4-fold above controls. No data on carcinogenicity. Dose not established, but should not be used without RTV boosting in pregnancy (FDA warning). Mean level decreased by 68% at 30–32 wks gestation compared to 6 wks postpartum.

Breastfeeding Compatibility
- Unknown breast milk excretion. Breastfeeding is not recommended in the US in order to avoid postnatal transmission of HIV to the child, who may not yet be infected.

DOSING.
Dosing for Decreased Hepatic Function
- Use with caution in ESLD.

Renal Dosing
- Dosing for GFR of >50: usual dose.
- Dosing for GFR of <50: usual dose likely HD.
- Dosing in hemodialysis: usual dose. Very small amount removed in HD.
- Dosing in peritoneal dialysis: no data: usual dose likely.
- Dosing in hemofiltration: no data.

COMMENTS
- **Pros:** long-term clinical data supporting durability and potency; multiple mutations required for resistance.

DRUGS

- **Cons:** variable PK and inconvenient dosing without RTV boosting; nephrolithiasis (unique to IDV); GI side effects; retinoid effects (unique to IDV); insulin resistance (more common than with other PIs). No longer recommended or widely used because of better alternatives.

SELECTED REFERENCES

Dragsted UB, Gerstoft J, Pedersen C, et al. Randomized trial to evaluate indinavir/ritonavir versus saquinavir/ritonavir in human immunodeficiency virus type 1-infected patients: the MaxCmin1 Trial. *J Infect Dis*, 2003; 188: 635–42.

Comments: Open-label trial involving 306 patients randomized to receive IDV 800 mg twice daily + RTV 100 mg twice daily or SQV (sgc but allowed to change to hgc) 1000 mg twice daily + RTV 100 mg twice daily. At 48 wks, virological failure in 43 (27%) of 158 and 37 (25%) of 148 patients in IDV/RTV and SQV/RTV arms, respectively. More patients in IDV/RTV arm experienced ADRs. Failure seen in 78 of 158 patients in the ADV/RTV arm vs 51 of 148 in the SQV/RTV arm when switching from randomized treatment counted as failure (P = 0.009).

Shulman N, Zolopa A, Havlir D, et al. Virtual inhibitory quotient predicts response to ritonavir boosting of indinavir-based therapy in human immunodeficiency virus-infected patients with ongoing viremia. *Antimicrob Agents Chemother*, 2002; 46: 3907–16.

Comments: This trial evaluated the effect of intensification with boosting with RTV. 37 HIV-infected subjects with chronic detectable viremia and receiving 800 mg of IDV 3 ×/day were switched to IDV 400 mg twice daily + RTV 400 mg twice daily for 48 wks. At wk 3, 58% (21 of 36) achieved VL <50 or a reduction from the baseline load of 0.5 log10.

Staszewski S, Morales-Ramirez J, Tashima KT, et al. Efavirenz plus zidovudine and lamivudine, efavirenz plus indinavir, and indinavir plus zidovudine and lamivudine in the treatment of HIV-1 infection in adults. Study 006 Team. *N Engl J Med*, 1999; 341: 1865–73.

Comments: Open-label study involving 450 patients naïve to 3TC, NNRTIs, and PIs: randomized to receive EFV + AZT/3TC, IDV + AZT/3TC, or EFV + IDV. At 48 wks, by ITT analysis, VL <50 achieved in more patients in EFV + AZT/3TC arm than in IDV + AZT/3TC arm (64% vs 43%, P <0.01). More patients discontinued treatment because of ADRs in IDV arm vs EFV arm (43% vs 27%, P = 0.005).

Gulick RM, Mellors JW, Havlir D, et al. Treatment with indinavir, zidovudine, and lamivudine in adults with human immunodeficiency virus infection and prior antiretroviral therapy. *N Engl J Med*, 1997; 337: 734–9.

Comments: One of earliest ART trials comparing IDV + AZT/3TC, IDV monotherapy, and AZT/3TC in 97 patients who had received AZT for >6 mos, had CD4 50–400, and VL >20,000. Decrease in VL over the 1st 24 wks was greater in 3-drug arm than in the other arms (90% vs 43% vs 0%, respectively; P <0.001 for each comparison). In an open-label continuation with up to 6-yr follow-up, 47% of patients on IDV + AZT/3TC arm maintained VL <50 (Gulick RM, Meibohm A, Havlir D, et al. *AIDS* 2003;17:2345-9).

LAMIVUDINE

Paul A. Pham, PharmD and John G. Bartlett, MD

INDICATIONS

FDA

- Treatment of HIV infection in combination with other antiretrovirals.
- Treatment of HBV (*Epivir HB*).

Non-FDA Approved Uses

- Treatment of hepatitis in HIV-HBV coinfected patients.

FORMS TABLE

Brand name (mfr)	Forms†	Cost*
Combivir (ViiV Healthcare)	Oral tablet 150 mg 3TC/ 300 mg AZT	$16.55
Epivir (ViiV Healthcare)	Oral tablet 150 mg, 300 mg Oral soln 10 mg/mL (240 mL)	$7.63; $15.27 $122.14
Epivir HB (for HBV infection) (ViiV Healthcare)	Oral tablet 100 mg Oral soln 5 mg/mL (240 mL)	$13.66 $163.97
Epzicom (ViiV Healthcare)	Oral tablet ABC 600 mg + 3TC 300 mg	$35.78

Brand name (mfr)	Forms†	Cost*
Kivexa (available in Europe) (ViiV Healthcare)	Oral tablet ABC 600 mg + 3TC 300 mg	Variable (not available in US)
Trizivir (ViiV Healthcare)	Oral tablet ABC 300 mg + AZT 300 mg + 3TC 150 mg	$26.81

*Prices represent cost per unit specified, are representative of Average Wholesale Price (AWP).
†Dosage is indicated in mg unless otherwise noted.

USUAL ADULT DOSING
- Pill burden: 1–2/day.
- As *Epivir*: 3TC 300 mg PO once daily or 150 mg PO twice daily.
- As *Combivir* or *Trizivir*: 1 tab PO twice daily.
- As *Epzicom*: 1 tab PO once daily.

ADVERSE DRUG REACTIONS
General
- One of the best tolerated NRTIs with side effect profile comparable to placebo in hepatitis trials.

Occasional
- Headache, nausea, diarrhea, abdominal pain, and insomnia (association unclear; may be due to coadministered ARVs).
- Hepatitis flare or fulminant hepatitis (in HBV coinfected patients if 3TC withdrawn or with development of 3TC-resistant HBV).

Rare
- Lactic acidosis: listed as NRTI class effect, but unlikely to be caused by 3TC. *In vitro*, 3TC, along with TDF, FTC, and ABC, are not associated with mitochondrial toxicity.
- Pancreatitis (reported in pediatric patients).

DRUG INTERACTIONS
- No pertinent drug interactions since it is not a substrate, inhibitor, or inducer of CYP450 isoforms.

DRUG-DRUG INTERACTIONS—See Appendix I, p. 552, for table of drug-drug interactions.

RESISTANCE
- 184V: selected by 3TC, resulting in high-level resistance to 3TC and FTC, slight decrease in susceptibility to ddI and ABC, and enhanced susceptibility to AZT, d4T, and TDF.
- TAMs (41L, 210W, 215Y/F, 219Q/E, 67N, 70R): resistance likely with multiple TAMs.
- T69S: high-level resistance.
- Q151M complex: high-level resistance.
- K65R: intermediate resistance.
- 44D and 119I: increase 3TC resistance in combination with TAMs.

PHARMACOLOGY
Mechanism
- Intracellular phosphorylation to active lamivudine triphosphate, which competitively inhibits HIV DNA polymerase.

Pharmacokinetic Parameters
- **Absorption:** 86%.
- **Metabolism and Excretion:** renal excretion accounts for 71%.
- **Protein Binding:** 36%.
- **Cmax, Cmin, and AUC:** Cmax = 3 mcg/mL; intracellular carbovir triphosphate 100 FM/ million cells.
- **$T_{\frac{1}{2}}$:** serum: 5–7 hrs; intracellular: 12 hrs.
- **Distribution:** widely distributed. Vd = 1.3 L/kg.

Pregnancy Risk
- Category C: negative carcinogenicity and teratogenicity studies in rodents. Placental passage ratio of 1.0 (newborn:mother). Well tolerated in pregnant patients.

DRUGS

Breastfeeding Compatibility

- No human data, breast milk excretion in animal studies. Breastfeeding is not recommended in the US in order to avoid postnatal transmission of HIV to the child, who may not yet be infected.

DOSING

Dosing for Decreased Hepatic Function

- Usual dose.

Renal Dosing

- Dosing for GFR of >50: 300 mg once daily or 150 mg PO twice daily.
- Dosing for GFR 30–49: 150 mg PO once daily.
- Dosing for GFR 15–29: 150 mg × 1 then 100 mg once daily.
- Dosing for GFR of <10: 150 mg × 1 then 25–50 mg once daily.
- Dosing in hemodialysis: 50 mg × 1, then 25–50 mg once daily (post-HD).
- Dosing in peritoneal dialysis: 150 mg × 1, then 25–50 mg once daily (limited data).
- Dosing in hemofiltration: no data; consider 150 mg PO once daily.

COMMENTS

- **Pros:** very well tolerated; active against HBV; convenient coformulations available; once-daily dosing with low pill burden (1 tab once daily); resistance (184V mutation) increases susceptibility to AZT, d4T, and TDF, and delays accumulation of TAMs; 3TC or FTC are essential components of all recommended initial regimens; coformulated with AZT (*Combivir*), ABC (*Epzicom*), and AZT + ABC (*Trizivir*). Decreased fitness with 184V mutation, which may result in partial antiviral activity.
- **Cons:** high-level resistance with single point mutation (184V); risk of hepatitis flare or fulminant hepatitis if 3TC withdrawn or if resistance develops in coinfected patients; high rate of HBV resistance with prolonged therapy if not used in combination with other anti-HBV agent (typically TDF); shorter intracellular half-life compared to FTC; more frequent emergence of 184V with AZT/3TC than TDF/FTC in GS934 study.

SELECTED REFERENCES

Fox Z, Dragsted UB, Gerstoft J, et al. A randomized trial to evaluate continuation versus discontinuation of lamivudine in individuals failing a lamivudine-containing regimen: the COLATE trial. *Antivir Ther*, 2006; 11: 761.

Comments: *In vitro* data suggest benefit of continuing 3TC after virological failure due to a decrease in viral fitness. This prospective randomized trial did not support this theory. At wk 48 the average decline in VL (AAUCMB) was comparable between the 2 groups (P = 0.65). However, continuing 3TC despite M184V mutation may be beneficial for resistance reasons, especially in patients taking AZT, d4T, or TDF. In patients who continued 3TC, 10.7 (95% CI: 7.5, 14.0) fewer nucleotide changes in viruses containing M184V (P <0.0001) were observed.

Castagna A, Danise A, Menzo S, et al. Lamivudine monotherapy in HIV-1-infected patients harbouring a lamivudine-resistant virus: a randomized pilot study (E-184V study). *AIDS*, 2006; 20: 795–803.

Comments: This open-label pilot study determined whether there was clinical or immunological benefit to continuing 3TC in patients harboring M184V mutation. Patients randomly assigned to monotherapy with 3TC 300 mg once daily or discontinuation of all ARV drugs (TI group). By wk 48, 20 of 29 (69%) patients in TI group (69%) and 12 of 29 (41%) in the 3TC group had discontinued study because of immunological (CD4 <350) or clinical failure, which was significantly delayed in 3TC group (P = 0.018).

Dienstag JL, Schiff ER, Wright TL, et al. Lamivudine as initial treatment for chronic hepatitis B in the United States. *N Engl J Med,*, 1999; 341: 1256–63.

Comments: Randomized, placebo-controlled trial in 34 centers in US with 66 untreated patients with HBV given 3TC 100 mg/day for 52 wks. Statistically significant histologic improvement with 3TC treatment (52% vs 23%), decreased levels of HBeAg (undetectable in 32% vs 11%), and suppression of HBV DNA (44% vs 16%). Rate of AEs same in both groups. Limitation of 3TC monotherapy is development of resistance, which occurred at rate of 15%–20% per yr.

Perry CM, Faulds D. Lamivudine. A review of its antiviral activity, pharmacokinetic properties and therapeutic efficacy in the management of HIV infection. *Drugs*, 1997; 53: 657–80.

Comments: Review article outlining therapeutic efficacy, pharmacokinetic properties, and antiviral activity.

LOPINAVIR/RITONAVIR

Paul A. Pham, PharmD and John G. Bartlett, MD

INDICATIONS

FDA

• Treatment of HIV infection in combination with other antiretrovirals.

FORMS TABLE

Brand name (mfr)	Forms†	Cost*
Kaletra (US); *Aluvia* (developing countries) (Abbott Laboratories)	Oral soln 400/100 mg per 5 mL (160-mL bottle)	$13.15 per 5 mL; $420.95 per 160 mL
	Oral tablet 200/50 mg; 100/25 mg	$7.02 per 200/50-mg tab; $3.51 per 100/25-mg tab

*Prices represent cost per unit specified, are representative of Average Wholesale Price (AWP).
†Dosage is indicated in mg unless otherwise noted.

USUAL ADULT DOSING

• 400/100 mg 2 tabs twice daily with or without food OR 5 mL twice daily with food.
• PI-naïve or treatment-experienced patients with <3 LPV-resistant mutations: consider 800/200 mg (4 tabs or 10 mL of liquid) once daily (tabs with or without food, liquid with food).
• With EFV: consider LPV/r 500/125 mg twice daily + EFV 600 mg at bedtime, especially in PI-experienced patients. Standard doses acceptable for PI naïve patients.
• With NVP: consider LPV/r 500/125 mg twice daily + NVP 200 mg twice daily, especially in PI-experienced patients. Standard doses acceptable for PI naïve patients.
• With IDV: LPV/r 400/100 mg (2 tabs) twice daily + IDV 600 or 666 mg twice daily.
• With SQV: LPV/r 400/100 mg (2 tabs) twice daily + SQV 1000 mg twice daily.
• With FPV: not recommended by some. Consider LPV/r 600/150 mg (3 tabs) with FPV 1400 mg twice daily (high rate of GI intolerance).
• With NFV: avoid coadministration.
• With ATV: LPV/r 400/100 mg (2 tabs) twice daily + ATV 300 mg once daily. Use with caution due to prolonged PR interval.
• With TPV/r: coadministration not recommended.
• With DRV/r: coadministration not recommended.
• With ETR: usual dose.
• With RAL: usual dose.
• With MVC: usual dose + MVC 150 mg twice daily.

ADVERSE DRUG REACTIONS

Common

• Diarrhea (any grade) 50% and 39% with LPV/r tabs administered once daily and twice daily, respectively. Moderate or severe drug diarrhea occurred in 14% and 11% in patients taking LPV/r once and twice daily, respectively.

Occasional

• Nausea, vomiting, abdominal pain, asthenia, and headache.
• Elevated triglycerides (12%–22%) and cholesterol (14%–22%). Significant triglyceride elevation more common when LPV/r is combined with EFV.
• Insulin resistance, hyperglycemia, and diabetes.
• Hepatitis (10%–12%).

Rare

• Pancreatitis (unclear association).
• Rash. Toxic epidermal necrolysis (TEN) has been reported.
• Nephrolithiasis (unclear association).
• QTc prolongation (5.3 msec [95% CI 8.1]). Use with caution with other drugs that can prolong QTc.

DRUGS

- PR interval prolongation (24.9 msec [95% CI 21.5, 28.3]). 2nd- and 3rd-degree AV block reported. Use with caution in patients with baseline cardiac conduction abnormalities.

DRUG INTERACTIONS

- Substrate, inhibitor, and likely an inducer of CYP3A4 and glucoronyl transferase. May also weakly induce CYP2C9 and CYP2C19 and weakly inhibit CYP2D6 (clinical significance unknown). LPV/r generally increases serum levels of drugs that are substrates of CYP3A4 (but reduction in serum levels have also occurred). Drugs that are inducers of CYP3A4 may decrease serum levels of LPV. Drugs that are inhibitors of CYP3A4 may increase serum levels of LPV.

DRUG-DRUG INTERACTIONS—See Appendix I, p. 553, for table of drug-drug interactions.

RESISTANCE

- Resistance develops from multiple PI mutations.
- Primary PI mutations (32I, 82A/F/T/S, 47V/A) and secondary PI mutations (10, 20, 24, 33, 46, 47, 50, 53, 54, 63, 71, 73, 76, 84, 90): >4 mutations: decrease potency of LPV/r.
- I50V: selected by APV; reduces susceptibility to LPV.
- 63P: reduced susceptibility to LPV when combined with other PI mutations.

PHARMACOLOGY

Mechanism

- Inhibition of HIV protease, which results in nonfunctional, immature, and noninfectious virions.

Pharmacokinetic Parameters

- **Absorption:** tabs: food increases bioavailability by 27%. Caps and oral soln: increase in bioavailability by 48% and 80%, respectively, when administered with moderate fat meal (23%–25% of calories from fat).
- **Metabolism and Excretion:** primarily biliary excretion with less than 3% excreted unchanged in the urine.
- **Protein Binding:** 98%–99%.
- **Cmax, Cmin, and AUC:** LPV/r 400 mg twice daily at steady state: mean Cmax = 9.8 (±3.7) mcg/mL; Cmin = 7.1 (±2.9) mcg/mL; AUC 92.6 (±36.7) mcg/mL hr.
- **$T_{\frac{1}{2}}$:** 5–6 hrs.

Pregnancy Risk

- Category C: no treatment-related malformation seen in animal studies. No embryonic and fetal development toxicities seen in rabbits. Pregnancy Registry shows birth defects in 5/267 (1.9%) 1st-trimester exposures: less than the expected rate of 3.1%. Consider increasing dose to 3 tabs twice daily in 3rd trimester and resume standard dose after delivery.

Breastfeeding Compatibility

- No data. Breastfeeding in HIV+ patients not recommended in US in order to avoid postnatal transmission of HIV to the child, who may not yet be infected.

DOSING

Dosing for Decreased Hepatic Function

- Use with caution in ESLD.

Renal Dosing

- Dosing for GFR of 50–80: usual dose.
- Dosing for GFR of 10–50: no data; usual dose likely.
- Dosing for GFR of <10: no data; usual dose likely.
- Dosing in hemodialysis: usual dose (not removed with HD).
- Dosing in peritoneal dialysis: no data; usual dose likely.
- Dosing in hemofiltration: no data.

COMMENTS

- **Pros:** coformulation with RTV may improve adherence in some patients. Preferred PI in pregnancy. Long-term efficacy as initial therapy; good PK profile that exceed IC_{50} by >25-fold throughout dosing interval, enabling LPV/r to have activity against some PI-resistant strains, though DRV/r or sometimes TPV/r now preferred for patients with PI resistance based on TITAN, POWER, and RESIST studies. Better CD4 response compared to EFV-containing regimens, and less resistance with failure.

- **Cons:** GI intolerance, hyperlipidemia, and/or insulin resistance in some patients. More GI toxicity than with some other boosted PIs. Virologically inferior to EFV-containing regimens in PI-naïve patients. DRV/r and TPV/r preferred for highly experienced patients, and DRV/r may have advantage even in LPV-susceptible, PI-experienced patients. For PI-naïve patients, other once-daily boosted PIs with lower RTV dose (e.g., ATV/r, DRV/r, and possibly FPV/r) have comparable or superior efficacy with better tolerability and less toxicity. May have lower potency in patients with baseline CD4 <50 compared to CD4 >200.

SELECTED REFERENCES

Molina J, Andrade-Villanueva J, Echevarria J, et al. Once-daily atazanavir/ritonavir versus twice-daily lopinavir/ritonavir, each in combination with tenofovir and emtricitabine, for management of antiretroviral-naive HIV-1-infected patients: 48 week efficacy and safety results of the CASTLE study. *Lancet*, 2008; 372: 646–55.

Comments: CASTLE trial compared ATV/r 300/100 mg daily vs LPV/r 400/100 mg (caps) twice daily both combined with TDF/FTC in 883 treatment-naïve patients. Results at 48 wks showed comparable rates of VL (<50 c/mL) suppression (78% for ATV/r vs 76% for LPV/r). Response rates comparable with VL >100K; however, there was lower rates of virologic suppression in LPV/r-treated patients with lower baseline CD4 counts (80% with CD4 >200 vs 63% with CD4 <50; P = 0.0085). Lower response rate observed with LPV/r-treated group may be due to higher discontinuation due to adverse events compared to ATV/r-treated patients. GI intolerance was higher in LPV/r-treated group (diarrhea [2% vs 11%] and nausea [4% vs 8%]). As expected, LPV/r-treated patients had greater lipid changes from baseline (12% vs 24% TC increase and 13% vs 51% TG increase).

Riddler SA, Haubrich R, DiRienzo G, et al. Class-sparing regimens for initial treatment of HIV-1 infection. (ACTG 5142). *N Engl J Med*, 2008; 358: 2095–106.

Comments: 757 ARV-naïve patients randomized to 3 regimens: LPV/r + NRTIs, EFV + NRTIs, and LPV/r + EFV. At a median follow-up of 112 wks, the time to virologic failure was longer in EFV-treated patients (P = 0.006). At 96 wks, 89% of patients in EFV + 2 NRTIs arm had VL <50 vs 77% in LPV/r + 2 NRTIs arm (P = 0.003). LPV/r + EFV arm had similar virologic efficacy compared to EFV + 2 NRTIs arm (83% vs 89%). No difference between 3 arms in time to 1st treatment-limiting toxicity, but significant triglycerides elevation was higher in EFV + LPV/r-treated patients. Despite superior virologic response in the EFV + 2 NRTIs regimen, LPV/r-containing regimen resulted in higher CD4 increase (241 vs 285, P = 0.01). In patients with virologic failure, development of resistance the highest in the EFV + LPV/r arm, followed by EFV + 2 NRTIs arm compared to LPV/r + 2 NRTIs. Any mutations (excluding minor PI mutations were observed in 70%, 48%, and 21% in EFV + LPV/r arm, EFV + 2 NRTIS, and LPV/r + 2 NRTIs, respectively.

Ortiz R, Dejesus E, Khanlou H, et al. Efficacy and safety of once-daily darunavir/ritonavir versus lopinavir/ritonavir in treatment-naive HIV-1-infected patients at week 48. *AIDS*, 2008; 22: 1389.

Comments: ARTEMIS evaluated DRV/r (800/100 mg once daily) vs LPV/r (once or twice daily, but majority received twice-daily dosing) both combined with TDF/FTC in treatment-naïve patients. Characteristics of patients (N = 689) comparable at baseline with median VL of ~70,000 and CD4 220. At wk 48 (ITT-TLOVR), 84% of DRV/r-treated patients and 78% of LPV/r-treated patients achieved VL <50; difference was 5.6% (P <0.0001) and within 12% margin of noninferiority, but missed claim of superiority (P = 0.062). However, in patients with baseline VL >100,000 c/mL, DRV/r superior (79% vs 67%; P <0.05), which was subsequently attributed to use of once-daily LPV/r. Median CD4 increase comparable between 2 groups (137 for DRV/r and 141 for LPV/r). GI intolerance was significantly higher in the LPV/r-treated patients (14% vs 7%) and moderate-to-severe diarrhea (10% vs 4%).

Madruga JV, Berger D, McMurchie M, et al. Efficacy and safety of darunavir-ritonavir compared with that of lopinavir-ritonavir at 48 weeks in treatment-experienced, HIV-infected patients in TITAN: a randomised controlled phase III trial. *Lancet*, 2007; 370: 49.

Comments: Evaluated DRV/r (600/100 mg twice daily) vs LPV/r (400/100 mg twice daily), both with OBT, in patients who had failed prior therapy and were naïve to LPV/r. Baseline patients characteristic (N = 595) comparable between 2 groups: median VL 4.31 log, CD4 232, 31% were PI-naïve; 82% were susceptible to 4 or more PIs. At wk 48, significantly more DRV/r- than LPV/r-treated patients had VL <400 c/mL (77% vs 68%; estimated difference 9%, 95% CI 2–16) and within 12% margin of noninferiority.

Johnson M, Grinsztejn B, Rodriguez C, et al. 96-week comparison of once-daily atazanavir/ritonavir and twice-daily lopinavir/ritonavir in patients with multiple virologic failures. *AIDS*, 2006; 20(5): 711–8.

Comments: 358 patients who had failed at least 2 ART regimens containing at least 1 PI, NNRTI, or NRTI randomized to ATV/r 300/100 mg once daily, ATV/SQV 400/1200 mg once daily, or LPV/r 400/100 mg twice daily each combined with TDF + 1 NRTI. Not all patients were heavily PI-experienced. At 48 wks, trend favoring LPV/r arm (46% vs 38% VL <50, P = NS). However, at 96 wks, virologic suppression comparable between ATV/r- and LPV/r-treated patients. Mean VL reduction L −2.29 and −2.08 login ATV/r and LPV/r groups, respectively. Virologic response higher with <4 PI mutations at baseline. In patients with 4+ PI mutations, undetectable VL achieved in only 20% and 23% in ATV/r and LPV/r, respectively. Total cholesterol (+9%) and fasting TG (+30%) higher in LPV/r-treated group. Grade 2–4 diarrhea less common in ATV/r patients (3%) vs LPV/r (13%) patients. Study limitations: unknown percentage of critical PI mutations, only 1/3 on PI-containing regimen at time of genotype analysis; post-hoc analysis of the truly PI-experienced underpowered to show differences between groups.

Dragsted UB, Gerstoft J, Youle M, et al. A randomized trial to evaluate lopinavir/ritonavir versus saquinavir/ritonavir in HIV-1-infected patients: the MaxCmin2 trial. *Antivir Ther*, 2005; 10: 735–43.

Comments: This trial compared LPV/r (400/100 mg twice daily) with SQV/r (1000/100 mg twice daily) + at least 2 NRTI/NNRTIs in 324 patients. Population heterogenous (33% naïve and 32% with virologic failure of at least 1 PI). At 48 wks, treatment failure occurred in 29/163 (18%) and 53/161 (33%) of patients in the LPV/r and SQV/r arms, respectively (ITT, P = 0.002, log rank test). Risk of discontinuation also higher in SQV arm (30% vs 14%, P = 0.0001). No overall difference in risk of Grade 3 and 4 ADRs in the 2 arms.

Cohen C, Nieto-Cisneros L, Zala C, et al. Comparison of atazanavir with lopinavir/ritonavir in patients with prior protease inhibitor failure: a randomized multinational trial. *Curr Med Res Opin*, 2005; 21: 1683–92.

Comments: Phase III trial comparing ATV (400 mg once daily) with LPV/r (400/100 mg twice daily), in combination with 2 NRTIs, in 300 experienced patients with virologic failure following single PI-based regimen. At 48 wks, LPV/r resulted in significantly greater reduction in VL than unboosted ATV (−2.02 vs −1.59 log, P <0.001). Unboosted ATV is inferior to LPV/r for salvage.

DeJesus E, LaMarca A, Sension M, Beltran C, Yeni P. The Context Study: efficacy and safety of GW433908/RTV in PI-experienced subjects with virological failure (24 week results). Presented at: 10th Conference on Retroviruses and Opportunistic Infections (CROI 2003); February 10–14, 2003: Boston, MA.

Comments: Open-label, randomized study of 315 patients who had experienced virologic failure to 1 or 2 prior PI-containing regimens. Median CD4 263 and VL 4.14 log. Time-average change in VL from baseline at 48 wks: −1.53 log for twice-daily FPV/r and −1.76 log for LPV/r, a difference of 0.244 (97.5% CI −0.017, 0.561). VL <50 through wk 48 in 37%, 46%, and 50% on once-daily FPV/r, twice-daily FPV/r, and LPV/r, respectively. Once-daily FPV/r performed poorly and should not be used in PI-experienced patients. Trend favoring LPV/r, although the time-average change in VL from baseline not statistically different from twice-daily FPV/r. In PI-experienced patients, FPV 700 mg twice daily + RTV 100 mg twice daily was not noninferior to LPV/r as defined by the time-average decline in VL from baseline. Study underpowered for secondary endpoint of VL <50 at 48 wks.

Bongiovanni M, Bini T, Adorni F, et al. Virological success of lopinavir/ritonavir salvage regimen is affected by an increasing number of lopinavir/ritonavir-related mutations. *Antivir Ther*, 2003; 8: 209–14.

Comments: Independent predictive factors related to virologic success with LPV/r regimens are VL and number of mutations at baseline; each additional log of VL reduced probability of virological success by 34.0% and each extra mutation by 14.5%.

Walmsley S, Bernstein B, King M, et al. Lopinavir-ritonavir versus nelfinavir for the initial treatment of HIV infection. *N Engl J Med*, 2002; 346: 2039–46.

Comments: Prospective, double-blind trial involving 653 naïve patients randomized to LPV/r + d4T + 3TC or NFV + d4T + 3TC. Patients well matched at baseline with median CD4 count of 232 and VL 5.01–4.98 log. At wk 48, more patients treated with LPV/r than NFV had HIV RNA <400 (75% vs 63%, P <0.001) and <50 (67% vs 52%, P <0.001). Discontinuation rate due to ADR was 3.4% among patients receiving LPV/r and 3.7% among patients receiving NFV. In patients with virologic failure, genotypic resistance was observed in 25 of 76 NFV-treated patients (33%) and none of 37 patients treated with LPV/r (P <0.001).

MARAVIROC

Maureen M. Forrestel, PharmD and Paul A. Pham, PharmD

INDICATIONS

FDA

- Used in combination with other ARVs in ART-experienced adult patients infected with CCR5 (R5)-tropic HIV-1.
- Used in combination with other ARVs in ART-naïve adult patients infected with CCR5 (R5)-tropic HIV-1 (not a DHHS preferred 1st-line agent).

FORMS TABLE

Brand name (mfr)	Forms†	Cost*
Selzentry (US); *Celsentri* (Europe) (ViiV Healthcare)	Oral tablet 150 mg; 300 mg	$18.36 for both 150-mg and 300-mg tabs

*Prices represent cost per unit specified, are representative of Average Wholesale Price (AWP).
†Dosage is indicated in mg unless otherwise noted.

USUAL ADULT DOSING
- Pill burden: 2 tabs/day (4/day if using 600 mg twice daily).
- MVC 300 mg PO twice daily with or without food.
- With all PIs (except TPV/r): MVC 150 mg PO twice daily (MVC 300 mg twice daily with TPV/r).
- With LPV/r + EFV: MVC 150 mg PO twice daily.
- With SQV/r + EFV: MVC 150 mg PO twice daily.
- With EFV (without PI coadministration): MVC 600 mg PO twice daily. Monitor for postural hypotension during the 1st 2 wks.
- With EFV (with PI coadministration): MVC 150 mg twice daily.
- With ETR (without PI coadministration): MVC 600 mg twice daily. Monitor for postural hypotension during the 1st 2 wks.
- With ETR (with PI coadministration): MVC 150 mg twice daily.
- With NVP: limited data, consider MVC 300 mg PO twice daily.
- With RAL: standard dose.

ADVERSE DRUG REACTIONS
General
- Generally well tolerated in clinical trials, with similar rates of study discontinuation vs placebo.

Common
- Diarrhea, nausea, headache, and fatigue at rates similar to or less than those of placebo.

Occasional
- Cough, fever, and upper respiratory tract infection (pneumonia uncommon).
- Rash.
- AST/ALT elevation.
- CK elevation.
- Myalgia.
- Abdominal pain.
- Dizziness.
- Orthostatic hypotension (dose dependent, uncommon at recommended dose, but patients with renal insufficiency and those treated with higher dose may be at increased risk).

Rare
- Hepatotoxicity with allergic features (rash, eosinophilia, elevated IgE).
- Cardiac events related to coronary artery disease (1.3%).

DRUG INTERACTIONS
- Does not inhibit or induce CYP3A4. As MVC is a substrate of CYP3A4 and Pgp, dose should be adjusted when coadministered with CYP3A4 and/or Pgp inhibitors or inducers. Drug-drug interactions are unlikely with NRTIs and enfuvirtide.

DRUG-DRUG INTERACTIONS—See Appendix I, p. 564, for table of drug-drug interactions.
RESISTANCE
- MVC-resistant viruses that emerged *in vitro* contained amino acid substitutions/deletions in the V3 loop of the HIV-1 envelope (gp120), with primary substitutions isolated being A19T and I26V. MVC failure can also be due to selection of preexisting X4- or dual/mixed-tropic virus, that is not inhibited by MVC.

PHARMACOLOGY
Mechanism
- MVC inhibits CCR5 receptors on the cell membrane, preventing the interaction of gp120 and CCR5 necessary for CCR5-tropic HIV-1 to enter cells.

Pharmacokinetic Parameters
- **Absorption:** rapid absorption with a 33% bioavailability.
- **Metabolism and Excretion:** 22% metabolized by CYP3A4 (N-dealkylation) and 11% hydroxylated. Both inactive metabolites and unchanged drugs are excreted via fecal route (>76%) with 20% excreted in the urine.
- **Protein Binding:** 76%.
- **Cmax, Cmin, and AUC:** Cmax = 266 ng/mL; Cmin = 54 ng/mL; AUC = 1681 ng h/mL.
- **T$_{\frac{1}{2}}$:** 14–18 hrs.
- **Distribution:** 194 L.

DRUGS

Pregnancy Risk
- Category B: no human data. Not teratogenic in rats or rabbits studies.

Breastfeeding Compatibility
- Based on animal studies, MVC is extensively secreted into rat milk. MVC is not recommended in breastfeeding mothers.

DOSING

Dosing for Decreased Hepatic Function
- Limited data; no dose adjustment likely with mild to moderate. A single-dose study in subjects with mild-to-moderate hepatic impairment has shown little impact on MVC pharmacokinetics, with less than a 50% increase in exposure to MVC.

Renal Dosing
- Dosing for GFR of 50–80: usual dose.
- Dosing for GFR of 30–50: usual dose.
- Dosing for GFR 10–30: consider MVC 150 mg twice daily if Sx of postural hypotension. Avoid MVC if coadministered with CYP3A4 inhibitors or inducers.
- Dosing for GFR of <10: consider MVC 150 mg twice daily if Sx of postural hypotension. Avoid MVC if coadministered with CYP3A4 inhibitors or inducers.
- Dosing in hemodialysis: MVC not significantly removed in HD. Consider MVC 150 mg twice daily if Sx of postural hypotension. Avoid MVC if coadministered with CYP3A4 inhibitors or inducers.
- Dosing in peritoneal dialysis: no data.
- Dosing in hemofiltration: no data.

COMMENTS

- 1st CCR5 antagonist. Well tolerated, with no cross-resistance to currently available drugs. Effective when used in combination with OBT in heavily treatment-experienced patients with R5-tropic virus and multiple resistance mutations who were failing therapy. Use of MVC in these patients resulted in mean VL reduction of almost 2 logs and VL suppression to <50 in 45% of treated patients.
- Not recommended in patients with dual/mixed (D/M)- or X4-tropic virus due to lack of efficacy.
- Tropism assay should be performed prior to initiation of treatment with MVC. *Trofile* (Monogram Biosciences, Inc.) coreceptor tropism assay is only commercially available assay that has been well studied; it detects presence of R5-, X4-, or D/M tropic *virus*.
- Tropism assay requires VL >1000, which means that MVC cannot be used to substitute for other drugs in a suppressive regimen.
- Sensitivity of former tropism assay to detect D/M or X4-tropic virus was 100% when it comprised at least 10% of total viral population, but 83% when it comprised 5% of population. In MOTIVATE trials, 7.6% of participants had R5-tropic virus at screening but D/M-tropic virus at baseline (4–6 wks later), presumably representing failure of initial assay to detect D/M- or X4-tropic virus present at low levels. Current enhanced sensitivity assay has sensitivity of 99.7%.
- Although MVC clearly has a role in management of treatment-experienced patients, lack of long-term safety data, nonviral target, high cost of tropism assay, inconvenience of twice-daily dosing, and failure to meet noninferiority threshold compared to EFV for <50 threshold in the MERIT trial means that MVC is unlikely be widely used in treatment-naïve patients in the near future, though approved for this indication.

SELECTED REFERENCES

Cooper DA, Heera J, Goodrich J, et al. Maraviroc versus efavirenz, both in combination with zidovudine-lamivudine, for the treatment of antiretroviral-naive subjects with CCR5-tropic HIV-1 infection. *J Infect Dis*, 2010; 201: 803.

Comments: Over 700 patients with mean baseline VL 4.8 logs and median CD4 of approximately 250 enrolled in this prospective randomized trial. Participants received AZT/3TC with either EFV or MVC for 48 wks. MVC (dosed twice daily) found to be noninferior to EFV in viral suppression to <400 (70.6% vs 73.1%, respectively), but did not meet noninferiority threshold using <50 assay (65.3% vs 69.3%). However, a subsequent analysis using enhanced sensitivity Trofile assay found that 3.5% (25 patients) with R5 virus at screening had D/M-virus visit, presumably reflecting sensitivity of the Trofile assay in use at the time. Elimination of these 25 patients would eliminate the difference in virologic suppression. Mean CD4 increases were 170 and 144 in MVC- and EFV-treated patients, respectively. Overall discontinuation rates similar between groups; however, patients on MVC less likely than patients on EFV to withdraw from study due to AEs (4.2% vs 13.6%, respectively), but more likely to withdraw due to lack of treatment effect (11.9% vs 4.2%, respectively). CNS side effects more common in EFV-treated group.

Gulick RM, Lalezari J, Goodrich J, et al. Maraviroc for previously treated patients with R5 HIV-1 infection. *N Engl J Med*, 2008; 359: 1429–41.

Comments: Heavily treatment-experienced patients who were failing their current ARV regimens, had at least 6 mos of prior treatment with at least 1 agent (2 agents for PIs) from 3 of 4 ARV drug classes, and/or documented resistance to 3 of the 4 ARV drug classes and VL >5000 were enrolled. patients enrolled had a median VL of 4.86 log and median CD4 of 167. 41% had baseline VL>100,000 and 58% had a baseline CD4 <200. Approximately 2/3 had an overall susceptibility score (OSS, number of active drugs in background regimen) of <3. Patients randomized to MVC once daily, MVC twice daily, or placebo, each with OBT. At 48 wks, mean decrease in VL greater with MVC than with placebo: ~1.66 and ~1.82 log with once-daily and twice-daily regimens, respectively, vs -0.80 with placebo. When stratified by ENF use, virologic suppression significantly greater in ENF-treated patients who had not previously used ENF (van der Ryst E, et al. 4th International Aids Society (IAS) Conference, Sydney, 2007, Abstract WEPEB115LB). As expected, virologic response better if OBR contained active drugs. VL<50 achieved in 32.7%, 46.7%, 55.7%, and 59% of MVC-treated patients when they had 0, 1, 2, 3 active drugs in OBR, respectively.

NELFINAVIR

Paul A. Pham, PharmD and John G. Bartlett, MD

INDICATIONS

FDA

- Treatment of HIV infection in combination with other antiretrovirals.

FORMS TABLE

Brand name (mfr)	Forms†	Cost*
Viracept (ViiV Healthcare [US and Canada] and Roche [outside the US and Canada])	Oral tablet 250 mg; 625 mg	$2.81 per 250-mg tablet; $7.03 per 625-mg tablet
	Oral powder 50 mg/g (144-g container)	$74.15

*Prices represent cost per unit specified, are representative of Average Wholesale Price (AWP).
†Dosage is indicated in mg unless otherwise noted.

USUAL ADULT DOSING

- Pill burden: 4 tabs/day (625-mg tab).
- NFV 1250 mg twice daily with fatty meal.
- With EFV or NVP: standard doses.
- With IDV: NFV 1250 mg twice daily + IDV 1200 mg twice daily (limited data, not recommended).
- With RTV: limited data, high rate of GI intolerance with marginal PK benefit, not recommended.
- With SQV: limited data; limited PK benefit; not recommended.
- With LPV/r: limited data; generally not recommended.
- With ATV, FPV, TPV, and DRV: no data, avoid coadministration.
- With MVC: no data; consider MVC 150 mg twice daily.
- With RAL: no data; standard doses likely.
- With ETR: no data, consider standard doses.

ADVERSE DRUG REACTIONS

Common

- Self-limited secretory diarrhea in 10%–30%. Typically responds to regular use of fiber supplements, calcium supplements, or loperamide.

Occasional

- Fat accumulation.
- Hyperlipidemia.

DRUGS

- Insulin resistance ± hyperglycemia or diabetes.
- Transaminase elevation.

Rare
- Urticaria.
- Severe hepatitis.

DRUG INTERACTIONS
- Substrate of 2C19 (major) and CYP3A4 (minor), inducer and inhibitor at CYP3A4, and inducer of glucuronosyl transferase. NFV active M8 metabolite is a substrate of CYP3A4 (major). Drugs that are inhibitors of CYP3A4 may increase levels of main NFV metabolite (N8). Drugs that are inducers of CYP2C19 may decrease NFV serum levels.

DRUG-DRUG INTERACTIONS—See Appendix I, p. 569, for table of drug-drug interactions.

RESISTANCE
- D30N: most common primary mutation selected by NFV, resulting in intermediate resistance to NFV, but no cross-resistance to other PIs.
- L90M: can also be selected by NFV, resulting in intermediate resistance to NFV and SQV, and low-level cross-resistance to other PIs.
- Other PI mutations (10F/I, L36I, 46I/L, 71V/T, 77I, 82A/F/T/S, 84V, 88D/S): multiple mutations will result in high-level resistance.

PHARMACOLOGY

Mechanism
- Inhibition of HIV protease, which results in nonfunctional, immature, and noninfectious virions.

Pharmacokinetic Parameters
- **Absorption:** variable absorption 20%–80%; high-fat food (20% and 50% fat content) increases absorption by 3–4-fold, respectively.
- **Metabolism and Excretion:** NFV is converted to its major active metabolite (M8) by CYP2C19; M8 is metabolized by CYP3A4. Both unchanged drug and metabolites are excreted in the feces.
- **Protein Binding:** 99%.
- **Cmax, Cmin, and AUC:** mean steady-state Cmax = 3–4 mcg/mL; Cmin = 1–3 mcg/mL; AUC = 53 mcg/mL hr.
- **$T_{\frac{1}{2}}$:** 3.5–5 hrs.

Pregnancy Risk
- Category B: placental passage unknown. Not teratogenic in rodent studies.

Breastfeeding Compatibility
- Unknown breast milk excretion. Breastfeeding not recommended in the US in order to avoid postnatal transmission of HIV to infant.

DOSING

Dosing for Decreased Hepatic Function
- Use with caution in ESLD.

Renal Dosing
- Dosing for GFR of 50–80: usual dose.
- Dosing for GFR of 10–50: usual dose likely.
- Dosing for GFR of <10: usual dose likely (PK unchanged in renal failure).
- Dosing in hemodialysis: usual dose. Removed with HD, must be given post-HD on days of dialysis.
- Dosing in peritoneal dialysis: no data: usual dose likely.
- Dosing in hemofiltration: no data.

COMMENTS
- **Pros:** extensive experience in pregnancy.
- **Cons:** the only unboostable PI; less potent than NNRTIs and boosted PIs; high variability in absorption with dependence on fatty foods; more diarrhea compared to other PIs; failure with L90M can occur (compared to little or no resistance with boosted PIs), leading to greater PI cross-resistance; twice-daily dosing.

SELECTED REFERENCES

Rodriguez-French A, Boghossian J, Gray GE, et al. The NEAT study: a 48-week open-label study to compare the antiviral efficacy and safety of GW433908 versus nelfinavir in antiretroviral therapy-naive HIV-1-infected patients. *J Acquir Immune Defic Syndr*, 2004; 35: 22–32.
Comments: Open-label, randomized study involving 249 naïve patients with median CD4 212 and VL 4.83 log. Patients received FPV 1400 mg twice daily + ABC/3TC or NFV 1250 mg twice daily + ABC/3TC. ITT analysis: VL <50 through wk 48 in 55% of FPV-treated patients vs 41% of NFV-treated patients, difference of 14% (95% CI 2%, 27%). FPV retained good viral potency in patients with HIV RNA >100,000 compared to NFV (55% vs 24% achieved VL <50, respectively). Mean VL comparable between treatment groups at wk 48: −2.41 log for FPV twice-daily group and −2.32 log for NFV twice-daily group. Mean treatment difference −0.082 (95% CI: −0.333–0.169). Only 24% of patients with VL >100,000 achieved VL <50 c/mL.

Rufo PA, Lin PW, Andrade A, et al. Diarrhea-associated HIV-1 APIs potentiate muscarinic activation of Cl-secretion by T84 cells via prolongation of cytosolic Ca2+ signaling. *Am J Physiol Cell Physiol*, 2004; 286: C998–C1008.
Comments: Prospective study showing that NFV induces a secretory form of diarrhea in HIV+ patients and has a secretagogue effect on intestinal epithelial cell lines.

Gathe JC, Ive P, Wood R, et al. SOLO: 48-week efficacy and safety comparison of once-daily fosamprenavir/ritonavir versus twice-daily nelfinavir in naive HIV-1-infected patients. *AIDS*, 2004; 18: 1529–37.
Comments: Open-label, randomized study involving 649 naïve patients with median CD4 of 170 and VL of 4.81 log10. Patients received FPV 1400 mg once daily + RTV 200 mg once daily + ABC 300 mg twice daily + 3TC 150 mg twice daily or NFV 1250 mg twice daily + ABC 300 mg twice daily + 3TC 150 mg twice daily. ITT analysis: VL <400 through wk 48 in 69% of FPV-treated patients and 68% of NFV-treated patients, difference of 1% (95% CI, −6%, 8%). VL <50 through wk 48 in 55% of FPV-treated patients vs 53% of NFV-treated patients. In a sub-analysis patients with VL >100,000, both FPV and NFV (66% vs 64%, respectively) achieved VL <400. Daily FPV/r was equivalent to NFV in PI-naïve patients. Unfortunately, this study compared FPV with NFV, a PI known to have an inferior PK profile compared to other agents in its class.

Robbins GK, De Gruttola V, Shafer RW, et al. Comparison of sequential three-drug regimens as initial therapy for HIV-1 infection. *N Engl J Med*, 2003; 349: 2293–303.
Comments: ACTG 384: 620 patients randomized to compare sequential 3-drug regimens in 4 groups: EFV-based ART combined with AZT/3TC or d4T/ddI or NFV + AZT/3TC or d4T/ddI. EFV outperformed NFV in all arms. Starting with a 3-drug regimen containing EFV combined with AZT and 3TC appeared to delay failure of 2nd regimen, compared with starting a regimen containing NFV (HR for failure of 2nd regimen, 0.71; 95% CI, 0.48–1.06).

Walmsley S, Bernstein B, King M, et al. Lopinavir-ritonavir versus nelfinavir for the initial treatment of HIV infection. *N Engl J Med*, 2002; 346: 2039–46.
Comments: Prospective, double-blind trial involving 653 naïve HIV+ patients. Patients randomized to LPV/r + d4T/3TC or NFV + d4T/3TC. At wk 48, greater proportions of patients treated with LPV/r than of patients treated with NFV had VL<400 (75% vs 63%, P <0.001) and <50 (67% vs 52%, P <0.001). Less variability in response across VL and CD4 spectra with LPV/r than NFV, and less resistance with failure.

Podzamczer D, Ferrer E, Consiglio E, et al. A randomized clinical trial comparing nelfinavir or nevirapine associated to zidovudine/lamivudine in HIV-infected naive patients (the Combine Study). *Antivir Ther*, 2002; 7: 81–90.
Comments: Prospective randomized trial comparing NVP/AZT/3TC to NFV/AZT/3TC. At 12 mos in the ITT analysis, proportion of patients with VL <200 was 60% in the NFV/AZT/3TC arm and 75% NVP/AZT/3TC arm (P = 0.06), and proportion <20 was 50% and 65%, respectively (P = 0.06). Trend favoring NVP, but not statistically significant.

DRUGS

NEVIRAPINE

Paul A. Pham, PharmD and John G. Bartlett, MD

INDICATIONS

FDA

- Treatment of HIV infection in combination with other antiretrovirals.
- Due to increased risk of hepatitis, avoid starting NVP in women with CD4 >250 and men with CD4 >400.

Non-FDA Approved Uses

- Single dose at time of delivery to prevent perinatal transmission (widely used in developing countries, but risk of NNRTI resistance; combination therapy preferred when available). Risk of hepatitis for women with CD4 >250 does not apply to single-dose NVP.

Brand name (mfr)	Forms†	Cost*
Viramune and	Oral tablet 200 mg	$10.24
Viramune XR	Oral suspension 50 mg/5 mL (240 mL)	$118.50 per 240 mL
(Boehringer Ingleheim)	Oral XR tablet 400 mg	$20.47

*Prices represent cost per unit specified, are representative of Average Wholesale Price (AWP).
†Dosage is indicated in mg unless otherwise noted.

USUAL ADULT DOSING

- Pill burden: 1 tab/day (*Viramune XR*).
- NVP 200 mg once daily ×14 days then 200 mg twice daily or 400 mg (XR tablet) once daily.
- If rash occurs during initial 14 days lead-in period of 200 mg/day, NVP dose should not be increased until the rash has resolved (BUT total duration of once-daily lead-in dosing period should not exceed 28 days).
- With LPV/r: consider NVP standard dose + LPV/r 600/150 mg (3 tabs) twice daily in PI-experienced patients. Standard doses of both drugs may be adequate in PI-naïve patients.
- With IDV: NVP standard dose + either IDV 1000 mg q8h or IDV 800 mg twice daily + RTV 100 mg twice daily.
- With SQV: NVP standard dose + SQV 1000 mg twice daily + RTV 100 mg twice daily.
- With NFV: NVP standard dose + NFV 1250 mg twice daily.
- With FPV: consider NVP standard dose + FPV 700 mg twice daily + RTV 100 mg twice daily (limited data).
- With ATV: avoid coadministration.
- With DRV: consider NVP standard dose + DRV/r 600/100 mg twice daily (limited data).
- With TPV: consider NVP standard dose + TPV/r 500/200 mg twice daily (limited data).
- With MVC: consider NVP standard dose + MVC 300 mg twice daily (limited data).
- With ETR or EFV: not recommended.
- With RAL: standard doses.
- Discontinuation of NVP-based regimen: continue NRTI for 7 days after NVP discontinuation or substitute PI/r for NVP × 1–4 wks before discontinuation.
- Switching from EFV to NVP: NVP dose escalation not necessary. Start with NVP 200 mg twice daily on day 1 (*AIDS* 2004;18:572).

ADVERSE DRUG REACTIONS

Common

- Maculopapular erythematous rash with or without pruritus in 17%; requires NVP discontinuation in 7%. Steroids not effective. Cross-reaction with EFV unlikely. D/C NVP if rash is blistering, involves mucous membranes, is accompanied by elevated transaminase levels, or fever.

Occasional

- Hepatitis (2 forms): (1) severe acute hepatitis (part of hypersensitivity reaction) reported in up to 11% of treatment-naïve women with CD4 >250 (12-fold increase compared to women with CD4 <250) and 6.4% of men with CD4 >400. This form of hepatitis occurs early in the course (6–8 wks) and is presumed to be immune-mediated; may accompany rash and fever; (2) hepatitis usually occurring after mos of therapy in up to 15% of patients, usually asymptomatic, resembling transaminatis seen with PIs and EFV, and may usually be "treated through." Rate is increased with HBV and HCV coinfection. Some recommend NVP discontinuation if ALT >5 or 10 × UNL.
- Hypersensitivity reaction presenting as rash, hepatitis, fever, arthralgias, and myalgias in 1st 6–8 wks of therapy; can be fatal if not recognized.
- Rhabdomyolysis observed in some patients with rash and hepatitis.

Rare

- Stevens-Johnson sydrome or toxic epidermal necrolysis (TEN) with 5 reported deaths.

DRUG INTERACTIONS

- CYP3A4 substrate and inhibitor. May significantly decrease serum levels of other CYP3A4 substrates. CYP3A4 inducers may decrease NVP levels.

DRUG-DRUG INTERACTIONS—See Appendix I, p. 578, for table of drug-drug interactions.

RESISTANCE

- K103N: high-level resistance (seen more when NVP is used with AZT); causes high-level cross-resistance to all available NNRTIs.
- 181C/I: high-level resistance to NVP, DLV; low-level resistance to EFV, though clinical data do not support use of EFV after NVP failure. 181C partially reverses TAM-mediated AZT and TDF resistance.
- 106A/M: 106A causes high-level NVP resistance, intermediate DLV resistance, and low-level EFV resistance; 106M causes high-level NVP and EFV resistance and intermediate DLV resistance; 106I is a polymorphism that does not cause NNRTI resistance.
- 188C/L/H: 188C causes high-level resistance to NVP and low-level resistance to EFV and DLV; 188H causes low-level resistance to NVP, DLV, EFV; 188L causes high-level resistance to NVP, EFV and low to intermediate resistance to DLV.
- 190A/S: 190A causes high-level resistance to NVP, intermediate resistance to EFV; susceptibility or hypersusceptibility to DLV (clinical significance unknown); 190S same as above, but high-level EFV resistance.
- 230L: high-level NVP resistance, intermediate EFV resistance, low-level DLV resistance.
- 108I: potential low-level resistance to NVP, EFV, and DLV.
- 100I: intermediate resistance to NVP, DLV, EFV.

PHARMACOLOGY

Mechanism

- Noncompetitive inhibition of HIV DNA polymerase resulting in disruption of catalytic site of the enzyme.

Pharmacokinetic Parameters

- **Absorption:** 93% absorption with or without food.
- **Metabolism and Excretion:** metabolized by CYP3A4 to several hydroxylated metabolites, which undergo subsequent glucuronidation. Both unchanged drug and metabolites are excreted in the feces.
- **Protein Binding:** 50%–60%.
- **Cmax, Cmin, and AUC:** median AUC: 55.95 mcg/mL hr; Cmax: 5.86 mcg/mL; Cmin 3.72 mcg/mL at steady state. NVP component in Triomune (NVP/d4T/3TC) and Duovir (NVP/AZT/3TC) met US bioequivalency standards but d4T, AZT, and 3TC did not.
- **$T_{\frac{1}{2}}$:** 25–30 hrs.
- **Distribution:** good CNS penetration. CSF: plasma ratio = 0.45.

Pregnancy Risk

- Category C: placental passage of 100% in humans. In HIVNET 006 trial NVP 200 mg given to 21 HIV-infected pregnant patients. NVP well tolerated and no fetal defects noted (*AIDS* 1999; 13: 479–86).

Breastfeeding Compatibility

- Breastfeeding not recommended in the US in order to avoid postnatal transmission of HIV to uninfected child.

DOSING

Dosing for Decreased Hepatic Function

- AUC may be increased up to 41%–100%; NVP should not be administered to patients with moderate (Childs Pugh B) or severe (Childs Pugh C) hepatic impairment.

Renal Dosing

- Dosing for GFR of 50–80: 200 mg once daily × 14 days then 200 mg twice daily or 400 mg once daily (XR).
- Dosing for GFR of 10–50: 200 mg once daily × 14 days then 200 mg twice daily or 400 mg once daily (XR).
- Dosing for GFR of <10: 200 mg once daily × 14 days then 200 mg twice daily or 400 mg once daily (XR).

DRUGS

- Dosing in hemodialysis: 200 mg once daily × 14 days then 200 mg twice daily or 400 mg once daily (XR); on days of dialysis dose post-dialysis.
- Dosing in peritoneal dialysis: no data. Consider standard dose.
- Dosing in hemofiltration: no data. Consider standard dose.

COMMENTS

- **Pros:** efficacy comparable to EFV at 1 yr in 2NN trial (though noninferiority not established); more favorable lipid profiles than EFV; no neuropsychiatric toxicity; safety and efficacy of single dose to prevent perinatal transmission established.
- **Cons:** less clinical data than for EFV; potential for severe hepatoxicity and sometimes lethal rash reaction; CD4 count restrictions; single-dose NVP used to prevent perinatal transmission associated with development of high-level resistance to NNRTIs; considered alternative in current US treatment guidelines. Inconclusive data on efficacy when combined with TDF + either FTC or 3TC.

SELECTED REFERENCES

van Leth F, Phanuphak P, Ruxrungtham K, et al. Comparison of first-line antiretroviral therapy with regimens including nevirapine, efavirenz, or both drugs, plus stavudine and lamivudine: a randomised open-label trial, the 2NN Study. *Lancet*, 2004; 363: 1253–63.

Comments: Large prospective randomized trial comparing NVP 400 mg once daily, NVP 200 mg twice daily, EFV 600 mg once daily, or NVP (400 mg) + EFV (800 mg) once daily + d4T and 3TC for 48 wks in 1216 naïve patients. EFV and NVP regimens comparable (but did not meet noninferiority criteria) with VL <50 at wk 48 in 65% vs 60%, respectively (P = 0.193). Contrary to earlier retrospective analyses showing EFV to be superior to NVP, this large prospective trial demonstrated comparability. Due to the higher rates of hepatotoxicity observed in NVP recipients (9.6% vs 3.5%) EFV is still the preferred NNRTI.

Jackson JB, Musoke P, Fleming T, et al. Intrapartum and neonatal single-dose nevirapine compared with zidovudine for prevention of mother-to-child transmission of HIV-1 in Kampala, Uganda: 18-month follow-up of the HIVNET 012 randomised trial. *Lancet*, 2003; 362: 859–68.

Comments: Single-dose intrapartum NVP was compared to AZT (intrapartum + 7 days postpartum) for prevention of perinatal transmission. Estimated risks of HIV transmission in AZT and NVP groups were 10.3% and 8.1% at birth (P = 0.35); 20.0% and 11.8% by age 6–8 wks (P = 0.0063); 22.1% and 13.5% by age 14–16 wks (P = 0.0064); and 25.8% and 15.7% by age 18 mos (P = 0.0023).

Podzamczer D, Ferrer E, Consiglio E, et al. A randomized clinical trial comparing nelfinavir or nevirapine associated to zidovudine/lamivudine in HIV-infected naive patients (the Combine Study). *Antivir Ther*, 2002; 7: 81–90.

Comments: Prospective randomized trial comparing NVP + AZT/3TC vs NFV + AZT/3TC. At 12 mos in ITT analysis, 60% and 75% in NFV and NVP arms had VL <200, respectively (P = 0.06), and 50% and 65% had VL <20 (P = 0.06). NVP was compared to NFV, a PI known to have inferior PK profile when compared to other agents in that class. It remains to be determined how NVP compares to LPV/r (the gold standard PI).

van der Valk M, Kastelein JJ, Murphy RL, et al. Nevirapine-containing antiretroviral therapy in HIV-1 infected patients results in an anti-atherogenic lipid profile. *AIDS*, 2001; 15: 2407–14.

Comments: Substudy of the ATLANTIC trial comparing lipid parameters in patients treated with d4T + ddI and either NVP, IDV or 3TC. LDL increased in both NVP and IDV arms but offset by a dramatic increase in HDL (49%) in NVP-treated patients. NVP may be the preferred NNRTI in patients with uncontrolled hyperlipidemia, but results from the switch study (PI regimen switch to NVP) have been conflicting.

RALTEGRAVIR

Paul A. Pham, PharmD

INDICATIONS

FDA

- Treatment of HIV-1 infection in combination with other ARV agents in ART-experienced patients with evidence of HIV replication despite ongoing ART.
- Treatment of HIV-1 infection in combination with other ARV agents in ART-naïve patients.

Non-FDA Approved Uses

- Substitution for other ARV agents due to drug toxicity or intolerance in patients on suppressive regimen (limited data).

FORMS TABLE

Brand name (mfr)	Forms†	Cost*
Isentress (Merck and Co., Inc.)	Oral tablet 400 mg	$17.91 per tab
	RAL 100 mg chewable tablet and 25 mg chewable tablet	tba

*Prices represent cost per unit specified, are representative of Average Wholesale Price (AWP).
†Dosage is indicated in mg unless otherwise noted.

USUAL ADULT DOSING
- Pill burden: 2 tabs/day.
- 400 mg film-coated tablet OR 300 mg (three 100 mg chewable tablets)* PO twice daily with or without food".
  (*Note: chewable tablets are not interchangeable with film-coated tablets. Avoid chewable tablets in patients with phenylketonuria)
- In combination with all PIs, NRTIs, and NNRTIs: use standard dose (400 mg PO twice daily).

PEDIATRIC DOSE
- > or = 12 years of age: 400 mg film-coated tab twice-daily.
- 6–11 years of age (must be at least 25 kg): 400 mg film-tab OR 300 mg (three 100 mg chewable tablets) twice daily.
- Weight base pediatric dosing for 2 to less than 6 years of age: 6 mg/kg/dose twice daily chewable tablets.
- 10–13 kg: 75 mg twice daily.
- 14–19 kg: 100 mg twice daily.
- 20–27 kg: 150 mg twice daily.
- 28–39 kg: 200 mg twice daily.
- >40 kg: 300 mg twice daily.

ADVERSE DRUG REACTIONS
General
- Generally well tolerated with comparable ADR rates to placebo. Rates of discontinuation of therapy due to AEs were 2% with RAL + optimized background therapy (OBT) and 1.4% with placebo + OBT.

Occasional
- Nausea, diarrhea, flatulence.
- Headache.
- Fever (unclear association).
- Pruritis.
- Creatine kinase elevation.
- Transaminase elevation.
- CNS side effects (e.g., depression, paranoia, and suicidal ideation and behaviors).

Rare
- Myopathy and rhabdomyolysis. CPK elevation (Grade 3–4) more common in patients treated with RAL compared to EFV.
- Malignancies (3.5% in RAL recipients at 48 wks vs 2.6% in placebo recipients); difference did not persist, but post FDA-approval surveillance for malignancies in progress.
- Severe rash (DRESS and Stevens Johnson Syndrome).
- Cerebellar ataxia.
- Thrombocytopenia.

DRUG INTERACTIONS
- Not a substrate, inhibitor, or inducer of CYP3A4; therefore, significant drug interactions with CYP3A4 substrates, inhibitors, and inducers are unlikely. RAL is primarily metabolized by glucuronidation via the enzyme, UDP-glucuronosyltransferase (UGT) 1A1.

DRUGS

DRUG-DRUG INTERACTIONS—See Appendix I, p. 586, for table of drug-drug interactions.

RESISTANCE

- 2 pathways to resistance with mutations in integrase gene: (1) N155H + (E92Q, V151I, T97A, G163R, L74M); (2) Q148K/R/H + (G140S/A, E138K).
- Other pathways may exist, e.g., Y143R/C + (L74A/I, E92Q, T97A, I203M, S230R).
- Evidence of cross-resistance with elvitegravir (investigational integrase inhibitor). Q148 pathway leads to cross-resistance to S/GSK1349572 (investigational integrase inhibitor).
- Integrase inhibitor genotypic and phenotypic resistance tests available. Genotype generally preferred, as it provides information about susceptibility/cross-resistance to investigational integrase inhibitors.

PHARMACOLOGY

Mechanism

- RAL inhibits integrase, an essential enzyme responsible for catalyzing the insertion of HIV DNA into the host genome.

Pharmacokinetic Parameters

- **Absorption:** absolute bioavailability not established.
- **Metabolism and Excretion:** eliminated mainly by metabolism via a UGT1A1-mediated glucuronidation pathway. RAL-glucuronide and RAL are eliminated excreted in feces (51%) and urine (32%).
- **Protein Binding:** 83%.
- **Cmax, Cmin, and AUC:** geometric mean AUC 0–12h and Cmin were 14.3 microM per hr and 142 nM, respectively. Efficacy not associated with Cmin, but *in vitro*, antiviral response associated with AUC/EC50.
- **T$_{\frac{1}{2}}$:** 9 hrs. RAL exhibited a long residence time on the integrase/DNA complexes. Clinical trials evaluating once-daily RAL are underway.
- **Distribution:** CNS to plasma ratio of 7.3%. RAL CSF concentrations exceeded IC$_{50}$ of wild-type HIV.

Pregnancy Risk

- Category C: no human data. Animal developmental studies found a higher incidence of supernumerary ribs compared to control.

Breastfeeding Compatibility

- No human data, but based on animal studies, RAL concentrated in breast milk.

DOSING

Dosing for Decreased Hepatic Function

- No dosage adjustment is necessary for patients with mild-to-moderate hepatic impairment. The effect of severe hepatic impairment on the pharmacokinetics of RAL has not been studied.

Renal dosing

- Dosing for GFR of 50–80: usual dose.
- Dosing for GFR of 10–50: no data. Usual dose likely.
- Dosing for GFR of <10: no data. Usual dose likely.
- Dosing in hemodialysis: no data. Dose post-HD on days of dialysis.
- Dosing in peritoneal dialysis: no data.
- Dosing in hemofiltration: no data.

COMMENTS

- **Pros:** 1st approved integrase inhibitor, with no cross-resistance to currently approved ARVs. Highly effective when used in combination with OBT in heavily treatment-experienced patients with extensive resistance to currently approved ARVs. Good short-term safety and few drug interactions. More rapid VL reduction at 4 and 8 wks vs EFV in treatment naïve-patients (clinical significance unknown) with comparable 96-wk results and superior at 192 weeks.
- **Cons:** unknown long-term safety. Lower barrier to resistance than boosted PIs. Cross-resistance with investigational integrase inhibitor elvitegravir and some cross-resistance with dolutegravir, which may limit ability to sequence within integrase inhibitor class.

SELECTED REFERENCES

Eron JJ, Young B, Cooper DA, et al. Switch to a raltegravir-based regimen versus continuation of a lopinavir-ritonavir-based regimen in stable HIV-infected patients with suppressed viraemia (SWITCHMRK 1 and 2): two multicentre, double-blind, randomised controlled trials. *Lancet*, 2010; 375: 396–407.

Comments: SWITCHMRK 1 and 2 evaluated switch to RAL in ART-experienced patients who were virologically controlled on stable LPVr-based regimen. Patients had median of 5 previous ARVs. Patients randomized to switch LPV/r to RAL (N = 350) or continue on LPV/r (N = 352) while remaining on same background ART, which included at least 2 NRTI. Switch to RAL resulted in lower cholesterol and triglycerides; however, at wk 24, RAL did not demonstrate noninferiority compared to LPV/r. 293 of 347 (84.4%) vs 319 of 352 (90.6%) patients had VL <50 in RAL and LPVr groups, respectively; treatment difference –6.2 % (95% CI, –11.2 to –1.3; NC = F). Demonstrates importance of evaluating ART history and resistance before switching to regimen with lower barrier to resistance.

Eron J, et al. CROI 2011. Abstract 150LB QDMRK, A Phase III Study of the Safety and Efficacy of Once Daily (QD) Versus Twice Daily (BID) Raltegravir (RAL) in Combination Therapy for Treatment-Naïve HIV-Infected Patients (Pts).
Comments: Randomized study of RAL 800 mg once daily vs RAL 400 mg twice daily, each with TDF/FTC, in 770 ART-naïve patients. At 48 wks, 83.2% taking RAL once daily vs 88.9% RAL twice daily achieved VL <50. Treatment difference of –5.7% (CI –10.7%, –0.83%) did not meet criteria for noninferiority. Difference was largely driven by patients with high VL. Among those with VL >100,000, 74.3% of once-daily group vs 84.2% of twice-daily group had undetectable VL.

Markowitz M, Nguyen BY, Gotuzzo E, et al. Sustained antiretroviral effect of raltegravir after 96 weeks of combination therapy in treatment-naive patients infected with HIV-1 infection. *J Acquir Immune Defic Syndr*, 2009; 52: 350–6.
Comments: Randomized, double-blind, study of RAL vs EFV, both combined with TDF/FTC, in 198 ART-naïve patients. At wk 96, 83% of RAL and 84% of EFV-treated patients achieved undetectable VL (<50). As expected, lower CNS adverse events observed in RAL-treated patients.

Steigbigel RT, Cooper DA, Kumar PN, et al. Raltegravir with optimized background therapy for resistant HIV-1 infection *N Engl J Med*, 2008; 359: 339–354.
Comments: Randomized, double-blind studies of RAL vs placebo, each with OBT, in 699 treatment-experienced patients failing ARTs with HIV resistant to PIs, NNRTIs, and NRTIs. In a combined analysis, at 48 wks, 62.1% taking RAL + OBT vs 32.9% taking placebo + OBT achieved VL <50 (P <0.001). CD4 increased by 84 in RAL group vs 37 in placebo group (P <0.001). In a sub-analysis, 1st use of ENF, DRV, or both in the OBT + RAL resulted in VL <50 in 82%, 68%, 80% of treated patients, respectively. In RAL-treated patients with genotypic sensitivity score (GSS) of 0 and ≥1, VL <50 achieved in 44% and 71%, respectively. No difference in virologic suppression between GSS score of 1 and 2 or greater in RAL-treated patients, but may have been due to partial activity of the OBT.

Grinsztejn B, Nguyen B, Katlama C, et al. Safety and efficacy of the HIV-1 integrase inhibitor raltegravir (MK-0518) in treatment-experienced patients with multidrug-resistant virus: a phase II randomized controlled trial. *Lancet*, 2007; 369: 1261–9.
Comments: Randomized, double-blind, multidose (200, 400, 600 mg twice daily) placebo-controlled trial of RAL in patients with multidrug-resistant HIV. All patients genotypically or phenotypically resistant to at least 1 drug in each of 3 classes (NNRTIs, NRTIs, PIs). Baseline characteristics comparable between the 2 groups. Of the 133 patients randomized to RAL + OBR, VL = 4.7 log, CD4 = 240, and 9.9 yrs of prior ARTs. OBR contained a median of 4 ARVs with 45 (36%) receiving ENF. At 24 wks, VL <50 achieved in 65%–67% and 13% of RAL and control patients, respectively. Due to the virologic benefit seen in the RAL arm, all patients (including those in placebo arm) were switched to RAL 400 mg twice daily after 24 wks. Overall, those who had achieved virologic suppression on RAL at 24 wks had largely maintained it to 48 wks; 54% taking any dose of RAL had VL <50.

DRUGS

RILPIVIRINE

Paul A. Pham, PharmD

Indications
FDA
- Rilpivirine is indicated for the treatment of HIV-1 infection in ART-naïve patients in combination with other antiretrovirals agents.

Forms Table

Brand name (mfr)	Forms[†]	Coast*
Edurant (Janssen Therapeutics)	Oral tablet 25 mg tablet	$25.21
Complera (Gilead Sciences)	Oral tablet RPV/TDF/FTC 25mg/300mg/200mg	tba

*Prices represent cost per unit specified, are representative of "Average Wholesale Price" (AWP).
†Dosage is indicated in mg unless otherwise noted.

USUAL ADULT DOSING
- RPV 25 mg (one tablet) taken once daily with a meal.
- RPV/TDF/FTC (*Complera*) 1 tablet once daily with meal.
- Concurrent ART agents: Standard RPV dose recommended with PI/r, MVC, RAL and NRTI. Co-administration with ddI is complicated by the need to take ddI on an empty stomach, and RPV must be taken with a meal.

ADVERSE DRUG REACTIONS
Common
Symptomatic
- Vomiting
- Headache
- Dizziness
- Insomnia
- Abnormal dreams
- Depression
- Rash
- Drug discontinuation

Laboratory Changes
- Creatinine elevation
- AST elevation
- LDL-C
- Total cholesterol
- Triglyceride

Occasional
- Fat redistribution including increased visceral fat with central obesity, dorsocervical fat enlargement, breast enlargement and peripheral fat wasting has been observed. The mechanism and causal role of RPV is unclear.
- Dose dependent QTc prolongation (QTc increased 4.8, 10.7, 23.3 milliseconds with 25 mg, 75 mg, 300 mg dose, respectively.)
- CNS (h/a, dizziness, insomnia, abnormal dreams). Incidence lower compared to EFV.
- Depressive disorders including depressed mood, major depression and suicidal ideation. During phase 3 trials the rate of depression, regardless of causality, was 8%; most were mild or moderate in severity. The rate of Grade 3 or 4 depression was 1%.
- LDL cholesterol and triglyceride elevation (lower compared to EFV)
- Rash (lower incidence compared to EFV)

DRUG INTERACTIONS
- RPV should not be co-administered with several **anticonvulsants** (phenytoin, phenobarbital, oxcarbazepine), rifabutin, rifampin, rifapentine, **proton pump inhibitors** (PPIs-omeprazole, pantoprazole, rabeprazole, lansprazole, esomeprazole), more than a single dose of **dexamethasone**, or **St. John's wort**. Use caution and dose separation with **H2 blockers, antacids**.
- PI: RPV concentrations increased (e.g DRV/r and LPV/r increase RPV AUC 130% and 52%, respectively; use standard dose.) PI or PI/r concentrations are not altered by co-administration. This applies to ATV, ATV/r, FPV, FPV/r, DRV/r, LPV/r, SQV/r, TPV/r. Use standard doses of RPV and the PI or PI/r. Consider monitoring QTc in patients at risk for QTc prolongation.
- Avoid co-administration with any other **NNRTI** (e.g. DLV, EFV, ETR, NVP).

DRUG-DRUG INTERACTIONS—See Appendix I, p. 597, for table of drug-drug interactions.
RESISTANCE
- High level resistance: 101P and 181L/V; mutations associated with virologic failure 90I, 101E/PT, 138K/G, 179I/L, 198I/C, 189I, 221Y, 227C/L and 230L. The most common mutation associated with failure is 138K, which increases resistance by 2.8-fold without 184I and 6.7-fold with 184I. With RPV resistance, there is cross-resistance to ETR in 89% and cross-resistance to NVP in 63%.

PHARMACOLOGY
Mechanism
- Rilpivirine is a diarylpyrimidine NNRTI. It inhibits HIV-1 replication by non-competitive inhibition of HIV-1 reverse transcriptase.

Pharmacokinetic Parameters

- **Absorption:** Food (500 kcal normal or high fat meal) improves RPV absorption. Fasted condition or high protein drink decreases RPV absorption by 40-50%.
- **Metabolism and Excretion:** RPV undergoes oxidative metabolism via CYP3A4. Parent drug and metabolite are primarily excreted in the feces (85%) and urine (6.1%).
- **Protein Binding:** High protein binding: 99.7%
- **Cmax, Cmin, and AUC:** Mean AUC = 2397 mcg/mL hr (+/− 1032 mcg/mL hr); Mean Cmin = 80 mcg/mL (+/− 37 mcg/mL)
- **$T_{\frac{1}{2}}$:** 50 hrs.

Pregnancy Risk

- Category B. No human data. No teratogenic or embryonic toxicity observed in animal studies.

Breast Feeding Compatibility

- No data.

DOSING

Dosing for Decreased Hepatic function

- No dose adjustment needed for mild to moderate (Child-Pugh A and B) hepatic impairment

Renal Dosing

- Dosing for GFR of 50-80: Usual dose
- Dosing for GFR of 10-50: Usual RPV dose. Avoid *Complera* co-formulation.
- Dosing for GFR of <10 mL/min: Usual RPV dose. Avoid *Complera* co-formulation.
- Dosing in hemodialys: Standard dose likely. Unlikely to be removed in HD.
- Dosing in peritoneal dialysis: Standard dose likely. Unlikely to be removed in PD.
- Dosing in hemofiltration: No data. Usual dose likely.

COMMENTS

- **Advantages:** Potent activity against HIV; well tolerated; once daily administration; relatively few drug interactions; minimal effect on blood lipids; small pill size and low pill burden; active against HIV strains with K103N mutation; single-tablet coformulation with TDF/FTC.
- **Disadvantages:** Relatively new so clinical experience limited; difficult transition from EFV-based ART due to induction of RPV metabolism; low genetic barrier to resistance; a major resistance mutation (138K) also confers resistance to ETR; increased rates of failure with baseline VL >100,000 c/mL and with suboptimal adherence compared to EFV; 500 kcal meal requirement; reduction in bioavilability without gastric acid; contraindicated with PPIs, and dose separation required with H2 blockers and antacids.

CLINICAL TRIALS

- The registration trials were ECHO and THRIVE, with comparison to EFV in 1,368 treatment-naïve patients randomized to receive RPV 25 mg or EFV 600 mg once daily in combination with TDF/FTC (ECHO) or combined with investigator's choice of TDF/FTC, AZT/3TC or ABC/3TC (THRIVE). Criteria for inclusion was a baseline VL >5000 c/mL, susceptibility to NRTIs and absence of specific NNRTI mutations.
- The rate of virologic failure was nearly the same, but there were significantly more failures with a baseline VL >100,000 c/mL.
- Caution or use of an alternative agent is recommended with a baseline VL >100,000 c/mL.
- RPV was better tolerated, with lower frequency of neurologic psychiatric and rash reactions.
- As expected virologic failure was associated with NNRTI and NRTI RAMs. For RPV the dominant RAM was 138K compared to K103N with EFV. This difference will influence NNRTI sequences, especially with ETR, which is active against 103N but has reduced activity with 138K (see resistance section).

SELECTED REFERENCES

Cohen CJ et al: Rilpivirine versus efavirenz with two background nucleoside or nucleotide reverse transcriptase inhibitors in treatment-naive adults infected with HIV-1 (THRIVE): a phase 3, randomised, non-inferiority trial. *Lancet*, 2011; 378:229.

Comment: Large registration trial randomized treatment-naïve patients to rilpivirine or efavirenz, both combined with investigator's choice of NRTIs (i.e ABC/3TC, TDF/FTC, AZT/3TC). The majority (60%) of patients were given TDF/FTC in combination with rilpivirine or efavirenz. Virologic response rate at 48 weeks was non-inferior between rilpivirine- and efavirenz-treated patients. Virologic failures were observed in 7% (24 of 340) of rilpivirine- and 5% (18 of 338) of efavirenz-treated patients. Compared to efavirenz, incidence of rash, dizziness, and cholesterol elevation was lower in rilpivirine-treated patients.

DRUGS

Molina JM et al: Rilpivirine versus efavirenz with tenofovir and emtricitabine in treatment-naive adults infected with HIV-1 (ECHO): a phase 3 randomised double-blind active-controlled trial. *Lancet*, 2011; 378:238.

Comment: Second large multicenter registration trial randomized treatment-naïve patients to rilpivirine or efavirenz, both combined with TDF/FTC. Virologic response rate at 48 weeks in rilpivirine-treated group was non-inferior to efavirenz-treated group. The incidence of virological failures was 13% in rilpivirine- versus 6% in efavirenz-treated patients. In the combined analysis (summarized above), high baseline viral load (>100,000 copies/mL) resulted in higher rates of virologic failure.

RITONAVIR

Paul A. Pham, PharmD and John G. Bartlett, MD

INDICATIONS
FDA
- Treatment of HIV-infection in combination with other antiretrovirals.
- Pharmacokinetic enhancement of APV, ATV, DRV, FPV, SQV, TPV, and LPV.

Non-FDA Approved Uses
- Pharmacokinetic enhancement of IDV.

FORMS TABLE

Brand name (mfr)	Forms†	Cost*
Norvir (Abbott Laboratories)	Oral soft gel capsule 100 mg Oral soln 80 mg/mL Oral tablet	$10.29 $216.03/80 mL $10.29

*Prices represent cost per unit specified, are representative of Average Wholesale Price (AWP).
†Dosage is indicated in mg unless otherwise noted.

USUAL ADULT DOSING
- Pill burden: 1–4 tabs/day (based on doses of 100 mg once daily to 200 mg twice daily to enhance PK of other PIs).
- RTV 600 mg PO twice daily (FDA approved dose; rarely used due to severe GI intolerance).
- With IDV: RTV 100 mg twice daily + IDV 800 mg twice daily (less GI intolerance but more nephrolithiasis), or RTV 200 mg twice daily + IDV 800 mg twice daily (highest incidence of nephrolithiasis, use only if EFV coadministered), or RTV 400 mg twice daily + IDV 400 mg twice daily (more GI intolerance, rarely used).
- With SQV: RTV 100 mg twice daily + SQV 1000 mg twice daily, or RTV 400 mg twice daily + SQV 400 mg twice daily or RTV 100 mg once daily + SQV 2000 mg once daily (dose being studied in ART-naïve patients) or RTV 400 mg twice daily + SQV 400 mg twice daily (high rate of GI intolerance, rarely used).
- With APV: RTV 100 mg twice daily + APV 700 mg twice daily (FPV liquid preferred), or RTV 200 mg once daily + APV 1400 mg once daily (FPV liquid preferred).
- With FPV: RTV 100 mg twice daily + FPV 700 mg twice daily, or RTV 100 or 200 mg once daily + FPV 1400 mg once daily (once-daily dosing for PI-naïve patients only) or RTV 300 mg once daily + FPV 1400 mg once daily when coadministered with EFV.
- With ATV: RTV 100 mg once daily + ATV 300 mg once daily (with EFV and ATV, use RTV 100 mg once daily + ATV 400 mg once daily: for patients without PI resistance).
- With NFV: not recommended. Combination of RTV 400 mg twice daily + NFV 500–750 mg twice daily has been studied, but limited data; high rate of GI intolerance with only marginal PK enhancement of NFV levels.
- With NVP: standard dose for both drugs, but rarely used due to high rate of GI intolerance.
- With TPV: RTV 200 mg twice daily + TPV 500 mg twice daily.
- With DRV: RTV 100 mg twice daily + DRV 600 mg twice daily OR RTV 100 mg once daily + DRV 800 mg once daily (PI-naïve patients only or without DRV-resistant mutation).
- With MVC: decrease MVC to 150 mg twice daily.

- With ETR: high dose RTV not recommended, but DRV/r, SQV/r, and LPV/r may be coadministered at standard dose.
- With RAL: no interaction; use standard doses of both drugs.

Adverse Drug Reactions

Common

- Severe GI intolerance (nausea, vomiting, and diarrhea).
- Abdominal pain, common with 600 mg twice-daily dosing.
- Taste perversion.
- Asthenia.
- Circumoral and peripheral paresthesias.
- Lower doses used for PI boosting better tolerated.

Occasional

- Lipodystrophy, especially fat accumulation.
- Insulin resistance, hyperglycemia, and diabetes.
- Hyperlipidemia: increased triglycerides and/or cholesterol.
- Transaminase elevation (more common with RTV 400–600 mg twice daily).
- Association between RTV (and other PIs) and osteonecrosis/avascular necrosis has not been confirmed.
- QTc and PR interval prolongation (with RTV 400 mg twice daily). Use with caution in patients with structural heart disease or at risk for conduction system abnormalities.

Drug Interactions

- Substrate, potent inhibitor, and inducer of CYP3A4, CYP1A2, possibly CYP2C19, and phase II glucuronidation and a mild CYP2D inhibitor. Generally increases serum levels of drugs that are CYP3A4 substrates although in some cases its inducing effects may also decrease serum levels of drugs that are substrate of CYP3A4, CYP1A2, and possibly CYP2C19. RTV may increase serum levels of drugs that are CYP2D6 substrates.

Drug-Drug Interactions—See Appendix I, p. 599, for table of drug-drug interactions.

Resistance

- 82A/F/T/S: intermediate resistance.
- PI mutations: 10, 20, 32, 33, 36, 46, 71, 77: secondary PI mutations that increase RTV resistance inpresence of primary mutations.
- 50V, 54V, 90M: low-level resistance when present as single mutations.
- Unclear whether low "boosting" doses select for resistance mutations. PI resistance uncommon in patients failing boosted PIs without preexisting PI mutations.

Pharmacology

Mechanism

- Inhibition of HIV protease, which results in nonfunctional, immature, and noninfectious virions.

Pharmacokinetic Parameters

- **Absorption:** 60%–80% absorption; levels increased 15% with food.
- **Metabolism and Excretion:** metabolized by CYP3A4 and 2D6 to several hydroxylated metabolite, which undergo subsequent glucuronidation. Both unchanged drug and metabolites are excreted in the feces.
- **Protein Binding:** 98%–99%.
- **Cmax, Cmin, and AUC:** mean steady-state AUC = 61 mcg hr/mL; Cmax = 11.2 mcg/mL; Cmin = 3 mcg/mL.
- **T$_\frac{1}{2}$:** 3–5 hrs.

Pregnancy Risk

- Category B: placental passage of 115% mid-term and 15%–64% late-term demonstrated in rodent studies. In human placental perfusion model, RTV showed little accumulation in the fetal compartment and no accumulation in placental tissue. Not teratogenic but cryptochidism reported in rodents studies. No data on carcinogenicity.

Breastfeeding Compatibility

- Unknown breast milk excretion. Breastfeeding is not recommended in the US in order to avoid postnatal transmission of HIV to the child.

DRUGS

DOSING

Dosing for Decreased Hepatic Function
- Use with caution in ESLD (especially at higher doses).

Renal Dosing
- Dosing for GFR of 50–80: 600 mg twice daily (FDA dose; rarely used).
- Dosing for GFR of 10–50: 600 mg twice daily (FDA dose; rarely used).
- Dosing for GFR of <10: 600 mg twice daily (FDA dose; rarely used).
- Dosing in hemodialysis: usual dose; dose post-HD (small amount removed in HD).
- Dosing in peritoneal dialysis: no data: usual dose likely, dose post-HD.
- Dosing in hemofiltration: no data.

COMMENTS

- **Pros:** the most reliable PI booster: typically used to enhance pharmacokinetics of all PIs except NFV, resulting in higher drug levels, longer half-lives, decreased dose and/or dosing frequency, greater activity against PI-resistant virus, and lower likelihood of resistance with failure.
- **Cons:** costly; dose-dependent GI side effects, hepatitis, cholesterol and triglyceride elevation; many drug interactions.

SELECTED REFERENCES

Kirk O, Mocroft A, Pradier C, et al. Clinical outcome among HIV-infected patients starting saquinavir hard gel compared to ritonavir or indinavir. *AIDS*, 2001; 15: 999–1008.
Comments: Analysis of 2708 patients who started RTV (21%), IDV (50%), or 810 SQV hgc (30%). After 12 mos, proportions of patients with VL <500 were 47%, 54%, and 41%, respectively. Due to poor GI tolerability, RTV was never prospectively studied as a sole PI against other PIs or NNRTIs. In this nonrandomized study, RTV appears to be equivalent to IDV. RTV is now exclusively used as a pharmacokinetic booster.

Florence E, Dreezen C, Desmet P, et al. Ritonavir/saquinavir plus one nucleoside reverse transcriptase inhibitor (NRTI) versus indinavir plus two NRTIs in protease inhibitor-naive HIV-1-infected adults (IRIS study). *Antivir Ther*, 2001; 6: 255–62.
Comments: Small open-label, randomized clinical trial comparing RTV + SQV and NRTI to IDV and 2 NRTIs in PI-naïve patients. At 48 wks, VL <400 achieved in 43% (39/90) in RTV/SQV arm and 63% (57/90) in the IDV arm (P = 0.005).

Hsu A, Granneman GR, Bertz RJ. Ritonavir: clinical pharmacokinetics and interactions with other anti-HIV agents. *Clin Pharmacokinet*, 1998; 35: 275–91.
Comments: A review of the pharmacokinetics and drug interactions with RTV.

SAQUINAVIR

Paul A. Pham, PharmD and John G. Bartlett, MD

INDICATIONS

FDA
- Treatment of HIV-infection in combination with other ARV agents.

FORMS TABLE

Brand name (mfr)	Forms†	Cost*
Invirase (Roche Pharmaceuticals)	Oral hard gel capsule 200 mg	$3.72
	Oral tablet 500 mg	$8.55

*Prices represent cost per unit specified, are representative of Average Wholesale Price (AWP).
†Dosage is indicated in mg unless otherwise noted.

USUAL ADULT DOSING

- Pill burden: min 6/day (based on 2 SQV 500-mg tabs twice daily + 1 RTV 100-mg cap twice daily). Storage: SQV cap and tab can be stored at room temperature.
- FDA approved dose: SQV 1000 mg twice daily + RTV 100 mg twice daily with or without food.

- Not recommended without RTV boosting.
- SQV 2000 mg once daily + RTV 100 mg once daily. Unapproved dose with limited clinical data.
- SQV 400 mg twice daily + RTV 400 mg twice daily (rarely used due to poor tolerability).
- With LPV/r: SQV 1000 mg twice daily + LPV/r 400/100 mg (2 tabs) twice daily.
- With NFV: SQV 1200 mg twice daily + NFV 1250 mg twice daily (large pill burden; rarely used).
- With ATV: use with caution. May increase risk of PR interval prolongation. Consider ATV 300 mg + RTV 100 mg + SQV 1500–2000 mg once daily (limited clinical data). SQV 1200 mg once daily + ATV 400 mg once daily (poor clinical outcome) OR SQV 2000 mg once daily + ATV 400 mg once daily (based on PK data).
- With NVP: SQV 1000 mg twice daily + RTV 100 mg twice daily + NVP 200 mg twice daily OR SQV 400 mg twice daily + RTV 400 mg twice daily (rarely used) + NVP 200 mg twice daily.
- With EFV: consider SQV 1000 mg twice daily + RTV 100 mg twice daily + EFV 600 mg once daily.
- With TPV: SQV AUC decreased by 76%. Coadministration not recommended.
- With IDV: insufficient data.
- With FPV: consider SQV 1000 mg twice daily + RTV 100 mg twice daily + FPV 700 mg twice daily.
- With DRV: avoid coadministration.
- With MVC: SQV 1000 mg twice daily + RTV 100 mg twice daily + MVC 150 mg twice daily.
- With ETR: SQV 1000 mg twice daily + RTV 100 mg twice daily + ETR usual dose, but avoid rifabutin coadministration.
- With RAL: usual doses likely.

ADVERSE DRUG REACTIONS
Common
- GI intolerance: nausea, diarrhea, abdominal pain.

Occasional
- Insulin resistance ± hyperglycemia ± diabetes.
- Hyperlipidemia: increased triglycerides and/or cholesterol (may be less common or severe than with other PIs except ATV).
- Transaminase elevation (comparable to other PIs).
- Fat accumulation.

Rare
- QTc prolongation. Avoid in patients at risk for QTc prolongation (e.g., structural heart disease, hypokalemia, and other drugs that prolong QTc).
- PR interval prolongation may occur. 2nd- and 3rd-degree AV block reported. Use with caution in patients with underlying structural heart disease, preexisting conduction system abnormalities, ischemic heart disease, or cardiomyopathies.

DRUG INTERACTIONS
- Substrate and weak inhibitor of CYP3A4. May modestly increase serum level of other CYP3A4 substrates. Drugs that are inducers of CYP3A4 may decrease SQV levels.

DRUG-DRUG INTERACTIONS—See Appendix I, p. 610, for table of drug-drug interactions.

RESISTANCE
- L90M: selected by SQV, resulting in intermediate SQV and NFV resistance, and partial cross-resistance to other PIs.
- G48V: selected by SQV, resulting in intermediate SQV resistance and low-level cross-resistance to other PIs.
- 54V/L, 71VT, 73S, 77I, 82A, 84V, others: multiple mutations increase resistance.

PHARMACOLOGY
Mechanism
- Inhibition of HIV protease, which results in nonfunctional, immature, and noninfectious virions.

Pharmacokinetic Parameters
- **Absorption:** only 4% absorption with food. Absorption not influenced by food when combined with RTV.

DRUGS

- **Metabolism and Excretion:** extensive 1st-pass metabolism; over 90% of SQV is metabolized by hepatic and intestinal CYP3A4 isoenzyme.
- **Protein Binding:** 98%.
- **Cmax, Cmin, and AUC:** mean steady-state (with SQV/RTV) AUC = 29,214 ng hr/mL; Cmax = 1420 ng hr/mL; Cmin = 371 ng/mL.
- **T$_\frac{1}{2}$:** 1–2 hrs.
- **Distribution:** 700 L.

Pregnancy Risk
- Category B: placental passage in humans unknown. Placental passage in rat and rabbit is minimal. No teratogenicity reported in rodent studies. No data on carcinogenicity. High variability in SQV pharmacokinetics in pregnancy. SQV/r 1000/100 mg twice daily is recommended dose in pregnancy.

Breastfeeding Compatibility
- Unknown breast milk excretion. Breast feeding is not recommended in the US in order to avoid postnatal transmission of HIV to the child, who may not yet be infected.

DOSING

Dosing for Decreased Hepatic Function
- Do not use in patients with severe liver hepatic impairment.

Renal Dosing
- Dosing for GFR of 50–80: usual dose likely.
- Dosing for GFR of 10–50: usual dose likely.
- Dosing for GFR of <10: usual dose likely.
- Dosing in hemodialysis: usual dose (not removed in HD).
- Dosing in peritoneal dialysis: no data: usual dose likely (unlikely to be removed in dialysis due to high protein binding and large volume of distribution).
- Dosing in hemofiltration: no data.

COMMENTS
- **Pros:** less effect on lipids and noninferior efficacy compared to LPV/r.
- **Cons:** inferior to LPV/r in PI-experienced patients; higher pill burden than the preferred or alternative PIs. Potential for QTc and PR interval prolongation.

SELECTED REFERENCES

Walmsley S, Avihingsanon A, Slim J, et al. Gemini: a noninferiority study of saquinavir/ritonavir versus lopinavir/ritonavir as initial HIV-1 therapy in adults. *J Acquir Immune Defic Syndr*, 2009; 50: 367–74.

Comments: Head-to-head trial compared SQV/r (1000 mg/100 mg twice daily with LPV/r [400/100 mg twice daily]), both combined with FTC/TDF in 337 ARV-naïve patients. At 48 wks, SQV/r was noninferior to LPV/r with 64.7% of SQV/r + TDF/ FTC and 63.5% of LPV/r + TDF/FTC-treated patients achieved VL <50. Patients treated with SQV/r had lower median increase in TG (increase of 14 vs 55 mg/dL) and numerically lower proportion of patients with total cholesterol levels above those recommended (31% vs 39%).

Johnson M, Grinsztejn B, Rodriguez C, et al. 96-week comparison of once-daily atazanavir/ritonavir and twice-daily lopinavir/ritonavir in patients with multiple virologic failures. *AIDS*, 2006; 20: 711–8.

Comments: 358 patients who failed >2 ART regimens containing >1 PI, NNRTI, and NRTI randomized to ATV 300 mg + RTV 100 mg once daily, ATV 400 mg + SQV 1200 mg once daily, or LPV/r 400/100 mg twice daily, each combined with TDF + 1 NRTI. ATV + SQV arm did not perform as well as the other 2 arms, with only 26% achieving VL <50 at 48 wks, which resulted in discontinuation of this arm. At 96 wks, virologic suppression comparable between ATV/r and LPV/r-treated patients. Mean VL reduction from baseline was −2.29 and −2.08 log in ATV/r and LPV/r groups, respectively. As expected, virologic response rates were higher with <4 PI mutations at baseline. In patients with 4 or more PI mutations, undetectable VL achieved in only 20% and 23% in ATV/r and LPV/r arms, respectively. Total cholesterol (+9%) and fasting triglycerides (+30%) higher in LPV/r-treated group. Grade 2–4 diarrhea less frequent in ATV/r patients (3%) vs LPV/r- (13%) treated patients.

Montaner JS, Schutz M, Schwartz R, et al. Efficacy, safety and pharmacokinetics of once-daily saquinavir soft-gelatin capsule/ritonavir in antiretroviral-naive, HIV-infected patients. *MedGenMed*, 2006; 8: 36.

Comments: EFV outperformed SQV sgc 1600 mg + RTV 100 mg in study involving 161 ART-naïve patients. At 48 wks, EFV arm outperformed boosted SQV arm for viral suppression to <50 (71% vs 51%, respectively; P = 0.008). Nausea and vomiting more frequent in PI arm, which may explain outcome. Dizziness, rash, and fatigue more common in the NNRTI arm. No differences in lipid changes between treatments.

Dragsted UB, Gerstoft J, Youle M, et al. A randomized trial to evaluate lopinavir/ritonavir versus saquinavir/ritonavir in HIV-1-infected patients: the MaxCmin2 trial. *Antivir Ther*, 2005; 10: 735–43.

Comments: Trial compared LPV/r (400/100 mg twice daily) with SQV sgc + RTV (1000/100 mg twice daily) + >2 NRTI/NNRTIs in 324 patients. Population was heterogenous and included 33% ART-naïve, 48% PI-naïve, and 32% who had experienced virologic failure of >1 PI. At 48 wks, treatment failure occurred in 18% and 33% of patients in the LPV/r and SQV/r arms, respectively (ITT, P = 0.002). Risk of treatment discontinuation also higher in SQV arm (29% vs 13%, P = 0.0001); however, no overall difference in risk of Grade 3 and 4 adverse events in the 2 arms.

Dragsted UB, Gerstoft J, Pedersen C, et al. Randomized trial to evaluate indinavir/ritonavir versus saquinavir/ritonavir in human immunodeficiency virus type 1-infected patients: the MaxCmin1 Trial. *J Infect Dis*, 2003; 188: 635–42.

Comments: 306 patients randomized to receive open-label IDV 800 mg + RTV 100 mg twice daily or SQV sgc but allowed to change to SQV hgc 1000 mg + RTV 100 mg twice daily At 48 wks, virological failure in 43 (27%) of 158 and 37 (25%) of 148 patients in IDV + RTV and SQV + RTV arms, respectively. More patients in IDV + RTV arm experienced adverse events. When switching from randomized treatment counted as failure, this was seen in 78 of 158 patients in IDV + RTV arm vs 51 of 148 patients in SQV + RTV arm (P = 0.009).

STAVUDINE

Paul A. Pham, PharmD and John G. Bartlett, MD

INDICATIONS

FDA

- Treatment of HIV infection in combination with other antiretrovirals.

FORMS TABLE

Brand name (mfr)	Forms†	Cost*
Zerit (Bristol-Myers Squibb)	Oral capsule 15 mg; 20 mg; 30 mg; 40 mg	$6.76; $7.03; $7.45; $7.60
	Oral liquid 1 mg/mL (200-mL bottle)	$84.72/bottle
Stavudine (Camber Pharmaceuticals and other generic manufacturers)	Oral capsule 15 mg; 20 mg; 30 mg; 40 mg	$6.09; $6.33; $6.73; $6.86

*Prices represent cost per unit specified, are representative of Average Wholesale Price (AWP).
†Dosage is indicated in mg unless otherwise noted.

USUAL ADULT DOSING

- Pill burden: 2/day.
- Wt >60 kg: 40 mg PO twice daily (data supporting 30 mg PO twice daily, less toxic and recommended by WHO, but limited efficacy data).
- Wt <60 kg: 30 mg PO twice daily.
- Package insert recommends dose reduction (wt >60 kg: 20 mg twice daily; wt <60 kg: 15 mg twice daily) for peripheral neuropathy; however, treatment with alternate agent preferred due to limited efficacy data with lower doses and potential for irreversible neuropathy with continued use.

ADVERSE DRUG REACTIONS

Common

- Peripheral neuropathy (5%–24%). Onset is usually 2–6 mos. Reversible with early discontinuation.
- Macrocytosis (inconsequential).
- Lipoatrophy: caused by mitochondrial toxicity. d4T most common cause; dose dependent—may be less common or severe with 30 mg twice daily.

Occasional

- GI intolerance with diarrhea.
- Lactic acidosis and/or hepatic steatosis caused by mitochondrial toxicity. Potentially life-threatening: d4T most common cause.
- Hyperlipidemia.

DRUGS

Rare
- HIV-associated neuromuscular weakness syndrome (HANWS): ascending motor weakness, generally accompanied by lactic acidosis.
- Esophageal ulcer (association unclear).

DRUG INTERACTIONS
- Few pharmacokinetic drug interactions.
- AZT: coadministration with AZT contraindicated due to *in vitro* and *in vivo* antagonism.
- ddI: avoid coadministration due to increased rate of lactic acidosis and peripheral neuropathy.
- Use with caution with any drug capable of causing peripheral neuropathy.

DRUG-DRUG INTERACTIONS—See Appendix I, p. 620, for table of drug-drug interactions.

RESISTANCE
- TAMs (41L, 67N, 70R, 210W, 215Y/F, 219 Q/E): selected by d4T and AZT; increasing d4T resistance (and NRTI cross-resistance) with increasing number of TAMs.
- 151M complex and 69S insertion confer high-level resistance to d4T in setting of multi-NRTI resistance.
- 184V: as with AZT, 184V mutation (associated with 3TC resistance) may increase susceptibility or delay resistance to d4T.
- 65R: can be selected by d4T, especially with non-subtype B virus; causes low-level d4T resistance.

PHARMACOLOGY
Mechanism
- Intracellular phosphorylation to active stavudine triphosphate, which competitively inhibits HIV DNA polymerase.

Pharmacokinetic Parameters
- **Absorption:** 86% absorption; not affected by food or fasting.
- **Metabolism and Excretion:** 50% excreted unchanged in the urine via glomerular filtration and tubular secretion.
- **Protein Binding:** <5%.
- **Cmax, Cmin, and AUC:** Cmax: 1.4 mcg/mL after a single dose of 70 mg. Cmax for the Triomune (NVP/3TC/d4T) formulation is 40% higher than Zerit (d4T).
- **$T_{\frac{1}{2}}$:** serum: 1.0 hrs; intracellular: 3.5 hrs.

Pregnancy Risk
- Category C: studies in rhesus monkeys demonstrated 76% placental passage. Not teratogenic in rodent studies (but sternal bone calcium decreases seen). Carcinogenic studies not completed. Pregnant patients may be at increase risk of lactic acidosis (FDA warns against its use in pregnancy).

Breastfeeding Compatibility
- No human data, breast milk excretion in animal studies. Breastfeeding not recommended in the US in order to avoid postnatal transmission of HIV to the child, who may not yet be infected.

DOSING
Dosing for Decreased Hepatic Function
- Usual dose, but an alternative NRTI should be considered.

Renal Dosing
- Dosing for GFR of 50–80: Wt >60 kg: 40 mg twice daily or 30 mg twice daily (WHO recommendation); wt <60 kg: 30 mg twice daily.
- Dosing for GFR 26–50: Wt >60 kg 20 mg twice daily; wt <60 kg: 15 mg twice daily.
- Dosing for GFR 10–25: Wt >60 kg 20 mg once daily; wt <60 kg 15 mg once daily.
- Dosing for GFR of <10: Wt >60 kg: 20 mg q24h; wt <60 kg: 15 mg q24h.
- Dosing in hemodialysis: Wt >60 kg dose: 20 mg q24h; wt <60 kg dose: 15 mg q24h; on days of dialysis dose post-dialysis.
- Dosing in peritoneal dialysis: Wt >60 kg dose: 20 mg q24h; wt <60 kg dose: 15 mg q24h, on days of dialysis dose post-dialysis.
- Dosing in hemofiltration: No data: consider half of standard dose.

COMMENTS
- **Pros:** well studied NRTI. Well tolerated in short term; gradual emergence of TAM-medicated resistance.
- **Cons:** NRTI most commonly associated with mitochondrial toxicity, including lipoatrophy, lactic acidosis, and hepatic steatosis; ddI + d4T + EFV inferior to AZT + 3TC + EFV in ACTG384; d4T + 3TC + EFV noninferior to TDF + 3TC + EFV in GS903, but with greater toxicity (neuropathy, lipoatrophy, hyperlipidemia). No longer a recommended drug in guidelines used in developed countries, and no longer preferred agent in resource-limited seettings (WHO Guidelines). Important to refrigerate (10°C or lower) oral liquid formulation since significant loss of stability was observed after 4 wks at 25°C.

SELECTED REFERENCES
Gallant JE, Staszewski S, Pozniak AL, et al. Efficacy and safety of tenofovir DF vs stavudine in combination therapy in antiretroviral-naive patients: a 3-year randomized trial. *JAMA*, 2004; 292: 191–201.

Comments: Randomized, double-blind, placebo-controlled trial with 600 patients to compare 2 initial ART regimens: TDF/3TC/EFV vs d4T/3TC/EFV. At wk 48, 239 (80%) of 299 patients receiving TDF and 253 (84%) of 301 patients receiving d4T (95% CI, −10.4%–1.5%) achieved a VL <400. Equivalence was also demonstrated in the secondary analyses (VL <50) at wk 48 and through 144 wks. d4T was associated with greater toxicity, including hyperlipidemia, neuropathy, and lipodystrophy.

Robbins GK, De Gruttola V, Shafer RW, et al. Comparison of sequential three-drug regimens as initial therapy for HIV-1 infection. *N Engl J Med*, 2003; 349: 2293–303.

Comments: 620 patients randomized to compare sequential 3-drug regimens in 4 groups: EFV-based ART combined with AZT/3TC or d4T/ddI or NFV + AZT/3TC or d4T/ddI. Not surprising, EFV outperformed NFV in all arms. With a median of 2.3 yr follow-up, EFV combined with AZT/3TC associated with virologic failure in 14% and 23% of patients with the 1st and 2nd regimen, respectively. Higher rate of virologic failure in the EFV/d4T/ddI arm, with 31% and 58% of patients with the 1st and 2nd regimen, respectively.

DRUGS

TENOFOVIR DF

Paul A. Pham, PharmD and John G. Bartlett, MD

INDICATIONS
FDA
- Treatment of HIV-infection in combination with other antiretroviral drugs.
- Treatment of HBV.

Non-FDA Approved Uses
- Treatment of hepatitis in HIV-HBV coinfected patients.

FORMS TABLE

Brand name (mfr)	Forms†	Cost*
Viread (Gilead Sciences)	Oral tablet 300 mg	$25.72
Truvada (Gilead Sciences)	Oral tablet TDF 300 mg/FTC 200 mg	$39.84
Atripla (Bristol-Myers Squibb and Gilead Sciences)	Oral tablet EFV 600 mg/TDF 300 mg/ FTC 200 mg	$61.09
Complera (Gilead Sciences)	TDF/FTC/RPV 300/200/25 mg tablet	$68.19/ tablet

*Prices represent cost per unit specified, are representative of Average Wholesale Price (AWP).
†Dosage is indicated in mg unless otherwise noted.

USUAL ADULT DOSING
- Pill burden: 1 tab/day.
- TDF: 1 tab once daily without regard to meals. Fatty meals improve absorption by 40% (clinical significance unknown but not thought to be significant).

- TDF/FTC (*Truvada*): 1 tab once daily without regard to meals.
- EFV/TDF/FTC (*Atripla*): 1 tab once daily. Evening dosing on an empty stomach recommended at first to decrease EFV-associated side effects.
- RPV/TDF/FTC (*Complera*): 1 tab once daily with a meal.

ADVERSE DRUG REACTIONS

General

- Generally well tolerated. For *Atripla*, see efavirenz (p. 277) for EFV-associated side effects. For *Complera*, see rilpivirine (p. 311) for RPV-associated side effects.
- Greater loss of bone density than with other ARVs.

Occasional

- Flatulence, nausea, and vomiting. Asymptomatic elevation of CPK in 12%; transaminase elevation in 4%–5%. Neutropenia in 3% and increased amylase in 9%.
- TDF associated with a decrease in bone density (higher rates compared to other NRTIs, but generally modest and nonprogressive).
- Patients with underlying renal insufficiency or other conditions predisposing to renal insufficiency may be at increased risk for nephrotoxicity.

Rare

- Case reports of nephrotoxicity with characteristic features of Fanconi syndrome (hypophosphatemia, hypouricemia, proteinuria, and normoglycemic glycosuria).
- Lactic acidosis and hepatic steatosis: causal relationship not established. *In vitro*, TDF is one of the NRTIs least associated with mitochondrial toxicity. In a clinical trial, d4T resulted in significantly more hyperlactemia (>2.2 mmol/L) compared to TDF (27% vs 4%, P <0.0001).

DRUG INTERACTIONS

- Low likelihood drug interactions with PIs (with the exception of ATV and LPV) and NNRTIs, since TDF is not a substrate, inhibitor, or inducer of CYP3A4.

DRUG-DRUG INTERACTIONS—See Appendix I, p. 621, for table of drug-drug interactions.

RESISTANCE

- TAMs (41L, 210W, 215Y/F, 219Q/E, 67N, 70R): selected by AZT, d4T; high-level resistance with 3 or more TAMs that include 41L and 210W.
- K65R: selected by TDF, causing intermediate tenofovir resistance, and intermediate resistance to ddI, 3TC, FTC, low-level resistance to ABC and possibly d4T. Susceptibility to AZT retained (may be hypersusceptible).
- M184V: increased susceptibility; may partially reverse 65R- or TAM-mediated resistance.
- T69 insertion: intermediate resistance in setting of multi-NRTI resistance.
- Q151M complex: tenofovir sensitivity retained.
- L74V: increased susceptibility to tenofovir (clinical significance unknown).

PHARMACOLOGY

Mechanism

- TDF inhibits the activity of HIV reverse transcriptase by competing with the natural substrate deoxyadenosine 5'-triphosphate causing DNA chain termination.

Pharmacokinetic Parameters

- **Absorption:** oral absorption: 30% (fasting) and 40% with fatty meal.
- **Metabolism and Excretion:** renal excretion by glomerular filtration and active tubular secretion by MRP4.
- **Protein Binding:** $<7.2\%$.
- **Cmax, Cmin, and AUC:** mean Cmax = 296 ± 90 ng/mL; AUC = 2287 ± 685 ng h/mL.
- **$T_{\frac{1}{2}}$:** serum: 11–14 hrs; intracellular: 12–50 hrs.
- **Distribution:** Vd = 1.2 ± 4 L/kg.

Pregnancy Risk

- Category B: gravid rhesus monkeys study showed normal fetal development, but reduction in body weight, insulin-like growth factor, and fetal bone porosity observed (*JAIDS* 2002; 29: 207). Lower TDF exposure during 3rd trimester than postpartum period. Because of lack of data on use in human pregnancy and concern regarding potential fetal bone effects, TDF should be used as component of a maternal ART regimen only after careful consideration of alternatives. In 1st-trimester exposure (N = 606) and 2nd- or 3rd-trimester exposure (N = 336), prevalence of birth defects was 2.3% and 1.5%, respectively (Pregnancy Registry). This was similar to overall rates in general population.

Breastfeeding Compatibility

• Not recommended.

DOSING

Dosing For Decreased Hepatic Function

• No data. Usual dose likely.

Renal Dosing

• Dosing for GFR of 50–80: usual dose.
• Dosing for GFR of 30–49: TDF 300 mg q48h or TDF/FTC (*Truvada*) 1 tab q48h.
• Dosing for GFR of 10–30: TDF 300 mg q72–96h. *Atripla* (TDF/FTC/EFV) or *Complera* (TDF/FTC/RPV) not recommended with GFR <50.
• Dosing for GFR of <10: TDF 300 mg q7 days. *Atripla* (TDF/FTC/EFV) and *Complera* (TDF/FTC/RPV) not recommended with GFR <50.
• Dosing in hemodialysis: TDF 300 mg q7 days following HD (may require more if more than three 4-hr HD sessions). *Atripla* (TDF/FTC/EFV) and *Complera* (TDF/FTC/RPV) not recommended with GFR <50.
• Dosing in peritoneal dialysis: no data. Consider dose reduction. *Atripla* (TDF/TDF/FTC) and *Complera* (TDF/FTC/RPV) not recommended with GFR <50.
• Dosing in hemofiltration: no data. Consider dose reduction.

COMMENTS

• **Pros:** once-daily administration; well tolerated with few short-term side effects and no clear mitochondrial or other long-term toxicity; few drug interactions; beneficial effect on lipids; activity against some NRTI-resistant strains; longer intracellular half-life than most NRTIs; active against HBV. Coformulations available, including a single-pill, once-daily regimen. TDF/FTC is now the preferred NRTI backbone for initial therapy in DHHS and IAS-USA guidelines.
• **Cons:** potential for nephrotoxicity (may be increased when coadministered with PIs); may decrease bone density more than other NRTIs (generally modest and nonprogressive); resistance with selection of K65R.

DRUGS

SELECTED REFERENCES

Sax PE, Tierney C, Collier AC, et al. Abacavir-lamivudine versus tenofovir-emtricitabine for initial HIV-1 therapy. *N Engl J Med*, 2009; 361: 2230–40.
Comments: Randomized controlled trial compared TDF/FTC and ABC/3TC in combination with EFV or boosted ATV. At a median follow-up of 60 wks, among patients with VL >100K c/mL, the time to virologic failure was significantly shorter in the ABC/3TC group than in the TDF/FTC group (HR, 2.33; 95% CI, 1.46–3.72; P <0.001). 57 virologic failures (14%) were observed in the ABC/3TC group vs 26 (7%) in the TDF/FTC group. In patients with VL <100K c/mL, there was no significant difference in time to virological failure between groups. Shorter time to Grade 3/4 safety event with ABC/3TC than TDF/FTC when combined with EFV, and shorter time to treatment modification with ABC/3TC vs TDF/FTC with either EFV or ATV/r. HLA B*5701 testing not routinely performed. Greater lipid increases with ABC/3TC than TDF/FTC, but total/HDL cholesterol ratios similar.

Arribas JR, Pozniak AL, Gallant JE, et al. Tenofovir DF, emtricitabine, and efavirenz compared with zidovudine, lamivudine, and efavirenz in treatment-naive patients: 144-week analysis. *J Acquir Immune Defic Syndr*, 2008; 47: 75.
Comments: 144-wk multicenter, open-label trial comparing TDF + FTC vs coformulated AZT/3TC, both administered in combination with EFV, in 509 treatment-naïve patients. Mean baseline VL 5.0 log. At 144 wks, significantly more patients in the TDF/FTC arm reached and maintained an HIV RNA level <400 c/mL (71% TDF/FTC/EFV vs 58% ZDV/3TC/EFV; P = 0.004). CD4 cell increase in the TDF/FTC arm was 312 vs 271 in the AZT/3TC arm; P=0.09). More patients in the ZDV/3TC arm discontinued therapy because of adverse events (11% vs 5%; P = 0.01). ZDV/3TC arm had significantly less limb fat than patients in the TDF/FTC arm (5.4 vs 7.9 kg; P=0.001) at 144 wks.

Gallant JE, Rodriguez AE, Weinberg WG, et al. Early virologic nonresponse to tenofovir, abacavir, and lamivudine in HIV-infected antiretroviral-naive subjects. *J Infect Dis*, 2005; 192: 1921–30.
Comments: High rates of virologic failure in the triple-NRTI arm (TDF + ABC/3TC) (49%) vs 5% in ABC/3TC + EFV arm, resulted in early termination of the trial. Genotype from subset with failure showed 184V (36%) and both 65R + 184V (64%). ABC/3TC + TDF not recommended as an optional 1st-line regimen for naïve patients.

Gallant JE, Staszewski S, Pozniak AL, et al. Efficacy and safety of tenofovir DF vs stavudine in combination therapy in antiretroviral-naive patients: a 3-year randomized trial. *JAMA*, 2004; 292: 191–201.
Comments: Virologic outcome similar in both groups at wk 48 analysis; 239 (80%) of 299 patients receiving TDF and 253 (84%) of 301 patients receiving d4T (95% CI, −10.4%–1.5%) achieved VL <400. However, TDF associated with better lipid profiles and less lipodystrophy.

TIPRANAVIR

Paul A. Pham, PharmD and John G. Bartlett, MD

INDICATIONS
FDA
- Treatment of HIV+ patients with evidence of viral replication who are highly treatment-experienced or have HIV resistant to multiple PIs.

FORMS TABLE

Brand name (mfr)	Forms†	Cost*
Aptivus (Boehringer Ingelheim Pharmaceuticals)	Oral capsule 250 mg Oral liquid 100 mg/mL (95 mL)	$9.89

*Prices represent cost per unit specified, are representative of Average Wholesale Price (AWP).
†Dosage is indicated in mg unless otherwise noted.

USUAL ADULT DOSING
- Pill burden: 8/day.
- TPV 500 mg + RTV 200 mg twice daily with food. RTV 200 mg twice daily required to achieve desired serum concentrations.
- ETR, LPV/r, SQV, APV, FPV, and ATV: coadministration not recommended due to potent inducing effects of TPV on Pgp and glucuronidation.
- EFV: standard TPV/r dose, but PK study conducted with TPV/r 750/200 mg twice daily.
- NVP: consider standard doses.
- IDV, NFV, DRV: no data, avoid coadministration.
- MVC: standard dose TPV/r + MVC 300 mg twice daily.
- RAL: consider standard doses.
- TPV liquid should not be refrigerated or frozen. Use within 60 days after opening.

ADVERSE DRUG REACTIONS
Common
- Transaminase elevation: grade 2–4 ALT and/or AST elevation reported in 17.5% of TPV/r-treated patients vs 10% in comparator group (LPV/r, IDV/r, SQV/r, and APV/r).
- Elevated serum triglycerides: grade 3–4 (TG >750 mg/dL) in 19% of TPV/r-treated patients vs 9% in comparator group (LPV/r, IDV/r, SQV/r, and APV/r).
- Elevated cholesterol: grade 3–4 (cholesterol >400 mg/dL) reported in 3% of TPV/r-treated patients vs 0.3% in comparator group (LPV/r, IDV/r, SQV/r, and APV/r).
- Incidence of diarrhea, nausea, vomiting, and abdominal pain comparable to other PIs.
Occasional
- Other PI class adverse effects: insulin resistance, including hyperglycemia, and fat accumulation.
- Headache.
- Rash reported in 8%–14%. Appears to be higher in women.
Rare
- Intracranial hemorrhage: avoid in patients with head trauma/surgery or bleeding diathesis.

DRUG INTERACTIONS
- *In vitro*, TPV/r inhibits CYP1A2, CYP2C9, CYP2C19, CYP2D6, and CYP3A4 and induces phase II glucuronidation and the drug transporter P-glycoprotein (Pgp).
- Based on a pharmacokinetic study: (1) moderate inducer of CYP1A2; (2) modest inhibitor of CYP2C19 at the 1st dose, but an inducer at steady state; (3) inhibitor of CYP2D6 and CYP3A4/5 after 1st dose and steady state.

DRUG-DRUG INTERACTIONS—See Appendix I, p. 622, for table of drug-drug interactions.
RESISTANCE
- In RESIST-1 and -2 trials, 50% response (VL reduction >0.5 log or wk 4 VL <50) with <12 PI mutations; 32% with >19. 41%–44% response with up to 5 primary PI mutations.

- Mutation score: the following mutations affect TPV susceptibility: 10V, 13V, 20M/R/V, 33F, 35G, 36I, 43T, 46L, 47V, 54A/M/V, 58E, 69K, 74P, 82L/T, 83D, 84V. >2 mutations = reduced susceptibility; >7 mutations = resistance.
- 30N, 48V, 50V/L, 82A, 90M do not contribute to TPV mutation score.
- Phenotypic resistance (PhenoSense assay): FC <1 = full susceptibility; FC 1–4 = partial susceptibility; FC >4 = resistance.

PHARMACOLOGY
Mechanism
- Inhibition of protease prevents cleavage of synthesized polyproteins, resulting in the maturation and release of immature, noninfectious viruses.

Pharmacokinetic Parameters
- **Absorption:** bioavailability improved by 31% with high-fat meal.
- **Metabolism and Excretion:** substrate and potent inducer of CYP3A4. Excreted primarily in feces (82.3%) with only 4.4% recovered in the urine.
- **Protein Binding:** >99.9%.
- **Cmax, Cmin, and AUC:** Cmax: approximately 120 mcg/mL; Cmin: approximately 35 mcg/mL (dose TPV/r 500/200mg twice daily at steady state).
- $T_{\frac{1}{2}}$: 6 hrs.

Pregnancy Risk
- Category C: no human data. Not teratogenic in rats and rabbits studies.
- Breastfeeding Compatibility.
- CDC does not recommend breastfeeding to avoid postnatal transmission of HIV.

DOSING
Dosing for Decreased Hepatic Function
- Child-Pugh Class A: usual dose. TPV/r should not be used in patients with moderate-to-severe hepatic insufficiency (Child-Pugh Class B and C).

Renal dosing
- Dosing for GFR of 50–80: usual dose.
- Dosing for GFR of 10–50: no data. Usual dose likely.
- Dosing for GFR of <10: no data. Usual dose likely.
- Dosing in hemodialysis: no data. Usual dose likely (dose post-HD).
- Dosing in peritoneal dialysis: no data. Usual dose likely.
- Dosing in hemofiltration: no data.

COMMENTS
- **Pros:** active against many PI-resistant strains. More active than other boosted PIs in PI-experienced patients in RESIST trials. Active against some DRV-resistant strains.
- **Cons:** requires boosting with RTV 200 mg twice daily. More transaminase and lipid elevation than with comparator PIs. Can't be combined with other PIs because of potent Pgp induction. DRV often active in these patients (and in some with TPV resistance), and is generally better tolerated. FDA black box warning of potential risk for fatal and nonfatal intracranial hemorrhage in patients treated with boosted TPV. 3 reports of hepatic cytolysis in patients on RAL + TPV/r.

SELECTED REFERENCES
Walmsley SL, Katlama C, Lazzarin A, et al. Pharmacokinetics, safety, and efficacy of tipranavir boosted with ritonavir alone or in combination with other boosted protease inhibitors as part of optimized combination antiretroviral therapy in highly treatment-experienced patients (BI Study 1182.51). *J Acquir Immune Defic Syndr*, 2008; 47: 429–40.
Comments: At steady state, TPV/r decreased plasma trough levels 52%, 80%, and 56% for LPV, SQV, and APV recipients, respectively.

Baxter JD, Schapiro JM, Boucher CA, et al. Genotypic changes in human immunodeficiency virus type 1 protease associated with reduced susceptibility and virologic response to the protease inhibitor tipranavir. *J Virol*, 2006; 80: 10794–801.
Comments: Genotypic correlates of TPV resistance, replacing older criteria for resistance based on TPV mutation score (see Resistance section on p. 328).

Hicks CB, Cahn P, Cooper DA, et al. Durable efficacy of tipranavir-ritonavir in combination with an optimised background regimen of antiretroviral drugs for treatment-experienced HIV-1-infected patients at 48 weeks in the Randomized Evaluation of Strategic Intervention in multi-drug reSistant patients with Tipranavir (RESIST) studies: an analysis of combined data from two randomised open-label trials. *Lancet*, 2006; 368: 466–75.

DRUGS

Comments: Patients with VL >1000 and >1 primary PI mutation, but <2 primary mutations at codons 33, 82, 84, and 90 randomized to receive TPV/r or other PIs. At 48 wks, 30.4% in the TPV/r group and 13.8% of participants in the CPI/r group achieved VL <400 and 23% vs 10% achieved <50 (P <0.001). Similar to the POWER studies, patients on ENF had better response rate. Discontinuation rate was comparable in both groups.

ZIDOVUDINE

Paul A. Pham, PharmD and John G. Bartlett, MD

INDICATIONS
FDA
- Treatment of HIV infection in combination with other antiretrovirals.

FORMS TABLE

Brand name (mfr)	Forms†	Cost*
Retrovir and generic zidovudine (ViiV Healthcare and generic manufacturers [Roxane Laboratories, Ranbaxy Laboratories, and Aurobindo Pharmaceuticals])	Oral tablet 100 mg; 300 mg	$2.97; $8.92 for Retrovir (100 mg; 300 mg); $0.95 for generic AZT. (300 mg)
	IV vial 10 mg/mL (20 mL)	$32.16
	Oral syrup 10 mg/mL (8 oz)	$71.34
	Oral tablet 60 mg	n/a (not available in US)
Combivir (ViiV Healthcare)	Oral tablet 300 mg AZT/150 mg 3TC	$14.55
Trizivir (ViiV Healthcare)	Oral tablet 300 mg AZT/150 mg 3TC/300 mg ABC	$23.58

*Prices represent cost per unit specified, are representative of Average Wholesale Price (AWP).
†Dosage is indicated in mg unless otherwise noted.

USUAL ADULT DOSING
- Pill burden: 2/day.
- AZT 300 mg PO twice daily (preferred) or 200 mg PO 3 ×/day with or without food (often better tolerated with food).
- Combivir (AZT 300 mg + 3TC 150 mg) 1 tab PO twice daily.
- Trizivir (ABC 300 mg + AZT 300 mg + 3TC 150 mg) 1 tab PO twice daily.
- Perinatal transmission protocol (ACTG 076) AZT 300 mg PO twice daily starting from wk 14 to delivery; intrapartum: AZT IV 2 mg/kg 1st hr, then 1 mg/kg/hr until delivery; postpartum: syrup 2 mg/kg q6h (or 1.5 mg/kg q6h IV) × 6 wks to the infant.

ADVERSE DRUG REACTIONS
General
- GI intolerance higher than with other NRTIs.
Common
- GI intolerance, headache (5%–10%).
- Insomnia, malaise, myalgia, and asthenia.
- Bone marrow suppression (anemia usually seen within 4–6 wks and neutropenia usually seen after 12–24 wks).
- Fingernail discoloration/hyperpigmentation.
- Benign macrocytosis (crude indicator of adherence).
Occasional
- Transaminase elevation with reversible hepatitis.
- Lipoatrophy.

Rare
- Myopathy (with LDH and CPK elevation with ragged red fibers on muscle biopsy).
- Cardiomyopathy.
- Lactic acidosis or hyperlactatemia ± hepatic steatosis (consider in patients with progressive fatigue, abdominal pain, N and V, weight loss, and/or dyspnea).

DRUG INTERACTIONS
- Extensive first-past liver metabolism to glucuronide AZT. Drugs that induce glucuronidation may decrease AZT plasma concentrations; clinical significance of these potential interactions is unknown since plasma concentrations of AZT do not correlate well with antiviral activity and it is the intracellular triphosphate that exerts antiviral activity.

DRUG-DRUG INTERACTIONS—See Appendix I, p. 634, for table of drug-drug interactions.

RESISTANCE
- TAMs: selected by AZT and d4T. Resistance (including NRTI cross-resistance) increases with number of TAMs. Greater resistance with 41L/L210W/T215Y pathway than withD67N/K70R/K219 pathway.
- E44D, V118I: accessory mutations that increase AZT resistance when combined with TAMs (especially M41L/L210W/T215Y).
- Q151M or T69 insertion: high-level AZT resistance and NRTI cross-resistance. Selected by AZT/ddI and ddI/d4T combinations.
- M184V: increases AZT susceptibility, partially reversing effect of TAMs, but cannot overcome effect of multiple TAMs.
- K65R and L74V: increase susceptibility to AZT (clinical significance unknown).

PHARMACOLOGY
Mechanism
- Intracellular phosphorylation to active zidovudine triphosphate, which competitively inhibits HIV DNA polymerase.

Pharmacokinetic Parameters
- **Absorption:** 60% absorption; high-fat meals may decrease absorption (clinical significance unknown).
- **Metabolism and Excretion:** metabolized by liver to glucuronide (G-ZVD) that is renally excreted.
- **Protein Binding:** 34%–38%.
- **Cmax, Cmin, and AUC:** mean steady-state Cmax = 1.5 mcg/mL. AZT triphosphate intracellular levels 0.19 mcg/mL.
- **$T_{\frac{1}{2}}$:** plasma: 1.1 hrs; intracellular: 3 hrs.

Pregnancy Risk
- Category C: human studies demonstrated 85% placental passage. No maternal toxicities or fetal defects noted with AZT during pregnancy. Long-term toxicity data (up to 3.9 yrs) for infants exposed to AZT *in utero* and postpartum did not show an increased risk of adverse effects or developmental abnormalities.

Breastfeeding Compatibility
- Mean concentration of AZT was similar in human milk and in serum. Breastfeeding is not recommended in the US in order to avoid postnatal transmission of HIV to the child, who may not yet be infected.

DOSING
Dosing For Decreased Hepatic Function
- 100 mg 3 ×/day.

Renal Dosing
- Dosing for GFR of 50–80: 300 mg twice daily.
- Dosing for GFR of 10–50: 300 mg twice daily.
- Dosing for GFR of <10: 300 mg once daily.
- Dosing in hemodialysis: 300 mg once daily.
- Dosing in peritoneal dialysis: 300 mg once daily.
- Dosing in hemofiltration: no data. Usual dose likely.

DRUGS

COMMENTS

- **Pros:** availability of generics; extensive long-term data and clinical experience; documented efficacy in preventing perinatal and occupational transmission; effective in treating thrombocytopenia. Crosses blood-brain barrier, and experience with treatment of dementia. High-level resistance requires multiple mutations: failure of AZT/3TC-containing combinations results in gradual accumulation of TAMs. When AZT used in a TDF- or ABC-containing regimen, K65R or L74V unlikely to occur.
- **Cons:** twice-daily dosing; GI intolerance (especially nausea), headaches, fatigue, asthenia, anemia, neutropenia; mitochondrial toxicity, including lipoatrophy, lactic acidosis, hepatic steatosis; high-level resistance with multiple TAMs leads to broad NRTI cross-resistance. AZT/3TC less effective than TDF/FTC at 48 wks, primarily because of greater drop-out due to anemia and other side effects.

SELECTED REFERENCES

Gallant JE, DeJesus E, Arribas JR, et al. Tenofovir DF, emtricitabine, and efavirenz vs. zidovudine, lamivudine, and efavirenz for HIV. *N Engl J Med*, 2006; 354: 251–60.
Comments: 509 treatment-naïve patients randomized to receive TDF + FTC + EFV or AZT/3TC + EFV. At 48 wks, 77% of TDF/FTC/EFV-treated patients and 68% of AZT/3TC/EFV-treated patients achieved a VL <50 cs/mL (ITT; P = 0.034). Discontinuation due to adverse events higher with AZT/3TC + EFV (9% vs 4%), with 6% experiencing severe anemia. NRTI resistance profiles between wks 8 and 48 for patients with HIV RNA >400 c/mL showed 1 TAM and 7 M184V/I mutations in AZT/3TC + EFV arm. In contrast to GS903, NRTI resistance was limited to only 2 M184V/I and no K65R mutations in patients w/ virologic failure on TDF + FTC + EFV. Patients in the TDF + FTC arm also had significantly greater limb fat by DXA at 48 wks than those in AZT/3TC arm.

Gulick RM, Ribaudo HJ, Shikuma CM, et al. Three- vs four-drug antiretroviral regimens for the initial treatment of HIV-1 infection: a randomized controlled trial. *JAMA*, 2006; 296: 769–81.
Comments: A continuation phase of ACTG 5095 compared AZT/3TC and AZT/ABC/3TC, each combined with EFV in treatment-naïve patients. There were no significant differences between the 3- and 4-drug antiretroviral regimens; approximately 80% of patients had VL <50 through 3 yrs.

Gulick RM, Ribaudo HJ, Shikuma CM, et al. Triple-nucleoside regimens versus efavirenz-containing regimens for the initial treatment of HIV-1 infection. *N Engl J Med*, 2004; 350: 1850–61.
Comments: Randomized, double-blind study comparing 3 regimens (AZT/3TC/ABC, AZT/3TC/EFV, AZT/3TC/ABC/EFV) as initial treatment in naïve patients. After median follow-up of 32 wks, 82 of 382 patients in the triple-nucleoside group (21%) and 85 of 765 of those in the combined EFV groups (11%) had virologic failure; time to virologic failure significantly shorter in the triple-nucleoside group (P <0.001). Based on results of this trial, triple-nucleoside regimens no longer recommended as first-line therapy in naïve patients.

Robbins GK, De Gruttola V, Shafer RW, et al. Comparison of sequential three-drug regimens as initial therapy for HIV-1 infection. *N Engl J Med*, 2003; 349: 2293–303.
Comments: ACTG 384: 620 patients randomized to compare sequential 3-drug regimens in 4 groups: EFV-based ART combined with AZT/3TC or d4T/ddI or NFV + AZT/3TC or d4T/ddI. Most effective and best tolerated combination was AZT/3TC + EFV, with virologic failure in 14% and 23% of patients with the 1st and 2nd regimen, respectively (median 2.3 yr follow-up). Higher rate of virologic failure in the EFV/d4T/ddI arm (31% and 58%).

Katzenstein DA, Hammer SM, Hughes MD, et al. The relation of virologic and immunologic markers to clinical outcomes after nucleoside therapy in HIV-infected adults with 200 to 500 CD4 cells per cubic millimeter. AIDS Clinical Trials Group Study 175 Virology Study Team. *N Engl J Med*, 1996; 335: 1091–8.
Comments: 391 HIV+ subjects with CD4 200–500 randomly assigned to receive AZT alone, ddI alone, AZT + ddI, or AZT + ddC. After 8 wks, the mean (± SE) decrease from baseline log HIV RNA was 0.26 ± 0.06 for patients treated with AZT alone, 0.65 ± 0.07 for ddI alone, and 0.93 ± 0.10 for AZT + ddI (p <0.001). One of the 1st studies to show that the risk of progression of HIV disease is strongly associated with viral load.

Fischl MA, Richman DD, Grieco MH, et al. The efficacy of azidothymidine (AZT) in the treatment of patients with AIDS and AIDS-related complex. A double-blind, placebo-controlled trial. *N Engl J Med*, 1987; 317: 185–91.
Comments: The 1st trial to show survival benefit with ART therapy. Of the 282 patients, 19 placebo recipients and 1 AZT recipient died during the study period (p<0.001).

DAUNORUBICIN CITRATE LIPOSOME INJECTION

Paul A. Pham, PharmD and John G. Bartlett, MD

INDICATIONS

FDA

- Treatment of advanced HIV-associated Kaposi sarcoma (KS).

FORMS TABLE

Brand name (mfr)	Forms†	Cost*
DaunoXome (Gilead)	IV vial 50 mg/50 mL	$340.00

*Prices represent cost per unit specified, are representative of Average Wholesale Price (AWP).
†Dosage is indicated in mg unless otherwise noted.

USUAL ADULT DOSING

- 40 mg/m^2, administer over 60 min via IV infusion q2 wks. Diluted 1:1 with D5W before administration. Each vial contains daunorubicin citrate equivalent to 50 mg daunorubicin base (concentration of 2 mg/mL). Recommended concentration after dilution = 1 mg daunorubicin/mL of solution. Do not mix with saline, bacteriostatic agents such as benzyl alcohol, or any other solution.

ADVERSE DRUG REACTIONS

Common

- Granulocytopenia.
- Nausea, vomiting.
- Alopecia.

Occasional

- Cardiotoxicity with cumulative dose >300 mg/square meter: hypertension, palpitation, syncope, pericardial effusion, pericardial tamponade, ventricular extrasystoles, cardiac arrest, sinus tachycardia, atrial fibrillation, pulmonary hypertension, myocardial infarction, supraventricular tachycardia, CHF, and angina pectoris.
- Triad of back pain, flushing, and chest tightness has been reported; generally occurs during the 1st 5 min of infusion. Symptoms subside with interruption of infusion, and usually do not recur if infusion resumed at a slower rate.

Rare

- Dyspnea and cough.
- Neuropathy.

DRUG INTERACTIONS

- AZT and other marrow suppressive drugs (e.g., ganciclovir, pyrimethamine): potential for additive bone marrow suppression.

PHARMACOLOGY

Mechanism

- Works through inhibition of topoisomerase-II at the point of DNA cleavage.

Pharmacokinetic Parameters

- **Metabolism and Excretion:** daunorubicin metabolized to daunorubicinol.
- **Protein Binding:** 63%.
- **T$_{\frac{1}{2}}$:** 4.4 hrs.
- **Distribution:** Vd = 6.4 L.

DRUGS

Pregnancy Risk
- Category D: not recommended.

Breastfeeding Compatibility
- Not recommended.

DOSING

Dosing for Decreased Hepatic Function
- Serum bilirubin 1.2 to 3 mg/dL, give 3/4 the normal dose; serum bilirubin >3 mg/dL, give 1/2 the normal dose.

Renal Dosing
- Dosing for GFR of 50–80: usual dose.
- Dosing for GFR of 10–50: SCr >3 mg/dL: administer 1/2 of normal dose.
- Dosing for GFR of <10: SCr >3 mg/dL: administer 1/2 of normal dose.
- Dosing in hemodialysis: no data.
- Dosing in peritoneal dialysis: no data.
- Dosing in hemofiltration: no data.

COMMENTS

- Effective for treatment of KS. Direct comparison between liposomal doxorubicin and liposomal daunorubicin has not been conducted. Liposomal daunorubicin substantially less expensive.
- Monitor cardiac function monitored regularly. Should be administered only under supervision of physician experienced in use of cancer chemotherapeutic agents.

SELECTED REFERENCES

Lichterfeld M, Qurishi N, Hoffmann C, et al. Treatment of HIV-1-associated Kaposi's sarcoma with pegylated liposomal doxorubicin and ART simultaneously induces effective tumor remission and CD4+ T cell recovery. *Infection*, 2005; 33: 140–7.
Comments: This observational study found that 81.5% of the patients had complete or partial responses within 8 wks of treatment with daunorubicin + ART.

Gill PS, Wernz J, Scadden DT, et al. Randomized phase III trial of liposomal daunorubicin versus doxorubicin, bleomycin, and vincristine in AIDS-related Kaposi's sarcoma. *J Clin Oncol*, 1996; 14: 2353–64.
Comments: Prospective trial comparing liposomal daunorubicin to ABV. Overall response rate (complete or partial) was 25% for the liposomal daunorubicin and 28% for the ABV group (not statistically significant).

Girard PM, Bouchaud O, Goetschel A, et al. Phase II study of liposomal encapsulated daunorubicin in the treatment of AIDS-associated mucocutaneous Kaposi's sarcoma. *AIDS*, 1996; 10: 753–7.
Comments: Phase II trial showed that 73% achieved partial response with median time of response 30 days and minimal ADRs. Granulocytoma seen in 53%.

DOXORUBICIN LIPOSOMAL

Paul A. Pham, PharmD and John G. Bartlett, MD

INDICATIONS

FDA
- Treatment of AIDS-related Kaposi sarcoma (KS).
- Ovarian cancer.

FORMS TABLE

Brand name (mfr)	Forms[†]	Cost[*]
Doxil (JOM Pharmaceutical)	IV vial 2 mg/mL (10 mL); 2 mg/mL (25 mL)	$1157.56 (10 mL); $2894.40 (25 mL)

[*]Prices represent cost per unit specified, are representative of Average Wholesale Price (AWP).
[†]Dosage is indicated in mg unless otherwise noted.

- 20 mg/m² IV over 30 min q3 wks (initial rate of 1 mg/min). Dilute in D5W; do not administer IM, SC, as bolus injection or undiluted solution; continue until response (use patients ideal weight to calculate body surface area).
- Local erythematous streaking along vein and/or facial flushing may occur with rapid infusion rate.

ADVERSE DRUG REACTIONS
Common
- Dose-dependent nausea and vomiting (30%–60%).
- Dose-dependent leukopenia (60%–80%).
- Alopecia.
- Mucositis.

Occasional
- Alkaline phosphatase increase.
- Cardiac toxicity (10%): cardiomyopathy, CHF, arrhythmia, pericardial effusion and tachycardia. Use with caution in patients with h/o cardiac disease, thoracic radiation, or exposure to high dose anthracyclines and cyclophosphamide. LVEF should be closely monitored when the total dose is 320 mg/m², 480 mg/m², and every 160 mg/m² thereafter.
- Palmar-plantar erythrodysesthesia.
- Rash.
- Stomatitis.
- Facial flushing.
- Tissue necrosis with extravasation during administration. If extravasation occurs, apply ice immediately for 30–60 min then alternate off/on every 15 min for 1d. Elevate and rest extremity. Consult plastic surgeon if pain, erythema, and/or swelling persist beyond 48 hrs.
- Acute infusion reactions (back pain, flushing, and chest tightness) may occur in 1st 5 min of infusion. Stop infusion and resume at lower rate.

DRUG INTERACTIONS
- CYP2D6 and CYP3A4 substrate. Moderate inhibition of CYP2B6.
- ETR, NVP, and EFV: may decrease serum levels of doxorubicin.
- MVC: interaction unlikely.
- PIs and DLV: may increase serum levels of doxorubicin but no apparent toxicity with coadministration observed in clinical trials (*HIV Clinical Trials* 2001; 2: 429).
- RAL: interaction unlikely.

PHARMACOLOGY
Mechanism
- Doxorubicin hydrochloride encapsulated in long-circulating STEALTH liposomes (microscopic vesicles composed of a phospholipid bilayer capable of encapsulating active drugs). Works through inhibition of topoisomerase-II at the point of DNA cleavage.

Pharmacokinetic Parameters
- **Metabolism and Excretion:** extensively metabolised in the liver todoxorubicinol, sulfate conjugate of 4-demethyl, 7-deoxyaglycones, and glucuronide conjugate of 4-demethyl, 7-deoxyaglycones.
- **T$_{\frac{1}{2}}$:** 45–55 hrs.
- **Distribution:** Vd = 2.8 L/m².

Pregnancy Risk
- Category D: not recommended.

Breastfeeding Compatibility
- Not recommended.

DOSING
Dosing for Decreased Hepatic Function
- Bilirubin 1.2–3 mg/dL –50% of normal dose; bilirubin of greater than 3 mg/dL –25% of normal dose.

DRUGS

Renal Dosing
- Dosing for GFR of 50–80: no data.
- Dosing for GFR of 10–50: no data, usual dose likely since only 5% of dose is renally excreted.
- Dosing for GFR of <10: no data, usual dose likely since only 5% of dose is renally excreted.
- Dosing in hemodialysis: no data.
- Dosing in peritoneal dialysis: no data.
- Dosing in hemofiltration: no data.

SELECTED REFERENCES

Martin-Carbonero L, Barrios A, Saballs P, et al. Pegylated liposomal doxorubicin plus highly active antiretroviral therapy versus highly active antiretroviral therapy alone in HIV patients with Kaposi's sarcoma. *AIDS*, 2004; 18: 1737–40.
Comments: In moderate–advanced KS, better response rates observed in ART plus liposomal doxorubicine group compared to ART alone group (76% vs 20%).

Cheung TW, Remick SC, Azarnia N, et al. AIDS-related Kaposi's sarcoma: a phase II study of liposomal doxorubicin. The TLC D-99 Study Group. *Clin Cancer Res*, 1999; 5: 3432–7.
Comments: Dose finding study confirmed dose-dependent response (5% response in 10 mg/m^2 group vs 24% in 20 mg/m^2 group). Neutropenia was major toxicity occurring in 68% and 81% of patients in low and high dose arms, respectively.

Northfelt DW, Dezube BJ, Thommes JA, et al. Pegylated-liposomal doxorubicin versus doxorubicin, bleomycin, and vincristine in the treatment of AIDS-related Kaposi's sarcoma: results of a randomized phase III clinical trial. *J Clin Oncol*, 1998; 16: 2445–51.
Comments: Randomized trial showed 46% response rate with pegylated-liposome doxorubicin vs 25% response rate for ABV. Liposomal doxorubicin less toxic than standard combination chemotherapy.

PACLITAXEL

Paul A. Pham, PharmD and John G. Bartlett, MD

INDICATIONS

FDA
- 2nd-line treatment of AIDS-related Kaposi sarcoma (KS).
- 2nd-line treatment of metastatic breast cancer.
- 1st-line treatment of non-small cell lung cancer (in combination with cisplatin or carboplatin).
- 2nd-line treatment of metastatic ovarian cancer.

FORMS TABLE

Brand name (mfr)	Forms†	Cost*
Taxol (ER Squibb and Sons)	IV vial 300 mg 50-mL vial (6 mg/mL)	$584.41
Paclitaxel (generic manufacturer)	IV vial 5 mL; 16.7 mL; 25 mL; 50-mL vial (6 mg/mL)	$17.70; $51.96; $79.20; $162.00

*Prices represent cost per unit specified, are representative of Average Wholesale Price (AWP).
†Dosage is indicated in mg unless otherwise noted.

USUAL ADULT DOSING
- AIDS-related KS: 135 mg/m^2 over 3 hrs q3 wks or 100 mg/m^2 over 3 hrs q2 wks.
- Paclitaxel should be diluted to a final concentration of 0.3–1.2 mg/mL with 0.9% NS or D5W; paclitaxel should be infused through an inline filter.
- Premedication with dexamethasone 20 mg PO or IV at 6 and 12 hrs before dose + diphenhydramine 50 mg IV + H2 blocker IV 30 min prior to dose recommended to prevent hypersensitivity reaction. Fatal reactions have occurred despite premedication.
- Patients with severe hypersensitive reaction should not be rechallenged.

- Do not give to patients with solid tumor with baseline ANC <1500 or to patients with KS and ANC <1000.

ADVERSE DRUG REACTIONS

Common

- Abnormal LFTs.
- Peripheral neuropathy.
- Nausea and vomiting.
- Myalgia and arthralgia.
- Myelosuppression-neutropenia with increased risk of infection (frequent CBC monitoring recommended).
- Bradycardia and hypotension.

Occasional

- Anaphylaxis (2%–4%) and hypersensitivity reactions.

Rare

- Hepatic encephalopathy/necrosis.
- Interstitial pneumonia.
- Neuroencephalopathy.

DRUG INTERACTIONS

- CYP2C8/9 and 3A4 substrate.
- ddI and d4T: potential for additive peripheral neuropathy with paclitaxel coadministration.
- EFV and NVP: may decrease paclitaxel levels.
- PIs and DLV: may increase paclitaxel levels.
- ETR: may ↑ or ↓ paclitaxel levels.

PHARMACOLOGY

Mechanism

- Promotes microtubule assembly by enhancing action of tubulin dimers, stabilizing existing microtubules, and inhibiting their disassembly, interfering with the late G2 mitotic phase, and inhibiting cell replication. Can distort mitotic spindles resulting in breakage of chromosomes.

Pharmacokinetic Parameters

- **Metabolism and Excretion:** extensively metabolized in the liver to inactive metabolites that are excreted in the urine and feces.
- **Protein Binding:** 89%–98%.
- **Cmax, Cmin, and AUC:** following continuous 6-hr paclitaxel infusions of 175 mg/m^2, mean Cmax were 3.2 micromol/L, respectively.
- **T$_\frac{1}{2}$:** 3.1–52.7 hrs.
- **Distribution:** Vd = 67,182 L/m^2.

Pregnancy Risk

- Category D: paclitaxel is embryotoxic, fetotoxic, and reduces fertility.

Breastfeeding Compatibility

- Not recommended.

DOSING

Dosing for Decreased Hepatic Function

- May require dose adjustment since grade III/IV myelosuppression is seen in patients with hepatic impairment. With bilirubin 2–4 × ULN: 135 mg/m^2, and >4 × ULN: 50 mg/m^2 or consider holding dose.

Renal Dosing

- Dosing for GFR of 50–80: usual dose.
- Dosing for GFR of 10–50: usual dose.
- Dosing for GFR of <10: usual dose.
- Dosing in hemodialysis: no data.
- Dosing in peritoneal dialysis: no data.
- Dosing in hemofiltration: no data.

COMMENTS

- Effective chemotherapeutic agent in patients who fail to respond to 1st-line treatment for KS.

SELECTED REFERENCES

Tulpule A, Groopman J, Saville MW, et al. Multicenter trial of low-dose paclitaxel in patients with advanced AIDS-related Kaposi sarcoma. *Cancer,* 2002; 95: 147–54.

Comments: Open-label study to assess safety and efficacy of paclitaxel in patients with AIDS-KS who failed to respond to previous chemotherapy. Complete or partial response in 56%, with median duration of response 8.9 mos. 77% were on a PI; response rate did not differ in patients on PI-based regimens.

Gill PS, Tulpule A, Espina BM, et al. Paclitaxel is safe and effective in the treatment of advanced AIDS-related Kaposi's sarcoma. *J Clin Oncol,* 1999; 17: 1876–83.

Comments: Phase II trial involving 56 patients with AIDS-related KS. Paclitaxel was given at dose of 100 mg/m² every 2 wks until complete remission, disease progression, or unacceptable toxicity. Median duration of response 10.4 mos. R 59% showed complete or partial response.

Lipid-Lowering Agents

FENOFIBRATE

Paul A. Pham, PharmD and John G. Bartlett, MD

INDICATIONS

FDA

- Hyperlipoproteinemia-type 4 and 5.

Non-FDA Approved Uses

- Treatment of hypertriglyceridemia, including ART-associated.

FORMS TABLE

Brand name (mfr)	Forms†	Cost*
Tricor (Abbott Laboratories)	Oral nanocrystal-lized tab 145 mg	$4.60 per 145-mg tab
Lofibra (Gate Pharmaceuticals)	Oral micronized cap 67 mg; 134 mg; 200 mg	$0.99 per 67-mg cap; $1.90 per 134-mg cap; $2.96 per 200-mg cap
	Oral micronized tab 54 mg; 160 mg	$0.99 per 54-mg tab; $2.96 per 160-mg tab
Triglide (Sciele Pharma, Inc.)	Oral tab 50 mg; 160 mg	$1.53 per 50-mg tab; $4.58 per 160-mg tab

*Prices represent cost per unit specified, are representative of Average Wholesale Price (AWP).
†Dosage is indicated in mg unless otherwise noted.

USUAL ADULT DOSING

- Fenofibrate (*Tricor*): 145 mg PO once daily with meals; start at lower dose in elderly. Lower dose formulations discontinued by manufacturer. Consider titrating with *Lofibra* (see below) on response (max 160 mg/day).
- Fenofibrate (*Lofibra*): start at 67 mg PO once daily with meals; increase by 67 mg/day q4–6 wks (max 200 mg/day).
- Fenofibrate (*Lofibra*) 67 mg micronized tab = fenofibrate (*Tricor*) 54 mg micronized cap.
- Should be discontinued if no response in 2–3 mos.

ADVERSE DRUG REACTIONS

Occasional

- Transaminase elevation (dose-related hepatotoxicity with ALT to >3 × ULN in 6% of those receiving 134–200 mg/day). LFTs return to normal range in most cases with discontinuation or continued treatment.
- Rash, urticaria, and pruritus.
- Myositis.
- Erectile dysfunction.

Rare

- Gallstones.
- Leukopenia.
- Rhabdomyolysis: increased risk when combined with "statins".
- Pancreatitis.
- Agranulocytopenia.
- Eczema.
- Thrombocytopenia.
- Influenza-like syndrome.

DRUGS

DRUG INTERACTIONS

- Bile acid binding agents (cholestyramine and colestipol): bind fenofibrate take fenofibrate >1 hr before or 4–6 hrs after bile acid binding agents.
- "Statins": may increase risk of rhabdomyolysis (no pharmacokinetic interaction with rosuvastatin).
- Warfarin: may increase INR.

PHARMACOLOGY

Mechanism

- Hydrolyzed to its active metabolite fenofibric acid, which increases lipoprotein lipase activity. This results in increased lipolysis of triglyceride and VLDL.
- 90% (micronized formulation); administer with food.

Pharmacokinetic Parameters

- **Absorption:** 90% (micronized formulation); administer with food.
- **Metabolism and Excretion:** extensive glucuronidation prior to renal excretion.
- **Protein Binding:** 99%.
- **T$_{\frac{1}{2}}$:** 22 hrs (active fenofibric acid).
- **Distribution:** Vd = 0.9 L/kg.

Pregnancy Risk

- Category C: no human data. Animal data using large doses reported teratogenicity.

Breastfeeding Compatibility

- No data.

DOSING

Dosing for Decreased Hepatic Function

- No data. Use with caution.

Renal Dosing

- Dosing for GFR of 50–80: usual dose.
- Dosing for GFR of 10–50: dose reduction should be considered.
- Dosing for GFR of <10: dose reduction should be considered.
- Dosing in hemodialysis: no data. Dose reduction should be considered.
- Dosing in peritoneal dialysis: no data.
- Dosing in hemofiltration: no data.

COMMENTS

- Not as potent as "statins" for decreasing LDL and increasing HDL cholesterol (*J Cardiovasc Risk* 1999; 6: 113–116). Fenofibrate equivalent to gemfibrozil in lowering triglycerides, but has more convenient dosing; may have slight benefit in lowering LDL.

SELECTED REFERENCES

Aberg JA, Zackin RA, Brobst SW, et al. A randomized trial of the efficacy and safety of fenofibrate versus pravastatin in HIV-infected subjects with lipid abnormalities: AIDS Clinical Trials Group Study 5087. *AIDS Res Hum Retroviruses*, 2005; 21: 757–67.
Comments: Randomized, open-label study compared fenofibrate 200 mg (N = 88) to pravastatin 40 mg (N = 86) daily for treatment of dyslipidemia in HIV+ patients. Subjects who failed to reach National Cholesterol Education Program (NCEP) composite goal on monotherapy by wk 12 received both drugs. Composite goal at wk 12 achieved in only 1% of fenofibrate and 5% of pravastatin subjects. Even with addition of alternative agent, <10% of patients achieved NCEP composite goal.

Rao A, D'Amico S, Balasubramanyam A, et al. Fenofibrate is effective in treating hypertriglyceridemia associated with HIV lipodystrophy. *Am J Med Sci*, 2004; 327: 315–8.
Comments: In this observational study, fenofibrate significantly decreased ART-associated triglyceride elevation. Baseline and 6 mos fasting triglyceride levels were 886 ± 172 mg/dL, and 552 ± 104, respectively (P <0.05). No change in LDH and HDL.

Insua A, Massari F, Rodríguez Moncalvo JJ, et al. Fenofibrate of gemfibrozil for treatment of types IIa and IIb primary hyperlipoproteinemia: a randomized, double-blind, crossover study. *Endocr Pract*, 2002; 8: 96–101.
Comments: Randomized, double-blind, crossover study to assess effects of gemfibrozil (900 mg) or fenofibrate (200 mg) in HIV-negative patients with hyperlipidemia. Percentage decrease in total cholesterol and LDL cholesterol greater with fenofibrate than with gemfibrozil (−22% vs −15%, P <0.02; and −27% vs −16%, P <0.02, respectively). Reductions in triglyceride levels (−54% vs −46.5%), apolipoprotein B, and fibrinogen, and increase in HDL (+9% for both drugs), showed no significant difference between treatment arms.

GEMFIBROZIL

Paul A. Pham, PharmD and John G. Bartlett, MD

INDICATIONS

FDA

• Treatment of hypertriglyceridemia.

FORMS TABLE

Brand name (mfr)	Forms†	Cost*
Lopid and generic (Pfizer and generic manufacturer)	Oral tab 600 mg	$1.25

*Prices represent cost per unit specified, are representative of Average Wholesale Price (AWP).
†Dosage is indicated in mg unless otherwise noted.

USUAL ADULT DOSING

• 600 mg PO twice daily 30 min before meals; discontinue if no reduction in triglycerides (TG) by 3 mos.
• May increase LDL and total cholesterol levels (return to pretreatment levels 6–8 wks after discontinuation).

ADVERSE DRUG REACTIONS

Common

• Dyspepsia.

Occasional

• Diarrhea, nausea, and vomiting.
• Transaminase elevation. Monitor transaminases at baseline, 3 and 6 mos, and yearly; discontinue if persistent unexplained grade 3/4 elevation (5–10 × ULN).
• Abdominal pain.

Rare

• Myositis, impotence, gallstones, and hypokalemia.
• Anemia.
• Leukopenia.
• Eosinophilia.
• Alkaline phosphatase elevation.

DRUG INTERACTIONS

• Gemfibrozil increased rosuvastatin AUC by 90% (use fenofibrate with rosuvastatin).
• HMG-CoA reductase inhibitors ("statins"): may increase risk of rhabdomyolysis.
• Repaglinide: gemfibrozil increases concentrations of repaglinide and may prolonged its hypoglycemic effects.
• Ursodiol efficacy may be decreased.
• Warfarin: increased INR.

PHARMACOLOGY

Mechanism

• Inhibition of peripheral lipolysis through reduced hepatic extraction of free fatty acids, which reduces hepatic TG production resulting in decreased TG and increased HDL.

Pharmacokinetic Parameters

• **Absorption:** well absorbed, 97%.
• **Metabolism and Excretion:** extensive hepatic metabolism with renal excretion of metabolite and unchanged drug.
• **Protein Binding:** 99%.
• **T$_{\frac{1}{2}}$:** 1.5 hr.

Pregnancy Risk

• Category C: some animal data show teratogenicity, other studies do not. Limited human data.

DRUGS

Breastfeeding Compatibility
• No data.

DOSING

Dosing for Decreased Hepatic Function
• Consider dose reduction. Use with caution.

Renal Dosing
• Dosing for GFR of 50–80: usual dose.
• Dosing for GFR of 10–50: 600–1200 mg once daily.
• Dosing for GFR of <10: 300–600 mg/day. Some recommend avoiding in renal failure.
• Dosing in hemodialysis: no data.
• Dosing in peritoneal dialysis: no data.
• Dosing in hemofiltration: no data.

COMMENTS
• Recommended for patients with TG >500. Dietary counselling, exercise, weight loss, and control of diabetes mellitus and hypothyroidism should be attempted before initiating therapy. Monitor transaminases and ask about muscle pain, especially with statin coadministration.
• Contraindicated in patients with preexisting gallbladder disease and hepatic or severe renal dysfunction. Fenofibrateoften used instead due to once-daily dosing with meals and potential for greater lipid reduction (Insua).

SELECTED REFERENCES

Insua A, Massari F, Rodríguez Moncalvo JJ, et al. Fenofibrate or gemfibrozil for treatment of types IIa and IIb primary hyperlipoproteinemia: a randomized, double-blind, crossover study. *Endocr Pract,* 2002; 8: 96–101.

Comments: Randomized, double-blind, crossover study to assess effects of gemfibrozil (900 mg) or micronized fenofibrate (200 mg) in HIV-negative patients with hyperlipidemia. Percentage decrease in total cholesterol and LDL cholesterol greater with fenofibrate than with gemfibrozil (−22% vs −15%, P <0.02; and −27% vs −16%, P <0.02, respectively). Reductions in triglycerides levels (−54% vs −46.5%), apolipoprotein B, and fibrinogen, as and increase in HDL (+9% for both drugs), showed no significant difference between treatment arms.

Schambelan M, Benson CA, Carr A, et al. Management of metabolic complications associated with antiretroviral therapy for HIV-1 infection: recommendations of an International AIDS Society-USA panel. *J Acquir Immune Defic Syndr,* 2002; 31: 257–75.

Comments: Although change in diet alone can markedly improve elevated triglyceride levels, it is unlikely to return patients to normal. The International Aids Society (IAS) guideline suggests a fibric acid if fasting triglycerides persistently >500 mg/dL (5.6 mmol/L).

Miller J, Brown D, Amin J, et al. A randomized, double-blind study of gemfibrozil for the treatment of protease inhibitor-associated hypertriglyceridaemia. *AIDS,* 2002; 16: 2195–200.

Comments: This randomized placebo-controlled trial found only modest 18% decrease in triglycerides levels in gemfibrozil-treated patients. SQV/r and IDV were most common PI used during study period. Mean changes in triglycerides from wk 4 to 16 were −1.22 mmol/l and +0.35 mmol/l for gemfibrozil and placebo groups respectively (P = 0.08).

NIACIN

Paul A. Pham, PharmD and John G. Bartlett, MD

INDICATIONS

FDA
• Hyperlipidemia.
• Atherosclerosis prevention and myocardial infarction prophylaxis.
• Niacin deficiency and pellagra.

FORMS TABLE

Brand name (mfr)	Forms†	Cost*
Niacin SR (Watson Lab) (generic manufacturer)	Oral SR tablet 250 mg; 500 mg	$0.12 per 250 mg; $0.28 per 500 mg

Brand name (mfr)	Forms†	Cost*
Niacin (generic manufacturer)	Oral IR tablet 50 mg; 100 mg; 125 mg; 250 mg; 500 mg; 1000 mg	$0.02–$0.10
Niaspan (Kos Pharmaceuticals)	Oral ER tablet 500 mg; 750 mg; 1000 mg	$2.54 per 500 mg; $3.62 per 750 mg; $4.49 per 1000 mg
Slo-Niacin (Upsher-Smith Laboratories)	250 mg ER tab 750 mg ER tab	$0.09 $0.18

*Prices represent cost per unit specified, are representative of Average Wholesale Price (AWP).
†Dosage is indicated in mg unless otherwise noted.

USUAL ADULT DOSING
- Slow release niacin: 500 mg qhs titrate to maintenance of 1–2 g 3 ×/day.
- Immediate release niacin: initiate with 100 mg 3 ×/day with gradual increase over 5–8 wks to average dose of 1 g 3 ×/day (max: 6 g/day).
- Extended release niacin (*Niaspan*) or controlled release (*Slo-Niacin*): 500 mg at bedtime (wks 1–4); increase to 1 g at bedtime (wks 5–8). May increase by 500 mg/4-wk (max: 2 g/day).
- Take with food to reduce GI distress and consider pre-treatment with ASA to prevent flushing.

ADVERSE DRUG REACTIONS
Common
- Facial flushing (occurs in the early course of therapy but generally improves with continued use). Pretreatment 30 min before niacin with ASA may help with flushing.
- GI: nausea, vomiting.

Occasional
- Pruritus (consider antihistamine).
- Hyperglycemia (loss of glycemic control in DM).
- Elevated uric acid.
- Elevation of alkaline phosphatase.
- Decreased phosphorous (mean 13% decrease).

Rare
- Hepatotoxicity (incidence may be higher with sustained release niacin).
- Thrombocytopenia.
- Myopathy.
- Rash.
- Elevation of direct bilirubin.

DRUG INTERACTIONS
- Alcohol and hot drinks: may increase flushing and pruritus. Avoid with niacin.
- Cholestyramine: may decrease niacin absorption. Separate administration time by 4–6 hrs.
- Lovastatin: may increase risk of myopathy with coadministration (do not exceed lovastatin 20 mg/day). Prospective trial did not find a higher incidence of myopathy when niacin 1 g was coadministered with lovastatin 40 mg/day. (*Am J Cardiol* 2003; 91: 667–72).
- Oral hypoglycemics: effect may be decreased by niacin. Monitor for therapeutic efficacy.
- Pravastatin, atorvastatin, rosuvastatin: may increase risk of myopathy with coadministration. Avoid or use with close monitoring.
- Simvastatin: may increase risk of myopathy with coadministration (do not exceed simvastatin 10 mg with coadministration).

PHARMACOLOGY
Mechanism
- Reduces hepatic synthesis of VLDL, which leads to a reduction in LDL synthesis. Niacin also increases HDL by reducing its catabolism.

DRUGS

Pharmacokinetic Parameters
- **Absorption:** 60%–76%.
- **Metabolism and Excretion:** extensively metabolized in the liver to active and inactive metabolites that are renally excreted.
- $T_{\frac{1}{2}}$: 45 min.

Pregnancy Risk
- Category C (when used in high doses): avoid high dose niacin in pregnancy.

Breastfeeding Compatibility
- Excreted in breast milk. No data on safety of high dose niacin during breastfeeding.

DOSING

Dosing for Decreased Hepatic Function
- Use with caution with past history of liver disease. Niaspan contraindicated with active liver disease.

Renal Dosing
- Dosing for GFR of 50–80: usual dose.
- Dosing for GFR of 10–50: no data. Use with caution in patients with renal disease.
- Dosing for GFR of <10: no data. Use with caution in patients with renal disease.
- Dosing in hemodialysis: no data.
- Dosing in peritoneal dialysis: no data.
- Dosing in CAVH: no data.

COMMENTS
- Niacin can have beneficial but modest effect on LDL, HDL, and triglycerides. Associated with high incidence of flushing early in the course of therapy.

SELECTED REFERENCES

Expert Panel on Detection, Evaluation, and Treatment of High Blood Cholesterol in Adults. Executive summary of the Third Report of the National Cholesterol Education Program (NCEP) Expert Panel on Detection, Evaluation, and Treatment of High Blood Cholesterol in Adults (Adult Treatment Panel III). *JAMA,* 2001; 285: 2486–97.
Comments: NCEP guidelines with updates at *www.nhlbi.nih.gov/guidelines/cholesterol/atp3upd04.htm.*

Capuzzi DM, Guyton JR, Morgan JM, et al. Efficacy and safety of an extended-release niacin (Niaspan): a long-term study. *Am J Cardiol,* 1998; 82: 74U–81U; discussion 85U–86U.
Comments: At 96 wks, LDL-cholesterol levels decreased by 20%, HDL increased by 28%, total cholesterol decreased by 13%, and triglyceride 28%. All changes from baseline were significant (P <0.001). Generally well tolerated, although flushing was common (75%). Elevation in liver enzymes was seen but no severe hepatoxicity reported.

OMEGA-3-FATTY ACID (FISH OIL)

Paul A. Pham, PharmD

INDICATIONS

FDA
- Indicated as an adjunct to diet to reduce very high (>500 mg/dL) triglyceride (TG) levels in adult patients.

FORMS TABLE

Brand name (mfr)	Forms†	Cost*
Lovaza (GlaxoSmithKline)	Oral soft gel capsule 1 g	$1.97 per cap
Fish oil (major pharmaceuticals)	Oral capsule 1 g	$0.10 per cap

*Prices represent cost per unit specified, are representative of Average Wholesale Price (AWP).
†Dosage is indicated in mg unless otherwise noted.

USUAL ADULT DOSING
- 4 g once daily OR 2 g twice daily with meals.

ADVERSE DRUG REACTIONS

General
- Generally well tolerated.

Occasional
- GI: nausea, abdominal pain, and eructation (belching).
- Taste perversion.
- Rash.
- Increase ALT levels without a concurrent increase in AST levels were observed.
- May increase LDL-C.

DRUG INTERACTIONS
- Limited data. Induction of cytochrome P450 enzymes in rat studies. No human studies.
- Aspirin: may increase bleeding time.
- Clopidogrel: may increase bleeding time.
- Lopinavir: did not affect LPV plasma concentrations.
- Propranolol: may enhance anti-hypertensive effect.
- Warfarin: may increase bleeding time. Although in clinical studies omega-3-fatty acid did not produce clinically significant bleeding episodes, patients should be closely monitored.

PHARMACOLOGY

Mechanism
- Unknown but may inhibit acyl CoA:1,2-diacylglycerol acyltransferase and increased peroxisomal oxidation in the liver.

Pregnancy Risk
- Category C: not teratogenic in animal studies.

Breastfeeding Compatibility
- No data.

DOSING

Dosing for Decreased Hepatic Function
- No data.

Renal Dosing
- Dosing for GFR of 50–80: usual dose.
- Dosing for GFR of 10–50: no data.
- Dosing for GFR of <10: no data.
- Dosing in hemodialysis: no data.
- Dosing in peritoneal dialysis: no data.
- Dosing in hemofiltration: no data.

COMMENTS
- *Lovaza* is a concentrate of omega-3, long chain, polyunsaturated fatty acids from fish oil (90% of the total content as opposed to an average of 35% in fish oil). In patients with TG >500 mg/dL, *Lovaza* can decrease serum TG by up to 45%, but may increase LDL compared to placebo. In combination with fibrate and/or "statins," *Lovaza* can further decrease serum TG levels.
- Study showed that fish oil is safe and effective treatment for hypertriglyceridemia in HIV+ patients treated with LPV/r-based regimen. A non-FDA approved fish oil formulation other than *Lovaza* was tested in that study.

SELECTED REFERENCES
Gerber JG, Kitch DW, Fichtenbaum CJ, et al. Fish oil and fenofibrate for the treatment of hypertriglyceridemia in HIV-infected subjects on antiretroviral therapy: results of ACTG A5186. *J Acquir Immune Defic Syndr*, 2008; 47(4): 459–66.
Comments: Open-labeled prospective study evaluating safety and efficacy of fish oil + fenofibrate. 100 HIV+ participants on LPV/r-containing regimen with hypertriglyceridemia randomized 1:1 to fish oil or fenofibrate × 8 wks (step 1). If TG ≥200, combination given from wk 10–18 (step 2). Only 4/47 and 8/48 of patients treated with fish oil and fenofibrate, respectively had TG <200. 75 (90.4%) of nonresponders were treated with combination of fenofibrate and fish oil. Response rate with combination therapy was 22.7% No effect on LPV levels. Fish oil was effective and safe, although majority did not reach TG ≤200.

DRUGS

Manfredi R, Calza L, Chiodo F. Polyunsaturated ethyl esters of n-3 fatty acids in HIV-infected patients with moderate hypertriglyceridemia: comparison with dietary and lifestyle changes, and fibrate therapy. *J Acquir Immune Defic Syndr,* 2004; 36: 878–80.

Comments: This was an open label observational study comparing Omacor to lifestyle changes or fibrate therapy in 156 HIV-infected patients treated with ART. Low dose Omacor (2 g/day) decreased triglyceride levels by a modest 15.3 mg/dL.

Durrington PN, Bhatnagar D, Mackness MI, et al. An omega-3 polyunsaturated fatty acid concentrate administered for one year decreased triglycerides in simvastatin treated patients with coronary heart disease and persisting hypertriglyceridaemia. *Heart,* 2001; 85: 544–8.

Comments: Omacor (4 g/day) was effective in lowering triglyceride by 20%–30% in patients who had persistent elevated triglyceride despite simvastatin treatment. No deleterious effect on low density or high density lipoprotein cholesterol, biochemical, and hematological safety tests.

HMG-CoA REDUCTASE INHIBITORS ("STATINS")

Paul A Pham, PharmD

INDICATIONS
FDA
- Atherosclerosis: fluvastatin, lovastatin.
- Cardiovascular events (secondary prevention): pravastatin; coronary heart disease (primary prevention): pravastatin, simvastatin, fluvastatin, lovastatin.
- Stroke/TIA (prophylaxis): simvastatin.
- Hypercholesterolemia, heterozygous familial: pravastatin (pediatrics), fluvastatin, atorvastatin, lovastatin; hypercholesterolemia, homozygous familial: simvastatin, atorvastatin, rosuvastatin.
- Hypercholesterolemia (primary): fluvastatin, rosuvastatin, lovastatin, atorvastatin; hypertriglyceridemia: atorvastatin, rosuvastatin.

Non-FDA Approved Uses
- Hyperlipidemia associated with ART.

FORMS TABLE

Brand name (mfr)	Forms†	Cost*
Pravachol (Bristol-Myers Squibb) and generic pravastatin	Oral tablet 5 mg; 10 mg; 20 mg; 40 mg; 80 mg	$2.00 per 5 mg; $3.18 per 10 mg; $3.24 per 20 mg; $4.79 per 40 mg; $4.92 per 80 mg
Mevacor; Altoprev (time release tablet) (Merck and Co.) and generic lovastatin	Oral tablet 10 mg; 20 mg; 40 mg Oral SR tablet 20 mg; 40 mg; 60 mg	$0.71 per 10 mg; $2.37 per 20 mg; $4.27 per 40 mg $6.61 per 20 mg; $6.97 per 40 mg; $7.68 per 60 mg
Zocor (Merck and Co.) and generic simvastatin	Oral tablet 5 mg; 10 mg; 20 mg; 40 mg; 80 mg	$2.40 per 5 mg; $3.22 per 10 mg; $5.61 for 20 mg, 40 mg, 80 mg
Lescol (Novartis Pharmaceuticals)	Oral XL tablet 80 mg Oral capsule 20 mg; 40 mg	$4.24 $3.31 per 20 and 40 mg

Brand name (mfr)	Forms†	Cost*
Lipitor (Pfizer US Pharmaceuticals) and generic atorvastatin	Oral tablet 10 mg; 20 mg; 40 mg; 80 mg	$3.44 per 10 mg; $4.90 per 20 mg; 40 mg; 80 mg; $3.85 per 10 mg; $5.49 for 20 mg, 40 mg, 80 mg
Crestor (AstraZeneca Pharmaceuticals)	Oral tablet 5 mg; 10 mg; 20 mg; 40 mg	$4.67 per tablet

*Prices represent cost per unit specified, are representative of Average Wholesale Price (AWP).
†Dosage is indicated in mg unless otherwise noted.

USUAL ADULT DOSING
Doses below are standard, but may not apply to patients on ART. See Drug Interactions that follow.
- Pravastatin: initial 40 mg PO once daily any time of the day (max 80 mg/day).
- Lovastatin: initial 20 mg PO once daily (at bedtime) with food (max 80 mg/day).
- Simvastatin: initial 20–40 mg PO once daily (at bedtime) (max 40 mg/day).
- Fluvastatin: initial 20–40 mg PO once daily (at bedtime) (max 80 mg/day).
- Atorvastatin: initial 10 mg PO once daily any time of day (max 80 mg).
- Rosuvastatin: initial 5–10 mg PO once daily any time of day (max 40 mg).
- Cerivastatin: recalled from the US market due to increased risk of rhabdomyolysis.

ADVERSE DRUG REACTIONS
Occasional
- GI intolerance: nausea, flatulence, diarrhea.
- Headache.
- Myositis.
- Hepatoxicity.
- Rhabdomyolysis.
- Insomnia.

DRUG INTERACTIONS
- Drug interactions with MVC and RAL unlikely.
- Atorvastatin also undergoes glucuronidation. CYP3A4 inhibitors can significantly increase serum levels of these statins.
- Atorvastatin: EFV decreases atorvastatin serum concentrations by 43%; no drug interaction data with NVP but potential to decrease atorvastatin concentrations. Dose may need to be increased. DVL: no data, but DLV may increase atorvastatin serum concentrations. Start with 10 mg/day and titrate to effect.
- Atorvastatin: FPV increases atorvastatin AUC by 130% (w/o RTV) and 150% (w/ RTV). Start with 10 mg/day and titrate to effect (max 40 mg/day).
- Atorvastatin: LPV/r increases atorvastatin AUC by 488%. Start with 10 mg/day and titrate to effect (max 40 mg/day).
- Atorvastatin: NFV increases atorvastatin AUC by 74%. Start with 10 mg/day and titrate to effect.
- Atorvastatin: RTV × SQV increases atorvastatin AUC by 450%. Start with 10 mg/day and titrate to effect (max 40 mg/day).
- Atorvastatin: TPV/r increased atorvastatin AUC by 9-fold. Start with 10 mg/day and titrate to effect (max 40 mg/day).
- Atorvastatin: DRV/r increased atorvastatin AUC by 4-fold. Start with 10 mg/day and titrate to effect (max 40 mg/day). No data for ATV and IDV.
- Cyclosporine, itraconazole, ketoconazole, voriconazole, posaconazole, erythromycin, clarithromycin, nefazodone, and grapefruit juice (>1 quart/day): may increase risk of myopathy with lovastatin or simvastatin coadministration.

DRUGS

- Fibrate and niacin: risk of statin-induced myopathy may be increased with fibrate and niacin coadministration.
- Fluvastatin: no drug interaction data. Metabolized primarily via CYP2C9; therefore, interaction unlikely with PIs, but ETR may increase fluvastatin serum concentrations. Rarely used due to low potency.
- Fluvastatin metabolized primarily by CYP2C9 and rosuvastatin minimally metabolized by the liver.
- Lovastatin: contraindicated with all PIs and DLV. No data for NVP and EFV, but NVP has potential of decreasing lovastatin concentrations.
- Pravastatin: EFV decreases pravastatin AUC by 40%; RTV + SQV decreases pravastatin AUC by 50% (may require pravastatin dose increase). DRV/r increased pravastatin AUC by 81%, but substantial interindividual variability (pravastatin exposure did not increase in most subjects; in a subset [6/14] exposure was increased by more than 200%). Consider starting with pravastatin 20 mg/day with close monitoring. No data with other PIs and NNRTIs.
- Pravastatin undergoes extensive 1st-pass metabolism via multiple metabolic pathways, particularly glucuronidation (independent of CYP3A4).
- Rosuvastatin: with TPV/r coadministration, rosuvastatin AUC and Cmax were increased by 37% and 123%, respectively. With coadministration start with rosuvastatin 5 mg/day.
- Rosuvastatin: with LPV/r coadministration, rosuvastatin AUC and Cmax were increased 2.1 to 4.7-fold, respectively. LPV and RTV PK parameters not significantly affected. With coadministration, start with rosuvastatin 5 mg/day. Use with close monitoring.
- Simvastatin: no drug interaction data with DLV but due to high potential for significant increase in simvastatin levels, simvastatin contraindicated with DLV coadministration. EFV decreases simvastatin AUC by 58% (may require simvastatin dose increase). No data for NVP, but potential for decreased simvastatin concentrations.
- Simvastatin: contraindicated with all PIs. RTV + SQV increases simvastatin AUC by 3059%; NFV increases simvastatin AUC by 506%.
- Simvastatin, lovastatin, and atorvostatin are CYP3A4 substrates.
- Avoid PIs with pitavastatin.

PHARMACOLOGY

Mechanism
- Inhibits HMG-CoA reductase.

Pharmacokinetic Parameters
- **Absorption:** pravastatin: 34% with 17% bioavailability. Lovastatin: 30% absorption with 5% bioavailability (take with food). Simvastatin: 5% bioavailability. Fluvasatin: 95% absorption with 20%–30% bioavailability. Atorvastatin: 14% bioavailability. Rosuvastatin: 50% absorption with 20% bioavailability.
- **Metabolism and Excretion:** pravastatin: extensive 1st-pass metabolism in liver with 20% renal and 71% in biliary excretion. Lovastatin: extensive liver hydrolysis to an active metabolite with 10% renal and 83% biliary excretion. Simvastatin: prodrug that undergoes extensive liver metabolism via CYP3A4 with 13% renal and 60% biliary excretion. Fluvastatin: metabolized by CYP2C9 (75%), 3A4 (20%), and 2D6 with 5% renal and 95% biliary excretion. Atorvastatin: metabolized by CYP3A4, and excreted in bile. Rosuvastatin: minimally metabolized by liver with 10% renal and 90% biliary excretion.
- **Protein Binding:** pravastatin: 43%–55%. Lovastatin: >95%. Simvastatin: 95%. Fluvastatin: 98%. Atorvastatin: 98%. Rosuvastatin: 88%.
- **Cmax, Cmin, and AUC:** Cmax: pravastatin: 15 ng/mL; lovastatin: 5.8 ng/mL; fluvastatin: 287 ng/mL; atorvastatin: 25 ng/mL; rosuvastatin: 37 ng/mL.
- **T$_{\frac{1}{2}}$:** pravastatin: 2.6–3.2 hrs. Fluvastatin: <3 hrs. Atorvastatin: 7–14 hrs. Rosuvastatin: 19 hrs. Lovastatin: 4.5 hrs. Rosuvastatin: 13–20 hrs.
- **Distribution:** pravastatin: 0.46 L/kg. Fluvastatin: 0.42 L/kg. Atorvastatin: 381 L. Rosuvastatin: 134 L.

Pregnancy Risk
- Category X: contraindicated.

Breastfeeding Compatibility
- Not recommended.

Dosing

Dosing for Decreased Hepatic Function
- Use with caution with all statins. No dose adjustment needed with rosuvastatin for mild-to-moderate hepatic insufficiency. Consider using the lowest dose with slow titration with other statins.

Renal Dosing
- Dosing for GFR of 30–80: usual dose for all "statins".
- Dosing for GFR of 10–30: of lovastatin >20 mg/day should be given with caution; rosuvastatin GFR initial dose 5 mg once daily. No dose adjustment with other statins, but slow titration with close monitoring recommended.
- Dosing for GFR of <10 mL/min: pravastatin initial dose 10 mg once daily; lovastatin GFR >20 mg/day should be given with caution; rosuvastatin GFR initial dose of 5 mg once daily. No dose adjustment with other statins, but slow titration with close monitoring recommended.
- Dosing in hemodialysis: atorvastatin not dialysed out; simvastatin 20 mg (max dose) once daily is safe and effective. No data with other statins; slow titration with close monitoring recommended.
- Dosing in peritoneal dialysis: atorvastatin not dialysed out (atorvastatin 10 mg once daily); simvastatin 20 mg once daily (max dose) is safe and effective. No data with other statins; slow titration with close monitoring recommended.
- Dosing in hemofiltration: no data for all statins.

Comments
- At recommended dose range the potency of statins is as follows: rosuvastatin > atorvastatin > lovastatin > simvastatin > pravastatin > fluvastatin, with mean LDL reduction of 55%–60%, 48%–52%, 48%, 39%–41%, 32%, and 23%, respectively. Due to lack of drug-drug interaction, pravastatin is often recommended in patients on a PI-containing ART regimen (except DRV/r that requires closer monitoring). However, in those who require a more potent agent, atorvastatin (use with caution at lowest dose of 10 mg with slow titration up to max of 40 mg/day) or rosuvastatin (start with 5 mg/day) may be considered with PI coadministration.
- Lovastatin and simvastatin contraindicated in patients taking DLV or any PIs. Patients treated with EFV may be treated with any statins with close monitoring. Patients should be counselled about Sx of rhabdomyolysis.

Selected References

Jones PH, Davidson MH, Stein EA, et al. Comparison of the efficacy and safety of rosuvastatin versus atorvastatin, simvastatin, and pravastatin across doses (STELLAR* Trial). *Am J Cardiol*, 2003; 92: 152–60.
Comments: 6-wk prospective randomized trial to evaluate efficacy of rosuvastatin, atorvastatin, pravastatin, and simvastatin. Rosuvastatin superior to all other HMG-CoA reductase inhibitors in terms of total cholesterol, LDL reduction, and HDL elevation.

Dubé MP, Stein JH, Aberg JA, et al. Guidelines for the evaluation and management of dyslipidemia in human immunodeficiency virus (HIV)-infected adults receiving antiretroviral therapy: recommendations of the HIV Medical Association of the Infectious Disease Society of America and the Adult AIDS Clinical Trials Group. *Clin Infect Dis*, 2003; 37: 613–27.
Comments: Current IDS and ACTG guidelines on the evaluation and management of dyslipemia in HIV+ patients receiving ARTs.

Schambelan M, Benson CA, Carr A, et al. Management of metabolic complications associated with antiretroviral therapy for HIV-1 infection: recommendations of an International AIDS Society-USA panel. *J Acquir Immune Defic Syndr*, 2002; 31: 257–75.
Comments: Based on drug interaction studies, IAS-USA guidelines recommend pravastatin and atorvastatin for use in HIV+ patients on PI-based ART who require therapy for cholesterol elevations.

Jones P, Kafonek S, Laurora I, et al. Comparative dose efficacy study of atorvastatin versus simvastatin, pravastatin, lovastatin, and fluvastatin in patients with hypercholesterolemia (the CURVES study). *Am J Cardiol*, 1998; 81: 582–7.
Comments: Review of the relative potency of HMG-CoA reductase inhibitors.

DRUGS

Miscellaneous

DARBEPOETIN ALFA

Paul A. Pham, PharmD and John G. Bartlett, MD

INDICATIONS

FDA

- Anemia due to chronic renal failure (CRF).
- Anemia due to chemotherapy-induced anemia.

Non-FDA Approved Uses

- Anemia-associated with HIV or ART in patients with low erythropoietin levels.

FORMS TABLE

Brand name (mfr)	Forms†	Cost*
Aranesp (Amgen)	SC injection 25 mcg; 40 mcg; 60 mcg; 100 mcg; 150 mcg; 200 mcg; 300 mcg; 500 mcg	$625.44 per 100 mcg

*Prices represent cost per unit specified, are representative of Average Wholesale Price (AWP).
†Dosage is indicated in mg unless otherwise noted.

USUAL ADULT DOSING

- CRF-associated anemia: start with 0.45 mcg/kg SC or IV qwk with target Hgb of 11.3 g/dL. Increase dose by 25% if Hgb response <1 g/dL during 4-wk period. Decrease dose by 25% if Hgb response >1 g/dL during 2-wk period.
- Chemotherapy-associated anemia: start with 2.25 mcg/kg SQ weekly. Increase dose to 4.5 mcg/kg if Hgb response <1 g/dL during 6-wk period. Decrease dose by 25% if Hgb >12 g/dL or response >1g/dL in a 2-wk time period. If Hgb >13 g/dL hold dose until Hgb <11 g/dL and restart at 25% of original dose.
- HIV-associated anemia: no data. Based on dose conversion recommended for patients with CRF, erythropoietin (Procrit) 40,000 units weekly = darbepoetin 100 mcg weekly.
- Increased Hgb not observed until 2–6 wks after initiating darbepoetin. Monitor Hgb weekly after initiation of therapy until stabilized and maintenance dose established. After dose adjustment, check Hgb weekly for >4 wks and at regular intervals.
- Evaluate iron status during treatment (supplemental iron recommended for patients with serum ferritin <100 mcg/L or transferrin saturation <20%).
- Contraindicated in uncontrolled HTN.
- In erythropoietin studies when Hgb target was 13.5 g/dL, there was increased risk of composite events (death, MI, hospitalization for CHF without HD, or CVA) 17.5% vs 13.5%; HR 1.34. Hold dose when Hgb >13 g/dL, and reinitiate with 25% reduction when Hgb <11 g/dL.

ADVERSE DRUG REACTIONS

General

- Generally well tolerated; ADRs comparable to placebo in clinical trials.

Common

- Injection site pain.
- HTN: BP monitoring and adherence with antihypertensive therapy and dietary restrictions essential. If BP difficult to control, dose should be reduced or withheld.

Occasional

- Peripheral edema.
- Vascular access thrombosis.
- Cardiac arrhythmias/arrest; congestive heart failure and anginal symptoms.

- Hypotension.
- Thrombosis (higher risk with Hgb >13).

Rare
- Headache, nausea, vomiting, dyspnea, myalgia, arthralgia, limb, and back pain (association unclear).

DRUG INTERACTIONS
- Thalidomide may increase risk of thromboembolism in patients with myelodysplastic syndrome.

PHARMACOLOGY
Mechanism
- Binds to the erythropoietin receptor on erythroid progenitor cells, stimulating production/differentiation of mature red cells.

Pharmacokinetic Parameters
- **Absorption:** bioavailability 37% after SC injection.
- **Metabolism and Excretion:** endogenous erythropoietin undergoes clearance primarily through hepatic metabolism.
- **Cmax, Cmin, and AUC:** Cmax >10 ng/mL and Cmin <1 ng/mL after 96 hrs. AUC 2 × that of equivalent dose of IV epoetin alfa (clinical significance unknown).
- **T$_{\frac{1}{2}}$:** 25–50 hrs.
- **Distribution:** limited to vascular space (about 60 mL/kg).

Pregnancy Risk
- Category C: human data are lacking. In animal studies, reduced fetal weight was observed after high doses, but there was no evidence of teratogenic effects.

Breastfeeding Compatibility
- No data.

DOSING
Dosing for Decreased Hepatic Function
- No data.

Renal Dosing
- Dosing for GFR of 50–80: usual dose.
- Dosing for GFR of 10–50: usual dose.
- Dosing for GFR of <10: usual dose.
- Dosing in hemodialysis: usual dose. Not dialyzable via HD.
- Dosing in peritoneal dialysis: usual dose. Not dialysable via peritoneal dialysis.
- Dosing in hemofiltration: no data. Usual dose likely.

COMMENTS
- Limited data on use of darbepoetin in HIV+ patients. Ongoing large clinical trial in HIV+ patients but results not available.
- Equivalent to erythropoietin in CRF.
- Price of darbepoetin and erythropoietin comparable. Some large institutions and buying groups may receive rebates with darbepoetin.
- Potential advantage of prolonged half-life with darbepoetin (less frequent dosing) may be clinically irrelevant, since erythropoietin can also be administered q2–3 wks (ICAAC 2003, abstract H1919).

SELECTED REFERENCES

Lucas C, Carrera F, Jorge C, et al. Effectiveness of weekly darbepoetin alfa in the treatment of anaemia of HIV-infected haemodialysis patients. *Nephrol Dial Transplant*, 2006; 21: 3202–6.
Comments: Amgen-sponsored open-label study that evaluated efficacy of switching from erythropoietin to darbepoetin in 12 HIV+ patients undergoing hemodialysis. An average darbepoetin dose of 40 mcg/wk was as effective as erythropoietin in maintaining Hgb >11g/dL.

Vansteenkiste J, Pirker R, Massuti B, et al. Double-blind, placebo-controlled, randomized phase III trial of darbepoetin alfa in lung cancer patients receiving chemotherapy. *J Natl Cancer Inst*, 2002; 94: 1211–20.
Comments: Placebo-controlled trial involving 320 anemic patients. 297 completed 1st 28d of study and were assessed for transfusions as primary endpoint. Patients receiving darbepoetin required fewer transfusions vs placebo (27%; 95% CI = 20%–35%). Similar ADRs between 2 groups.

DRUGS

Nissenson AR, Swan SK, Lindberg JS, et al. Randomized, controlled trial of darbepoetin alfa for the treatment of anemia in hemodialysis patients. *Am J Kidney Dis*, 2002; 40: 110–8.

Comments: Randomized, double-blind, noninferiority study to determine whether darbepoetin as effective as erythropoietin for treatment of anemia in patients with CRF on hemodialysis when administered at reduced dosing frequency. Mean changes in Hgb levels from baseline equivalent between the 2 groups. Safety profile of darbepoetin similar to that of erythropoietin.

ERYTHROPOIETIN

Paul A. Pham, PharmD and John G. Bartlett, MD

INDICATIONS

FDA

- Anemia secondary to chronic renal failure.
- Anemia secondary to AZT and low erythropoietin levels in HIV+ patients.
- Anemia secondary to chemotherapy.
- Reduction of allogenic blood transfusion in patients with significant blood loss during surgery.

Non-FDA Approved Uses

- Anemia without correctable cause in HIV+ patients w/ low erythropoietin levels (<500 IU/L).

FORMS TABLE

Brand name (mfr)	Forms†	Cost*
Procrit (Ortho Biotech); *Epogen* (Amgen)	SC 1-mL vial 2000 U/mL; 3000 U/mL; 4000 U/mL; 10,000 U/mL; 20,000 U/mL; 40,000 U/mL	$36.36 per 2000; $54.54 per 3000; $72.72 per 4000; $181.80 per 10,000; $346.56 per 20,000; $727.20 per 40,000

*Prices represent cost per unit specified, are representative of Average Wholesale Price (AWP).
†Dosage is indicated in mg unless otherwise noted.

USUAL ADULT DOSING

- 40,000 U SQ qwk (preferred) or 10,000 U 3 ×/wk with increase to 60,000 U/wk if Hgb increase <1 g/dL over 8 wks. Onset of action 1–2 wks; desired Hct in 8–12 wks. Discontinue if Hgb does not increase by >1 g/dL after additional 4 wks (reasons for lack of response: occult blood loss, iron, folic acid, and/or B12 deficiency, hemolysis, or underlying hematologic disease).
- Evaluate iron stores prior to initiation (transferrin saturation should be >20% and ferritin >100 ng/mL). Some recommend routine iron supplementation.
- Decrease dosage in monthly 10,000–20,000 U increments to minimum dose necessary to maintain adequate Hgb (target 11.3 gm/dL). When dosed to target of 13.5 gm/dL, there is an increased risk of composite events (death, myocardial infraction, hospitalization for CHF without HD, or stroke) 17.5% vs 13.5%; HR, 1.34; 95% CI 1.03–1.74; P = 0.03). Hold dose when Hgb >13 g/dL, and reinitiate w/ a 25% reduction or when Hgb is <11 g/dL. Monitor Hct q1–2 wk until maintenance dose established. Dosing q2–3 wks may also be effective.

ADVERSE DRUG REACTIONS

General

- In clinical studies of patients with breast, non-small cell lung, head and neck, lymphoid, and cervical cancers, overall survival and/or time to tumor progression was shorter when EPO was dosed to target a hemoglobin of 12 g/dL or greater.

Common
- Generally well tolerated.

Occasional
- Injection site reaction.
- HTN (contraindicated in patients with uncontrolled HTN).
- GI intolerance: nausea and diarrhea.
- Headache.
- Arthralgia.
- Thrombosis (associated with Hct >42% and cardiovascular diseases).

Rare
- Rash.
- Seizure.
- Edema.
- May be associated with an increased risk of tumor growth and shortened survival in patients with cancer.
- May increase risk of heart attack, heart failure, stroke, or thrombosis.

DRUG INTERACTIONS
- None.

PHARMACOLOGY

Mechanism
- Recombinant human erythropoietin (rHU EPO) mimics endogenous erythropoietin produced by the kidney in response to hypoxia and anemia.

Pharmacokinetic Parameters
- **Absorption:** well absorbed at injection site (IV or SQ administration; SQ preferred).
- **Metabolism and Excretion:** renally excreted. Minimally affected by renal failure.
- **$T_{\frac{1}{2}}$:** 4–16 hrs.
- **Distribution:** low volume of distribution.

Pregnancy Risk
- Category C: teratogenic in animal studies; no human data.

Breastfeeding Compatibility
- No data.

DOSING

Dosing for Decreased Hepatic Function
- Usual dose.

Renal Dosing
- Dosing for GFR of 50–80: usual dose.
- Dosing for GFR of 10–50: usual dose.
- Dosing for GFR of <10: usual dose.
- Dosing in hemodialysis: usual dose post-HD.
- Dosing in peritoneal dialysis: usual dose.
- Dosing in hemofiltration: no data. usual dose likely.

COMMENTS
- Efficacy demonstrated in HIV+ patients with serum erythropoietin <500 IU/L. Useful in management of anemia attributed to HIV and to drugs commonly used in this population (e.g., AZT, INF, ribavirin, ganciclovir, amphotericin B). However, preferred management of AZT-induced anemia is to use an alternative to AZT.
- Mortality benefit associated with EPO vs transfusion. Lack of response often due to low iron stores. Iron deficiency can be precipitated by use of EPO. Can cause HTN; BP should be monitored.
- Hgb target 11.3 gm/dL. Increased risk of death, MI, CHF, or stroke with target of 13.5 gm/dL.

SELECTED REFERENCES
Singh AK, Szczech L, Tang KL, et al. Correction of anemia with epoetin alfa in chronic kidney disease. *N Engl J Med*, 2006; 355: 2085–2098.

DRUGS

Comments: In this open-label study, 1432 patients with CKD randomized to receive EPO targeted to achieve 13.5 g/dL (N = 715) or 11.3 g/dL (N = 717). When dosed to target of 13.5 g/dL, there was increased risk of composite events (death, myocardial infraction, hospitalization for CHF without HD, or stroke) compared to target of 11.3 g/dL (17.5% vs 13.5%; HR 1.34; 95% CI, 1.03–1.74; P = 0.03). Authors concluded that new Hgb target should be 11.3 g/dL since there is higher morbidity without incremental improvement in the quality of life with target of 13.5 g/dL.

Levine AM, Salvato P, Leitz GJ; Champs 2 Study Group. Efficacy of epoetin alfa administered every 2 weeks to maintain hemoglobin and quality of life in anemic HIV-infected patients. *AIDS Res Hum Retroviruses,* 2008; 24(2): 131–9.

Comments: These preliminary data suggest that majority of anemic, HIV+ patients in this study maintained target Hgb level of 13 g/dL with the more convenient q2wk or q3wk dosing regimens.

Moore RD. Human immunodeficiency virus infection, anemia, and survival. *Clin Infect Dis*, 1999; 29: 44–9.

Comments: Mortality benefit associated with EPO vs transfusion. Unclear if benefit independent of EPO levels or selection bias in patients who required transfusions.

Henry DH, Beall GN, Benson CA, et al. Recombinant human erythropoietin in the treatment of anemia associated with human immunodeficiency virus (HIV) infection and zidovudine therapy. Overview of four clinical trials. *Ann Intern Med*, 1992; 117: 739–48.

Comments: Combined analysis of 4 double-blind, randomized, controlled trials of treatment of HIV-associated anemia with erythropoietin. In patients with low erythropoietin levels (<500 IU/L), EPO decreased need for transfusion and increased mean Hct by 4.6% points (P <0.001). Important to note that patients with erythropoietin level >500 IU/L showed no benefit.

FILGASTRIM (G-CSF)

Paul A. Pham, PharmD and John G. Bartlett, MD

INDICATIONS
FDA
- Chemotherapy-induced neutropenia in patients with cancer.
- Neutropenia following bone marrow transplantation.
- Mobilization of hemapoietic progenitor cells for collection by leukopheresis.
- Idiopathic, cyclic, or congenital neutropenia.

Non-FDA Approved Uses
- Severe neutropenia associated with HIV and/or opportunistic infections.
- Drug-induced neutropenia (AZT, ganciclovir, pyrimethamine, TMP-SMX, and others).

FORMS TABLE

Brand name (mfr)	Forms†	Cost*
Neupogen (Amgen)	SC vial 300 mcg/0.5 mL SC vial 480 mcg/0.8 mL	$275.04 $437.94
Neulasta (Amgen)	SC syringe 6 mg/0.6 mL	$3871.20

*Prices represent cost per unit specified, are representative of Average Wholesale Price (AWP).
†Dosage is indicated in mg unless otherwise noted.

USUAL ADULT DOSING
- Starting dose: 5–10 mcg/kg/dose SQ once daily (based on lean body weight), or approximate calculated dose using volume of 1cc (300 mcg), 0.5 cc (150 mcg), 0.25 (75 mcg), or 0.2 cc (60 mcg). Titrate dose by 50%/wk to maintain ANC >1000–2000. If unresponsive after 7 days at 10 mcg/kg/day, discontinue treatment.
- Rotate sites of injection. Monitor CBC 2 ×/wk. Maintenance dose 100–300 mcg 3–7 ×/wk.

ADVERSE DRUG REACTIONS
Common
- Bone pain (reported in up to 10%–20% of patients).
- Leukocytosis (when CBC not monitored properly).

Rare
- Myelodysplastic syndrome or acute myeloid leukemia in patients with congenital neutropenia.
- Dyspnea and pulmonary toxicity including alveolar hemorrhage manifesting as pulmonary infiltrates and hemoptysis.
- Sweet's Syndrome (acute febrile neutrophilic dermatosis).

DRUG INTERACTIONS
- Lithium: possible increase in leukocytosis; use with caution.
- Vincristine: additive peripheral neuropathy with G-CSF seen in a clinical trial (*J Clin Oncol* 1996;14:935–940).

PHARMACOLOGY

Mechanism
- Promotes proliferation and maturation of granulocytes.

Pharmacokinetic Parameters
- **Absorption:** predictable absorption after SQ administration.
- **Metabolism and Excretion:** renal excretion of 0.5–0.7 mL/min/kg.
- **Protein Binding:** no data.
- **Cmax, Cmin, and AUC:** 3.45 mcg/kg and 11.5 mcg/kg resulted in a Cmax of 4 and 49 ng/mL, respectively.
- **T$_\frac{1}{2}$:** 3.5 hrs.
- **Distribution:** Vd = 0.15 L/kg. 4 ng/mL (after 3.45 mcg/kg).

Pregnancy Risk
- Category C.

Breastfeeding Compatibility
- No data.

DOSING

Dosing for Decreased Hepatic Function
- No data, usual dose likely.

Renal Dosing
- Dosing for GFR of 50–80: usual dose.
- Dosing for GFR of 10–50: no data, usual dose likely.
- Dosing for GFR of <10: no data, usual dose likely.
- Dosing in hemodialysis: HD: no data, usual dose administered post-HD on days of HD.
- Dosing in peritoneal dialysis: PD: no data, usual dose likely.
- Dosing in hemofiltration: no data, usual dose likely.

COMMENTS
- 2002 USPHS/IDSA guidelines for OI prophylaxis do not recommend routine use of G-CSF in neutropenic HIV-infected patients. Most authorities feel that patients with AIDS can tolerate low ANC better than patients with cancer. Nevertheless, patients with AIDS and low ANC (<500) have 2–3-fold increase in bacterial infection rates. Therefore, reasonable to use G-CSF in neutropenic patients with an active infection.
- Neulasta is a pegylated formulation of G-CSF with advantage of prolonged serum half-life of 15–80 hrs vs 3.5 hrs for recombinant G-CSF. Advantage is reduced dosing frequency, primarily for neutropenia-associated with cancer chemotherapy. Drug supplied as single 6-mg vial for SQ injection at $3629/dose. Comparable cost of G-CSF for 11 days for a 70-kg patient is $2835.
- Use and efficacy of this product for indications other than cancer chemotherapy currently unknown. Some recommend that patients discard unused portion of single-dose vial; however, refrigeration of syringes with unused portion appears to be safe and effective.

SELECTED REFERENCES
Kuritzkes DR, Parenti D, Ward DJ, et al. Filgrastim prevents severe neutropenia and reduces infective morbidity in patients with advanced HIV infection: results of a randomized, multicenter, controlled trial. G-CSF 930101 Study Group. *AIDS*, 1998; 12: 65–74.
Comments: Prospective, randomized, controlled trial involving 258 patients showed that G-CSF-treated patients developed 31% fewer bacterial infections, 54% fewer severe bacterial infections, and had 26% less hospital days compared to control group. No mortality difference between groups. Routine use of MAC prophylaxis was not standard of care at the time this study was conducted, so incidence of MAC bacteremia, which was most common cause of severe infection, may now be much lower.

DRUGS

Moore RD, Keruly JC, Chaisson RE. Neutropenia and bacterial infection in acquired immunodeficiency syndrome. *Arch Intern Med*, 1995; 155: 1965–70.
Comments: Retrospective analysis of 118 neutropenic patients (ANC <1000) and 118 nonneutropenic patients. Adjusted relative risk for occurrence of bacterial infection 2.33 (95% CI 1–5.4; P = 0.05) in HIV-infected neutropenic patients.

GLUCOCORTICOIDS

Paul A. Pham, PharmD and John G. Bartlett, MD

INDICATIONS

FDA

- Adrenal insufficiency.
- TB meningitis.
- Idiopathic thrombocytopenic purpura (ITP).
- Cerebral edema (secondary to CNS toxoplasmosis).
- Numerous allergic, inflammatory, immunosuppressive conditions; trichinosis with neurologic or myocardial involvement; seasonal and perennial allergic and nonallergic rhinitis (intranasal steroid sprays); asthma (steroid inhalers); COPD (steroid inhalers in combination with beta-2 agonist).

Non-FDA Approved Uses

- Immune reconstitution inflammatory syndrome (IRIS).
- PCP with PO <70 mm Hg or A-a gradient >35 mm.
- HIV-associated nephropathy (HIVAN): limited data. Not routinely recommended.
- Bacterial meningitis (especially *S. pneumoniae*).
- TB pericarditis.

FORMS TABLE

Brand name (mfr)	Forms†	Cost*
Deltasone and generics (Roxane; generic manufacturers)	Oral tablet 1 mg; 2.5 mg; 5 mg; 10 mg; 20 mg; 50 mg tablet Oral liquid 1 mg/mL; 5 mg/mL	$0.03–$0.31 per tablet 1 mg/mL: $0.17/mL; 5 mg/mL: $1.17/mL
Decadron and generics (Roxane; generic manufacturers)	Oral tablet 0.5 mg; 0.75 mg; 1 mg; 1.5 mg; 2 mg; 4 mg; 6 mg Oral liquid 0.5 mg/5 mL IV vial 4 mg/mL; 10 mg/mL	$0.19–$0.97 per tablet $48.66 per 500 mL $1.09–$2.34 per vial
Cortef, Solu-Cortef, and generics (Pfizer; generic manufacturers)	Oral tablet 5 mg; 10 mg; 20 mg IV vial 100 mg; 250 mg; 500 mg; 1 g	$0.21–$1.11 per tablet $4.85 per 100 mg; $9.32 per 250 mg; $20.76 per 500 mg; $35.71 per 1 g
Medrol, Solu-Medrol, and generics (Pfizer; generic manufacturers)	Oral tablet 2 mg; 4 mg; 8 mg; 16 mg; 32 mg IV vial 40 mg; 125 mg; 500 mg; 1 g; 2 g Oral tablet 4 mg (Dosepak 21 tabs)	$0.84–$5.13 per tablet $4.32 per 40-mg vial; $5.80 per 125-mg vial; $12.90 per 500-mg vial; $24.43 per 1-g vial; $53.36 per 2-g vial $10.71 per Dosepak
Aerobid (Forest Pharmaceuticals)	Metered dose inhaler (MDI) 250 mcg/actuation	$98.03 per inhaler

Brand name (mfr)	Forms†	Cost*
Omnaris (Sepracor)	Nasal spray 120 mcg	$100.03
Asmanex (Schering-Plough)	Inhalation MDI 110 mcg and 220 mcg/actuation	$121.76/30 actuation
Advair (GlaxoSmithKline)	Disk inhaler (DSK) 100/50 mcg; 250/50 mcg; 500/50 mcg Inhalation MDI 45/21 mcg, 115/21 mcg, 230/21 mcg	$97.94, $97.94, $150.61 45/21 $129.38; 115/21 $217.57; 230/21 $203.40
Nasacort (Abbott Laboratories)	Intranasal spray 16.5 g	$111.83
QVAR (MDI); Beconase (intranasal) (Teva Pharmaceuticals and GlaxoSmithKline)	Inhalation MDI 40 mcg; 80 mcg Intranasal spray 42 mcg	$82.86; $104.82 $148.74
Pulmicort (AstraZeneca)	Inhalation powder 90 mcg; 180 mcg	$117.29; $157.06
Flovent (GlaxoSmith-Kline)	Inhalation nebs 0.25 mg/2 mL; 0.5 mg/2 mL; 1mg/2 mL Inhalation DSK 50 mcg; 100 mcg; 250 mcg Inhalation MDI 44 mcg; 110 mcg; 220 mcg	$7.55; $8.89; $17.77 $104.22; $109.88; $147.13 $109.88; $147.13; $228.53
Flonase (GlaxoSmith-Kline and generic manufacturer)	Intranasal nasal spray 50 mcg	$90.95

*Prices represent cost per unit specified, are representative of Average Wholesale Price (AWP).
†Dosage is indicated in mg unless otherwise noted.

DRUGS

USUAL ADULT DOSING

- Bacterial meningitis (especially pneumococcal meningitis): dexamethasone 10 mg q6h × 4 days in conjunction with ABx. Start 15 mins before or with 1st dose of ABx.
- Cerebral edema (mass effect secondary to CNS toxoplasmosis or other mass lesion): dexamethasone 4 mg PO or IV q6 hrs in conjunction with toxoplasmosis treatment.
- ITP: prednisone 30–60 mg/day with rapid taper to 5–10 mg/day.
- PCP with PO <70 mmHg or A-a gradient >35: prednisone 40 mg PO twice daily × 5 days, then 40 mg PO once daily × 5 days, then 20 mg/day to completion of treatment (IV methylprednisolone can be given as 75% of prednisone dose).
- TB meningitis grade I (Glasgow Coma Scale [GCS] of 3–15 with no focal neurologic signs): dexamethasone IV 0.3 mg/kg/day × 1 wk, then 0.2 mg/kg/day × 1 wk, and then 4 wks of PO therapy (0.1 mg/kg/day for wk 3, then a total of 3 mg/day, decreasing by 1 mg/wk).
- TB meningitis grade II and III (GCS of 11–14 or of 15 with focal neurologic signs for grade II; and patients with grade III had a score of <10 with focal neurologic signs). Dose same as above.

- MAC IRIS: treat for MAC combined with NSAIDs; if Sx persist give prednisone 20–60 mg/day for 4–8 wks, then slow taper over wks to mos. Surgical drainage may be required for focal abscesses or lymphadenitis.
- TB IRIS: for severe reaction after TB infection: prednisone 1 mg/kg/day × 1–2 wks, then slow taper over wks to mos. Continue TB and HIV therapy.
- IRIS, other pathogens: 40–60 mg daily with slow taper.
- Acute adrenal insufficiency: hydrocortisone succinate: 100 mg IV q8h. Once stable change to hydrocortisone 50 mg PO q8h × 6 doses then taper to 30–50 mg/day in divided doses.
- Chronic adrenal insufficiency: hydrocortisone 20 mg qam and 10 mg qpm.
- HIVAN: prednisone 60 mg/day (encouraging observational study but no prospective trials evaluating its safety and efficacy). ART preferred.
- Relative potency of corticosteroid: prednisone 5 mg = hydrocortisone 20 mg = dexamethasone 0.5–0.75 mg.

ADVERSE DRUG REACTIONS
Common
- Insomnia, agitation, nervousness.
- Hyperglycemia.
- Increased appetite.
- Leukocytosis.

Occasional
- Hypokalemia.
- Hypertension.
- CNS: delirium, euphoria, hallucination.
- Peptic ulcers (consider PPIs in high risk patients).
- OIs.
- Osteoporosis.
- Superinfection (i.e., thrush).
- Acne.
- Cushing's syndrome.
- Lipid abnormalities.
- Increase infection risk (with long-term administration).

Rare
- Osteonecrosis.
- Hirsutism.
- Hyperpigmentation.
- Skin atrophy.
- Amenorrhea.
- Hyperuricemia.
- Hypercalcemia.
- Pancreatitis.
- Cataracts.
- Papilledema.
- Reversible myopathy.

DRUG INTERACTIONS
- ASA: corticosteroids increases risk of gastrointestinal ulceration. Consider PPI coadministration.
- Cholestyramine: decreased absorption of corticosteroid. Separate administration time by 4–6 hrs.
- CYP3A4 enzyme inducers (i.e., phenytoin, phenobarbital, NVP, EFV, and rifamycin): may increase metabolism of dexamethasone and methylprednisolone. Clinical significance unknown.
- Dexamethasone and methylprednisolone are CYP3A4 substrates.
- Dexamethasone is a CYP3A4 inducer.

- Digoxin: monitor for toxicity secondary to corticosteroid induced hypokalemia.
- Fluoroquinolones: may increase risk of tendon rupture. Use with caution.
- Loop diuretics: may result in additive hypokalemia with corticosteroids.
- Neuromuscular blockers: may increase risk and/or severity of myopathy resulting in prolonged flaccid paralysis. Use with caution.
- PIs: inhaled or intranasal fluticasone. Increased risk of Cushing's syndrome and adrenal suppression. Avoid long-term coadministration. May apply to other steroids. Beclomethasone can be considered.
- PIs and NNRTIs: dexamethasone increases CYP3A4 activity by 25% and therefore may lower serum levels of PIs and NNRTIs. Clinical significance of these potential interactions unknown since there is substantial intersubject variability.
- PIs, DLV macrolides, azoles, and other CYP3A4 inhibitors: may increase serum levels of dexamethasone and methylprednisolone. Itraconazole: dexamethasone AUC increased by 3.7-fold. Methylprednisolone AUC increased by 2.5-fold but had no effect on prednisolone (*Br J Clin Pharmacol* 2001;51:443–50).
- RTV: increased prednisolone AUC 30%–41%. Interaction may apply to other boosted PI (PI/r). Prednisone dose adjustment may be needed with long-term coadministration of RTV.
- Vancomycin: corticosteroids decrease vancomycin CNS penetration, which may result in therapeutic failure (target vancomycin trough of 20 mcg/mL w/ CNS disease).

PHARMACOLOGY
Mechanism
- Decreases inflammation by suppression of migration of PMNs and reversal of increased capillary permeability.

Pharmacokinetic Parameters
- **Absorption:** hydrocortisone: 96%; dexamethasone: 60%–80%; prednisone: 92%; methylprednisolone: well absorbed.
- **Metabolism and Excretion:** hydrocortisone: hepatic metabolism to inactive glucuronide and sulfates metabolites that are renally excreted; dexamethasone: metabolized via CYP3A4 with renal and biliary excretion; prednisone: reduced in the liver to prednisolone, active metabolite excreted via renal and biliary route. Methylprednisolone: reversible oxidation of the 11-hydroxyl group to active metabolite that is renally excreted.
- **Protein Binding:** hydrocortisone: 90%; prednisone: 65%–91%.
- **$T_{\frac{1}{2}}$:** hydrocortisone: 1–2 hrs; dexamethasone: 2 hrs; prednisone: 2.6–3 hrs; methylprednisolone: 2–3 hours.
- **Distribution:** hydrocortisone: 34 L; dexamethasone: 2 L/kg; prednisone: 0.4–1 L/kg; methylprednisolone: 1.4 L/kg.

Pregnancy Risk
- Category C: dexamethasone, hydrocortisone; category B: prednisone.

Breastfeeding Compatibility
- No data.

DOSING
Dosing for Decreased Hepatic Function
- Usual dose.

Renal Dosing
- No dose adjustment for renal impairment, hemodialysis, or hemofiltration.

COMMENTS
- Long-term complications and infection risk are concerns with corticosteroid use in immunocompromised patients. However, short-term use safe and improves survival as adjunctive treatment of TB meningitis, pneumococcal meningitis, and severe PCP in HIV+ patients.

DRUGS

OTHER
TABLE 2-3. EQUIVALENCY CHART

INHALED CORTICOSTEROIDS

Agent	Dosing			Metabolism		Comments
	Low Dose	Medium Dose	High Dose	Frequency	Interaction with PIs	
Beclomethasone	80–240 mcg	240–480 mcg	>480 mcg	Twice daily	No	Prodrug; rapid conversion to 17-BMP by pulmonary esteraces during absorption (90%); CYP3A4 metabolism to less active metabolites (21-BMP, BOH)
Budesonide	180–600 mcg	600–1200 mcg	>1200 mcg	Twice daily	Potentially yes	Major CYP3A4 substrate; metabolites are relatively inactive (16α-hydroxyprednisolone, 6β-hydroxybudesonide)
Flunisolide	320 mcg	320–640 mcg	>640 mcg	Twice daily	Potentially yes	Major CYP3A4 substrate; 1st-pass metabolism: loss of 6α-fluorine, addition of 6β-hydroxy group Metabolites: 6β-hydroxy, glucuronide, and sulfate conjugates
Fluticasone	88–167 mcg	176–440 mcg	>440 mcg	Twice daily	yes	Extensive CYP3A4 metabolism to 17β-carboxylic acid (negligible activiy)
Mometasone	110 mcg	220–440 mcg	>440 mcg	Once daily	Potentially yes but minimal systemic absorption	Major CYP3A4 substrate; extensive 1st-pass metabolism
Triamcinolone	400–800 mcg	800–1200 mcg	>1200 mcg	2–4 puffs twice daily	Potentially yes	Mostly hepatic, some renal metabolism. Metabolites: 6β-hydroxytriamcinolone acetonide, 21-carboxytriamcinolone, 21-carboxy-6β-hydroxytriamcinolone

Potency: fluticasone >budesonide, beclomethasone >triamcinolone, flunisolide
DOSES IN SAME COLUMN HAVE COMPARABLE EFFICACY.

Adapted from the National Heart, Lung, and Blood Institute National Asthma Education and Prevention Program. *Expert Panel Report 3: Guidelines for the Diagnosis and Management of Asthma*, Full Report 2007. Defines step-wise approach for management of asthma in adults and children. Data included in table is for patients >11 yrs old.

SELECTED REFERENCES

Foisy MM, Yakiwchuk EM, Chiu I, et al. Adrenal suppression and Cushing's syndrome secondary to an interaction between ritonavir and fluticasone: a review of the literature. *HIV Med*, 2008; 9: 389–96 (Epub May 4, 2008).
Comments: Review of literature found total of 25 cases (15 adults and 10 children) of significant Cushing syndrome and adrenal suppression secondary to PI-fluticasone drug interaction.

Thwaites GE, Nguyen DB, Nguyen HD, et al. Dexamethasone for the treatment of tuberculous meningitis in adolescents and adults. *N Engl J Med*, 2004; 351: 1741–51.
Comments: Prospective randomized, double-blind, placebo-controlled trial in 545 patients found that treatment with dexamethasone associated with reduced risk of death (RR 0.69; 95% CI 0.52–0.92; P = 0.01).

de Gans J, van de Beek D, European Dexamethasone in Adulthood Bacterial Meningitis Study Investigators. Dexamethasone in adults with bacterial meningitis. *N Engl J Med*, 2002; 347: 1549–56.
Comments: Prospective double-blind study in 301 adults with acute bacterial meningitis found that early administration of dexamethasone led to reduction in mortality (RR of death 0.48; 95% CI 0.24–0.96; P = 0.04). In patients with pneumococcal meningitis, there were unfavorable outcomes in 26% of dexamethasone group compared with 52% of placebo group (RR 0.50; 95% CI, 0.30–0.83; P = 0.006). Dexamethasone should be used in patients with pneumococcal meningitis.

Bozzette SA, Sattler FR, Chiu J, et al. A controlled trial of early adjunctive treatment with corticosteroids for *Pneumocystis carinii* pneumonia in the acquired immunodeficiency syndrome. California Collaborative Treatment Group. *N Engl J Med*, 1990; 323: 1451–7.
Comments: Prospective double-blind, placebo-controlled trial in patients with AIDS with severe PCP found decrease in respiratory failure and improved survival with adjunctive corticosteroids. ADRs were not higher in corticosteroid treated group.

INTERFERON ALFA

Paul A. Pham, PharmD and John G. Bartlett, MD

INDICATIONS

FDA

- Hepatitis C and AIDS-related KS (interferon [IFN] alfa 2a and IFN alfa 2b).
- CML and hairy cell leukemia (IFN alfa 2a).
- Hepatitis B (IFN alfa 2b) (pegylated IFN alfa 2a).
- Condyloma acuminata, hairy cell leukemia, malignant melanoma, follicular lymphoma (IFN alfa 2b).
- Hepatitis C (pegylated IFN 2a and 2b) including treatment of HCV-HIV coinfected patients (*Pegasys* and *Copegus*).

FORMS TABLE

Brand name (mfr)	Forms†	Cost*
Intron A (Schering)	SC vial 10 million U; 18 million U; 50 million U	$178.00; $320.41; $890.10 per vial
	SC pen injection kit 3 million U; 5 million U; 10 million U	$394.21; $652.06; $1068.12 (6 pens per kit)
	SC vial kit 10 million U	$1048.45 (6 vials per kit)
Peg-Intron (Schering)	SC vial kit 50 mcg; 80 mcg; 120 mcg; 150 mcg	$553.41; $581.03; $610.12; $640.00 (4 vials per kit)
Pegasys (Roche Pharmaceuticals)	SC vial 180 mcg/mL	$633.30
	SC vial kit 180 mcg/0.5 mL	$2533.20 per vial kit (4 vials per kit)

*Prices represent cost per unit specified, are representative of Average Wholesale Price (AWP).
†Dosage is indicated in mg unless otherwise noted.

USUAL ADULT DOSING

- **HBV:** pegylated interferon alfa-2a (*Pegasys*) 180 mcg SQ qwk for 48 wks.
- **HBV:** 10 million U SQ or IM 3 ×/wk or 5 million U once daily × 16–24 wks (HBeAg+). Patients with negative HBeAg may require >12 mos treatment.
- **KS:** *Intron* A 30–36 million U 3–7 ×/wk until lesion resolution.
- **Condylomata:** *Intron* A 1 million U intralesional 3 ×/wk. 2–4 million U IM 3 ×/wk × 6 wks has also been effective, but associated with ADRs.
- **HCV (genotype I and 4):** *Peg-Intron* 1.5 mcg/kg SC qwk + ribavirin 1000 mg (<75 kg) or 1200 mg (>75 kg) × 48 wks + telaprevir (1st 12 wks). Dose reduction to 0.5 mcg/kg for ANC <750 or PLT <80K; D/c if ANC <500 or PLT <50K. Monotherapy with 1 mcg/kg q wk and lower ribavirin doses of 800 mg in combination with *Peg-Intron* is indicated by FDA but not recommended.
- **HCV (genotype I and 4):** *Pegasys* 180 mcg SC qwk + ribavirin 1000 mg (<75 kg) or 1200 mg (>75 kg) × 48 wks + telaprevir (1st 12 wks) (may reduce ribavirin to 800 mg/day and shorten treatment duration to 24 wks for genotype 2 and 3). For ANC <750: dose reduce to *Pegasys* 135 mcg/wk. For PLT <50K: dose *Pegasys* 90 mcg/wk. D/c if ANC <500 or PLT <25K.
- **HCV:** 3 million U SQ or IM 3 ×/wk in combination w/ ribavirin × 48 wks (pegylated IFN preferred).

ADVERSE DRUG REACTIONS

General

- Most patients experience dose-related side effects (more common with >18 million U).

Common

- Flu-like syndrome (50%–98%): fever, chills, fatigue, headache, arthralgias, usually within 6 hrs of administration, lasting 2–12 hrs. NSAIDs may alleviate Sx.
- GI intolerance (20%–65%): anorexia, abdominal pain, nausea, vomiting, diarrhea.
- Neuropsychiatric toxicity (20%–50%): irritability, depression, confusion, anxiety.
- Hepatitis (dose related in up to 40% receiving high doses).
- Marrow suppression.
- Rash and alopecia (up to 25%).
- Proteinuria.
- Metallic taste.

Occasional

- Dyspnea and cough.
- Elevations of bilirubin and alkaline phosphatase.
- Insomnia.
- Rash.

Rare

- Suicidal ideation or behavior.
- Thyroiditis with hyperthyroidism or hypothyroidism.
- Retinopathy.
- Rare cases of erythema multiforme, toxic epidermal necrolysis (TEN), and Stevens-Johnson syndrome reported.
- Injection site necrosis.
- Myositis.
- ITP and TTP.
- Decrease or loss of vision (case reports when used in combination with ribavirin).
- Reversible hearing loss and/or tinnitus.

DRUG INTERACTIONS

- ACE inhibitors (captopril and enalapril): case reports of neutropenia and thrombocytopenia with coadministration. Monitor closely.
- AZT, ganciclovir, pyrimethamine, cancer chemotherapy, and 5-FC: additive bone marrow suppression with INF coadministration. Monitor CBC closely.
- Phenobarbital: phenobarbital serum levels may be increased. Monitor levels closely.
- Theophylline: theophylline serum levels may be increased. Monitor levels closely.

PHARMACOLOGY

Mechanism

- Glycoprotein cytokine (intracellular messenger) with complex immunomodulating, antineoplastic, and antiviral properties after binding new cellular RNA and effector proteins are synthesized, mediating antiviral effect.

Pharmacokinetic Parameters
- **Absorption:** 80% absorption from SQ and IM site.
- **Metabolism and Excretion:** IFN: undergoes rapid proteolytic degradation during tubular reabsorption with only minor hepatic metabolism. Reabsorption of intact compound is minimal, and parent compound does not appear in urine. Peg-IFN: liver metabolism by nonspecific proteases (no renal metabolism). Excreted primarily in the bile (with little renal clearance).
- **Protein Binding:** no data.
- **Cmax, Cmin, and AUC:** mean concentration levels at steady state: peg-IFN-a2a: 20,000 pg/mL > Peg-IFN-a2b: 1000 pg/mL hrs >> IFN-a: 100 pg/mL.
- **T$_{\frac{1}{2}}$:** Peg-IFN-a2a: 77 hrs > Peg-IFN-a2b: 40 hrs >> IFN-a: 2–5 hrs.
- **Distribution:** no data.

Pregnancy Risk
- Category C: abortifacient in animal studies at high doses. In case reports of maternal administration does not appear to pose significant risk to the fetus; however, due to antiproliferative activity of interferon, should be avoided during gestation.

Breastfeeding Compatibility
- Avoid during breastfeeding.

DOSING

Dosing for Decreased Hepatic Function
- Usual dose.

Renal Dosing
- Peg-IFN-alfa 2a (*Pegasys*) dosing for GFR<30: 135 mg/d; HD: 135 mg/d.
- Peg-IFN-alfa 2b (*PegIntron*) dosing for GFR 30–50: decrease dose by 25%.
- Peg-IFN-alfa 2b (*PegIntron*) dosing for GFR 10–29 and HD: decrease dose by 50%.
- Dosing in peritoneal dialysis: no data. Consider dose reduction.
- Dosing in hemofiltration: no data. Consider dose reduction.

COMMENTS
- For parenteral treatment of hepatitis C (in combination with ribavirin), peg-IFN now preferred due to superior efficacy and more convenient weekly dosing. *Pegasys* has more prolonged half-life and reaches higher serum levels compared to *Peg-Intron*. Despite these differences, 2 products have comparable efficacy.
- Lower rate of SVR for genotype 1 in HIV-coinfected compared to non-HIV infected patients. Patients with <2 log drop in HCV RNA after 12-wk treatment with peg-IFN unlikely to achieve virological suppression. Consider d/c if there is <2 log drop in HCV RNA after 12 wks. Obtain CBC and chemistries (baseline, wk 2, and q6 wks) and TSH (baseline and q12 wks). Obtain EKG (baseline and PRN) for patients with cardiac disease and pregnancy test (4–6 wks) for women of childbearing potential.
- For hepatitis B treatment, *Pegasys* is preferred over standard IFN due to superior efficacy and more convenient dosing. 48 wks of *Pegasys* may be more efficacious than approved nucleoside/nucleotide analogues for treatment of HBV, but side effect profile, including flu-like Sx and depression, may complicate treatment. HBV genotypes A and D respond better to *Pegasys* than other genotypes.
- Uncontrolled psychiatric illness and decompensated liver disease are contraindications to IFN therapy. Rapid virological response (RVR) obtained at wk 4 of therapy is a very good positive predictive factor of sustained virologic response (PPV at 97%).

SELECTED REFERENCES

Sulkowski MS, Benhamou Y. Therapeutic issues in HIV/HCV-coinfected patients. *J Viral Hepat*, 2007; 14(6): 371–86.
Comments: Review of management of HCV in HIV coinfected patients.

Payan C, Pivert A, Morand P, et al. Rapid and early virological response to chronic hepatitis C treatment with IFN alpha2b or PEG-IFN alpha2b plus ribavirin in HIV/HCV co-infected patients. *Gut*, 2007; 56: 1111–6.
Comments: Rapid virologic response (RVR) was studied in 323 patients from the ANRS HC02 RIBAVIC trial, comparing interferon a2b 3 million U 63/wk with pegylated interferon a2b 1.5 mg/kg/wk, each combined with ribavirin 800 mg/day over 48 wks. RVR obtained at wk 4 of therapy had a very good positive predictive factor of sustained virologic response (PPV at 97%).

Chung RT, Andersen J, Volberding P, et al. Peginterferon alfa-2a plus ribavirin versus interferon alfa-2a plus ribavirin for chronic hepatitis C in HIV-coinfected persons. *N Engl J Med*, 2004; 351: 451–9.
Comments: Randomized trial with 133 patients with chronic hepatitis C and HIV-coinfection. Peginterferon alfa-2a (*Pegasys* 180 mcg) weekly for 48 wks was compared to IFN alfa-2a (6 million IU) 3 × wkly for 12 wks followed by 3 million IU

3 × wkly for 36 wks. Both groups received RBV. Treatment with peg-IFN and RBV associated with significantly higher rate of SVR than treatment with IFN and RBV (27% vs 12%, P = 0.03). In group given peg-IFN and RBV, only 14% of subjects with genotype 1 infection had sustained virologic response vs 73% with genotype other than 1 (11 of 15, P <0.001). Histologic responses observed in 35% of patients with no virologic response who underwent liver biopsy. Rate of SVR was disappointing and significantly lower than those observed in previous trials involving HIV-negative patients.

Fried MW, Shiffman ML, Reddy KR, et al. Peginterferon alfa-2a plus ribavirin for chronic hepatitis C virus infection. *N Engl J Med*, 2002; 347: 975–82.

Comments: Randomized trial involving 1121 HIV-negative subjects with chronic hepatitis C demonstrated that peg-IFN alfa-2a + ribavirin (RBV) resulted in more sustained virologic response vs peg-IFN alfa-2a monotherapy or IFN alfa-2b + ribavirin. In multivariate analysis factors that independently increased odds treatment success were non-genotype 1 disease, age <40 yrs, and body weight <75 kg.

Manns MP, McHutchison JG, Gordon SC, et al. Peginterferon alfa-2b plus ribavirin compared with interferon alfa-2b plus ribavirin for initial treatment of chronic hepatitis C: a randomised trial. *Lancet*, 2001; 358: 958–65.

Comments: Randomized trial involving 1530 patients with chronic hepatitis C (HIV-negative); peg-IFN alfa-2b + RBV compared with IFN alfa-2b + RBV. Peg-IFN superior to IFN in patients with genotype 1 (sustained virologic response rates 42% and 33% in the peg-IFN+ RBV and IFN+RBV, respectively), but for genotype 2 and 3, virologic response rates comparable.

INTRAVENOUS IMMUNE GLOBULIN (IVIG)

Paul A. Pham, PharmD and John G. Bartlett, MD

INDICATIONS
FDA
- Bone marrow transplant (to prevent graft versus host disease) CLL.
- Primary immunoglobulin deficiency.
- ITP.
- HIV (prevention of bacterial infections in HIV-infected children who are not receiving prophylaxis) but generally not recommended; Kawasaki disease.
- VZV postexposure prophylaxis.

Non-FDA Approved Uses
- Anemia due to parvovirus B19 infection.
- Indications with established efficacy: Guillain-Barre syndrome; steroid resistant dermatomyositis; multifocal motor neuropathy.
- Indications that are controversial: patients with streptococcal toxic shock syndrome treated with IVIG had trend toward a lower mortality rate; severe *C. difficile* colitis (case reports).

FORMS TABLE

Brand name (mfr)	Forms†	Cost*
Gammagard SD (FFF Enterprises, Inc.)	IV vial 2.5 g; 5 g; 10 g	$137.92/g
Gamunex (Talecris)	IV vial 1 g; 2.5 g; 5 g; 10 g; 20 g	$115.99/g
Gammagard Liquid (FFF Enterprises, Inc.)	IV vial 1 g; 2.5 g; 5 g; 10 g; 20 g	$124.10/g
Gamastan S/D (Talecris)	IV vial 2 mL; 10 mL	$48.88/2 mL; $223.30/10 mL

*Prices represent cost per unit specified, are representative of Average Wholesale Price (AWP).
†Dosage is indicated in mg unless otherwise noted.

USUAL ADULT DOSING
- ITP: 0.4–1 g/kg on day 1, 2, 14, then q2–3 wks. Consider ART and/or maintenance dosing.
- Anemia due to parvovirus B19 infection: 0.4 g/kg × 5 days. Consider ART and/or maintenance dosing of 0.4 g/kg q4 wks for relapse.

ADVERSE DRUG REACTIONS

Occasional

- Nonspecific infusion related side effects (hypotension, flushing, fever, chills, headache, back pain, and chest tightness).
- ARF (only with high sucrose formulations).
- Precipitation of rash and joint symptoms of fifth disease when treating parvovirus B19.

Rare

- Hemolysis.
- Transient neutropenia.
- Aseptic meningitis.
- Thrombosis.
- Hyponatremia.
- Anaphylaxis.

DRUG INTERACTIONS

- May affect immunogenicity of some live vaccines (i.e., rubella). If possible, defer vaccination until 3 mos after IVIG administration.

PHARMACOLOGY

Mechanism

- Blockade of the Fc receptor on macrophages of reticuloendothelial system in patients with immune cytopenia (e.g., ITP).

Pharmacokinetic Parameters

- **Metabolism and Excretion:** degradation rate of IgG concentration dependent, with higher concentration resulting in more rapid catabolism.
- $T_{\frac{1}{2}}$: 3–5 wks. 3 wks in patients with primary immunodeficiencies and healthy volunteers, 5 wks in patients with CLL. $T_{\frac{1}{2}}$ may be shorter in bone marrow transplant recipients.
- **Distribution:** rapid distribution with relatively small Vd.

Pregnancy Risk

- Category C: no risk to the fetus has been reported. Use in pregnant women considered acceptable.

Breastfeeding Compatibility

- No data.

DOSING

Dosing for Decreased Hepatic Function

- No data. Usual dose likely.

Renal Dosing

- Dosing for GFR of 50–80: usual dose.
- Dosing for GFR of 10–50: no data. Usual dose likely.
- Dosing for GFR of <10: no data. Usual dose likely.
- Dosing in hemodialysis: no data. Usual dose likely.
- Dosing in peritoneal dialysis: no data. Usual dose likely.
- Dosing in hemofiltration: no data. Usual dose likely.

COMMENTS

- Effective treatment for ITP. Advantage over steroids and ART is quick onset of action (generally within 24–48 hrs).
- Acute kidney failure secondary to sucrose load in some preparations has been reported, but currently available formulations *Gammagard S/D*, *Gama-STAN*, and *Gamunex* do not contain sucrose.
- Treatment of choice for anemia due to parvovirus B19. Expensive: $80–$120 per gram.

LEUCOVORIN (FOLINIC ACID)

Paul A. Pham, PharmD and John G. Bartlett, MD

INDICATIONS

FDA

- Prophylaxis for drug induced bone marrow toxicity (e.g., methotrexate, pyrimethamine, or trimethoprim).

DRUGS

- Antidote to the toxic effects of folic acid antagonists such as methotrexate, pyrimethamine, and trimethoprim.
- Megaloblastic anemias associated with sprue, nutritional deficiency, pregnancy, and infancy when oral folic acid therapy cannot be given.

FORMS TABLE

Brand name (mfr)	Forms†	Cost*
Leucovorin (Several generic manufacturers [Quad Pharmaceutical, Abbott Laboratories, American Pharmaceutical, and others])	Oral tab 5 mg; 10 mg; 15 mg; 25 mg	$2.03 per 5-mg tab; $2.36 per 10-mg tab; $4.46 per 15-mg tab; $8.02 per 25-mg tab
	IV vial 50 mg; 100 mg; 350 mg	$3.60 per 50-mg vial; $4.80 per 100-mg vial; $13.80 per 350-mg vial

*Prices represent cost per unit specified, are representative of Average Wholesale Price (AWP).
†Dosage is indicated in mg unless otherwise noted.

USUAL ADULT DOSING

- Toxoplasmosis induction therapy: 20 mg once daily × 6 wks (in combination with pyrimethamine and either sulfadiazine or clindamycin).
- Toxoplasmosis maintenance therapy: 15 mg once daily (in combination with pyrimethamine and either sulfadiazine or clindamycin).
- Therapy usually oral, but administer IV if vomiting or NPO status.

ADVERSE DRUG REACTIONS
General
- Generally well tolerated.

Rare
- Frequency not defined: anaphylactoid reactions, rash, erythema, pruritus, and thrombocytosis.

DRUG INTERACTIONS
- Does not antagonize activity of antifolate antimicrobials (i.e., trimethoprim or pyrimethamine).

PHARMACOLOGY
Mechanism
- A reduced form of folic acid, leucovorin supplies the necessary cofactor blocked by pyrimethamine and trimetrexate to prevent hematologic toxicity.

Pharmacokinetic Parameters
- **Absorption:** up to 97%. However at high doses >25 mg, absorption is decreased (e.g., 31% with 200 mg); therefore, administer IV if dose >25 mg/day.
- **Metabolism and Excretion:** rapidly converted in intestinal mucosa and hepatically by dihydrofolate reductase to 5-methyl-tetrahydrofolic acid which is the normal plasma folate. Metabolite is largely eliminated unchanged in urine.
- **Cmax, Cmin, and AUC:** oral doses of 15 mg result in mean folate level of 0.268 mcg/mL
- **$T_{\frac{1}{2}}$:** reduced folate parent drug: 6.2 hrs.

Pregnancy Risk
- Category C.

Breastfeeding Compatibility
- Excreted in breast milk.

DOSING
Renal Dosing
- Dosing for GFR of 50–80: usual dose.
- Dosing for GFR of 10–50: no data. Usual dose likely, but may need to be increased if coadministered folate antagonist antimicrobial $T_{\frac{1}{2}}$ is increased.

- Dosing for GFR of <10: no data. Usual dose likely, but may need to be increased if coadministered folate antagonist antimicrobial $T_{\frac{1}{2}}$ is increased.
- Dosing in hemodialysis: no data. Usual dose likely, but may need to be increased if coadministered folate antagonist antimicrobial $T_{\frac{1}{2}}$ is increased.
- Dosing in peritoneal dialysis: no data.
- Dosing in hemofiltration: no data.

COMMENTS
- Used to prevent pyrimethamine-induced hematologic toxicity in HIV+ patients. Must be administered when using pyrimethamine (+ either sulfadiazine or clindamycin) to prevent severe bone marrow suppression. Does not interfere with antimicrobial activity of trimethoprim or pyrimethamine (protozoa unable to utilize leucovorin). Normal folate levels are 0.005–0.015 mcg/mL (but fluctuates rapidly); consider checking RBC folate levels (if <0.1 mcg/mL, supplement).

SELECTED REFERENCES
Katlama C, De Wit S, O'Doherty E, et al. Pyrimethamine-clindamycin vs. pyrimethamine-sulfadiazine as acute and long-term therapy for toxoplasmic encephalitis in patients with AIDS. *Clin Infect Dis*, 1996; 22: 268–75.
Comments: One of many trials that used leucovorin with pyrimethamine (with either sulfadiazine or clindamycin) showed good response with minimal bone marrow suppression.

RHO (D) IMMUNE GLOBULIN

Paul A. Pham, PharmD and John G. Bartlett, MD

INDICATIONS
FDA
- Suppression of Rh isoimmunization in nonsensitized, Rho (D)-negative women to reduce likelihood of hemolytic disease in Rho (D)-positive fetus in present and future pregnancies.
- Treatment of ITP (including ITP secondary to HIV) in nonsplenectomized, Rho (D)-positive patients.

FORMS TABLE

Brand name (mfr)	Forms†	Cost*
WinRho (Baxter Bioscience)	IV vial 1500 IU; 5000 IU	$403.01 (1500 IU); $1351.72 (5000 IU)
HyperRho (Talecris)	IV syringe 300 mcg	$110.07 (300 mcg)

*Prices represent cost per unit specified, are representative of Average Wholesale Price (AWP).
†Dosage is indicated in mg unless otherwise noted.

USUAL ADULT DOSING
- ITP: 50 mcg/kg (250 IU/kg) IV over 3–5 min (may repeat dose up to 80 mcg/kg at 3–4 days). Reduce dose of 25–40 g/kg (125–200 IU/kg) if patient has Hgb <10. Maintenance dose: 25–60 mcg/kg.
- Vial should not be shaken (causes protein damage).

ADVERSE DRUG REACTIONS
Common
- Hemolysis with decrease in hemoglobin of approximately 2 g/dL. Monitor CBC.
Occasional
- Fever and chills (5%–10%). Premedicate with acetaminophen and diphenhydramine. Consider decrease infusion rate to 15–20 min.
- Severe hemolysis (Hgb >2 g/dL decrease).
Rare
- Anaphylactic reaction in patients with IgA deficiency. Avoid use in these patients.

DRUGS

DRUG INTERACTIONS
- May affect immunogenicity of some live vaccines (i.e., rubella). Defer vaccination for 3 mos after IVIG administration.

PHARMACOLOGY
Mechanism
- Anti-D globulin when given to Rh-positive patients with ITP coats patients D+ RBCs with antibodies, which prevents splenic clearance of antibody-coated platelets.

Pharmacokinetic Parameters
- **Absorption:** good absorption from IM site.
- **Metabolism and Excretion:** degradation rate of IgG is concentration dependent, with higher concentration resulting in more rapid catabolism.
- **Cmax, Cmin, and AUC:** Cmax: 36–48 ng/mL after 600 IU IV administration.
- **T$_{\frac{1}{2}}$:** 24 days.
- **Distribution:** rapid distribution with relatively small volume of distribution.

Pregnancy Risk
- Category C: routinely given to Rh-negative pregnant patients with Rh-positive fetus to prevent isoimmunization.

Breastfeeding Compatibility
- Rho antibodies present in human colostrum and milk, but none absorbed from infant's gut.

DOSING
Dosing for Decreased Hepatic function
- No data. Usual dose likely.

Renal Dosing
- Dosing for GFR of 50–80: usual dose.
- Dosing for GFR of 10–50: no data. Usual dose likely.
- Dosing for GFR of <10: no data. Usual dose likely.
- Dosing in hemodialysis: no data. Usual dose likely.
- Dosing in peritoneal dialysis: no data. Usual dose likely.
- Dosing in hemofiltration: no data.

COMMENTS
- Alternative treatment regimen for ITP. Advantages over IVIG include short infusion time and cost reduction, but onset of action slower than IVIG. Patients must have intact spleen, be Rho (D)-positive, and not severely anemic. Average increase in PLT count is 50,000. Effect lasts approximately 3 wks.
- Case reports of severe intravascular hemolysis. Monitor patients for 8 hrs after end of infusion. Perform dipstick U/A at baseline, 2 hrs, 4 hrs after administration, and prior to end of monitoring period (8 hrs).

SELECTED REFERENCES
Bussel JB, Graziano JN, Kimberly RP, et al. Intravenous anti-D treatment of immune thrombocytopenic purpura: analysis of efficacy, toxicity, and mechanism of effect. *Blood*, 1991; 77: 1884–93.
Comments: In this open label trial, mean increase in PLTs was 95,000 in nonsplenectomized patients with ITP. HIV status and duration of thrombocytopenia did not affect response.

Oksenhendler E, Bierling P, Brossard Y, et al. Anti-RH immunoglobulin therapy for human immunodeficiency virus-related immune thrombocytopenic purpura. *Blood*, 1988; 71: 1499–502.
Comments: 9/14 Rh+ HIV-infected patients responded (PLT >50,000) to anti-Rh immunoglobulin in this small open label trial.

Psychiatric

BENZODIAZEPINES

Paul A. Pham, PharmD

INDICATIONS

FDA

- Anxiety (alprazolam, chlordiazepoxide, diazepam, lorazepam, and oxazepam).
- Insomnia (estazolam, flurazepam, quazepam, temazepam, and triazolam).
- Alcohol withdrawal (oxazepam, alprazolam, and chlordiazepoxide).
- Seizure control (clorazepate, clonazepam, and diazepam).
- Skeletal muscle relaxant (diazepam); sedation-amnesia-anxiolytic for procedures (midazolam).

FORMS TABLE

Brand name (mfr)	Forms†	Cost*
Xanax, Niravam, and generic alprazolam (Pfizer, Schwarz, and generic manufacturers)	Oral tab 0.25 mg; 0.5 mg; 1 mg; 2 mg	0.25 mg: $0.70; 0.5 mg: $0.76; 1 mg: $1.16; 2 mg: $1.96
	Oral sustained-release tab 0.5 mg; 1 mg: 2 mg: 3 mg	0.5 mg: $2.93; 1 mg: $2.67; 2 mg: $3.55, 3 mg: $5.59
	Oral disintegrating tab 0.25 mg; 0.5 mg; 1 mg; 2 mg	0.25 mg: $2.43; 0.5 mg: $1.89; 1 mg: $2.52; 2 mg: $3.55
	Oral liquid 1 mg/mL	$2.23 per mL
Librium and generic chlordiazepoxide (Valeant Pharmaceutical and generic manufacturers)	Oral capsule 5 mg; 10 mg; 25 mg IV ampule 100 mg	5 mg: $0.35; 10 mg: $0.40; 25 mg: $0.43 $26.30 per ampule
Klonopin and generic clonazepam (Roche and generic manufacturers)	Oral tab 0.5 mg; 1 mg; 2 mg Oral disintegrating wafer 0.125 mg; 0.25 mg; 0.5 mg; 1 mg; 2 mg	0.5 mg: $0.75; 1 mg: $0.86; 2 mg: $1.18 0.125 mg: $1.84; 0.25 mg: $1.94; 0.5 mg: $2.08; 1 mg: $2.10; 2 mg: $3.06
Tranxene and generic clorazepate (Ovation Pharmaceutical and generic manufacturers)	Oral tab 3.75 mg; 7.5 mg; 15 mg	3.75 mg: $3.21; 7.5 mg: $3.99; 15 mg: $5.41
Valium and generic diazepam (Roche and generic manufacturers)	Rectal gel 5 mg/mL Oral tablet 2 mg: 5 mg: 10 mg Oral liquid 5 mg/mL IM vial 5 mg/mL (10 mL)	20-mg twin pak: $334.04 2 mg: $0.24; 5 mg: $0.32; 10 mg: $0.38 5 mg/mL: $2.22 per 5 mL $7.61 per 10-mL vial
ProSom and generic estazolam (Abbott Laboratories and generic manufacturers)	Oral tablet 1 mg and 2 mg	1 mg: $0.89; 2 mg: $0.99

(Continued)

DRUGS

FORMS TABLE *(CONT.)*

Brand name (mfr)	Forms†	Cost*
Dalmane and generic flurazepam (Valeant Pharmaceutical and generic manufacturers)	Oral capsule 15 mg and 30 mg	15 mg: $0.35; 30 mg: $0.28
Ativan and generic lorazepam (Biovail Pharmaceutical and generic manufacturers)	IM or IV vial 2 mg/mL Oral tablet 0.5 mg; 1 mg; 2 mg; 4 mg Oral liquid 2 mg/mL	$7.68 per mL 0.5 mg: $0.63; 1 mg: $0.84; 2 mg: $1.28; 4 mg: $4.68 $1.32 per mL
Versed (brand no longer available) and generic midazolam (Hospira Worldwide and generic manufacturers)	IM or IV vial 1 mg/mL or 5 mg/mL Oral liquid 2 mg/mL	1 mg/mL: $2.30 per 10-mL vial; 5 mg/mL: $7.19 per 10-mL vial $1.10 per mL
Serax (brand no longer available) and generic oxazepam (Faulding Laboratories)	Oral capsule 10 mg; 15 mg; 30 mg	10 mg: $0.87; 15 mg: $1.09; 30 mg: $1.64
Doral (generic quazepam) (Questcor Pharmaceuticals)	Oral tablet 15 mg	$4.42
Restoril and generic temazepam (Mallinckrodt and generic manufacturers)	Oral tablet 7.5 mg; 15 mg; 22.5 mg; 30 mg	7.5 mg: $0.58; 15 mg: $0.71; 22.5 mg: $0.79; 30 mg: $0.88
Halcion and generic triazolam (Pfizer and generic manufacturers)	Oral tablet 0.125 mg; 0.25 mg	0.125 mg: $0.65; 0.25 mg: $0.63

*Prices represent cost per unit specified, are representative of Average Wholesale Price (AWP).
†Dosage is indicated in mg unless otherwise noted.

USUAL ADULT DOSING
- Titrate to effect. The following are usual adult dosing ranges; dose may vary based on tolerance and indication for use.
  – Alprazolam: 0.25–0.5 mg 2–3 ×/day or 0.5–2 mg SR tab once daily.
  – Chlordiazepoxide: 10–20 mg 2–3 ×/day.
  – Clonazepam: 1.5–2 mg once daily.
  – Clorazepate: 5–30 mg twice daily.
  – Diazepam: 2–15 mg twice daily.
  – Estazolam: 0.5–2 mg at bedtime.
  – Flurazepam: 15–30 mg at bedtime.
  – Lorazepam: 0.5–2 mg once to twice daily.
  – Midazolam: 0.03–0.06 mg/kg IV for procedural sedation. Avoid with PIs, DLV, and EFV coadministration.
  – Oxazepam: 15–30 mg 3–4 ×/day.
  – Quazepam: 7.5–15 mg at bedtime.
  – Temazepam: 10–30 mg at bedtime.
  – Triazolam: 0.125–0.5 mg at bedtime. Avoid with PIs, DLV, and EFV coadministration.
- Gradual tapering recommended to decrease the potential for rebound, relapse, and withdrawal, especially with long-term use (>4 wks of daily use). Tapering will vary greatly

from one patient to the next. General recommendation is 25% dose reduction weekly until at 50% of original dose followed by 1/8 dose reduction q4–7 days.

ADVERSE DRUG REACTIONS

Common

• CNS: drowsiness, sedation, ataxia, confusion, dysarthria.

Occasional

• GI: nausea, vomiting, diarrhea.
• Potential for abuse and dependence (avoid high dose and long-term use).
• Confusion.

Rare

• Psychiatric: paradoxical excitement, paranoia, rage, disinhibition, and bizarre behavior.
• Incontinence, constipation.
• Fatigue.

DRUG INTERACTIONS

• Barbiturates: additive CNS depression with benzodiazepine coadministration.
• Clonazepam, clorazepate, diazepam, estazolam, flurazepam, quazepam, and chlordiazepoxide: no data with ART but all undergo oxidative metabolism with potential for interactions with PIs and NNRTIs.
• Inducers of CYP 3A4 (rifamycins, phenytoin, etc.): may significantly decrease serum level of triazolam and midazolam. Midazolam AUC decreased 37% with ETR coadministration.
• Interaction with MVC unlikely. Use standard dose.
• Midazolam and triazolam are pure CYP3A4 substrates. Inhibitors of CYP3A4 substrates (i.e., PIs, DLV, erythromycin, clarithromycin, cimetidine) may significantly prolong its half-life. Avoid coadministration of oral midazolam. Small doses of IV midazolam may be considered with LPV/r and TPV/r coadministration with close monitoring. *In vitro* RTV increased triazolam half-life by 14-fold. RTV decreased alprazolam clearance by 59% (single-dose study), however at steady state, alprazolam AUC decreased by 12%. No significant drug interaction between midazolam and RAL.
• Oxazepam, lorazepam, and temazepam (undergo phase II glucuronidation): no significant interaction with PIs and NNRTIs likely.

PHARMACOLOGY

Mechanism

• Binds to the GABA (A) receptor in the CNS and facilitates the action of GABA, an inhibitory neurotransmitter.

Pharmacokinetic Parameters

• **Absorption:** well absorbed (generally >90%).
• **Metabolism and Excretion:** lorazepam, oxazepam, temazepam undergo phase II glucuronidation to inactive glucuronide metabolite. Other benzodiazepines are dependent on CYP3A4 for oxidation with excretion primarily via hepatobiliary route but alprazolam, clorazepate, and diazepam (parent drug and active metabolite) are primarily renally excreted.
• **Protein Binding:** alprazolam and lorazepam: 80%–85%. All other benzodiazepines >90%.
• **$T_{\frac{1}{2}}$:** alprazolam: 11 hrs; chlordiazepoxide: 10–48 hrs (14–95 hr for active metabolite); clonazepam: 30–40 hrs; clorazepate: 8–25 hrs; diazepam: 19–54 hrs (40–100 hrs for active metabolite); estazolam: 10–24 hrs; flurazepam: 2–3 hrs (16–100 hrs for active metabolite); lorazepam: 12 hrs; midazolam: 1–5 hrs; oxazepam: 3–6 hrs; quazepam: 25–41 hrs (28–48 hrs for active metabolite); temazepam: 10–13 hrs; triazolam 2–5 hrs.
• **Distribution:** high volume of distribution for all benzodiazepines.

Pregnancy Risk

• Category D: not recommended. Risk for withdrawal symptoms during the neonatal period.

Breastfeeding Compatibility

• No data, likely to be excreted in breast milk (avoid).

DOSING

Dosing for Decreased Hepatic Function

• Lorazepam, temazepam, and oxazepam levels not significantly affected in liver disease. Other benzodiazepines may need dose adjustment in liver disease.

DRUGS

Renal Dosing

- Dosing for GFR of 50–80: usual dose.
- Dosing for GFR of 10–50: usual dose likely for all benzodiazepines, but alprazolam, clorazepate, and diazepam may need to be decreased.
- Dosing for GFR of <10: usual dose likely for all benzodiazepines, but alprazolam, clorazepate, and diazepam may need to be decreased.
- Dosing in hemodialysis: no data. Usual dose likely.
- Dosing in peritoneal dialysis: no data. Usual dose likely.
- Dosing in hemofiltration: no data.

COMMENTS

- To decrease risk of dependence, give smallest effective dose for shortest period of time. Withdrawal Sx occur 18 hrs to 3 days after abrupt discontinuation. Choose agents based on desired onset and duration of action, comorbid conditions (i.e., liver disease), and potential for drug interactions.
- Onset of action: alprazolam, clonazepam, diazepam, flurazepam, lorazepam, and midazolam <30 min; clorazepate, estazolam, oxazepam, quazepam, temazepam, triazolam, and chlodiazepoxide >30 min. With coadministration of PIs or DLV, temazepam, oxazepam, or lorazepam are recommended benzodiazepines.

SELECTED REFERENCES

Iwamoto M, Kassahun K, Troyer MD, Hanley WD, et al. Lack of a pharmacokinetic effect of raltegravir on midazolam: in vitro/in vivo correlation. *J Clin Pharmacol*, 2008; 48: 209–14.
Comments: No significant drug-drug interaction between raltegravir and midazolam.

Chouinard G. Issues in the clinical use of benzodiazepines: potency, withdrawal, and rebound. *J Clin Psychiatry*, 2004; 65 (suppl 5), 7–12.
Comments: A review of clinical issues of benzodiazepine use.

Greenblatt DJ, von Moltke LL, Harmatz JS, et al. Differential impairment of triazolam and zolpidem clearance by ritonavir. *J Acquir Immune Defic Syndr*, 2000; 24: 129–36.
Comments: An example of enzyme inhibition by a PI on a pure CYP3A4 substrate such as triazolam. RTV reduced triazolam clearance to <4% of control values, prolonged elimination half-life (41 vs 3 hrs; P <0.005), and magnified benzodiazepine agonist effects such as sedation and performance impairment.

BUPROPION

Paul A. Pham, PharmD and John G. Bartlett, MD

INDICATIONS

FDA

- Depression (*Wellbutrin*).
- Smoking cessation (*Zyban*).

FORMS TABLE

Brand name (mfr)	Forms†	Cost*
Wellbutrin and generics (GlaxoSmithKline and generic manufacturer)	Oral tablet 75 mg; 100 mg	75 mg: $0.72; 100 mg: $0.96
	Oral SR 12-hr tablet 100 mg; 150 mg	$1.68; $1.87
	Oral XL 24-hr tablet 150 mg; 300 mg	$5.22; $6.30
Zyban (GlaxoSmithKline)	Oral 12-hr tablet 150 mg	$3.70

*Prices represent cost per unit specified, are representative of Average Wholesale Price (AWP).
†Dosage is indicated in mg unless otherwise noted.

USUAL ADULT DOSING
- Immediate release: 100 mg 3 ×/day; begin at 100 mg twice daily (max 450 mg/day). Allow 4 days between each dose increase.
- SR tab: initial dose 150 mg/day in AM; may increase to 150 mg twice daily by days 4. Target dose: 150 mg twice daily (max 400 mg/day).
- XL tab: initial dose 150 mg/day in AM; may increase on days 4 to 300 mg/day (max 450 mg/day).
- Antidepressant effect may require up to 4 wks.
- Smoking cessation (*Zyban*): initiate with 150 mg/day × 3 days; increase to 150 mg twice daily. Treatment should continue for 7–12 wks with counseling.

ADVERSE DRUG REACTIONS
Common
- Dizziness, headache, insomnia, agitation.
- Nausea, vomiting, anorexia, weight loss.

Occasional
- Hypertension or hypotension.
- Somnolence.
- Tremor.
- Seizure (risk increases with doses >450 mg/day or with sudden or large increments in dose).

Rare
- Seizure (risk is 0.4% with doses of 300–450 mg/day).
- Psychosis, paranoia, and depersonalization (e.g., hostility, agitation). Depressed mood and possible increased risk of suicide-related events.
- Sexual dysfunction with decreased libido (less common than with SSRIs).

DRUG INTERACTIONS
- CYP2B6 and CYP3A4 (minor) substrate.

DRUG-DRUG INTERACTIONS — See Appendix I, p. 490, for table of drug-drug interactions.
PHARMACOLOGY
Mechanism
- Aminoketone antidepressant structurally different from all other antidepressants; exact mechanism of action not fully understood. Weak inhibitor of neuronal uptake of serotonin, norepinephrine, and dopamine, and does not inhibit monoamine oxidase.

Pharmacokinetic Parameters
- **Absorption:** 5%–20%.
- **Metabolism and Excretion:** extensive hepatic metabolism to 3 active metabolites that are excreted in the urine (87%) and feces (10%).
- **Protein Binding:** 82%–88%.
- **$T_{\frac{1}{2}}$:** 8–24 hrs (active metabolite may have longer $T_{\frac{1}{2}}$).
- **Distribution:** 19–21 L/kg.

Pregnancy Risk
- Pregnancy Category B: use with caution.

Breastfeeding Compatibility
- No data. Avoid with breastfeeding.

DOSING
Dosing for Decreased Hepatic Function
- Do not exceed 75 mg/day in ESLD.

Renal Dosing
- Dosing for GFR of 50–80: usual dose.
- Dosing for GFR of 10–50: reduce dosage initially with slow titration and close monitoring.
- Dosing for GFR of <10: reduce dosage initially with slow titration and close monitoring.
- Dosing in hemodialysis: limited data. Unlikely to be removed. Reduce dosage initially with slow titration and close monitoring.

COMMENTS
- Antidepressant of choice for patients with SSRI-induced sexual dysfunction. Effective for smoking cessation when combined with counseling.

DRUGS

SELECTED REFERENCES

Coleman CC, King BR, Bolden-Watson C, et al. A placebo-controlled comparison of the effects on sexual functioning of bupropion sustained release and fluoxetine. *Clin Ther*, 2001; 23: 1040–58.

Comments: Buproprion has significantly fewer sexual side effects (delayed orgasm, decreased libido) compared to fluoxetine.

Jamerson BD, Nides M, Jorenby DE, et al. Late-term smoking cessation despite initial failure: an evaluation of bupropion sustained release, nicotine patch, combination therapy, and placebo. *Clin Ther*, 2001; 23: 744–52.

Comments: Smoking cessation rates for bupropion alone were 19%, 11%, and 10% at 9 wks, 6 mos, and 1 yr, respectively. Rates for combination group similar to those for bupropion alone group and significantly better than placebo group.

BUSPIRONE

Paul A. Pham, PharmD and John G. Bartlett, MD

INDICATIONS

FDA

- Anxiety.

FORMS TABLE

Brand name (mfr)	Forms†	Cost*
BuSpar (generic manufacturer)	Oral tab 5 mg; 10 mg; 15 mg; 30 mg	$0.77; $1.42; $3.02; $3.64

*Prices represent cost per unit specified, are representative of Average Wholesale Price (AWP).
†Dosage is indicated in mg unless otherwise noted.

USUAL ADULT DOSING

- 5–10 mg 3 ×/day with food. Start with 5 mg PO 3 ×/day with an increase of 5 mg/day q2–4 days (max: 60 mg/day). Most patients require 30–60 mg/day.
- Should be taken with food.

ADVERSE DRUG REACTIONS

General

- Generally well tolerated.

Occasional

- Nausea and diarrhea.

Rare

- Sleep disturbances, nervousness, headache.
- Paresthesia.
- Depression.

DRUG INTERACTIONS

- Alcohol: unlike benzodiazepines, buspirone does not potentiate CNS depression with alcohol.
- Azoles, macrolides, PIs, DLV, and other CYP3A4 inhibitors may increase buspirone serum concentrations. Start with 5 mg 3 ×/day and titrate slowly.
- MVC: interaction unlikely.
- Phenytoin, phenobarbital, rifamycin, carbamazepine, NVP, EFV, ETR, and other CYP3A4 inducers. May significantly decrease buspirone serum concentrations. May require higher doses, titrate to effect.
- RAL: interaction unlikely.
- Rifampin: decreases buspirone AUC by 90%. Avoid coadministration.

PHARMACOLOGY

Mechanism

- Not well understood but may involve a decrease in serotonergic neuron activity.

Pharmacokinetic Parameters

- **Absorption:** >90% with food.

- **Metabolism and Excretion:** rapid and extensive hepatic metabolism via CYP3A4 to partially active metabolites. Less than 0.1% of parent compound excreted in urine.
- **Protein Binding:** 86%.
- **Cmax, Cmin, and AUC:** no data.
- **T$_{\frac{1}{2}}$:** 2.5 hrs.
- **Distribution:** 5.3 L/kg.

Pregnancy Risk
- Category B: not teratogenic at high doses in animal studies. A surveillance study involving 42 1st trimester exposures did not result in significant increase risk of birth defects.

Breastfeeding Compatibility
- Excreted in breast milk. Long-term effect unknown.

DOSING

Dosing for Decreased Hepatic Function
- Dose reductions should be considered in severe hepatic insufficiency.

Renal Dosing
- Dosing for GFR of 10–50: usual dose.
- Dosing for GFR of <10: 25%–50% reduction.
- Dosing in hemodialysis: 50% of usual dose. No supplementation needed.
- Dosing in peritoneal dialysis: no data.
- Dosing in hemofiltration: no data.

COMMENTS
- Nonbenzodiazepine, nonbarbiturate anxiolytic with no abuse potential, no additive sedation with alcohol, and potentially less rebound anxiety. Generally well tolerated with less fatigue, confusion, and decrease in libido. Slow onset of action (1–4 wks) limits its use to prevention of anxiety attacks rather than acute treatment. In a retrospective analysis, prior benzodiazepine use decreased efficacy of buspirone (*J Clin Psychiatry* 2000;61:91-4).

SELECTED REFERENCES

Laakmann G, Schüle C, Lorkowski G, et al. Buspirone and lorazepam in the treatment of generalized anxiety disorder in outpatients. *Psychopharmacology* (Berlin), 1998; 136: 357–66.

Comments: Buspirone comparable to lorazepam in treatment of generalized anxiety.

TRAZODONE

Paul A. Pham, PharmD and John G. Bartlett, MD

INDICATIONS

FDA
- Depression.

Non-FDA Approved Uses
- Insomnia.

FORMS TABLE

Brand name (mfr)	Forms†	Cost*
Desyrel and generics (Bristol-Myers Squibb and generic manufacturers)	Oral tablet 50 mg; 100 mg; 150 mg; 300 mg	$0.57; $0.73; $1.47; $5.44

*Prices represent cost per unit specified, are representative of Average Wholesale Price (AWP).
†Dosage is indicated in mg unless otherwise noted.

USUAL ADULT DOSING
- Depression: 50 mg 3 ×/day (may increase by 50 mg/day q3–7 days); maximum: 400 mg/day (outpatient) and 600 mg/day (inpatient).
- Insomnia: 25–150 mg at bedtime.

DRUGS

ADVERSE DRUG REACTIONS

Common
- Sedation.
- Dizziness.
- Nausea.
- Headache.

Occasional
- Anticholinergic side effects (dry mouth, blurred vision, urinary retention, and constipation).
- Fatigue.
- Orthostatic hypotension, syncope (not recommended in patients during acute recovery phase of MI).
- Tremor.
- Confusion.

Rare
- Priapism (1/6000). Cases of permanent dysfunction have been reported.
- Extrapyramidal symptoms.
- Hepatitis.
- Rash.

DRUG INTERACTIONS
- CNS depressant (e.g., ethanol, barbiturates, benzodiazepines, narcotic analgesics): additive sedation. Monitor for sedation.
- CYP3A4 substrate.
- CYP3A4 inducers (rifamycin, NVP, EFV, MVC, etc.): may decrease trazodone levels.
- CYP3A4 inhibitors (including PIs, DLV, macrolide, azoles, etc.): may increase trazodone levels. Avoid or use low-dose trazodone with close monitoring.
- Digoxin: case reports of increased digoxin serum levels with coadministration. Monitor for signs and symptoms of digoxin toxicity.
- Fluoxetine and fluvoxamine: may increase trazodone serum levels. Start with low-dose trazodone. Monitor for trazodone side effects.
- IDV: increased trazodone levels. Use low-dose trazodone with close monitoring. All other PIs may increase trazodone levels.
- Linezolid: theoretical risk of serotonin syndrome; avoid coadministration.
- MAO inhibitors: concurrent use may lead to serotonin syndrome; avoid concurrent use or use within 14 days.
- Phenytoin: case reports of increased phenytoin serum levels. Monitor phenytoin serum level.
- SSRIs and venlafaxine: rare potential for serotonin syndrome.
- Titrate dose to effect.

PHARMACOLOGY

Mechanism
- Mechanism of action not well understood but inhibits serotonin reuptake, causes adrenoreceptor subsensitivity, and induces significant changes in 5-HT presynaptic receptor adrenoreceptors. Trazodone also significantly blocks histamine (H1) and alpha1-adrenergic receptors.

Pharmacokinetic Parameters
- **Absorption:** >90%, improved with meals.
- **Metabolism and Excretion:** extensive metabolism to both active and inactive metabolites that are excreted in the urine.
- **Protein Binding:** 85%–95%.
- **$T_{\frac{1}{2}}$:** 6 hrs.
- **Distribution:** 0.47–0.84 L/kg.

Pregnancy Risk
- Category C: use with caution.

Breastfeeding Compatibility
- Excreted in breast milk; use with caution.

DOSING

Dosing for Decreased Hepatic Function
- Usual dose with close monitoring in ESLD.

Renal Dosing
- Dosing for GFR of 10–80: usual dose.
- Dosing for GFR of <10: usual dose with close monitoring.
- Dosing in hemodialysis: no data. use with close monitoring.
- Dosing in peritoneal dialysis: no data.
- Dosing in hemofiltration: no data.

COMMENTS
- Effective antidepressant, especially for patients with anxiety or insomnia.
- Orthostatic hypotension can be problematic. Less cardiotoxic in overdose compared to TCAs. Useful nonhabit-forming sedative, but delayed onset, morning sedation, anticholinergic effects may be problematic. Start at low dose and increase as tolerated.

SELECTED REFERENCES

Angelino AF, Treisman GJ. Management of psychiatric disorders in patients infected with human immunodeficiency virus. *Clin Infect Dis*, 2001; 33: 847–56.
Comments: Review outlining treatment issues for depression and other psychiatric illness seen in HIV infected patients.

Patten SB. The comparative efficacy of trazodone and imipramine in the treatment of depression. *CMAJ*, 1992; 146: 1177–82.
Comments: Meta-analysis of 6 studies demonstrating that trazodone efficacy comparable to TCAs.

Perry PJ, Garvey MJ, Kelly MW, et al. A comparative trial of fluoxetine versus trazodone in outpatients with major depression. *J Clin Psychiatry*, 1989; 50: 290–4.
Comments: Trazodone equivalent to SSRIs for the treatment of depression.

DRUGS

TRICYCLIC ANTIDEPRESSANTS

Paul A. Pham, PharmD and John G. Bartlett, MD

INDICATIONS

FDA
- Depression.
- Enuresis (imipramine only).

Non-FDA Approved Uses
- Postherpetic neuralgia.
- Peripheral neuropathy.
- Panic disorder (imipramine only).

FORMS TABLE

Brand name (mfr)	Forms†	Cost*
Amitriptyline (generic manufacturers)	Oral tablet 10 mg; 25 mg; 50 mg; 75 mg; 100 mg; 150 mg	$0.18; $0.34; $0.60; $0.88; $1.11; $1.16
Nortriptyline (generic manufacturers)	Oral capsule 10 mg; 25 mg; 50 mg; 75 mg Oral liquid 10 mg/5 mL	$0.44; $0.80; $1.46; $2.21 $1.46 per 5 mL
Imipramine (generic manufacturers)	Oral capsule 75 mg; 100 mg; 125 mg; 150 mg Oral tablet 10 mg; 25 mg; 50 mg	$16.86; $16.86; $15.17; $16.86 $0.43; $0.72; $1.22

*Prices represent cost per unit specified, are representative of Average Wholesale Price (AWP).
†Dosage is indicated in mg unless otherwise noted.

Brand name (mfr)	Forms†	Cost*
Doxepin (generic manufacturers)	Oral capsule 10 mg; 25 mg; 50 mg; 75 mg; 100 mg; 150 mg	$0.31; $0.42; $0.60; $0.90; $1.00; $3.33
	Oral liquid 10 mg/mL	$23.70 per 4 oz
Norpramin (Aventis) and generic desipramine	Oral tablet 10 mg; 25 mg; 50 mg; 75 mg; 100 mg; 150 mg	$0.96; $1.33; $2.51; $2.77; $4.20; $5.28

*Prices represent cost per unit specified, are representative of Average Wholesale Price (AWP).
†Dosage is indicated in mg unless otherwise noted.

USUAL ADULT DOSING
- Amitriptyline for depression: 50–100 mg at bedtime with weekly dose titration. Dose range: 25–150 mg/day (max: 300 mg/day).
- Nortriptyline for depression: 25 mg at bedtime initially with 25 mg dose increase q3–7 days (max: 150 mg/day). Consider serum level monitoring (target: 100–150 ng/dL).
- Imipramine for depression: 25 mg at bedtime with weekly dose titration of 25 mg (max: 100 mg/day).
- Doxepin for depression: 25 mg at bedtime with weekly dose titration (max: 300 mg/day). Administer twice daily with doses >150 mg/day.
- Desipramine for depression: 25 mg at bedtime with weekly dose increase (max: 200 mg/day).
- Lower doses may be used for peripheral neuropathy: amitriptyline or nortriptyline 25–75 mg at bedtime; increase dose over 2–3 wks.
- Consider lower starting doses in elderly patients.

ADVERSE DRUG REACTIONS
- TCAs are 2nd-line antidepressants due to higher incidence of side effects compared to SSRIs.

Common
- Sedation.
- Anticholinergic side effects (blurred vision, constipation, urinary retention, and dry mouth).

Occasional
- Orthostatic hypotension.
- Weight gain.

Rare
- Refractory arrhythmias with overdose.
- Heart block. Use with caution in patients with a history of cardiovascular disease (including previous MI, stroke, tachycardia, or conduction abnormalities).
- Seizure.
- Extrapyramidal symptoms (EPS) symptoms.
- Hallucinations.
- Rash.
- Alopecia.
- Sexual dysfunction.

DRUG INTERACTIONS
- Amitriptyline and clomipramine: 2D6 and 2C19 substrates. Desipramine and imipramine: 2D6 substrates.
- Anticholinergics (i.e., antipsychotics, diphenhydramine, atropine): additive anticholinergic effects. Consider alternative agent.
- Carbamazepine: TCAs may increase carbamazepine levels; monitor carbamazepine levels and dose adjust.
- Cholestyramine and sulcralfate: may bind TCAs and reduce their absorption; separate administration time by 4–6 hrs.

- Cisapride, type Ia and type III antiarrhythmics agents, selected quinolones (moxifloxacin): may increase risk of QTc prolongation and/or arrhythmia; concurrent use contraindicated in patients with baseline QTc prolongation or at risk for QTc prolongation.
- Clonidine: may inhibit antihypertensive response to clonidine. Monitor BP; consider alternative antihypertensive agent.
- CNS depressants (benzodiazepines, barbiturates, opiates, antipsychotics, ethanol, etc.): sedative effects may be additive; monitor for increased effects. Consider alternative agents.
- DLV, APV, FPV, and ATV: interaction unlikely (unless boosted with RTV). Interaction unlikely with EFV and NVP.
- ETR: may increase amitriptyline and desipramine serum concentrations. Monitor for TCA toxicities; consider dose reduction.
- Fluconazole: case reports of increased TCA serum concentrations. Monitor for TCA toxicities.
- LPV/r: may increase TCA serum levels. Clinical significance unknown; monitor TCA concentrations closely.
- MAO inhibitor (and theoretically linezolid): serotonin syndrome (hyperpyrexia, hypertension, tachycardia, confusion, seizures, and death) have been reported with MAO inhibitors. Avoid combination.
- MVC: TCA drug interactions unlikely.
- RAL: TCA drug interactions unlikely.
- RTV: increases desipramine AUC by 145%. RTV also has potential for increasing levels of other TCAs. Monitor TCA concentrations closely. Dose of TCAs may need to be decreased.
- SQV, IDV, NFV: weak CYP2D6 inhibitors. May increase TCA serum concentrations. Clinical significance unknown; monitor TCA serum levels closely.
- Tramadol: risk of seizures may be increased with TCAs. Monitor for seizures.
- Valproic acid: may increase TCA serum concentrations. Monitor for TCA toxicities.
- Warfarin: may increase INR. Monitor closely.

PHARMACOLOGY
Mechanism
- Increases synaptic concentration of serotonin and/or norepinephrine in CNS by inhibiting their reuptake by presynaptic neuronal membrane.

Pharmacokinetic Parameters
- **Absorption:** all TCAs well absorbed.
- **Metabolism and Excretion:** extensive metabolism via CYP2D6; active and inactive metabolite are primarily excreted in urine.
- **Protein Binding:** 80%–95%.
- **Cmax, Cmin, and AUC:** target serum level at steady state: nortriptyline (100–150 ng/dL); amitriptyline (200–250 ng/dL); imipramine ($>$225 ng/dL); doxepin (100–250 ng/dL); desipramine ($>$125 ng/dL). Correlation between serum level and efficacy has been established with nortriptyline.
- **T$_{\frac{1}{2}}$:** amitriptyline: 15 hrs, nortriptyline: 28–31 hrs, imipramine: 6–18 hrs, doxepin: 6–8 hrs, desipramine: 17 hrs. T$_{\frac{1}{2}}$ may be increased in the elderly.
- **Distribution:** large volume of distribution.

Pregnancy Risk
- amitriptyline, doxepin, desipramine: category C; nortriptyline, imipramine: category D (avoid in pregnancy).

Breastfeeding Compatibility
- Excreted in breastmilk. Breastfeeding is not recommended.

DOSING
Dosing for Decreased Hepatic Function
- Usual dose. Monitor closely in ESLD.

Renal Dosing
- No dose adjustment for renal impairment.
- Dosing in hemodialysis: not removed in HD.
- Dosing in peritoneal dialysis: limited data. Unlikely to be affected.
- Dosing in hemofiltration: no data.

DRUGS

COMMENTS
- Drug interactions, ADR profile, and potential for lethal refractory arrhythmias in overdose are reasons why TCAs have fallen to 2nd- to 3rd-line therapy behind SSRIs and atypical antidepressants (e.g., venlafaxine [*Effexor*], duloxetine [*Cymbalta*], mirtazapine [*Remeron*], bupropion [*Wellbutrin*].
- Nortriptyline may be better tolerated than other TCAs. Effective in diabetic peripheral neuropathy but results have been disappointing in HIV-associated neuropathy. With HIV+ patients, TCAs may result in weight gain.

SELECTED REFERENCES
Guaiana G, Barbui C, Hotopf M. Amitriptyline for depression. *Cochrane Database Syst Rev*, 2007:(3): CD004186.
Comments: Cochrane database review indicates that amitriptyline is at least as efficacious as other tricyclics, heterocyclic compounds, or SSRIs but associated with more side effects. When responder analysis stratified by study setting, amitriptyline more effective than control antidepressants in inpatients (OR 1.22, 95% CI 1.04–1.42), but not in outpatients.

Angelino AF, Treisman GJ. Management of psychiatric disorders in patients infected with human immunodeficiency virus. *Clin Infect Dis*, 2001; 33: 847–56.
Comments: Review of treatment issues for major depression and other psychiatric illness in HIV.

Kieburtz K, Simpson D, Yiannoutsos C, et al. A randomized trial of amitriptyline and mexiletine for painful neuropathy in HIV infection. AIDS Clinical Trial Group 242 Protocol Team. *Neurology*, 1998; 51: 1682–8.
Comments: Randomized, double-blind, placebo controlled trial concluded that TCAs did not relieve pain in patients with HIV-associated peripheral neuropathy.

SECTION 3
MANAGEMENT

Antiretroviral Therapy

ADHERENCE

Jeffrey Hsu, MD

DEFINITION
- Extent to which patient follows prescribed healthcare regimen.

INDICATIONS

Importance of Adherence
- <95% adherence associated w/ increased risk of virologic failure in early studies of unboosted PI-based regimens. May not apply to NNRTI- or boosted PI-based regimens.
- Adherence strongly correlated with viral suppression.
- Adherence results in better CD4 response to therapy.
- Nonadherence associated with resistance. In some studies, risk of resistance highest with good but incomplete adherence (e.g., 80%–90%). Little selective pressure with very poor adherence. Link between adherence and resistance also depends on potency/pharmacokinetics of regimen.
- Nonadherence limits future treatment options if it results in resistance.
- Nonadherence increases risk of HIV transmission.
- Behavioral intervention strategies addressing adherence are successful; approach should be tailored to address individual patient needs.

Factors Affecting Treatment Adherence
- Complexity of medication regimen (pill burden, food restrictions, dosing frequency).
- Active substance or alcohol abuse.
- Untreated psychiatric disorders (e.g., depression, anxiety, personality disorders).
- Side effects.
- Poor patient-provider relationship.
- Busy, chaotic lifestyle.
- Patient lack of knowledge about HIV and rationale for therapy.
- Cognitive problems (especially poor executive functioning, memory, attention, psychomotor speed).
- Lack of social support and concerns about social stigma.
- Most studies show no relationship with race, sex, age, socioeconomic status, or educational level.

CLINICAL RECOMMENDATION

Provider Strategies to Improve Adherence
- Determine patient readiness to begin ART by assessing beliefs about therapy, social support, use of drugs or alcohol, mental health issues, daily routine, and ability to meet basic needs.
- Identify possible barriers to adherence prior to beginning treatment and identify ways to remove them (transportation to clinic, childcare issues, need for stable housing).
- Refer patient for substance abuse/mental health treatment prior to beginning ART (active substance use, depression, and anxiety disorders are strong predictors of nonadherence).
- Consider using techniques such as motivational interviewing (MI) to improve patient readiness to begin treatment.
- Establish trusting clinician-patient alliance and invite patient collaboration in treatment decisions.
- Educate patient about treatment regimen, anticipated side effects, importance of adherence, and risk of resistance.
- Appropriately manage medication side effects as they emerge.
- Use written materials and audiovisual aides to help reinforce knowledge.
- If ART not urgent, consider "trial run" using vitamins or prophylactic medications prior to beginning ART to assess patient's ability to adhere to medication regimen.
- Schedule regular visits to monitor adherence.
- Questions about adherence should be asked in an open-ended, nonthreatening manner.
- Provide available contacts between visits for questions/problems with side effects.

- Provide social support by enlisting help of family members, friends, peer counselors, patient role models, and members of the healthcare team to reinforce/monitor adherence.
- Simplify regimen as much as possible (high pill burden, food restrictions, and increased dosing frequency correlated with lower adherence).
- Choose tolerable medications and be prepared to change drugs if needed.
- Monitor patient adherence with different measures (see below).

Patient Strategies to Improve Adherence
- Keep medication diary.
- Establish set time and place for taking medication.
- Identify medication-taking cues linked to daily routine (e.g., prior to brushing teeth, eating a meal).
- Use of cell phones, pagers, and alarms as reminders.
- Use of pillboxes.
- Plan ahead for changes in routine (vacations, holidays).
- Notify provider of side effects that may interfere with adherence or if considering discontinuation of therapy.
- Anticipate need for medication refills in advance.

Methods to Measure/Monitor Adherence
- Patient self-report assessed through questionnaires, interviews, diaries, pill identification test (PIT).
- Pill counts.
- Prescription refill monitoring.
- Use of electronic devices that measure patient adherence (e.g., MEMS cap).
- Directly observed therapy (DOT).
- Therapeutic drug monitoring (not routinely recommended, but may be helpful in selected cases).
- Viral load/CD4 count (crude and late measures).

SELECTED REFERENCES

Simoni JM, Pearson CR, Pantalone DW, et al. Efficacy of interventions in improving highly active antiretroviral therapy adherence and HIV-1 RNA viral load: A meta-analytic review of randomized controlled trials. *J Acquir Immune Defic Syndr*, 2006; 43 (Suppl 1): S23–35.
Comments: Meta-analytic review examining 19 randomized controlled trials of behavioral interventions with ART adherence as outcome measure. Across studies, patients receiving intervention were 1.5× more likely to achieve 95% adherence than the control group.

Simoni JM, Frick PA, Pantalone DW, et al. Antiretroviral adherence interventions: a review of current literature and ongoing studies. *Top HIV Med*, 2004; 11: 185–98.
Comments: Good review article summarizing published studies of adherence intervention strategies. Includes appendix listing ongoing research studies.

Chesney M. Adherence to HAART regimens. *AIDS Patient Care STDS*, 2003; 17: 169–77.
Comments: Article reviews adherence barriers, assessment, and interventions.

Sethi AK, Celentano DD, Gange SJ, et al. Association between adherence to antiretroviral therapy and human immunodeficiency virus drug resistance. *Clin Infect Dis*, 2003; 37: 1112–8.
Comments: Prospective 1-yr study showing that patients with 70%–89% adherence are the most likely to develop viral rebound w/ clinically significant resistance.

ANTIRETROVIRAL THERAPY: TREATMENT-EXPERIENCED PATIENTS

Lisa A. Spacek, MD, PhD

DEFINITION
- Use of ART in patients who have failed previous regimen(s).

INDICATIONS
General Guidelines
- Virologic suppression = confirmed VL below limit of assay detection (e.g., VL <20, 48, 50, or 75 depending on assay).

MANAGEMENT

- Virologic failure = confirmed VL >200.
- Immunologic failure = failure to achieve and maintain adequate CD4 increase despite viral suppression.
- Clinical failure = occurrence or recurrence of HIV-related event after >3 mos therapy, excluding immune reconstitution inflammatory syndrome (IRIS).
- Confirm detectable VL with repeat test. Rule out effect of intercurrent illness or recent vaccination.
- Assess and optimize adherence (reduce pill burden, simplify regimens, Rx substance abuse, review comprehension, Rx depression), addess ART side effects, pharmacokinetics (drug interactions, food effects), and comorbidities.
- Obtain resistance test while on failing regimen or within 4 wks of ART discontinuation.
- Consider ART Hx and all prior resistance test results when assessing resistance.
- Fully active agent = agent with expected activity based on patient's ART hx, drug resistance testing, or novel mechanism of action.
- Reestablish viral suppression to prevent accumulation of mutations in patients with discordant CD4 and VL, base therapeutic decisions on VL.

Prior Treatment Without Drug Resistance
- Goal: resuppress.
- Assess adherence. Consider variability in VL assays, measurement error, and self-resolving low-level viremia.
- Low level viremia (<1000), follow VL to determine need to change ART. If VL >500, check for drug resistance.
- If repeated viremia without drug resistance, consider resuming same or new regimen and recheck for emergence of resistance with genotypic testing after 2–4 wks on ART.

Limited Prior Treatment and Drug Resistance
- Goal to resuppress to VL <50 with ideally 3, but at least 2, fully active drugs. Avoid adding single, active agent. Drug potency, genetic barrier to resistance, and viral susceptibility more important than number of drugs in regimen.
- Use tropism testing (*Trofile*) to identify candidates for MVC therapy.
- Assess ETR susceptibility with resistance testing, review genotypes performed at time of previous NNRTI failure if available.
- Some drugs may offer partial activity despite class resistance (NRTIs, PIs). Other drugs do not offer partial activity (ENF, NNRTIs, RAL).
- If resistance detected, discontinue regimen promptly to optimize efficacy of newer NNRTIs (ETR) and RTV-boosted PIs (DRV, TPV) and to decrease risk of new mutations and preserve drug activity (ENF, NNRTIs, RAL).

Extensive Prior Treatment and Drug Resistance
- Phenotyping or virtual phenotyping in patients with extensive resistance may identify agents with greatest partial activity, especially among PIs.
- Agents from newer classes (INSTI, CCR5 antagonists, fusion inhibitors, or 2nd generation PIs and NNRTIs) should be used in combination with at least 1 other fully active drug whenever possible.
- In patients without 2 fully active agents, continue some form of therapy with goal to decrease risk of disease progression.
- Expert consultation advised.
- Patients without ART options may be candidates for research studies, expanded access programs, or investigational new drugs (INDs).

Professional Society Treatment Guidelines
- IAS-USA at *http://www.iasusa.org/guidelines/index.html.*
- DHHS at *http://www.aidsinfo.nih.gov/Guidelines/Default.aspx.*
- British HIV Association at *http://www.bhiva.org/PublishedandApproved.aspx.*
- European AIDS Clinical Society at *http://europeanaidsclinicalsociety.org/index. php?option=com_content and view=article and id=59 and Itemid=41.*

CLINICAL RECOMMENDATION
Extensive Prior Treatment
- Choice of drugs depends on toxicity and resistance profile.

- DRV: approved for ART-experienced patients with resistance to multiple PIs (POWER studies). Once-daily DRV/r 800/100 mg noninferior to twice-daily DRV/r 600/100 mg in patients without DRV resistance in open-label study (ODIN), and now approved for patients without DRV mutations Superior tolerability and toxicity profile compared to LPV/r and TPV/r. Resistance mutations: V11I, V32I, L33F, I47V, I50V, I54L/M, T74P, L76V, I84V, L89V. ≥3 mutations associated with diminished virologic response.
- TPV: approved for ART experienced patients. Resistance mutations: L10V, L33F, M36I/L/V K43T, M46L, I47V, I54A/M/V, Q58E, H69K/R, T74P, V82L/T, N83D, I84V, L89I/M/V. More hepatotoxicity and hyperlipidemia than other PIs, and increases risk for intracranial hemorrhage or bleeding in patients with risk factors, including bleeding diatheses. Assess relative susceptibility of DRV and TPV with resistance testing. Use DRV/r unless TPV shows greater susceptibility.
- ENF: injectable fusion inhibitor increases viral suppression as component of optimized background regimen (OBR) combined with agents in new classes. Patients with D/M- or X4-virus and cross-resistance to DRV, TPV, and ETR may benefit from salvage regimen that includes ENF and RAL. Adverse events include injection site reactions (98%) and hypersensitivity (<1%).
- RAL: oral integrase inhibitor; important to maintain strong ART-backbone, usually including a PI/r. Superior to placebo in combination with OBR in ART-experienced patients (BENCHMRK 1 and 2 studies). RAL resistance mutations: E92Q, Y143R/H/C, Q148K/R/H, N155H.
- ETR: 2nd generation NNRTI with activity against NNRTI-resistant virus, used in combination with a PI/r and consider inclusion of RAL or MVC. Superior to placebo in ART-experienced patients on DRV/r-containing OBR (DUET-1 and 2). Cannot be used with TPV. Adverse effects include rash, diarrhea and nausea.
- MVC: oral CCR5 antagonist that inhibits entry of HIV into CD4 cells. Confirmation of pure R5 tropism with tropism assay (*Trofile*) required before treatment. Superior to placebo in R5-tropic, ART-experience patients in combination with OBR (MOTIVATE 1 and 2). Failure occurs through selection of preexistent D/M- or X4-tropic virus or mutations in gp120 region of V3 loop.
- 3TC or FTC may be used in non-suppressive holding regimens or suppressive salvage regimens due to tolerability, partial activity, and decreased fitness benefits of M184V.
- Treatment interruption, not recommended, may increase risk for disease progression (CD4 decline, risk of HIV-related clinical events, including death).
- Consider TDM to verify whether adequate therapeutic levels are being achieved (See *www.hivpharmacology.com*).

SELECTED REFERENCES

Panel on Antiretroviral Guidelines for Adults and Adolescents. Guidelines for the use of antiretroviral agents in HIV-1-infected adults and adolescents. Department of Health and Human Services; January 1, 2011; 68–76. *http://aidsinfo.nih.gov/contentfiles/AdultandAdolescentGL.pdf*. Accessed March 30, 2011.
Comments: Viral load is most important indicator of response to ART. Virologic failure defined as confirmed VL >200. This threshold accounts for blips and assay variability.

Thompson MA, Aberg JA, Cahn P, et al. Antiretroviral treatment of adult HIV infection: 2010 Recommendations of the International AIDS Society-USA panel. *JAMA*, 2010; 304: 321–33.
Comments: Guidelines recognize that VL of 20–50 has unclear clinical significance. Recommendations include confirmation of viral load rebound on 2 separate tests at least 2–4 wks apart with review of regimen tolerability, drug-drug interactions, and patient adherence.

Johnson VA, Brun-Vezinet F, Clotet B, et al. Update of the drug resistance mutations in HIV-1: December 2010. *Top HIV Med*, 2010; 18: 156–63.
Note: Accessed at: *www.iasusa.org/resistance_mutations/mutations_figures.pdf*. Accessed March 30, 2011.
Comments: Nine new mutations: E138G and E138K for etravirine, E92Q for raltegravir, and M36L, M36V, H69R, L89I, L89M and L89V for tipranavir/ritonavir.

Marcelin AG, Flandre P, Descamps D, et al. Factors associated with virological response to etravirine in nonnucleoside reverse transcriptase inhibitor-experienced HIV-1-infected patients. *Antimicrob Agents Chemother*, 2010; 54: 72–7.
Comments: Better virologic response to ETR seen in 243 NNRTI-experienced patients using active new drugs (ENF, DRV or RAL) for the 1st time in combination with ETR and presence of K103N mutation at baseline. Mutations Y181V and E138A associated with poor viral response to ETR.

MANAGEMENT

Wilkin TJ, Ribaudo HR, Tenorio AR, Gulick RM. The relationship of CCR5 antagonists to CD4+ T-cell gain: a meta-regression of recent clinical trials in treatment-experienced HIV-infected patients. *HIV Clin Trials*, 2010; 11: 351–8.
Comments: Meta-analysis of 46 treatment groups from 17 trials on new ART (11 groups from 5 trials used CCR5 antagonists) showed additional CD4 gain of 30 after 24 wks in those groups using CCR5 antagonist after controlling for baseline VL and % achieving VL<50.

Hill AM, Cho M, Mrus JM. The costs of full suppression of plasma HIV RNA in highly antiretroviral-experienced patients. *AIDS Rev*, 2011; 13: 41–48.
Comments: Based on data from DUET (ETR), BENCHMRK (RAL) and MOTIVATE (MVC) clinical trials, costs per patient with viral suppression showed treatment of highly treatment-experienced patients were lower using combinations of newer ART compared to recycled NRTIs and ENF.

Eron JJ, Young B, Cooper DA, et al. Switch to a raltegravir-based regimen versus continuation of a lopinavir-ritonavir-based regimen in stable HIV-infected patients with suppressed viremia (SWITCHMRK 1 and 2); two multicentre, double-blind, randomized controlled trials. *Lancet*, 2010; 375: 396–407.
Comments: Study of 702 patients were randomized to continue LPV/r (N = 352) or switch to RAL (N = 350), lipids were lower in those who switched to RAL, but viral suppression was seen less frequently than expected on RAL. Studies were terminated at 24 wks; RAL was NOT non-inferior to LPV-r.

Scherrer AU, von Wyl V, Fux CA, et al. Implementation of raltegravir in routine clinical practice: selection criteria for choosing this drug, virologic response rates, and characteristics of failures. *J Acquir Immune Defic Syndr*, 2010; 53: 464–71.
Comments: Swiss HIV Cohort study patients on salvage Rx, especially ENF, switched to regimen containing RAL and had overall increase in CD4. Risk factors associated with virologic failure were genotypic sensitivity score ≤1, very low RAL plasma levels, poor adherence, and high baseline VL.

Dinoso JB, Kim SY, Wiegand AM, et al. Treatment intensification does not reduce residual HIV-1 viremia in patients on highly active antiretroviral therapy. *PNAS*, 2009; 106: 9403–08.
Comments: Two prospective studies of HIV viral kinetics and residual viremia (VL<1c/mL) detected by single-copy assay (SCA) found that levels of viremia were not reduced by ART intensification (at JHH: ATV/r or at NIH: EFV or LPV/r) in setting of susceptible virus and adequate drug concentrations. Residual viremia appears to be virus output from genetically stable reservoirs lacking new resistance mutations.

Wilson LE, Gallant JE. HIV/AIDS: the management of treatment-experienced HIV-infected patients: new drugs and drug combinations. *Clin Infect Dis*, 2009; 48: 214–21.
Comments: Review of ART in treatment-experienced patients.

DRUG INTERACTIONS

Paul A. Pham, PharmD

DEFINITION
- Pharmacodynamics and/or pharmacokinetics of a drug are altered by interacting substances (food, drugs, and herbals).

INDICATIONS

General Facts About Drug Interactions Involving ARV Therapy
- Liver is main organ involved in drug metabolism.
- Hepatic drug metabolism involves phase I oxidation/reduction (cytochrome P450 enzymes; CYP450) and phase II enzymes (conjugation enzymes).
- CYP450 enzymes are major metabolic pathway for PIs, NNRTIs, and MVC.
- Drugs can be CYP450 substrates, inhibitors, and/or inducers.
- Inhibition of CYP450 enzymes leads to accumulation of parent drug, while induction results in reduction of parent drug; substrates are drugs metabolized by >1 CYP450 enzyme.
- CYP3A4, the most abundant hepatic CYP450 isoenzyme, is main metabolic pathway for many PIs, most NNRTIs, and MVC. In addition, large number of commonly prescribed medications are CYP3A4 substrates.
- PIs are substrates and inhibitors of CYP450 enzymes (primarily CYP3A4). At steady state, some PIs (e.g., LPV/r, FPV/r, RTV) are mild inducers of CYP450. NVP, ETR, and to lesser extent EFV are CYP3A4 substrates and moderate inducers of CYP3A4. These pharmacologic properties of PIs and NNRTIs make them susceptible to drug interactions involving other CYP450 substrate, inhibitors, and inducers.
- NNRTIs can potentially alter plasma concentrations PIs (e.g., EFV reduces LPV concentrations).

- NRTIs, RAL, and ENF are not substrates, inhibitors, or inducers of the CYP450 enzymes. NRTIs are eliminated by renal route, although AZT and ABC undergo phase II metabolism. ENF is not metabolized. RAL undergoes phase II metabolism. Therefore, NRTIs, MVC, ENF are not prone to drug interactions involving CYP450 enzymes.
- Drug interactions can be beneficial (use of low-dose RTV to enhance plasma concentrations of other PIs), harmful, or not clinically significant. Table 3-1 shows some examples of clinically significant drug interactions.

Mechanisms of Drug Interactions

- **Pharmacodynamic drug interactions** result in a change in pharmacologic response without change in serum concentrations. Pharmacodynamic interactions can be a result of: (1) synergism: response from drug combination greater than predicted; (2) additive response from combination equal to that predicted; (3) antagonism: response less than predicted (e.g., d4T + AZT).
- **Pharmacokinetic drug interactions** result from altered drug absorption, distribution, metabolism, and/or excretion.
  - **Drug absorption** can be affected by: (1) alteration of GI motility; (2) inhibition and/ or induction of drug transporters (P-glycoprotein); (3) metabolism (CYP450 enzyme induction and/or inhibition); (4) change in intestinal blood flow; (5) change in gastric pH and/or emptying time; (6) drug absorption or complexation; (7) GI pathology.
  - **Drug distribution** can be affected by: (1) displacement of drugs from binding sites; (2) displacement of plasma proteins (albumin and alpha acid glycoprotein), but the clinical significance of this interaction in unknown.
  - **Drug metabolism** can be affected by: inhibition or induction of drug metabolizing enzymes (e.g., CYP450) leading to altered metabolism of the substrate drug metabolized by that enzymatic pathway. Clinical significance of change in affected drug concentration depends on its therapeutic index (safety/efficacy profile).
  - **Drug excretion** can be affected by: alteration of GFR, tubular secretion and/or reabsorption.

Possible Outcomes of ARV Pharmacokinetic and Pharmacodynamic Interactions

- Elevated drug exposure can lead to increase in adverse events (e.g., TDF increases ddI exposure leading to ddI-induced toxicity).
- Elevated drug exposure can lead to improved therapeutic outcomes (e.g., use of low-dose RTV to inhibit CYP3A4 activity and enhance plasma concentrations of other PIs).
- Diminished drug exposure can lead to therapeutic failure (e.g., CYP3A4 induction by rifampin lowers exposure of PIs, compromising therapeutic response).
- Some drug interactions not clinically significant and thus have no impact on pharmacokinetics or pharmacodynamics of ARV agents (e.g., TMP increases concentrations of 3TC).

CLINICAL RECOMMENDATION

Prevention and Management of Drug Interactions

- If possible, avoid polypharmacy.
- Be aware of food effects on ARV absorption.
- Be familiar with contraindicated drug combinations (see Table 3-1).
- Be familiar with "red flag" drugs. These drugs have high likelihood of drug interactions (e.g., potent CYP3A4 inhibitors: PIs, macrolides, many azole antifungals; CYP3A4 inducers: rifamycins, many anticonvulsants; CYP3A4 substrates with high risk of toxicity due to supratherapeutic concentrations: many antiarrhythmics, warfarin, QTc prolonging drugs, ergotamines, erectile dysfunction agents, many benzodiazepines, and some opiates).
- Ask about use of complementary and alternative medications, since some are known to lower plasma concentrations of PI agents (e.g., St. Johns wort).
- Many drug interactions can be managed by dose modifications, staggered administration, or use of an alternative agent.
- Use up-to-date literature resources to identify drug interactions involving ARV agents (refer to Table 3-1).
- If no PK data available, use alternative agents with lower likelihood of drug interaction based on pharmacologic principles.
- Consider using TDM when combining agents known to undergo CYP450 metabolism and also inhibit/induce these enzymes (e.g., patients on dual PI + NNRTI therapy).

MANAGEMENT

TABLE 3.1: CLINICALLY SIGNIFICANT DRUG-DRUG INTERACTIONS

Affected Drug	Interacting Drug	Effect	Recommendations
Alfuzosin	PIs, DLV	May significantly increase alfuzosin serum concentrations	Contraindicated. Consider tamsulosin or doxazosin.
Antacid	APV, ATV, DLV, TPV/r	May interfere with absorption	Separate dosing by 2 hrs before or 1 hr after to avoid reduced ARV bioavailability.
Antiarrhythmics (amiodarone, bepridil, flecainide, propafenone, quinidine)	PIs, DLV	May significantly increase antiarrhythmic serum concentrations	Contraindicated. Lidocaine, mexiletine, disopyramide, and dofetilide should also be avoided
Antifungal (itraconazole, ketoconazole, voriconazole)	PIs, NNRTI	Boosted PIs may increase itraconazole and ketoconazole, but decrease voriconazole serum concentrations	Use a max dose of itraconazole 200 mg twice daily or ketoconazole 200 mg once daily with boosted PIs and DLV coadministration. High-dose RTV contraindicated with voriconazole. Monitor voriconazole concentrations closely with boosted PI and NNRTI coadministration. See specific drug-drug interaction section for dose modifications.
ATV, DLV, itraconazole, ketoconazole	PPI and antacids	ATV AUC decreased by 75%. DLV, itraconazole, and ketoconazole AUC may be significantly decreased.	Coadministration not recommended. ATV may be given 2 hrs before or 10 hrs after H-2 blockers.
Benzodiazepines (alprazolam, midazolam, triazolam)	PIs, DLV	May significantly increase alprazolam, midazolam, triazolam, and serum concentrations	Contraindicated. Consider lorazepam.
Bosentan	PIs	Significant increase in bosentan serum concentrations	Coadminister bosentan (62.5 mg q24–48h) only after PIs have reached steady state (10 days). Avoid unboosted ATV.

Clarithromycin, erythromycin	PIs, DLV	Clarithromycin AUC increased by 94% with ATV coadministration	QTc prolongation observed. Use 50% of clarithromycin dose. Alternative: azithromycin.
Calcium channel blockers (amlodipine, diltiazem, nifedipine)	PIs, DLV	Diltiazem AUC increased by 125%	Increase in PR interval observed. Start with 50% diltiazem dose and titrate slowly.
Clopidogrel	ETR, azoles	Biotransformation to active clopidogrel metabolite may be inhibited	Avoid coadministration
ddI	TDF, allopurinol, and ribavirin	May increase risk of mitochondrial toxicity	Avoid coadministration. With TDF coadministration decrease ddI dose.
Erectile dysfunction agents (sildenafil, tadalafil, vardenafil)	PIs, DLV	Significant increase in serum concentrations of erectile dysfunction agents	Do not exceed the following doses: sildenafil 25 mg q48h; tadalafil 10 mg q72h; vardenafil 2.5 mg q72h.
Ergotamine	PIs, DLV	May significantly increase ergotamine serum concentrations	Contraindicated. Consider sumatriptan.
Fentanyl	PIs, DLV	May significantly increase fentanyl serum concentrations	Avoid coadministration. Alternative: morphine.
Fluticasone	PIs, DLV	May significantly increase fluticasone serum concentrations	Avoid coadministration. Consider beclomethasone.
Immunosuppressants (tacrolimus, sirolimus, cyclosporine)	PIs, DLV, azoles, macrolides	May significantly increase immunosuppressive agents	Monitor immunosuppressive agents serum concentrations closely. Significant dose adjustment needed.
Irinotecan	ATV; caution with other PIs, especially IDV	May increase irinotecan serum concentrations	Contraindicated

(Continued)

MANAGEMENT

385

TABLE 3.1: CLINICALLY SIGNIFICANT DRUG-DRUG INTERACTIONS *(cont'd.)*

Affected Drug	Interacting Drug	Effect	Recommendations
Methadone	PIs, NNRTI, ddI (buffered)	EFV, NVP (but not ETR), and buffered ddI may significantly decrease methadone concentrations. Some boosted PIs (TPV, LPV/r, SQV/r, FPV/r) may decrease methadone serum concentrations, but clinical significance unknown.	Monitor for methadone withdrawal symptoms and titrate methadone to effect
MVC	PIs, NNRTI, rifampin	EFV, ETR, and rifampin decrease MVC serum concentrations. Boosted PIs (except TPV/r) increase MVC serum concentrations.	With NVP and TPV/r: MVC 300 mg twice daily. With EFV, ETR, rifampin, and possibly rifabutin: use 600 mg twice daily. With other boosted PIs: MVC 150 mg twice daily.
PIs and NNRTIs	Phenytoin, carbamazepine, phenobarbital	PIs and NNRTIs concentrations may be decreased. LPV AUC decreased by 33% and phenytoin AUC decreased by 31%	Levels of all PIs and NNRTI may be decreased. Alternative: valproic acid, levetiracetam, and topiramate.
PIs (except NFV)	EFV, NVP, and ETR	Significant decrease PI's serum concentrations when not coadministered with ritonavir	Coadminister PI with ritonavir with NNRTI coadministration.
Prednisone	PIs, DLV	May increase prednisone serum concentration	May require dose adjustment with long-term coadministration
QTc prolongation agents (cisapride, astemizole, terfenadine, pimozide)	PIs, DLV	QTc prolongation with coadministration	Contraindicated. Antihistamines: loratadine, cetirizine, fexofenadine, desloratadine can be considered. GI or motility agent: metoclopramide. Antipsychotic: olanzapine can be considered.
Ranolazine	PIs, DLV	May significantly increase ranolazine serum concentrations	Contraindicated

Drug	ARVs	Effect	Management
Rifabutin	Ritonavir-boosted PIs	Rifabutin AUC increased 3–4 fold	Decrease rifabutin to 150 mg qod with boosted PIs coadministration
Rifampin, St. John's wort	All PIs, DLV, NVP, ETR, MVC, and RAL	Significant decrease in ARVs serum concentrations	Avoid coadministration. Consider rifabutin with coadministration or use EFV-based regimen with rifampin. RAL 800 mg twice daily and MVC 600 mg twice daily can be considered with rifampin, but no clinical data.
Salmeterol	PIs	May increase QTc prolongation	Avoid coadministration. Consider formoterol.
Statins (simvastatin, lovastatin)	PIs, DLV	May significantly increase simvastatin and lovastatin serum concentrations	Contraindicated. Consider pravastatin, atorvastatin, or rosuvastatin.
Statins (atorvastatin, rosuvastatin)	PIs, DLV	Increase in atorvastatin serum concentrations	Start with low dose atorvastatin (10 mg) and rosuvastatin
Telaprevir	FPV/r, DRV/r, and LPV/r	Telaprevir AUC decreased by 32%, 35%, and 54%, respectively. APV and DRV AUC decreased by 47% and 40% respectively.	Avoid FPV, DRV/r, LPV/r coadministration. Consider ATV/r with telaprevir (only 20% decrease in telaprevir exposure)
Warfarin	PIs, NNRTI	ETR may increase warfarin concentrations. EFV and NVP may decrease warfarin concentrations. RTV may increase or decrease (at steady state) warfarin serum concentrations.	Monitor INR closely with coadministration

MANAGEMENT

SELECTED REFERENCES

Sterling TR, Pham PA, Chaison RD. Treatment of HIV-related tuberculosis. *Clin Infect Dis*, 2010; S223.
Comments: Drug interactions involving rifamycins and antiretroviral agents are summarized.

Panel on Antiretroviral Guidelines for Adults and Adolescents. Guidelines for the use of antiretroviral agents in HIV-1-infected adults and adolescents. Department of Health and Human Services; January 1, 2011; 1–166. *http://www.aidsinfo. nih.gov/contentfiles/AdultandAdolescentGL.pdf*. Accessed July 17, 2011.
Comments: DHHS guidelines for management of drug interaction involving ARV agents.

Flexner CW, Pham PA. Pharmacology and drug interactions of HIV protease inhibitors. In: *Drug Interactions and Administrations in AIDS Therapy*. 3rd ed. New York: Basel; 2009:.
Comments: Review of pharmacokinetic and pharmacodynamic interactions involving ARVs.

INDUCTION-MAINTENANCE

Richard D. Moore, MD, MHS

DEFINITION

- Initiation of intensive ART regimen followed by simplification or deintensification after virologic suppression to improve convenience and tolerability and to decrease toxicity. Switches from standard 3-drug regimens to 1- or 2-drug regimens also studied.

INDICATIONS

- Aggressive induction regimens have been used to achieve more rapid initial suppression, but without supporting evidence.
- Switch to maintenance regimens to minimize long-term toxicity; fewer ADRs and drug-drug interactions with fewer drugs.
- Switch to maintenance regimens to optimize long-term tolerability/adherence; fewer drugs associated with better adherence and fewer side effects.
- Induction-maintenance, not standard of care.

CLINICAL RECOMMENDATION

- Induction-maintenance approach not recommended based on available evidence: variability in drug regimens, duration of time for induction, variable baseline VL and CD4, inconsistent results.
- Approach 1: 3-drug induction with 2 NRTIs + 1 PI; 2-drug maintenance with 2 NRTIs or 1 NRTI + 1 PI. Not effective.
- Approach 2: 3-drug induction with 3TC/TDF/EFV; then 2-drug maintenance with TDF/EFV. No clear advantage to maintenance arm, and less effective.
- Approach 3: 4-drug induction; 3-drug maintenance with 3 NRTIs. Some evidence of efficacy as maintenance after 4-drug induction in patients without prior NRTI resistance; however high rate of AEs with induction; AZT/3TC/ABC + EFV induction associated with higher VL failure than AZT/3TC/ABC + LPV/r induction.
- Approach 4: 4-drug induction with 2 NRTIs + 1 NNRTI + 1 PI; 3-drug maintenance with 2NRTIs + 1 NNRTI. 4 drugs no better than standard 3-drug regimen over 3 yrs in ARV-naive (see ACTG 5095, ref.). Four-drug induction better at 48 wks in another trial (*Antivir Ther*; 12: 47–54).
- Approach 5: 3-drug induction with LPV/r and 2 NRTIs, then LPV/r monotherapy. Some supportive evidence, but may not be as effective as 3-drug maintenance, and LPV/r no longer preferred PI. Suppression typically achieved with NRTI intensification in those with incomplete suppression.
- Approach 6: switching to DRV/r monotherapy was non-inferior to DRV/r +2 NRTI after VL <50 for >24 wks on 2 NRTI+PI. Not guideline recommended currently.

SELECTED REFERENCES

Arribas JR, Horban A, Gerstoft J, et al. The MONET trial: darunavir/ritonavir with or without nucleoside analogues, for patients with HIV RNA below 50 copies/ml. *AIDS*, 2010; 24: 223–30.
Comments: DRV/r monotherapy non-inferior to continuing 2 NRTI+PI after 24 wks of VL <50.

Arribas JR, Delgado R, Arranz A. Lopinavir-ritonavir monotherapy versus lopinavir-ritonavir and 2 nucleosides for maintenance therapy of HIV: 96-week analysis. *J Acquir Immune Defic Syndr*, 2009; 51: 147–52.
Comments: Patients on PI + NRTIs randomized to LPV/r monotherapy (with reintroduction of NRTIs if needed) or continued 3-ARV therapy. At 96-wks, 87% on LPV/r monotherapy and 78% on 3-ARVs had VL <50 (NS). AEs lower with monotherapy.

Mallolas J, Pich J, Penaranda M, et al. Induction therapy with Trizivir plus efavirenz or lopinavir/ritonavir followed by Trizivir alone in naive HIV-1 infected adults. *AIDS*, 2008; 22: 377–84.
Comments: AZT/3TC/ABC + EFV or LPV/r induction, followed by AZT/3TC/ABC alone as maintenance. High rate of adverse events during induction, relatively low rate of viral suppression during maintenance.

Cameron D, da Silva B, Arribas J et al. A randomized trial comparing lopinavir–ritonavir, zidovudine and lamivudine induction followed by lopinavir–ritonavir monotherapy with efavirenz, zidovudine, and lamivudine in antiretroviral-naive subjects: 96 week results. *J Infect Dis*, 2008; 198: 234–40.
Comments: LPV/r monotherapy after LPV/r + ZDV + 3TC vs EFV + ZDV + 3TC in ARV-naïve. At 96 wks, 48% of LPV/r and 61% of EFV with VL <50 (NS).

Gulick R, Ribaudo H, Shikuma C, et al. Three- vs four-drug antiretroviral regimens for the initial treatment of HIV-1 infection. *JAMA*, 2006; 296: 769–81.
Comments: RCT in ARV-naïve; no differences between 3- and 4-drug regimen (AZT/3TC/ABC + EFV vs AZT/3TC + EFV) in VL suppression <50 through 3 yrs at all VL, CD4 strata.

Girard PM, Cabie A, Michelet C, et al. EFV/TDF vs EFV/3TC/TDF as maintenance regimen in virologically controlled patients under HAART: a 6-month analysis of the COOL trial. Program and Abstracts of the 15th International AIDS Conference. July 11–16, 2004. Bangkok, Thailand.
Comments: Short (6-month) follow-up suggests that EFV/TDF as effective as EFV/3TC/TDF, but insufficient follow-up to recommend currently. May make no sense to do this since TDF/FTC now coformulated, 3TC and FTC are safe and well tolerated, and both increase genetic barrier to resistance for TDF.

Asboe D, Williams IG, Goodall RL, et al. A virological benefit from an induction/maintenance strategy: the Forte trial. *Antivir Ther*; 12: 47–54.
Comments: Virological benefit found with induction with 2 NRTIs + NNRTI + PI/r followed by 2 NRTIs + NNRTI compared to initial and continued therapy with 2 NRTIs + NNRTI.

INITIAL REGIMEN

Joel E. Gallant, MD, MPH

DEFINITION
- First drug regimen in ART-naïve patient.

INDICATIONS

DHHS Guidelines (10/14/11): Preferred Regimens
- 2-NRTI backbone + NNRTI or PI (preferably RTV-boosted) or INSTI (integrase strand transfer inhibitor).
- Regimens with optimal and durable efficacy, favorable tolerability and toxicity profile, and ease of use. Preferred regimens for nonpregnant patients listed in order of FDA approval of non-NRTI components, thus, by duration of clinical experience.
- **NNRTI-based regimen:** EFV/TDF/FTC. Do not use EFV during 1st trimester of pregnancy or in women trying to conceive or not using effective and consistent contraception.
- **PI-based regimens** (alphabetical order): (1) ATV/r + TDF/FTC or (2) DRV/r + TDF/FTC. ATV/r should not be used in patients who require >20 mg omeprazole equivalent per day. Use with caution in patients on PPIs (any dose), H2-blockers, antacids.
- **INSTI-based regimen:** RAL + TDF/FTC.
- **Preferred regimen for pregnant women:** LPV/r (twice daily) + AZT/3TC. 3TC may be substituted for FTC and vice versa.

DHHS Guidelines (10/14/11): Alternative Regimens
- Regimens that are effective and tolerable but have potential disadvantages compared with preferred regimens. May be the preferred for some patients.
- **NNRTI-based regimens** (alphabetical order): (1) EFV + ABC/3TC or (2) RPV/TDF/FTC or (3) RPV + ABC/3TC.
- **PI-based regimens** (alphabetical order): (1) ATV/r + ABC/3TC; or (2) DRV/r + ABC/3TC; or (3) FPV/r + AZT/3TC; or (4) FPV/r (once or twice daily) + (ABC/3TC or TDF/FTC); or (4) LPV/r (once or twice-daily) + (ABC/3TC or TDF/FTC).
- **INSTI-based regimens:** RAL + ABC/3TC.

MANAGEMENT

- 3TC may be substituted for FTC and vice versa.
- Use RPV with caution in patients with pre-treatment VL >100,000.
- Use of PPIs contraindicated with RPV.

DHHS Guidelines (10/14/11): Acceptable Regimens
- Regimens that may be selected for some patients but are less satisfactory than preferred or alternative regimens.
- **NNRTI-based regimens:** (1) EFV + AZT/3TC or (2) NVP + (ABC/3TC or TDF/FTC).
- **PI-based regimens:** ATV + (ABC or AZT)/3TC (ATV/r generally preferred. Unboosted ATV may be used when RTV boosting not possible. Do not use unboosted ATV with TDF).
- **CCR5 antagonist-based regimens:** MVC + AZT/3TC.

DHHS Guidelines (10/14/11): Regimens that May Be Acceptable but More Definitive Data Are Needed
- **NNRTI-based regimens:** (1) NVP + ABC/3TC or (2) RPV + AZT/3TC.
- **PI-based regimen:** DRV/r + AZT/3TC.
- **INSTI-based regimen:** RAL + AZT/3TC.
- **CCR5 antagonist-based regimen:** MVC + ABC/3TC.

DHHS Guidelines (10/14/11): Regimens that May Be Acceptable but Should Be Used with Caution
- **PI-based regimen:** SQV/r + TDF/FTC and ABC or AZT)/3TC.

DHHS Guidelines (10/14/11): Notes on Specific Agents
- 3TC may be substituted for FTC and vice versa.
- ATV/r should not be used in patients who require >20 mg omeprazole equivalent per day. Use with caution in patients on PPIs (any dose), H2-blockers, antacids.
- Do not use EFV during 1st trimester of pregnancy or in women trying to conceive or not using effective and consistent contraception.
- ABC should not be used in patients who test positive for HLA-B*5701; use with caution in patients with high risk of cardiovascular disease or with pretreatment VL >100,000.
- LPV/r + AZT/3TC is the preferred regimen for pregnant women. Once-daily LPV/r not recommended in pregnant women.
- Use RPV with caution in patients with pretreatment VL >100,000. Use of PPIs contraindicated with RPV.
- NVP should not be used (1) in patients with moderate-to-severe hepatic impairment (Child-Pugh B or C); (2) in women with pre-ART CD4 >250; or (3) in men with pre-ART CD4 >400.
- ATV/r generally preferred over unboosted ATV, which may be used when RTV boosting not possible. Do not use unboosted ATV with TDF.
- AZT can cause bone marrow suppression, lipoatrophy, and rarely lactic acidosis with hepatic steatosis.
- Perform troprism test before initiation of MVC therapy. MVC may be considered in patients who have only CCR5-tropic virus.
- Use NVP and ABC together with caution because both can cause HSRs within the first few weeks of therapy.
- SQV/r associated w/ PR and QTc prolongation in healthy volunteer study; see DHHS guidelines regarding ECG criteria for use.

IAS-USA Guidelines (7/21/10)
- **2-NRTI backbone**
  - **Recommended:** TDF/FTC: renal dysfunction, decreased bone mineral density affect choice.
  - **Alternative:** ABC/3TC: screen with HLA B*5701 assay to reduce risk of hypersensitivity reaction; may have less activity than TDF/FTC in patients w/ VL >100,000; may increase cardiovascular risk.
- **3rd agent**
  - **Recommended:** EFV: major psychiatric illness, 1st trimester pregnancy, or intention to become pregnant affect choice.
  - **Recommended:** ATV/r (300/100 mg once daily): hyperbilirubinemia, need for acid-reducing agents, and risk of nephrolithiasis affect choice.
  - **Recommended:** DRV/r (800/100 mg once daily): limited experience in naïve patients, availability of other options, and efficacy in experienced patients with multidrug resistant virus affect choice.
  - **Recommended:** RAL (400 mg twice daily): limited experience in naïve patients, availability of other options, and efficacy in experienced patients with multidrug resistant virus affect choice.

- **Alternatives:** LPV/r (200/50 mg tabs, 4 once daily or 2 tabs twice daily), FPV/r (700/100 mg twice daily or 1400/200 or 1400/100 mg once daily), or MVC (300 mg twice daily if used only with NRTIs).

CLINICAL RECOMMENDATION
NNRTI-Based Regimens

- **Advantages:** simplicity, tolerability, relative lack of long-term toxicity, single tablet regimens available, better virologic suppression with EFV than LPV/r in ACTG 5142, efficacy at all VL and CD4 strata.
- **Disadvantages:** lower genetic barrier to resistance: greater resistance consequences with failure than with PI/r; CNS side effects (EFV); hepatotoxicity and skin rash (NVP); lower CD4 response with EFV than LPV/r in ACTG 5142 despite superior virologic suppression.
- **EFV: Advantages:** the gold standard; coformulated with TDF/FTC; antiviral activity as good or better than all comparators to date. **Disadvantages:** CNS side effects, rash, likelihood of NNRTI resistance with failure, teratogenicity. Avoid EFV in pregnant women (especially 1st trimester) or women with pregnancy potential.
- **RPV: Advantages:** coformulated with TDF/FTC; better tolerated than EFV with fewer CNS effects, less rash and lipid effects. **Disadvantages:** less effective at VL >100,000 with greater resistance at failure, including cross-resistance to ETR.
- **NVP:** an acceptable NNRTI in women with CD4 <250 and men with CD4 <400. **Advantages:** well tolerated; safe in pregnancy; less lipid effects than with EFV; **Disadvantages:** risk of serious skin reactions and hepatotoxicity, especially in women, and at higher pretreatment CD counts; not as well studied as EFV with TDF/FTC or ABC/3TC.
- **ETR: Advantages:** well tolerated; active against most NNRTI-resistant viruses, including K103N mutations. **Disadvantages:** minimal data in ART-naïve patients, though may eventually have role for patients infected with EFV/NVP-resistant virus.

PI-Based Regimens

- **Advantages:** typically no PI resistance with failure of PI/r-based regimen; ATV/r had similar efficacy to EFV in ACTG 5202; greater CD4 increase w/ LPV/r than EFV in ACTG 5142; once-daily regimens with 100 mg/day of RTV (ATV/r, FPV/r, DRV/r); better tolerated with less hyperlipidemia than regimens with higher doses of RTV. **Disadvantages:** greater pill burden than with EFV or RPV coformulations; more GI side effects.
- **ATV ± RTV: Advantages:** lowest pill burden (2/day); well tolerated; less hyperlipidemia than LPV/r; does not require RTV boosting. Best choice if RTV boosting not possible (with ABC/3TC, not TDF/FTC). **Disadvantages:** potential for jaundice; requirement for gastric acidity (decreased absorption with proton pump inhibitors, H2 blockers, antacids); food requirement. RTV boosting preferred, and essential with TDF or EFV; cannot be combined with NVP.
- **DRV/r: Advantages:** DRV/r 800/100 mg once daily noninferior to LPV/r, and superior in patients with VL >100,000; well tolerated, with less hyperlipidemia than LPV/r; no jaundice or gastric acid concerns (vs ATV/r). **Disadvantages:** greater pill burden than ATV/r (3 vs 2); potential for rash.
- **LPV/r: Advantages:** convenience (coformulated with RTV); no food restriction with tablet formulation; preferred PI/r in pregnancy. **Disadvantages:** GI side effects; hyperlipidemia requires 200 mg/day of RTV.
- **FPV ± RTV: Advantages:** once- or twice-daily dosing (once daily with FPV/r 1400/100–200 mg only for PI-naïve patients); FPV/r twice daily equivalent to LPV/r twice daily in KLEAN study; no food restrictions. **Disadvantages:** no clear advantage of 700/100 mg twice daily over coformulated LPV/r; less clinical data with better tolerated FPV/r 1400/100 mg once-daily dose compared to ATV/r and DRV/r; potential for rash.
- **SQV/r: Advantages:** well tolerated with less diarrhea and more favorable lipid effects than LPV/r. **Disadvantages:** higher pill burden than other PIs (6/day); no clear advantages over PI/r regimens that include only 100 mg/day of RTV; black box warning for PR and QTc prolongation.
- **IDV ± RTV: Advantages:** none. **Disadvantages:** not recommended in DHHS guidelines; minimal data; nephrotoxicity; fluid requirement; elevated indirect bilirubin; dermatologic changes.
- **NFV: Advantages:** acceptable in pregnancy (LPV/r preferred). **Disadvantages:** not recommended in DHHS or IAS-USA guidelines; higher failure rate than other PIs; diarrhea; food requirement; inability to effectively boost with RTV; potential for PI resistance with failure (including L90M).
- **TPV/r:** not recommended for initial therapy.

MANAGEMENT

Integrase Inhibitor-Based Regimens
- RAL: **Advantages:** RAL + TDF/FTC noninferior to EFV/TDF/FTC and better tolerated in STARTMRK trial (Lennox) through 156 wks, with more rapid virologic suppression. **Disadvantages:** twice-daily dosing, barrier to resistance more similar to NNRTI- than PI/r-based regimens.

Choice of NRTI Backbone (as Component of HAART Regimen)
- TDF/FTC: **Advantages:** well tolerated; 1 tab once daily; no food restrictions; no mitochondrial toxicity; superior to AZT/3TC in GS934 with less toxicity, failure, and resistance (M184V); less K65R with TDF/FTC than TDF/3TC, increased AZT susceptibility w/ M184V and/or K65R. **Disadvantages:** nephrotoxicity, especially in patients with preexisting renal dysfunction and in patients on PI-based regimen; cross-resistance to ABC and ddI with K65R/M184V; greater loss of bone mineral density during initial therapy than with other NRTIs.
- ABC/3TC: **Advantages:** well tolerated; 1 tab once daily; no food restrictions; no mitochondrial toxicity. **Disadvantages:** need for HLA B*5701 testing to decrease risk of ABC hypersensitivity; decreased activity (vs TDF/FTC) in patients with baseline VL >100,000 in ACTG 5202; possible association with increased risk of MI; cross-resistance to ddI (L74V, K65R), TDF (K65R).
- AZT/3TC: **Advantages:** well studied; resistance to AZT (TAMs) occurs gradually; M184V increases AZT activity. **Disadvantages:** anemia; GI intolerance; mitochondrial toxicity; including lipoatrophy, twice-daily dosing, extensive NRTI cross-resistance when multiple TAMs present; inferior to TDF/FTC in GS934 with more toxicity, failure, and resistance (M184V).
- d4T + (3TC or FTC): **Advantages:** well studied; well tolerated; resistance to d4T (TAMs) occurs gradually; M184V increases d4T activity. **Disadvantages:** more toxic than other NRTIs (neuropathy, lipoatrophy, hyperlipidemia, lactic acidosis/hyperlactatemia, hepatic steatosis). Not recommended.
- AZT/3TC/ABC: potential for use in combination with 4th agent. In ACTG 5095 (Gulick) AZT/3TC/ABC + EFV not more effective than AZT/3TC + EFV. Therefore, triple NRTI backbone + NNRTI not recommended for initial regimen in patients w/ wild-type virus.
- ABC + ddI, TDF + ddI, ABC + TDF: avoid in naïve patients (minimal data, possible increased selective pressure for resistance). Sometimes used in patients with NRTI resistance, but minimal data; TDF increases ddI levels and toxicity and may decrease CD4 count: if used, reduce ddI dose.
- ddI + d4T: avoid (toxicity, lower efficacy).
- AZT + d4T: avoid (antagonism).

Use of Other Agents
- MVC: **Advantages:** R5 virus more common among ART-naïve patients; well tolerated; efficacy similar to EFV in MERIT study when enhanced sensitivity tropism assay used. **Disadvantages:** baseline tropism testing required; twice-daily dosing (once-daily dosing under study); lack of long-term safety data; studied only with AZT/3TC.
- ENF: no role for initial therapy due to high cost, need for twice-daily injection, and lack of data.

TREATMENT CONSIDERATIONS

Chronic Liver Disease/Viral Hepatitis
- No regimen contraindicated. Use caution with PIs (especially TPV), NNRTIs (especially NVP), d4T. Severe liver disease: decrease dose of some PIs (APV, FPV, ATV, IDV) (DHHS Guidelines).
- Chronic HBV: use regimen that includes TDF/FTC (or TDF + 3TC) for dual anti-HBV therapy.

Renal Insufficiency
- Avoid IDV, TDF, or use with caution. Dose adjust some NRTIs (ddI, 3TC, FTC, AZT, d4T, TDF).
- ART recommended for all patients with HIVAN, regardless of CD4 and VL.

Pregnancy or Child-Bearing Potential
- ART recommended for all pregnant women with HIV, regardless of VL and CD4. Transmission is less likely, but still possible, with VL <1000.
- If ART indicated for woman's health, start ART as soon as possible. If indicated only to prevent perinatal transmission, consider delaying until after 1st trimester.
- AZT/3TC preferred NRTI backbone (established efficacy with AZT, experience with AZT/3TC), but use regimen most likely to suppress viral load. TDF appears safe in pregnancy registry.

- LPV/r preferred PI in pregnant women. Always use twice-daily dosing; consider increasing dose (3 tabs twice daily) in 3rd trimester due to decreased LPV levels. ATV/r also approved in pregnancy (class B).
- Avoid EFV, especially in 1st trimester (teratogenicity).
- Avoid ddI/d4T (toxicity); DLV (teratogenicity in animals); liquid APV (contains propylene glycol).
- Avoid NVP in women with CD4 >250 (hepatotoxicity). Single-dose NVP not associated with hepatotoxicity.
- RPV class B, but no clinical data.
- Little experience with ENF, MVC, RAL, ETR in pregnancy.
- See Perinatal Guidelines (Perinatal HIV-1 Guidelines Working Group) for information on prevention of perinatal transmission.

KEYWORDS
Other
- Antiretroviral therapy.
- HAART.
- Starting therapy.
- Initial therapy.
- ART.

SELECTED REFERENCES
Panel on Treatment of HIV-Infected Pregnant Women and Prevention of Perinatal Transmission. Recommendations for use of antiretroviral drugs in pregnant HIV-1-infected women for maternal health and interventions to reduce perinatal HIV transmission in the United States. May 24, 2010; 1–117. *http://www.aidsinfo.nih.gov/ContentFiles/PerinatalGL.pdf*. Accessed August 5, 2011.
Comments: PHS guidelines on prevention of maternal-to-child transmission and use of ART in pregnant women.

Thompson MA, Aberg JA, Cahn P, et al. Antiretroviral treatment of adult HIV infection: 2010 recommendations of the International AIDS Society-USA panel. *JAMA*, 2010; 304: 321–33.
Comments: IAS-USA guidelines on antiretroviral therapy, including when to start, choice of initial regimen, monitoring therapy, changing therapy, etc.

Panel on Antiretroviral Guidelines for Adults and Adolescents. Guidelines for the use of antiretroviral agents in HIV-1-infected adults and adolescents. Department of Health and Human Services; January 1, 2011; 1–161. *http://www.aidsinfo. nih.gov/contentfiles/AdultandAdolescentGL.pdf*. Accessed July 17, 2011.
Comments: DHHS guidelines on antiretroviral therapy, including when to start, choice of initial regimen, monitoring therapy, changing therapy, etc.

Riddler SA et al. Class-sparing regimens for initial treatment of HIV-1 infection. *N Engl J Med*; 2008 May 15;358(20): 2095–106.
Comments: ACTG 5142: landmark study comparing EFV vs LPV/r (both + 2 NRTIs) vs EFV+LPV/r, demonstrating superior virologic efficacy with EFV + 2 NRTIs, but statistically better CD4 response and less resistance with failure with LPV/r.

Eron J et al: The KLEAN study of fosamprenavir-ritonavir versus lopinavir-ritonavir, each in combination with abacavir-lamivudine, for initial treatment of HIV infection over 48 weeks: a randomised non-inferiority trial. *Lancet*; 2006 Aug 5;368(9534): 476–82.
Comments: KLEAN study: open-label, randomized trial comparing FPV/r (700/100 mg twice-daily) vs LPV/r (soft-gel caps 400/100 mg twice-daily) in combination w/ ABC/3TC in 878 naïve pts. No difference in efficacy, tolerability, or toxicity, including hyperlipidemia, at 48 wks. Note that gel-cap formulation of LPV/r used; tolerability with tablet formulation appears better.

MONITORING THERAPY

Richard D. Moore, MD, MHS

DEFINITION
- Assessment recommended while on ART to monitor efficacy and toxicity of therapy viral load (VL).

CLINICAL RECOMMENDATION
Viral Load (VL)
- Key goal of ART is undetectable VL (<50 by *Amplicor*, <75 by *VERSANT*, <80 by *NucliSens*, <48 by *TaqMan*). Should be achieved by 16–24 wks.

- Virologic failure now defined as confirmed VL >200.
- Measure 2–8 wks after starting ART. Should decline by >1 log (10-fold) from baseline. Measure every 4–8 wks until undetectable.
- Stable ART regimen: measure every 3–6 mos (6 mos interval for adherent patients with longstanding virologic suppression).
- Change in ART motivated by drug toxicity or regimen simplification (not by resistance): measure after 2–8 wks to confirm potency of new regimen.

CD4 Count

- CD4 count: 3 mos after ART start, every 3–6 mos thereafter. If clinically stable with suppressed VL, consider every 6–12 mos.
- Average increase of ~100/yr until plateau. Plateau lower with low baseline CD4.
- Lack of CD4 response not evidence of treatment failure if VL undetectable.

Other Laboratory Tests

- **Fasting lipid panel:** measure pre-ART baseline; consider 4–8 wks after starting new ART regimen. If abnormal at last measurement, repeat after 6 mos. If normal at last measurment, repeat annually. Use to monitor if lipid-specific therapy started.
- **Chemistry panel:** at 2–8 wks after starting new ART regimen, then every 3–6 mos. ATV can increase indirect and total bilirubin (not clinically significant unless overt jaundice or scleral icterus present). Most PIs, NNRTIs, and some NRTIs can increase AST/ALT. AST/ALT every 2 wks (for 8–12 wks) after NVP and TPV start. If on TDF, consider 1st creatinine at 1 mo. Calculate CrCl (Cockcroft-Gault) or GFR (MDRD) Consider more frequent GFR monitoring if diabetes, hypertension or comorbidity with increased CKD risk.
- **CBC:** every 3–6 mos (more often on AZT).
- **Resistance assays:** measure if VL >500–1000 on therapy or within 4 wks after discontinuation.
- **Urinalysis:** if abnormal creatinine or history of abnormal urine protein. Consider routine monitoring in patients on TDF.
- **Lactate:** if suggestive Sx and on AZT, ddI, d4T.
- **TDM:** not routine. Consider only for PIs, NNRTIs (not NRTIs) if increased VL and significant drug-drug or drug-food interactions, GI, liver or renal absorption/metabolism issues, pregnancy, lack of expected response in ART-naïve, ART-experienced, and HIV with reduced susceptibilities. Significant limitations to interpretation.
- **HLA-B*5701:** before use of ABC. Hypersensitivity unlikely if negative. If positive, don't use ABC.
- **Tropism assay:** assess tropism if VL >1000 (Monogram *Trofile*) or lower VL (Monogram *Trofile DNA*), and considering therapy with MVC. If dual/mixed (D/M)- or X4-tropic virus present, don't use MVC. No indication for repeat testing once D/M or X4 virus detected.

Other Considerations

- **Adherence assessment:** non-judgmental questions. Side effects, daily schedules, food/ fasting requirements, OTCs, dietary supplements, depression, substance/alcohol use, social situation.
- **Behaviors:** sexual practices and partner HIV status, barrier and contraceptive use every 6 mos. Risk of HIV superinfection.
- Assess lipodystrophy by exam (pictures helpful). Certain NRTIs (AZT, ddI, d4T) associated with lipoatrophy (extremities, face, buttocks). PIs may be associated with fat accumulation (abdomen, neck, breasts). DEXA scan optional for further evaluation. Anthropomorphic measures (skin-fold, extremity/neck/abdomen circumference).
- Osteopenia can occur. Association w/ ART unclear. Routine screening not recommended. Consider in those ≥50 if high-risk (early menopause, steroids, hypogonadism). Maybe more common with TDF.
- Hip pain. Assess by MRI for AVN. Association w/ ART unclear. Hip X-ray not sensitive.
- Extremity pain. Consider neuropathy if on ddI or d4T.
- Nerve conduction studies to further assess. Other causes: HIV infection, B12 deficiency, thyroid disease, alcoholism, INH therapy.
- PPD: repeat after increased CD4 count on ART if previously negative with low CD4; repeat annually in patients at high risk for TB.

SELECTED REFERENCES

Hirsch MS, Günthard HF, Schapiro JM, et al. Antiretroviral drug resistance testing in adult HIV-1 infection: 2008 recommendations of an International AIDS Society-USA panel. *Clin Infect Dis*, 2008; 47: 266–85.
Comments: Up-to-date guidelines on ART resistance testing.

Aberg JA, Kaplan JE, Libman H, et al. Primary care guidelines for the management of persons infected with human immunodeficiency virus: 2009 update by the HIV Medicine Association of the Infectious Diseases Society of America. *Clin Infect Dis*, 2009; 49: 651–81.
Comments: Updated guidelines for primary care of HIV-infected patients.

Panel on Antiretroviral Guidelines for Adults and Adolescents. Guidelines for the use of antiretroviral agents in HIV-1-infected adults and adolescents. Department of Health and Human Services; January 1, 2011; 1–161. *http://aidsinfo.nih.gov/contentfiles/AdultandAdolescentGL.pdf*. Accessed July 17, 2011.
Comments: Up-to-date guidelines for evaluation of the HIV-infected adult and adolescent.

POSTEXPOSURE PROPHYLAXIS

Michael Melia, MD and Amita Gupta, MD, MHS

DEFINITION
- Use of ART following exposure or potential HIV exposure to prevent HIV infection.

INDICATIONS
Risk of Occupational Transmission
- Estimated 600,000–800,000 percutaneous injuries within US hospitals annually.
- Estimated risk of transmission: 0.3% per needlestick exposure; 0.09% per mucous membrane exposure.
- Risk for seroconversion: source with acute or late-stage HIV infection (high viral load), deep injury, needle placement in vein or artery, visible blood on device, contact of mucous membrane or non-intact skin with potentially infected tissue, blood, or other bodily fluid.
- Potentially infectious fluids: blood and/or visibly bloody fluids > cerebrospinal, synovial, pleural, peritoneal, pericardial, and amniotic fluids.
- Fluids extremely unlikely to be infectious (unless visibly bloody): feces, nasal secretions, saliva, sputum, sweat, tears, urine, vomitus.

Testing Source
- Rapid test: preferred. Use when source pt HIV status unknown. Result available in <1 hr, highly reliable in ruling out HIV, cost effective, and reduces HCW anxiety. Discontinue PEP if negative.
- Standard testing: ELISA usually available within 72 hrs. Discontinue PEP if negative.
- If acute seroconversion suspected in source, check viral load. This approach should be needed infrequently.

Risk of Transmission from Nonoccupational Exposure
- Risk of transmission in pre-HAART era: due to needle sharing IDU 67/10,000 exposures; receptive anal intercourse 50/10,000 exposures; receptive vaginal intercourse 10/10,000 exposures; insertive anal intercourse 6–7/10,000 exposures; receptive oral intercourse 1/10,000 exposures; insertive oral intercourse 0.5/10,000 exposures.

CLINICAL RECOMMENDATION
Efficacy and Duration of PEP (Post-Exposure Prophylaxis)
- Animal data show that PEP initiated <24 hrs after exposure and extended for 28 days effective in preventing transmission of SIV in macaques. One-wk PEP less effective than 4 wks course; treatment duration is therefore four wks.
- Retrospective case-control study showed 81% reduction in HIV transmission risk with AZT monotherapy. Currently available combination therapy likely more effective, although no data to substantiate this.
- Six PEP failures have been reported as of the most recent (2005) CDC guidelines.

Use and Selection of Occupational PEP
- 3-drug (2 NRTI + boosted PI) regimen: high-risk percutaneous exposure (e.g., large-bore hollow needle, deep puncture, visible blood on device, needle used in patient's artery or vein) to any patient known to have HIV OR a lower-risk percutaneous exposure or a large-volume

MANAGEMENT

mucous membrane or non-intact skin exposure to any patient with symptomatic HIV, AIDS, acute HIV seroconversion, or a high viral load.

- 2-drug (2 NRTI) regimen: less severe percutaneous injury or large-volume mucous membrane or non-intact skin exposure AND source has asymptomatic HIV infection or known HIV viral load of <1500; small-volume mucous membrane or non-intact skin exposure to any patient with symptomatic HIV, AIDS, acute HIV seroconversion, or a high viral load; consider if percutaneous injury or large-volume mucous membrane exposure and source has HIV-risk factors but HIV status is unknown; consider if percutaneous injury or large-volume mucous membrane exposure and source unknown (e.g., sharps container exposure) if local HIV prevalence high; consider if small-volume mucous membrane or non-intact skin exposure and source has asymptomatic HIV infection or known HIV viral load of <1500.
- No PEP: HIV-negative source; HIV status or source unknown; as above, consider 2-drug PEP if exposure to HIV+ person likely. Recommend HIV rapid testing of source in such cases and stop PEP if test negative.
- If concern for drug resistance: initiate 3-drug prophylaxis without delay and consult HIV expert to assist in selection of drugs to which source's virus unlikely to be resistant. Important to rapidly obtain source information on treatment history and any genotypes.
- NRTI backbone (author opinion): based on tolerability, once-daily dosing, and animal data, fixed-dose combination TDF/FTC is backbone of choice. AZT/3TC has long been standard backbone based on clinical data, but requires twice-daily dosing and is associated with more side effects. Consider d4T/3TC if TDF/FTC and AZT/3TC contraindicated or not tolerated. Do not use ABC/3TC because of possibility of life-threatening abacavir hypersensitivity reaction and inadequate time for HLA B*5701 testing. ddI/d4T should not be used given toxicities.
- 3rd agent (author opinion): although data limited, DRV/r and ATV/r are both relatively well-tolerated and can be dosed once-daily; DRV/r may also be more active than other boosted PIs for PI-resistant virus. LPV/r recommended in 2005 CDC guidelines but requires twice-daily dosing and causes more GI side effects. FPV/r can also be considered. NFV used in older PEP literature but aforementioned PIs likely better. Although single-tablet regimen is convenient, prefer PI over EFV because of relatively high rates of CNS side effects during 1st 2–4 wks of EFV use. NVP should NOT be used because of risk of serious hepatotoxicity in patients with normal CD4 counts.
- EFV should be avoided in pregnancy because of teratogenicity. TDF often avoided because of concern about fetal bone densitiy.

Use and Selection of Non-Occupational PEP (nPEP)

- Only consider for persons with infrequent exposures (e.g., not a commercial sex worker or someone who continuously shares injection drug use equipment).
- Recommend if patient seeks care within 72h of exposure of genitals, mucous membranes, non-intact skin, or percutaneous contact to blood, genital secretions, breast mild, or other blood-contaminated fluids of a person known to be HIV-infected.
- Consider (case-by-case basis) for patients who seek care within 72h of a high-risk exposure (e.g., MSM, IDU, commercial sex worker) of unknown HIV status.
- Do not use for patients who seek care >72h after exposure or if no HIV risk, although nPEP might be offered in certain (e.g., very high transmission risk) circumstances even if >72h after exposure.
- If nPEP is to be started, do so ASAP.
- Source patient HIV information should be secured, if possible.
- Duration of treatment is 28 days.
- Although no data to support recommendations, three-drug regimens viewed as superior to two-drug regimens. Three-drug nPEP is recommended (as listed above in Occupational PEP).
- Selection of medications is driven by same considerations as for PEP; EFV is listed as a preferred 3rd agent in CDC guidelines, but same caveats apply as previously.

Drugs for PEP

- AZT: established efficacy for PEP; high rates of GI intolerance, headache. Monitor CBC.
- 3TC: used in most PEP regimens: potent, well tolerated, available in co-formulation with AZT.
- d4T: long-term toxicity, but good short-term tolerability; do not combine with AZT.

- ABC: well tolerated but rarely used because of risk of hypersensitivity reaction (HSR); co-formulated with AZT/3TC or 3TC. HLA B*5701 testing can be used to screen for HSR, but this would delay institution of PEP.
- ddI: must be taken on empty stomach; GI intolerance, especially with buffered form; enteric coated ddI preferred.
- TDF: potent, well tolerated, once-daily dosing; effective for PEP in primate studies.
- FTC: daily, similar to 3TC, available coformulated with TDF.
- EFV: potent, but early CNS toxicity makes this a less desirable option.
- NVP: avoid in PEP as 22 HCWs had serious adverse reactions (12 hepatotoxicity including 1 liver transplant, 14 skin reactions including Stevens-Johnson syndrome) (US Public Health Service).
- LPV/r: potent, often active against PI-resistant virus, but may cause GI side effects.
- ATV ± RTV: potent, well tolerated with once-daily dosing, lowest pill burden among PIs; food requirement, indirect hyperbilirubinemia w/ occasional jaundice; requires RTV boosting with TDF coadministration.
- NFV: diarrhea, twice-daily dosing, fatty food requirement.
- FPV ± RTV: low pill burden, once- or twice-daily dosing, no food restrictions.
- DRV + RTV : may be most active against PI-resistant virus.

Monitoring and Counseling: All
- HIV serology (ideally via rapid test) at presentation and again at 6 wks, 3 mos, and 6 mos. Perform at 12 mos if HCV acquired with injury.
- PEP does not guarantee protection against infection. Success rates are likely ~80%.
- Medication side effects: 74% of HCWs experience side effects, including nausea, fatigue, headache, vomiting. Major reason for discontinuation before 4 wks. AZT may be major contributor; TDF better tolerated.
- Drug-drug interactions must be carefully considered, as many antiretroviral drugs are metabolized by the cytochrome p450 system.
- Clinical assessment and laboratory tests (CBC and metabolic profile, including assessment of glucose and renal and hepatic functions) prior to initiation of PEP and at wks two and four of PEP.
- Clinical assessment 3–5 days after starting PEP. Prescribe supportive-care meds (e.g., anti-emetics) if needed.
- Pregnancy: does not preclude PEP. AZT, 3TC, LPV/r considered safest in pregnancy. Avoid EFV in the first trimester due to teratogenicity. TDF often avoided because of concern about fetal bone density.
- Breastfeeding: consider temporary discontinuation for 6–12 wks after exposure.
- Blood and tissue donation: avoid for 6–12 wks after exposure.
- Prevent sexual transmission: safe sex or abstain until negative serology at 6 mos. Greatest risk in 1st 6–12 wks post injury.
- HIV resistance testing: not recommended as it takes too long to obtain results. Instead, obtain source patient's VL, ART history, and prior genotypes if available. Consult expert.
- Advise HCW to seek medical care for any new symptoms while on PEP and/or for any acute illness that occurs during follow-up period (1st 6 mos post injury). Risk of seroconversion highest within 1st 6–12 wks post injury.
- Do not neglect the possibility that the patient may need mental health care regarding his/her exposure.

Adjunctive Treatment, Monitoring and Counseling: HCW
- Employee/occupational health service should be contacted regarding all exposures to potentially contaminated fluids.
- For cutaneous exposures, the exposed skin should be cleansed with soap and water. Alcohol-based cleansers (virucidal) should also be used for small wounds and punctures.
- Exposed mucous membranes should be flushed with water or saline.
- Initiation of PEP: as quickly as possible, ideally with 1–2 hrs of injury. Benefits likely diminish significantly >24–36 hrs after exposure.

Adjunctive Treatment, Monitoring and Counseling: nPEP Patients
- Risk reduction strategies (e.g., sexual abstinence, consistent condom use, avoidance of sharing injection drug use paraphernalia) should be stressed.

MANAGEMENT

- Consider emergency contraception as appropriate.
- Pregnancy test at baseline and then 6 wks and 3 mos after exposure.
- Screening for HBV at baseline, during PEP, and then 6 wks after exposure.
- Screening for HCV at baseline and then 3 and 6 mos after exposure. Confirm positive serology with PCR.
- Screening for other STIs (syphilis, gonorrhoeae, chlamydia) at baseline, during PEP, and then 6 wks after exposure. Treat/prophylaxis empirically as appropriate.

Hepatitis B Post-Exposure Prophylaxis

- Exposed individual unvaccinated and source HBsAg+: recommend HBIG + vaccine series (3 doses).
- Exposed individual unvaccinated and source unknown: vaccine series (3 doses).
- Exposed individual vaccinated and known to be a responder (antibody to HBsAg >10 mIU/mL): no treatment.
- Exposed individual nonresponder and source HBsAg+ or high risk: HBIG × 1 + vaccine series or HBIG × 2.
- Exposed individual antibody status unknown: test for anti-HBs and no Rx if anti-HBs >10 mIU/mL. If <10, then HBIG × 1 and vaccine booster if source HBsAg+ or HBV vaccine series and titer at 1–2 mos if source unknown.

Hepatitis C Occupational Exposure

- 1.9% transmission rate from sharps injury from HCV infected source (review of 25 studies US Public Health Service).
- Source testing: (if possible): anti-HCV; confirm positives with quantitative HCV PCR.
- HCW: Baseline HCV Ab, HCV RNA, and ALT followed by HCV RNA at 4–6 wks (to detect acute HCV prior to seroconversion; usually have asymptomatic elevation of ALT); followed by HCV Ab, HCV RNA, and ALT at 4–6 mos.
- Currently no prophylaxis with immune globulin or antivirals recommended.
- If HCV transmitted, refer to an expert because early treatment usually curative.

Useful Management Resources

- National Clinician's PEP hotline (HRSA, CDC, AETC): 1-888-448-4911 or at *www.ucsf.edu/ hivcntr/Hotlines/PEPline.html*.
- Hepatitis hotline: 1-888-443-7232 or at *www.cdc.gov/hepatitis*.

SELECTED REFERENCES

Landovitz RJ, Currier JS. Clinical practice. Postexposure prophylaxis for HIV infection. *N Engl J Med*, 2009; 361(18): 1768–75.

Comments: Nice contemporary review of nPEP that highlights TDF/FTC or AZT/3TC PLUS ATV/r, DRV/r, or LPV/r as the medication combinations of choice for post-exposure prophylaxis. The authors favor use of nPEP if there is ≥0.1% risk of HIV transmission from an HIV+ person or a person of unknown HIV-status at high risk for infection.

Young TN, Arens FJ, Kennedy GE, et al. Antiretroviral post-exposure prophylaxis (PEP) for occupational HIV exposure. *Cochrane Database Syst Rev*, 2007; CD002835.

Comments: Cochrane systematic review of occupational PEP through Jan 2005, which found no direct evidence to support the use of multidrug antiretroviral regimens following occupational exposure to HIV. However, due to the success of combination therapies in treating HIV-infected individuals, the authors conclude that a combination of antiretroviral drugs should be used for PEP.

Smith DK, Grohskopf AL, Black RJ, et al. Antiretroviral postexposure prophylaxis after sexual, injection-drug use, or other nonoccupational exposure to HIV in the United States: recommendations from the U.S. Department of Health and Human Services. Atlanta: Centers for Disease Control and Prevention, 2005. *MMWR Recomm Rep*, 2005; 54: 1–20.

Comments: DHHS guidelines on nPEP that provide an excellent, detailed discussion of the risks and benefits of nPEP followed by a recommended approach to persons seeking nPEP. These contain more background information that the 2005 Occupational Exposures guidelines.

Panlilio AL, Cardo DM, Grohskopf AL, Heneine W, Ross CS; US Public Health Service. Updated U.S. Public Health Service Guidelines for the management of occupational exposures to HIV and recommendations for postexposure prophylaxis. *MMWR Recomm Rep*, 2005; 54: 1–17.

Comments: DHHS guidelines on the approach to the use of PEP for HCW. Provides recommendations on when two- or three-drug combinations should be used, as well as other useful tips on management and follow-up.

PREGNANCY AND PERINATAL TRANSMISSION

Christopher J. Hoffmann, MD, MPH

DEFINITION

- Approximate risk of mother-to-child transmission (MTCT) of HIV is 15%–30% for live births (mostly intrapartum) and 15% during breastfeeding. Taken together risk of HIV transmission during pregnancy, delivery, and breastfeeding is approximately 20%–40% without prevention of MTCT (PMTCT). Risks include higher maternal VL, lower CD4 count, severe prematurity (<33 wks), multiple gestation (twin A at higher risk), smoking, active HSV, genital ulcer disease. Risk lower with low VL, effective ART, Cesarean section delivery, intrapartum ART, formula feeding. Antenatal and postnatal PMTCT can decrease transmission to <1%. Uncontrolled HIV decreases fertility (30%) (correlated with VL and disease state), increases still birth, low birth weight, intrauterine growth retardation, chorioamnionitis, and maternal mortality (5 × increase). Control of HIV restores fertility. Pregnancy does not increase HIV progression, risk of OIs, or HIV-related survival. Hemodilution of pregnancy may cause apparent decrease in absolute CD4 (not CD4 %).

CLINICAL RECOMMENDATION

Preconception Counseling

- Discuss patient's reproductive plan.
- Efficacy of combined oral contraceptive pills (OCPs) decreased by some PIs and NNRTIs; minimal information on drug interactions with newer hormonal methods (patch, vaginal ring, estrogen-progestin injection) and with progestin-only methods. Reinforce dual protection with condom use. OCPs and FPV should not be coadministered, as antiretroviral levels decreased.
- Counsel all HIV+ women of reproductive age about HIV and pregnancy early and at intervals throughout care; offer preconception counseling for those who desire pregnancy (including impact of pregnancy on HIV progression, minimizing risk of transmission to uninfected partners, and vertical transmission and prevention).
- Avoid use of known teratogens in ART regimens in women trying to conceive or sexually active with men and not using contraception.
- Discuss risk of breastfeeding and importance of replacement feeding to prevent transmission.
- Assess for HIV resistance if no prior testing.
- Initiate folate supplementation preconception.

General Screening During Pregnancy

- Glucose tolerance testing (50 g glucose load) at 24–48 wks, especially if on PI.
- Check CD4 count initially and every 3 mos.
- Check VL initially, every 2 mos, and at 34–36 wks gestation.
- Liver enzyme elevations and drug hepatotoxicity more common during pregnancy.
- All women should be screened for HIV during pregnancy (regardless of perceived risk).
- At-risk women are at risk for acute HIV during pregnancy and should be retested during 3rd trimester. Consider HIV RNA to identify primary HIV infection in high-risk women, as up to 1/3 of MTCT in US may be from acute infection around or after conception.
- Invasive antenatal diagnostic techniques (amniocentesis and chorionic villus sampling) associated with increased risk of vertical transmission; avoid or perform in setting of maximally suppressed VL on ART. In addition, higher false + rate for serum screen for fetal aneuploidy among pregnant HIV+ women on PIs. HIV cannot be Dx'd antenatally in fetus.
- 2nd trimester fetal ultrasound recommended (especially if mother was on EFV during 1st trimester).
- If an infant is born to a mother of unknown HIV status, the infant can be tested by ELISA at birth to assess maternal HIV status.

General ART Guidelines During Pregnancy

- Use of ART reduces risk of MTCT even among women with low VL (possibly due to discordance between plasma and genital tract VL) and should be a part of antenatal care for ALL HIV+ women.
- No evidence of increased risk of fetal anomalies or intrauterine growth retardation associated with 1st-trimester exposure to AZT, 3TC, NVP, d4T, SQV, RTV, LPV, ddI, FTC, ABC, IDV, ATV (even in 1st trimester).

MANAGEMENT

- Evidence of increased risk of neural tube defects with use of EFV during 1st trimester. FDA pregnancy Category D.
- TDF should only be used in special circumstances, such as intolerance to other agents or chronic hepatitis B because of concerns regarding bone growth (evidence from animal studies). Birth registry data has not indicated increased birth defects. There are limited data on the effect of gestational exposure to TDF on bone growth post-partum.
- Insufficient data: ETR, DRV, FPV, RPV.
- NFV was briefly not recommended because of presence of a process-related impurity, ethyl methane sulfonate (EMS), that is teratogenic in animal studies; however, no human impact has been observed. Manufacturing has been changed and, as of March 2008, levels of EMS have been reduced and NFV is considered safe for use during pregnancy.
- Combination of d4T + ddI contraindicated, especially during pregnancy, due to high risk of pancreatitis and lactic acidosis.
- Recommended agents: AZT, 3TC, NVP, SQV, LPV/r, RTV, NFV, ATV. Try to include AZT in all regimens, unless contraindication or suppressed VL and compelling reason not to add. Benefit believed to exist beyond reducing VL.
- If HBsAg +, optimal regimen includes TDF + either 3TC or FTC.
- Alternative agents: ddI, FTC, d4T, ABC, TDF, IDV, RTV.
- Do not start NVP if CD4 >250 due to increased risk of serious hepatotoxicity/hepatic necrosis.
- Consider redosing PIs during 3rd trimester because of increased volume of distribution (avoid unboosted IDV). However, currently no clear guidelines for dose adjustment of PIs. LPV/r is most commonly used PI: dose often increased to 3 tabs twice daily in 3rd trimester, especially if PI experienced. If using ATV consider ATV/r 400/100 mg once-daily during 3rd trimester.
- Used as a boosting agent, RTV is effective, demonstrates minimal transplacental passage, and has good safety profile.
- Documented good placental passage: AZT, TDF, 3TC, FTC, d4T, EFV, NVP, LPV/r.
- Register all pregnant women receiving ART in Antiretroviral Pregnancy Registry (*www.APRegistry.com*) to track pregnancy outcomes.

Patient on ART at Conception

- Continue current regimen unless it includes EFV, ddI + d4T. Consider switch to either LPV/r or NVP if on EFV. Create new regimen if on ddI + d4T.
- With significant hyperemesis, strongly consider holding all ART until after 1st trimester to decrease risk of development of resistance due to missed doses.
- Continue ART after delivery.

Patient Not on ART at Conception

- Counsel regarding role of ART in reducing vertical transmission and discuss potential for risk to infant with any drug.
- Obtain resistance testing if not previously obtained.
- If patient is willing and appropriate ART candidate, start ART after wk 14 (in 2nd trimester) to decrease risk of intolerance from nausea and emesis and to decrease teratogenesis risk. Association between longer duration of ART prior to delivery and reduced HIV transmission among mothers with VL<400. Ideally start NO LATER than 28 wks gestation.
- In general, use standard combinations recommended for nonpregnant adults with the following considerations:
    1. Tailor to known resistance and prior ART exposure.
    2. Avoid EFV, especially in 1st trimester (see previous General Guidelines) and do not use NVP if pretreatment CD4 >250.
    3. Include AZT when not contraindicated (severe anemia, resistance) or strong reason to use alternative agents (such as TDF/FTC in setting of chronic HBV) because AZT has excellent passage into placenta and there is extensive clinical experience in pregnancy.
    4. LPV/r generally preferred among PIs; consider dose increase in 3rd trimester as noted previously.
- If patient does not meet criteria for ART and does not want to continue, discontinue ART after delivery. Consider substitution of PI for NNRTI for 2–4 wks before stopping to prevent NNRTI resistance.
- If woman refuses ART, can use antenatal AZT and single-dose NVP (sdNVP) antepartum: AZT (300 mg PO twice daily) starting at 28 wks + AZT 600 mg at onset of labor + sdNVP 200 mg at

onset of labor. Postpartum: AZT/3TC 300/150 mg twice daily × 7–14 days (can also use TDF 300 mg + either FTC 300 mg or 3TC 300 mg once daily × 7–14 days).

- If viral load <1000, some experts recommend antenatal AZT as above, but most prefer combination ART.

Patient Presents in Labor Without Antepartum ART

- Efficacy of AZT and of NVP have both been demonstrated; however, no trials of NVP + AZT vs AZT alone. One option is to use AZT alone; however, combining AZT with NVP may be more effective. Drawback is high risk of inducing NVP resistant HIV in the mother. Continuation of AZT/3TC for 1 wk postpartum in the mother has been shown to decrease risk of resistance.
- Intrapartum IV AZT (loading dose 2 mg/kg over 1 hr, then 1 mg/kg) until delivery with 3TC 150 mg PO twice daily and NVP 200 mg PO at onset of labor. If not in labor start AZT/3TC 300/150mg twice daily. If cesarean, start IV AZT 3 hrs pre-op.
- Continue AZT/3TC 300/150 mg PO twice daily for 1 wk postpartum.

Intrapartum Care

- Route of delivery depends on VL prior to delivery (at 36–38 wks gestation) and general obstetrical considerations. If VL >1000, labor has not started and ROM has not occurred, schedule elective cesarean section (no evidence of benefit after onset of labor or ROM). Data support vaginal delivery when VL <1000 and on ART, unless other obstetrical indications. May consider cesarean section with VL 50–1000; although not based on evidence of reduced risk of transmission. No HIV indication for cesarean section if maternal VL<50.
- If cesarean section planned, start AZT infusion 3 hr before procedure (loading 2 mg/kg IV over 1 hr followed by 1 mg/kg/hr until delivery) and use routine ABx prophylaxis.
- If planned vaginal delivery, start AZT at onset of labor (loading 2 mg/kg IV over 1 hr followed by 1 mg/kg/hr until delivery). Use for all patients even if on ART or with history of AZT resistance. (Hold d4T if patient regularly receiving this agent because of antagonism with AZT, but continue other ART agents).
- Avoid fetal scalp electrodes, fetal scalp sampling, and artificial rupture of membranes (increased HIV transmission risk).
- **NOTE:** methergine contraindicated if patient receiving PI or EFV because of decreased methergine metabolism leading to risk of severe ergot toxicity. If treatment needed for uterine atony/hemorrhage, misoprostol, oxytocin, and prostaglandin F2 alpha are all safe. If no alternatives exist, methergine should be used in a low dosage and for as short as possible.

Care of Infant

- The National Perinatal HIV Hotline (1-888-488-8765) provides free clinical consultation on all aspects of perinatal HIV care.
- Start AZT 6–12 hrs postpartum and continue for 6 wks (4 wks may be sufficient).
- Standard AZT dose: 2 mg/kg q6hr or 4 mg/kg q12hr.
- Premature infant AZT dose (hepatic glucuronidation is impaired with <35 wks gestation): 2 mg/kg q12hr × 2 wks then 2 mg/kg q8hr after 2 wks in 30 wks at delivery or after 4 wks if <30 wks gestational age at delivery.
- If HIV status remains unknown at 6 wks, initiate PCP prophylaxis in infant with TMP/SMX (should be able to be determined by 2 wks in most infants).
- Breastfeeding contraindicated where safe alternatives exist (even if mother has HIV RNA <50 and is receiving ART); replacement feeding essential to reduce transmission risk in industrialized countries. However, formula feeding increases mortality in resource-limited settings, thus breastfeeding with infant prophylaxis or maternal ART recommended in those settings.
- Mothers and others with HIV should not pre-masticate food as this has been associated with HIV transmission.
- Infant HIV testing: nucleic acid testing required if age <18 mos because of placental antibody transfer. Age >2–4 wks, HIV DNA testing >90% sensitive (for subtype B, current HIV DNA assays less sensitive for non-B subtypes). Age >2–3 mos, HIV RNA >90% (less subtype impact). Test (1) 14–21 days, (2) 1–2 mos, (3) 4–6 mos. Repeat any positive nucleic acid test on a separate blood sample. Dx with (1) 2 positive nucleic acid tests, (2) HIV Ab reactive with positive confirmatory Western blot or IFA, age >18 mos. HIV can be excluded with (1) 2 negative nucleic acid tests age >14 days, (2) 1 negative nucleic test, age >2 mos, (3) negative HIV Ab test, age >18 mos.

MANAGEMENT

HIV and HBV Coinfection
- Risk of HBV transmission correlated with plasma HBV DNA concentration; HBV DNA significantly higher in HIV coinfection making transmission much more likely.
- HIV-HBV coinfected women should receive regimen active against HBV (ideally TDF/FTC).
- Infants born to women with chronic HBV should receive HBIG and start 3-dose HBV vaccination series within 12 hrs of birth.

SELECTED REFERENCES
Panel on Treatment of HIV-Infected Pregnant Women and Prevention of Perinatal Transmission. Recommendations for the use of antiretroviral drugs in pregnant HIV-1-infected women for maternal health and interventions to reduce perinatal transmission in the United States. September 14, 2011; 1–117. *http://www.aidsinfo.nih.gov/ContentFiles/PerinatalGL.pdf*. Accessed September 14, 2011.
Comments: Excellent resource. Comprehensive and regularly updated with descriptions of all major clinical trials, specific guidelines, and approaches for complex cases.

Gray GE, McIntyre JA. HIV and pregnancy. *BMJ*, 2007; 334: 950–3.
Comments: Good review on impact of HIV on maternal health.

THERAPEUTIC DRUG MONITORING

Paul A. Pham, PharmD

DEFINITION
- Therapeutic drug monitoring (TDM): adjustment of drug doses based on measured plasma concentrations to attain values within a therapeutic range, an established range of concentrations in clinical studies associated with maximal virologic suppression and/or minimal adverse drug reactions.

INDICATIONS
Scenarios in Which TDM May Be Considered (DHHS Guidelines, 01/2011)
- When food-drug and drug-drug interactions could lead to decreased therapeutic efficacy.
- In pathophysiological conditions that may significantly impair GI, hepatic function, and renal function, thereby affecting drug absorption, distribution, metabolism, or elimination (e.g., cirrhosis, bariatric surgery).
- In treatment-experienced patients with virus with reduced susceptibility to ARVs (higher concentrations may be required).
- In treatment-naïve patients with suboptimal virologic response (exclude other causes of treatment failure such as poor adherence, incorrect dosing or dosing frequency, poor adherence to food requirements, drug-drug interactions).
- In pregnant women due to metabolic and physiological changes that can affect PK (including absorption, distribution, metabolism, elimination, blood flow, plasma protein concentrations, intestinal transit, etc).
- For prevention of ARV-induced concentration-dependent toxicity.
- When using unconventional ARV regimens or dosing not studied in clinical trials.
- Consider in pediatric patients when there are limited dosing data.

CLINICAL RECOMMENDATION
Facts About TDM of ARV Drugs
- Rational for TDM: (1) plasma concentration for PIs and NNRTIs associated with treatment response; and (2) high inter-patient variability in plasma concentrations of PIs and NNRTIs.
- Although small pharmacokinetic substudies suggest a relationship between drug exposure and virologic suppression, two prospective studies found no benefit with TDM.
- Methodological limitations of these studies: small sample size, low target concentrations and lag time between "subtherapeutic" concentrations and change of dose.
- Boosted-PI regimen may benefit less from TDM due to higher achievable concentrations.
- Limited data correlating plasma concentrations of NRTIs with their intracellular triphosphate active drug; thus TDM not practical for NRTIs.
- Limited data on utility of TDM for ENF; association between ENF plasma concentration (>2.2 mcg/mL) and VL suppression in treatment-experienced patients.

- Higher RAL trough and C_{all} (geometric mean of all sparse PK samples) associated with a greater probability of a successful treatment outcome.
- NVP TDM did not improve virologic success or adverse drug reaction rate.
- EFV TDM associated with treatment response and CNS side effects.
- PIs, EFV, and MVC target trough concentrations may be associated with improved virologic response (see Table on p. 404).

Limitations to Implementation of TDM in Clinical Practice

- Lack of large randomized prospective studies showing that TDM improves clinical outcome.
- Minimum target plasma concentrations for PIs and NNRTIs based on studies with wild type virus (*AIDS Res Hum Retroviruses*; 2002 Aug 10; 18: 825); limited data for treatment-experienced patients with resistant virus (*Antimicrob Agents Chemother*; 2003; 47: 594). No consensus on how plasma protein binding of drugs should be factored into target concentrations.
- Proposed minimum target concentration range based on monotherapy exposure, even though ART comprises >3 drugs; effect of other ARVs in the regimen on target plasma concentrations remains unknown.
- Lack of established concentration ranges that correlate with therapeutic response.
- Poor quality control for TDM drug assays (concerns with accuracy). Slow turnaround time in many centers resulting in a delay of dose adjustment.
- Numerous confounders affect TDM interpretation (including poor or intermittent adherence, patient not reporting precise time of last dose, incorrect dosing or dosing frequency, lack of adherence to food requirements, sampling/processing errors, unmeasured active metabolites, effects of circadian rhythm, etc).
- Interpretation requires expertise and assays are costly.
- Lack of agreement about best PK parameter to predict therapeutic response (AUC vs Cmin [trough] vs Cmax); trough more commonly used for convenience.
- High intra-patient variability of plasma concentration of ARV agents (a single sample might not be representative; clinical decisions should be made after two or more trough samples collected).

Recommendations

- Outside clinical trials, consider TDM for specific scenarios listed above.
- Trough concentrations for TDM should be measured at 8 hrs for 3 × daily dosing, 12 hrs for twice-daily, and 24 hrs for once-daily.
- Provide: (1) dose and frequency of the ARVs; (2) time sample obtained; (3) time of last dose; (4) indication for TDM; (5) concomitant medications.
- Send specimens to a laboratory that participates in QA/QC programs.
- Consult an expert clinical pharmacologist or clinical pharmacist in interpretation of ARV concentrations and need for dose adjustments.
- TDM should be used as part of an integrated approach and not in isolation.
- Trough concentrations should be within or above the recommended minimum trough concentration ranges generated from *in vivo* and *in vitro* studies (see Table on p. 404).

ESTIMATED MINIMUM TARGET CONCENTRATION RANGES FOR WILD-TYPE VIRUS

Drug	Concentration Range (ng/mL)
ATV	150
EFV	1000 (CNS toxicity associated with Cmin >4000 ng/mL)
FPV	400 (measured as APV concentration)
IDV	100
LPV/r	1000
MVC	>50
NFV[a]	800

(Continued)

ESTIMATED MINIMUM TARGET CONCENTRATION RANGES
FOR WILD-TYPE VIRUS (cont'd.)

Drug	Concentration Range (ng/mL)
NVP	3000
RTV	2100 (RTV given as a single PI)
SQV	100–250
TPV	20,5000 (for treatment experienced patients with resistant virus)

aMeasurable active (M8) metabolite.
NOTE: higher concentrations may be required in treatment-experienced patients with resistant virus.
Source: 2011 DHHS Guidelines for the Use of Antiretroviral Agents in HIV-Infected Adults and Adolescents. Available at http://aidsinfo.nih.gov/ContentFiles/AdultandAdolescentGL.pdf.

Median (range) trough concentrations from clinical trials	
Pharmacokinetic exposure-response relationship data for DRV, ETR, and RAL are accumulating but are not sufficient to recommend minimum trough concentrations. The following are median trough concentrations observed in clinical trials.	
DRV/r (600/100 mg twice daily)	3300 (1255–7368)
ETR	275 (81–2980)
RAL	72 (29–118)

SELECTED REFERENCES

Panel on Antiretroviral Guidelines for Adults and Adolescents. Guidelines for the use of antiretroviral agents in HIV-1-infected adults and adolescents. Department of Health and Human Services; January 1, 2011; 1–181. http://aidsinfo.nih.gov/contentfiles/AdultandAdolescentGL.pdf. Accessed July 17, 2011.
Comments: DHHS guidelines on TDM for ARV drugs.

Best B, Goicoechea M, Witt M, et al. A randomized controlled trial of therapeutic drug monitoring in treatment-naive and experienced HIV-1-infected patients. JAIDS, 2007; 46: 433.
Comments: Prospective open-label 48-wk study randomized patients to TDM vs standard of care. TDM group received sparse pharmacokinetic sampling at wk 2. 64% of patients had nontarget exposure at least once during the 48-wk study period. Among patients with below-target concentrations, there was a trend favoring TDM-arm (viral load reduction 2.4 vs 1.9 log P = 0.09).

Thompson MA, Aberg JA, Cahn Pm, et al. Antiretroviral treatment of adult HIV infection: 2010 recommendations of the International AIDS Society-USA panel. JAMA, 2010; 304: 321–33.
Comments: IAS-USA guidelines do not recommend TDF for routine care but use of TDM of PIs and NNRTI s maybe useful in selected cases (e.g., pregnant women, children, and patients with renal or liver failure), When managing potential drug-drug interactions, or in virologic failure in the absence of resistance when adherence excellent.

LaPorte CJL, Black D, Blaschke T, et al. Updated guidelines to perform therapeutic drug monitoring for antiretroviral agents Rev Antivir Ther, 2006; 3: 4–14.
Comments: Guidelines for TDM.

Slish JC, Catanzaro LM, Ma Q, et al. Update on the pharmacokinetic aspects of antiretroviral agents: implications in therapeutic drug monitoring. Curr Pharm Des, 2006; 12: 1129–45.
Comments: Review article about TDM for ARV drugs.

Nettles RE, Kieffer TL, Kwon P, et al. Intermittent HIV-1 viremia (blips) and drug resistance in patients receiving HAART. JAMA, 2005; 293: 817–29.
Comments: Frequent PK sampling revealed significant variability in plasma concentrations of PIs and NNRTIs. Results challenge utility of TDM and suggest that single samples to access ARV plasma concentrations may have limited value.

Burger D et al. Therapeutic drug monitoring of nelfinavir and indinavir in treatment-naive HIV-1-infected individuals. AIDS; 2003 May 23; 17: 1157.
Comments: In a pharmacokinetic sub-study of ATHENA cohort, ARV-naive pts prescribed IDV- (N=55) or NFV(N=92)-containing regimens were randomized to TDM (plasma concentrations reported to clinicians in addition to expert advice)

or no TDM (clinicians given only expert advice). Expert advice included increase or reduction of PI dose, addition of low dose RTV, discussion of food requirements. Results: 81% and 59% of NFV treated pts and 75% and 48% of IDV treated pts in the TDM and no TDM groups, respectively, achieved VL < 500. After one year of follow-up, 17.4% and 39.7% of pts discontinued therapy in the TDM group and control group, respectively. The significant differences in discontinuation rate were due to virologic failure in the NFV- treated pts and toxicity in the IDV-treated pts. However, in a sub-analysis of the study, pts who received RTV-boosted IDV did not benefit from TDM. Limitations: small sample size, use of PIs no longer widely used, and uncertainty about number of clinicians who followed expert advice.

Durant J et al. Importance of protease inhibitor plasma levels in HIV-infected patients treated with genotypic-guided therapy: pharmacological data from the Viradapt Study. *AIDS*; 2000 July 7; 14: 1333.
Comments: In a pharmacologic substudy of Viradapt (a prospective, randomized study of ARV-experienced pts evaluating impact genotype on virologic response). PI (NFV , SQV , IDV , and RTV) trough concentrations were independent predictors of change in VL. Limitation is that adherence not measured.

Rating: Important

Clevenbergh P et al. PharmAdapt: a randomized prospective study to evaluate the benefit of therapeutic monitoring of protease inhibitors: 12 week results. *AIDS*; 2002 Nov 22; 16: 2311.
Comments: PHARMADAPT: Prospective, randomized study comparing TDM vs. no TDM in experienced pts failing current regimen. Pts randomized to TDM (84 pts) vs. no TDM (96 pts). Target trough PI concentration was protein binding-corrected IC50 of wild type virus. Pts in TDM group had PI dose modification at wk 8 based on wk 4 trough concentrations. Results: VL change equivalent in control and intervention groups. Limitations: small sample size, low target concentrations, 4-wk lag time between sampling and reporting of PI concentrations (time between sampling and reporting of PI concentrations might had been too long, leading to development of resistance that could have affected study findings). In addition, modification of PI therapy due to "subtherapeutic" troughs occurred for only 23.5% of pts receiving PI TDM. It was interesting to note that due to the wide inter- and intra-pt variability in concentrations, 14% of pts spontaneously changed from 1 "category" to the other between wk 4 and 8 without any intervention.

Rating: Important

Bossi P et al: GENOPHAR: a randomized study of plasma drug measurements in association with genotypic resistance testing and expert advice to optimize therapy in patients failing antiretroviral therapy. *HIV Med*; 2004; 5: 352.
Comments: GENOPHAR: Randomized 134 ART experienced-pts to expert recommended therapy based on genotypic resistance only vs. genotypic resistance plus TDM. No difference in virologic response rate observed between the 2 groups at 12 wks; in the multivariate analysis, only prior exposure to ≥2PIs predicted response. Limitations: similar trial design limitations as PHARMADAPT. In addition, both trials had large proportion of patients on RTV-boosted PI regimens that may have made TDM intervention less critical.

Rating: Important

Acosta EP, Gerber JG, Adult Pharmacology Committee of the AIDS Clinical Trials Group: Position paper on therapeutic drug monitoring of antiretroviral agents. *AIDS Res Hum Retroviruses*; 2002 Aug 10; 18: 825.
Comments: ACTG position paper provides guidelines for use of TDM for ARV drugs in clinical setting.

Marcelin AG et al: Genotypic inhibitory quotient as predictor of virological response to ritonavir-amprenavir in human immunodeficiency virus type 1 protease inhibitor-experienced patients. *Antimicrob Agents Chemother*; 2003; 47: 594.
Comments: Discusses clinical utility of the genotypic inhibitory quotient (ratio of Cmin to the number of PI mutations) in TDM, to define plasma concentrations needed to control PI resistant viruses.

MANAGEMENT

TOXICITY AND SIDE EFFECTS: SWITCHING THERAPY

Lisa A. Spacek, MD, PhD and Joseph Cofrancesco, Jr., MD, MPH

DEFINITION
- Modification of ART regimen due to, or to prevent, adverse events (AEs), including short-term side effects and long-term clinical or lab toxicities.

INDICATIONS
DHHS Guidelines (10/14/2011)
- Rates of treatment-limiting AEs are declining in ART-naïve patients enrolled in trials (<10%); however, this may underestimate long-term toxicity.
- Risk factors for AEs: women have higher risk of Stevens-Johnson syndrome, rashes, hepatotoxicity from NVP, and lactic acidosis from NRTIs; comorbid conditions: alcohol or drug use, viral hepatitis; drug-interactions; and genetic factors.

IAS-USA Guidelines (7/10)
- Single-agent switches to reduce toxicity, avoid drug interaction, or improve convenience are endorsed. Goal to maintain virologic suppression.
- Avoid treatment interruptions. If planned surgery or severe toxicity, prior to interruption, consider drug half-lives (NNRTIs) and D/C drugs in staggered manner.

CLINICAL RECOMMENDATION

General
- Evaluate clinical and lab data to identify drug, rule out other causes, consider single drug switch or treat the adverse effect. If severe toxicity, may need to D/C all drugs.

Cardiovascular Disease (CVD)
- HIV infection itself increases risk of CVD, interruption of ART not recommended to improve lipid profile.
- SQV/r can prolong PR and QT intervals on EKG. ATV/r and LPV/r associated with increased PR interval.
- ABC and ddI associated with increased risk of MI, especially in patients with multiple traditional cardiac risk factors. Causal association not established.
- RTV-boosted PIs increase risk of hyperlipidemia, DRV/r and ATV/r better lipid profile than LPV/r.
- NNRTIs increase TG, HDL, LDL (EFV > NVP).

Gastrointestinal Effects
- Diarrhea: associated with PIs: NFV, LPV/r > DRV/v and ATV/r. Control with fiber supplementation or anti-motility agents, consider change to different PI or switch drug class.
- Hepatotoxicity: severe hepatic toxicity seen with NVP, contraindicated in women with CD4 >250, men with CD4 >400, and Child-Pugh Class B and C, never use for post-exposure prophylaxis; steatosis seen with NRTIs; non-cirrhotic portal hypertension, ddI; drug-induced hepatitis seen with all PIs, TPV/r has more hepatic events than other PIs.
- Nausea/vomiting: ddI and ZDV > other NRTIs.
- Pancreatitis: ddI and associated with PI-induced hypertriglyceridemia.
- Hyperbilirubinemia: ATV and IDV cause indirect hyperbilirubinemia.
- HBV coinfected patients may experience flare if TDF, FTC, or 3TC are withdrawn or HBV resistance develops.
- IRIS-associated hepatitis: TB, MAC, HBV, HCV coinfection.

Hypersensitivity Reaction (HSR)
- ABC: systemic HSR in 5%–8%, progressive with each dose: fever, rash, malaise, dyspnea, N/V, HA; median onset, 9 days; 90% in 1st 6 wks of exposure to ABC. Substitute other NRTI (usually TDF or AZT) once Dx established. DO NOT rechallenge with ABC.
- HLA-B*5701 testing should be performed prior to initiating ABC; those + for haplotype should not receive ABC.
- NVP: hepatotoxicity and rash with fever, malaise, fatigue, oral lesions, conjunctivitis, facial edema and granulocytopenia. Two-wk dose escalation reduces risk.
- Stop or switch for severe rash, systemic Sx, or rash with hepatotoxicity.

Metabolic Abnormalities
- DM/insulin resistance: DM reported in up to 6% of HIV+; impaired glucose tolerance, 15%–20%. 4-fold increased risk of DM in men on ART (MACS). IDV greatest risk of impaired insulin sensitivity. ATV and ATV/r not found to alter insulin sensitivity. Insulin-sensitizing agents preferred Rx.
- Lactic acidosis: NRTIs (ddI, d4T, ZDV). Less often seen as use of TDF and ABC has increased. Fatigue, N/V, diarrhea, abdominal pain. Elevated liver enzymes in hepatic steatosis. Check serum lactate, bicarbonate, arterial pH. Severe lactic acidosis, stop NRTIs. If mild-moderate, consider non-thymidine analog NRTIs.
- Lipoatrophy: NRTIs = d4T > ZDV. May be slowly and partially reversible. Switch to TDF or ABC. Polylactic acid (e.g., *Sculptra*) and calcium hydroxylapatite (e.g., *Radiesse*) approved for facial lipoatrophy. Lipohypertrophy seen in EFV, PI and RAL-containing regimens. Liposuction may be useful in disfiguring cases.

Rash
- NNRTIs, ATV, DRV, FPV, and MVC. Mild-moderate rash common and does not require discontinuation.
- Stop or switch for severe rash (mucosal involvement or desquamation), systemic symptoms (ABC), or rash with hepatotoxicity (NVP).

- DRV and FPV: sulfa-allergic patients may be at increased risk (but not contraindicated for mild-moderate sulfa allergy).
- Use caution when starting NNRTIs, ABC, and/or TMP/SMX simultaneously.

Nervous System Effects

- CNS: common with EFV therapy during 1st days-weeks; usually improves with time. If no improvement after 3–4 wks, may not resolve. Take EFV in evening on empty stomach during early therapy. Consider switch to NVP or PI or another class for depression, psychosis, hallucinations, or prolonged or intolerable side effects (>3–4 wks).

Peripheral Neuropathy

- Most often associated with d4T or ddI, but can also occur with HIV itself. Switch to TDF, ABC, or ZDV or another class. Renal effects.
- Renal insufficiency: switch from IDV to other PI or NNRTI. Adjust TDF dose based on calculated creatinine clearance, or switch from TDF to ABC or ZDV or to NRTI-sparing regimen. Investigate underlying cause.
- Nephrolithiasis: switch from IDV or ATV to other PI or NNRTI.
- TDF: rare reports of Fanconi syndrome and acute renal insufficiency.

Bone Marrow Effects

- Anemia: rule out other causes. If ZDV-related, switch to another agent.
- Leukopenia: rule out other causes. If ZDV-related, switch to another agent.

Bone

- Osteonecrosis/avascular necrosis: rule out other causes (e.g., steroid use, diabetes mellitus, hyperlipidemia). Role of ART unclear. Hip replacement often required.
- Osteopenia/osteoporosis: TDF associated with loss of bone mineral density. Baseline bone densitometry >50 yo. Rule out hypogonadism and vitamin D deficiency. Rx includes bisphosphonates, adequate calcium, and vitamin D.

SELECTED REFERENCES

Panel on Antiretroviral Guidelines for Adults and Adolescents. Guidelines for the use of antiretroviral agents in HIV-1-infected adults and adolescents. Department of Health and Human Services; January 1, 2011; 126–9. *http://aidsinfo.nih.gov/contentfiles/AdultandAdolescentGL.pdf*. Accessed March 31, 2011.
Comments: Table 13 (in Guidelines) lists side effect profiles and comments on each drug class.

European AIDS Clinical Society. Guidelines: prevention and management of non-infectious co-morbidities in HIV. Version 5-4. November 1, 2009. *www.europeanaidsclinicalsociety.org/images/stories/EACS-Pdf/2_non_infectious_co_morbidities_in_hiv.pdf*. Accessed April 13, 2011.
Comments: Clinically-oriented document includes table of frequent and severe side effects.

Molina JM, Andrade-Villanueva J, Echevarria J, et al. Once-daily atazanavir/ritonavir compared with twice-daily lopinavir/ritonavir, each in combination with tenofovir and emtricitabine, for management of antiretroviral-naive HIV-1-infected patients: 96-week efficacy and safety results of the CASTLE study. *J Acquir Immune Defic Syndr*, 2010; 53: 323–32.
Comments: Randomized trial, 96-wk data on 883 ART-naïve patients found ATV/r 300/100 q day associated with less GI disturbance and a better lipid profile compared to LPV/r 400/100 twice daily.

Post FA, Moyle GJ, Stellbrink HJ, et al. Randomized comparison of renal effects, efficacy, and safety with once-daily abacavir/lamivudine versus tenofovir/emtricitabine, administered with efavirenz, in antiretroviral-naive, HIV-1-infected adults: 48-week results from the ASSERT study. *J Acquir Immune Defic Syndr*, 2010; 55: 49–57.
Comments: Randomized, prospective study of 385 ART-naïve patients evaluated adverse events in ABC/3TC/EFV versus TDF/FTC/EFV followed 48 wks. Increase in markers of tubular dysfunction seen in TDF/FTC/EFV arm, unclear significance. Better efficacy in TDF/FTC/EFV arm.

Aberg JA, Kaplan JE, Libman H, et al. Primary care guidelines for the management of persons infected with human immunodeficiency virus: 2009 update by the HIV Medicine Association of the Infectious Diseases Society of America. *Clin Infect Dis*, 2009; 49: 651–81.
Comments: Evidence-based guidelines for the management of HIV+ patients includes discussion of ART adverse effects.

Worm SW, Sabin C, Weber R, et al. Risk of myocardial infarction in patients with HIV infection exposed to specific individual antiretroviral drugs from the 3 major drug classes: the data collection on adverse events of anti-HIV drugs (D:A:D) study. *J Infect Dis*, 2010; 201: 318–30.
Comments: D:A:D study examined 178,835 PY of follow-up. Increased risk of MI was associated with ABC, ddI, IDV, and LPV/r.

MANAGEMENT

TREATMENT INTERRUPTION

Joel E. Gallant, MD, MPH

DEFINITION
- Planned interruption of therapy, with resumption based on clinical rationale or pre-determined time schedule.

INDICATIONS

CD4-Guided Treatment Interruption
- Goal: to decrease total time on therapy with prolonged interruptions while maintaining CD4 in safe range.
- Early studies demonstrated that CD4 nadir was strongest predictor of time off therapy. Best candidates for treatment interruption (TI) were those with high CD4 nadir and good response to ART, especially those who did not meet current guidelines for ART at initiation.
- SMART and Trivacan studies found greater morbidity and mortality in patients who stopped with CD4 >350 and resumed with CD4 <250.
- Differences between TI and continuous therapy in SMART partially but not entirely explained by CD4 count, leaving possible role for inflammation and/or immune activation due to viral rebound or untreated viremia.
- Not recommended in guidelines outside of clinical trial.

INTERVAL-GUIDED TREATMENT INTERRUPTION
- Goal: to decrease total time on therapy with scheduled interruptions.
- Candidates: patients with good CD4 and VL response to therapy.
- Risk of drug resistance with repeated interruptions, especially with NNRTI-based regimens.
- Increased morbidity with TI strategy in DART trial (Africa).
- "Short-cycle" therapy (e.g., 1 wk on/1 wk off or 5 days on/2 days off) safe in some small studies, but associated with increased failure and resistance in others.
- Not recommended in guidelines outside of clinical trial.

Structured Treatment Interruption (STI) to Improve Immune Response ("Autoimmunization")
- Goal: to improve HIV-specific immunity through periodic reexposure of immune system to HIV viremia.
- Candidates: patients with good CD4 and VL response to therapy treated during chronic or primary infection.
- No evidence of improved long-term virologic control in patients treated during primary or chronic infection.
- Minimal data supporting this approach.
- Possible rationale with primary but not chronic infection.
- Not recommended outside of clinical trials.

Salvage STI
- Goal: to allow reemergence of wild-type virus to improve response to salvage therapy.
- Candidates: patients failing ART with no suppressive options.
- Conflicting results in clinical trials, but several studies show rapid CD4 decline, increased OIs and other complications, and no virologic benefit after resumption of ART.
- Potential risk of marked CD4 decline, adverse clinical outcomes.
- Resistance permanent; resistant virus expected to reemerge with reintroduction of ART.
- Conflicting data: best results have been with STI followed by aggressive salvage therapy ("mega-HAART"), but several studies suggest that interruption in patients with advanced disease can be dangerous.
- Not recommended.

Partial Treatment Interruption (PTI)
- Goal: to maintain clinical and immunologic stability and decrease toxicity or risk of resistance by stopping some but not all drugs.
- Candidates: patients failing ART with no suppressive options.
- Supportive data from small observational studies only.
- Response to continued NRTI therapy better than continued PI therapy, but no comparison with standard therapy.
- Observational study: better results with stopping PIs than NRTIs.

- Safety in patients with advanced disease unclear; may be associated with more rapid progression than continued therapy with >1 drug class.
- Monitor CD4, VL.
- Role of replication capacity (RC) assay uncertain.
- PTI was sometimes used to continue ART while preserving drug classes for later use, but rarely necessary now because of availability of suppressive options for most patients.

CLINICAL RECOMMENDATION

CD4-Guided Treatment Interruption

- Data from early studies supported interruption of therapy in selected patients, but larger SMART trial found increase in morbidity and mortality. Unclear whether this was due to interruption itself or to specific CD4 thresholds used (resumption with CD4 <250), though differences not entirely explained by CD4.
- Not recommended. Probably safest in those who did not meet current guidelines for therapy when they started, but current guidelines now recommending earlier initiation.
- VL after interruption correlates with pretreatment VL, though initial rebound may be higher.
- Use caution with NNRTI-containing regimens. Consider substitution of PI for 1–4 wks before stopping.
- Counsel patients about (1) increased risk of HIV transmission, and (2) potential for symptomatic viremia with rebound.
- Consider resistance testing when VL >1000 (2–3 wks).

Structured Treatment Interruption (STI) to Improve Immune Response ("Autoimmunization")

- Minimal data supporting this approach.
- Possible rationale with primary but not chronic infection.
- Not recommended outside of clinical trials.

Interval-Guided Treatment Interruption

- Minimal data supporting this approach, and potential risk for resistance.
- Risk of resistance increases with repeated interruptions, especially with NNRTI-based regimens and with "off intervals" long enough to allow viral rebound (e.g., >2–7 days).
- Not recommended outside of clinical trials.

Salvage STI

- Potential risk of marked CD4 decline, adverse clinical outcomes.
- Resistance permanent; resistant virus expected to re-emerge with reintroduction of ART.
- Conflicting data: best results have been with STI followed by aggressive salvage therapy ("mega-ART"), but several studies suggest that interruption in patients with advanced disease can be dangerous.
- Not recommended.

PARTIAL TREATMENT INTERRUPTION (PTI)

- Observational study: better results with stopping PIs than NRTIs.
- Safety in patients with advanced disease unclear; may be associated with more rapid progression than continued therapy with >1 drug class.
- Monitor CD4, VL.
- Role of replication capacity (RC) assay uncertain.
- PTI was sometimes used to continue ART while preserving drug classes for later use, but rarely necessary now because of availability of suppressive options for most patients.

SELECTED REFERENCES

Danel C, Moh R, Chaix ML, et al. Two-months-off, four-months-on antiretroviral regimen increases the risk of resistance, compared with continuous therapy: a randomized trial involving West African adults. *J Infect Dis*, 2009; 199: 66–76.
Comments: Resistance analysis from Trivacan study (Danel, 2006 below) demonstrating unacceptable risk for resistance with intermittent treatment strategy.

Strategies for Management of Antiretroviral Therapy (SMART) Study Group, El-Sadr WM, Lundgren JD, et al. CD4+ count-guided interruption of antiretroviral treatment. *N Engl J Med*, 2006; 355: 2283–96.
Comments: Large randomized, multicenter trial (N >5000) comparing continuous ART with CD4-guided treatment interruption (stop with CD4 >350, resume with CD4 <250). Study stopped early because of greater morbidity and mortality in TI arm, including greater incidence of treatment complications at all CD4 strata.

Ananworanich J, Gayet-Ageron A, Le Braz M, et al. CD4-guided scheduled treatment interruptions compared with continuous therapy for patients infected with HIV-1: results of the Staccato randomised trial. *Lancet*, 2006; 368: 459–65.

Comments: 430 patients (mostly Thais on SQV/r) with CD4 >350 and VL <50 randomised to continue therapy (N = 146) or scheduled TIs (N = 284). ART resumed if CD4 <350. Patients in TI group spent 61.5% of time on therapy. VL <50 in 90% of TI group vs 92% of continued treatment group (P = NS). Diarrhea and neuropathy more common with continuous treatment; candidiasis more common with TI. No significant differences in resistance between groups. Supported CD4-guided TI strategy, though SMART studies larger and more powerful.

Danel C, Moh R, Minga A, et al. CD4-guided structured antiretroviral treatment interruption strategy in HIV-infected adults in west Africa (Trivacan ANRS 1269 trial): a randomised trial. *Lancet*, 2006; 367: 1981–9.

Comments: Trial comparing continuous ART, intermittent ART (2 mos off/4 mos on), and CD4-guided treatment interruption (criteria as with SMART trial). Latter arm stopped early because of greater morbidity and mortality, including higher incidence of TB and invasive bacterial infections.

VIROLOGIC FAILURE: WHEN TO MODIFY THERAPY

Richard D. Moore, MD, MHS

DEFINITION
• Incomplete VL suppression or virologic rebound after complete suppression.

INDICATIONS
• Virologic failure is defined as the inability to achieve or maintain VL <200 (confirmed), which eliminates most cases of apparent viremia caused by blips or assay variability. For adherent patients who do not have resistance to prescribed drugs, VL suppression generally achieved in patients 24 wks, but may take longer.
• No consensus on optimal time to change therapy. By current guidelines, aggressive would be for 2 consecutive VL >200 after 24 wks on ARV regimen.
• For extensively treated patients without suppressive options: partial suppression (e.g., decline in VL of >0.5 log). Goal: to preserve immunologic function as long as possible. Current guidelines (DHHS, IAS-USA) state that goal of therapy for all patients is VL <50 due to availability of multiple new agents.

CLINICAL RECOMMENDATION
• Before change, assess reason for failure: adherence, tolerability (e.g., side effects), pharmacokinetic issues (food/fasting requirements, drug-drug interactions, potency of current ARTs), prior ART experience, and potential for or known resistance.
• Get genotype before change if VL high enough (VL >500–1000).
• Limited prior exposure with no resistance: consider adherence, pharmacokinetic issues.
• TDM for PIs or NNRTIs (not NRTIs). No clear guidelines, but consider if suspected absorption issues (e.g., GI disease, pregnancy) or unpredictable drug interactions.
• Consider regimen change with repeated VL 200–1000 to minimize development of resistance, especially if on ART with low genetic barrier (e.g., NNRTI). If continuing same regimen, follow VL closely; ongoing viremia can lead to accumulation of mutations.
• Change regimen ASAP with repeated VL >1000.
• New regimen should contain at least 2, and preferably 3, fully active drugs based on treatment history, resistance testing, or new class. Change ART guided by current and previous therapy and resistance testing. Consider class change (e.g., PI to NNRTI, NNRTI to PI, PI or NNRTI to CCR5, INSTI, 2nd generation NNRTI or PI - if not resistant), NRTI with different resistance pattern. Goal is VL suppression to <50.
• If VL > 1000 and no drug resistance found, resume regimen (if patient off > 4 wks and/or nonadherent) or start new regimen based on treatment history and repeat genotype in 2–4 wks.
• Treatment interruption never indicated.
• Extensive treatment experience: if no suppressive options (uncommon scenario now), continuing therapy reduces risk of progression. Continuing therapy NRTI provides better control than continuing PI, though new mutations develop with both classes over time.
• New agents: ETR active against most NNRTI-resistant virus, but cross-resistance can occur; MVC (only if R5-tropic by tropism assay) and RAL (active in most integrase inhibitor-naive patients). DRV/r and/or TPV/r may be active if PIs used previously, but cross-resistance can occur.

- 3TC alone superior to treatment discontinuation if M184V present (in patients with high CD4 nadirs).
- Immunologic failure only (CD4 < 200 with VL <200). Associated factors: low CD4 at ART start, older age, coinfection, other meds (e.g., AZT and bone marrow suppression), immune activation and loss of regenerative potential, other comorbidity). No consensus on need for ART change. Immune-based therapies not recommended currently.

Selected References

Hirsch MS, Gunthard HF, Schapiro JM, et al. Antiretroviral drug resistance testing in adult HIV-1 infection: 2008 recommendations of an international AIDS Society-USA panel. *Clin Infect Dis*, 2008; 47: 266–85.
Comments: Up-to-date IAS-USA resistance testing recommendations.

Panel on Antiretroviral Guidelines for Adults and Adolescents. Guidelines for the use of antiretroviral agents in HIV-1-infected adults and adolescents. Department of Health and Human Services; January 1, 2011; 68–76. *http://aidsinfo.nih.gov/contentfiles/AdultandAdolescentGL.pdf*. Accessed March 31, 2011.
Comments: Summary of current guidelines for treatment regimen failure, clinical criteria, and options for subsequent regimens.

Ribaudo H, Lennox J, Currier J, et al. Virologic failure endpoint definition in clinical trials: is using HIV-1 RNA threshold <200 copies/mL better than <50 copies/mL? An analysis of ACTG studies. Paper presented at: 16th Conference on Retroviruses and Opportunistic Infections; February 8–11, 2009; Montreal, Canada. Abstract 580.
Comments: Study showing that VL <200 clinically relevant for monitoring ART.

Moore RD, Keruly JC. CD4+ cell count 6 years after commencement of highly active antiretroviral therapy in persons with sustained virologic suppression. *Clin Infect Dis*, 2007; 44: 441–6.
Comments: Observational study showing that CD4 counts do not increase as much and morbidity is higher if the CD4 at ART start is low.

Siliciano JD, Kajdas J, Finzi D, et al. Long-term follow-up studies confirm the stability of the latent reservoir for HIV-1 in resting CD4+ T cells. *Nat Med*, 2003; 9: 727–8.
Comments: Demonstrates that viral resistance does not occur from archived HIV.

WHEN TO START THERAPY: CHRONIC HIV INFECTION

Joel E. Gallant, MD, MPH

Definition
- Initiation of ART in a previously naïve-patient.

Indications

DHHS Guidelines (10/14/11)
- ART should be initiated in patients with history of AIDS-defining illness or with CD4 <350 (AI).
- ART should be initiated, regardless of CD4 count, in patients with following conditions: pregnancy (AI), HIVAN (AII), and HBV coinfection when treatment of HBV is indicated (AIII).
- ART recommended for patients with CD4 350–500. Panel was divided on the strength of recommendation: 55% voted for strong recommendation (A), and 45% voted for moderate recommendation (B) (A/B-II).
- For patients with CD4 >500, panel was evenly divided: 50% favored starting ART (B), 50% viewed therapy as optional (C) (B/C-III).

DHHS Guidelines Rating Criteria
- Strength Recommendation:
- A: Strong recommendation for treatment.
- B: Moderate recommendation for treatment.
- C: Optional recommendation for treatment.
- Quality of Evidence for Recommendation.
- I: One or more randomized trials with clinical outcomes and/or validated laboratory endpoints.
- II: One or more well-designed, nonrandomized trials or observational cohort studies with long-term clinical outcomes.
- III: Expert opinion.

MANAGEMENT

IAS-USA Guidelines (7/21/10)

- Asymptomatic: CD4 ≤500: ART recommended (<350 AI, 350–500 AII).
- Asymptomatic: CD4 >500: consider ART unless elite controller (VL <50) or stable CD4 and low VL without ART (CIII).
- ART recommended regardless of CD4: symptomatic HIV disease (AI), pregnancy (AI), VL >100,000 (AII), yearly CD4 decline >100 (AII), active HBV (BII) or HCV (AII) infection, active or high risk for cardiovascular disease (BII), HIVAN (BII), symptomatic primary HIV infection (BII), high transmission risk (e.g., seronegative partner) (BII), age >60 (BII, mentioned in text but not table).

WHO Guidelines (11/09)

- Start ART in all patients with CD4 <350 irrespective of clinical symptoms (AII).
- CD4 testing required to determine if patients with HIV and WHO clinical stage 1 or 2 disease need to start ART (AIII).
- Start ART in all patients with HIV and WHO clinical stage 3 or 4 irrespective of CD4 count (AIII).

Ratings for strength of recommendation: A: strong recommendation; B: moderate recommendation; C: optional recommendation.

Ratings for quality of evidence for a recommendation: I: one or more randomized trials with clinical outcomes and/or validated laboratory endpoints; II: one or more well-designed, nonrandomized trials or observational cohort studies with long-term clinical outcomes; III: expert opinion.

CLINICAL RECOMMENDATION

Data Summary

- Symptomatic infection: strong data supporting treatment.
- CD4 <350: strong data supporting treatment.
- CD4 350–500: growing body of data from large clinical cohorts supporting treatment. DHHS and IAS-USA guidelines now recommend ART at this level.
- CD4 >500: data equivocal, with 1 large observational cohort showing survival advantage.
- VL criteria: some cohorts show VL >100,000 as independent indicator of need for therapy, though CD4 remains stronger indicator. VL no longer a criterion in DHHS guidelines, but is consideration in IAS-USA guidelines.

Other Considerations

- Patient readiness critical. Patients should understand rationale for therapy and need for adherence before starting. Urgency of therapy lower at higher CD4 counts.
- Risk factors for nonadherence include active substance abuse, mental illness, inadequate housing, though these are not contraindications to ART. Address these issues before starting if therapy not urgent.
- Immediate ART beneficial during some acute OIs. Greatest urgency with conditions for which ART is primary therapy (e.g., PML, cryptosporidiosis, dementia, HIVAN) or for which CD4 count strongly affects prognosis (e.g., lymphoma, KS). Evidence of benefit for early ART with PCP (ACTG 5164) and TB.
- Despite risk of IRIS, ART should not be delayed more than 2–3 wks after initiation of Rx for TB or MAC.
- IRIS with cryptococcal or TB meningitis may be severe or life threatening. Delay of ART may be warranted, at least until intracranial pressure controlled.
- ART decreases transmission (HPTN 052). Consider ART in patients with HIV-negative partners or engaging in high-risk behavior.

Rationale for Early Initiation of Therapy

- Availability of simpler, more effective, less toxic, and better-tolerated regimens.
- Data from cohort studies demonstrating benefit to earlier therapy with longer follow-up.
- Theoretical risk of prolonged exposure to high VL, regardless of CD4 count (e.g., lymphoma, KS, neuro complications).
- SMART study: increased morbidity and mortality (including from nonopportunistic complications) in patients who interrupted therapy compared to continuous therapy, regardless of CD4 count. Substudy of SMART found 5-fold greater risk in patients not on ART at enrollment who delayed ART rather than starting immediately (Emery).
- Decreased risk of HIV transmission.
- Greater likelihood of CD4 normalization, with clinical benefits.

- Reduction in HIV-associated inflammation and immune activation may have long-term benefits (e.g., decreased risk of cardiovascular disease, malignancy, neurocognitive decline, bone loss).
- Unclear to what degree early ART will prevent "early aging" associated with HIV infection, and which components of aging it will affect.

Special Populations

- HIV/HBV coinfection: if HBV therapy indicated, initiate ART regardless of CD4 as it allows easy treatment of both HIV and HBV (with regimen containing TDF + either FTC or 3TC). Treating HBV alone more complicated and not as well tolerated.
- HIV/HCV coinfection: ART may decrease progression of HCV-related liver disease (data equivocal).
- Discordant couples: treatment of HIV+ partner may decrease risk of transmission to negative partner.
- Pregnant women: treat with ART beginning in 2nd trimester (or continue ongoing ART). Can consider d/c of ART after delivery if no indications for therapy, though rationale waning for interrupting therapy in adherent patient with VL <50 and no side effects. If indicated for health of the mother, ART should be initiated in 1st trimester.
- Patients at risk for cardiovascular disease: growing evidence that ART decreases risk.
- Older patients: generally have poorer CD4 responses, so starting earlier ensures higher CD4 count.

SELECTED REFERENCES

Thompson MA, Aberg JA, Cahn P, et al. Antiretroviral treatment of adult HIV infection: 2010 recommendations of the International AIDS Society-USA panel. *JAMA*, 2010; 304: 321–33.
Comments: IAS-USA guidelines on antiretroviral therapy, including when to start, choice of initial regimen, monitoring therapy, changing therapy, etc. Also available at *www.iasusa.org*.

Panel on Antiretroviral Guidelines for Adults and Adolescents. Guidelines for the use of antiretroviral agents in HIV-1-infected adults and adolescents. Department of Health and Human Services; January 1, 2011; 128–9. *http://aidsinfo.nih.gov/contentfiles/AdultandAdolescentGL.pdf*. Accessed August 5, 2011.
Comments: DHHS guidelines on antiretroviral therapy, including when to start, choice of initial regimen, monitoring therapy, changing therapy, etc. Updated regularly.

Kitahata MM, Gange SJ, Abraham AG, et al. Effect of early versus deferred antiretroviral therapy for HIV on survival. *NEJM*, 2009; 360: 1815–26.
Comments: NA-ACCORD: a large North American cohort study demonstrating improved survival among patients who started ART at CD4 350–500 or >500 compared to those who deferred ART.

Zolopa A, Andersen J, Powderly W, et al. Early antiretroviral therapy reduces AIDS progression/death in individuals with acute opportunistic infections: a multicenter randomized strategy trial. *PLoS One*, 2009; 4: e5575.
Comments: Randomized trial comparing early vs deferred initiation of ART in patients with OIs, demonstrating 50% reduction in risk of disease progression or death in patients who began ART early vs those who delayed ART. Results most applicable to patients with PCP (representing 2/3 of study population, most of whom were on steroids).

Emery S, Neuhaus JA, Phillips AN, et al. Major clinical outcomes in antiretroviral therapy (ART)-naive participants and in those not receiving ART at baseline in the SMART study. *J Infect Dis*, 2008; 197: 1133–44.
Comments: Analysis of subset of SMART (treatment interruption) participants who were ART-naïve or not on ART at entry, demonstrating better outcomes with immediate than deferred therapy.

Cohen MS, Chen YQ, McCauley M, et al. Prevention of HIV-1 infection with antiretroviral therapy. *N Engl J Med* 2011; 365:493–505.
Comments: HPTN 052, a large, randomized, multinational study of serodiscordant couples demonstrating 96% reduction in sexual transmission when HIV+ partner treated with ART.

Neaton J, Grund B. Earlier initiation of antiretroviral therapy in treatment-naive patients: implications of results of treatment interruption trials. *Curr Opin HIV/AIDS*, 2008; 3: 1–117.
Comments: Discussion of the implications of treatment interruption trials, especially SMART, on the timing of initiation of ART in naïve patients.

WHO HIV/AIDS Programme. Rapid advice: antiretroviral therapy for HIV infection in adults and adolescents. November, 2009. *www.who.int/hiv/pub/arv/rapid_advice_art.pdf*. Accessed August 5, 2011.
Comments: New WHO recommendations for ART in developing countries, now recommending therapy with CD4 <350.

MANAGEMENT

BASELINE AND ROUTINE TESTING

Joel E. Gallant, MD, MPH

DEFINITION
- Baseline and follow-up studies for HIV-infected patients.

CLINICAL RECOMMENDATION

Baseline Tests
- HIV serology: repeat if Dx based on single serology without inconsistent VL results (e.g., undetectable or very low).
- HIV RNA (VL): assess baseline VL, predict rate of CD4 decline, assess need for ART. Repeat if clinical decision to be based on result.
- CD4 count and percent: assess immune function, determine need for ART and OI prophylaxis.
- Resistance test: recommended at baseline for all naïve patients, regardless of need for ART. Genotype preferred. Test as soon as possible after Dx, regardless of need for ART.
- CBC: anemia, leukopenia, thrombocytopenia common.
- Chemistry panel: assess liver status and renal function.
- Syphilis serology: coinfection common.
- HBsAg: Dx chronic HBV infection. Check HBeAg if positive. Consider HBV DNA if HBsAg negative but unexplained AST, ALT elevations, or if HBcAb positive with negative HBsAb.
- HBsAb and/or anti-HBc: assess for immunity and vaccine efficacy or eligibility.
- Anti-HCV Ab: coinfection common. Check HCV RNA if anti-HCV + or if negative with abnormal AST, ALT, HCV risk factors, or CD4 <200.
- HAV total or IgG Ab: assess for immunity and vaccine efficacy or eligibility, especially in patients with chronic HBV or HCV.
- Anti-*Toxoplasma* IgG: Dx latent infection. Seropositive: use primary prophylaxis when indicated. Seronegative: counsel on avoidance of exposure.
- Anti-CMV IgG: recommended for those at low risk of CMV (non-MSM, non-IDU). Seropositive: risk for CMV with CD4 <50. Seronegative: counsel on avoidance of exposure. Use CMV-negative or WBC-reduced blood products.
- Pap smear: higher rates of cervical dysplasia and cancer in HIV+ women. Consider anal Pap also, especially in women and MSM.
- Tuberculin skin test (TST) or interferon-gamma releasing assay (IGRA): detect latent M. Tb infection. TST: Mantoux method skin test using 5 TU. Positive test = 5 mm induration in HIV+ patients. Anergy testing not recommended. IGRA preferred if Hx of BCG vaccination.
- G6-PD level: consider in patients at risk: African or Mediterranean descent. Avoid oxidant agents (e.g., dapsone, primaquine) if deficient.
- Chest X-ray: Consider to look for asymptomatic TB and to establish baseline. DHHS does not recommend routine CXR in asymptomatic patients with negative PPD.
- Screening for *N. gonorrhea* and *C. trachomatis*: detect asymptomatic infection.
- Fasting lipid profile: to establish baseline before initiating ART.
- Tetanus vaccine (dT or Tdap): if last >10 yrs ago.
- Pneumococcal vaccine: if CD4 >200 and no previous vaccination or a single vaccination >5 yrs ago.
- General preventive care (if providing primary care to the patient): (e.g. mammogram, hemoccult, BP screening, fasting glucose, PSA, colonoscopy as recommended for HIV-negative patients).
- HLA B*5701 assay: if treatment with ABC being considered.
- Tropism (*Trofile*) assay: if treatment with MVC being considered.

Routine Tests
- HIV RNA (VL): repeat q2–4 mos in untreated patients or stable treated patients. After starting or changing ART, repeat at 1–4 wks, at 12–16 wks, and at 16–24 wks. Some test monthly until VL <50. Can consider testing q6 mos in adherent patients w/ VL suppression >2–3 yrs and stable clinical and immunologic status.

- CD4 count/percent: repeat q3–6 mos in untreated patients and stable treated patients. In patients on suppressive ART with CD4 well above OI threshold, CD4 may be monitored q6–12 mos.
- Resistance testing: repeat as indicated, primarily for virologic failure (treated patients) (see Resistance Testing: Genotype [p. 42] and Resistance Testing: Phenotype [p. 43]).
- CBC: repeat at q3–6mos, more often in patients on marrow suppressive drugs (e.g., AZT), patients with Sx of anemia, or patients with low/borderline counts.
- Chemistry panel: repeat annually. Repeat more often (e.g., q3mos) in patients on hepatotoxic or nephrotoxic drugs, including most ART regimens.
- HBsAg: repeat in seronegative patients as clinically indicated or if ongoing risk for infection.
- HBsAb: repeat as clinically indicated or to assess response to vaccination.
- Tropism (*Trofile*) assay: if treatment with MVC being considered.
- Anti-HCV Ab: repeat as clinically indicated or if ongoing risk for infection. Use HCV RNA if suspicion of acute HCV infection.
- HAV total or IgG Ab: repeat to assess response to vaccination.
- Anti-*Toxoplasma* IgG: repeat if seronegative at baseline, CD4 <100, and unable to take TMP-SMX prophylaxis.
- Pap smear: repeat at 6 mos, then annually if normal. Repeat "inadequate" specimens. Refer patients with atypia for colposcopy.
- TST or IGRA: consider annual testing if at ongoing risk for TB exposure. Repeat if CD4 <200 at time of initial negative test and CD4 now >200.
- Screening for *N. gonorrhea* and *C. trachomatis*: repeat annually in sexually active patients.
- Fasting lipid profile and fasting glucose: when switching ART, 3–6 mos after starting/switching ART, then annually if OK.
- Tetanus vaccine (dT or Tdap): every 10 yrs.
- Influenza vaccine: annually.
- Pneumococcal vaccine: booster after 5 yrs if CD4 >200.
- HLA B*5701 assay: if treatment with ABC being considered.
- General preventive care (if providing primary care to the patient): as recommended for HIV-negative patients.

SELECTED REFERENCES

Kaplan JE, Benson C, Holmes KH, et al. Guidelines for prevention and treatment of opportunistic infections in HIV-infected adults and adolescents: recommendations from CDC, the National Institutes of Health, and the HIV Medicine Association of the Infectious Diseases Society of America. *MMWR Recomm Rep*, 2009; 58: 1–207. Accessed 9/1/11.
Comments: USPHS/IDSA guidelines on OI prevention and treatment, which include recommendations on baseline and routine testing.

US Preventive Services Task Force (USPSTF). *Guide to Clinical Preventive Services*, 2010-2011. Available at *www.ahrq.gov/clinic/pocketgd1011/*. Accessed August 4, 2011.
Comments: Recommendations for preventive screening for men and women. HIV care providers who provide primary care should follow these recommendations for general preventive care in addition to HIV-specific recommendations.

NHLBI/NIH National Cholesterol Education Program (NCEP). Third Report of the Expert Panel on Detection, Evaluation, and Treatment of High Blood Cholesterol in Adults (Adult Treatment Panel III). 2004. *www.nhlbi.nih.gov/guidelines/cholesterol/*. Accessed August 5, 2011.
Comments: Does not have HIV-specific guidelines, but general guidelines that are helpful to the HIV clinician.

Aberg JA, Kaplan JE, Libman H, et al. Primary care guidelines for the management of persons infected with human immunodeficiency virus: 2009 update by the HIV Medicine Association of the Infectious Diseases Society of America. *Clin Infect Dis*, 2009; 49: 651–81.
Comments: IDSA/HIVMA guidelines for primary care of HIV-infected patients. Includes recommendations for baseline and routine testing, as well as healthcare maintenance interventions and monitoring.

Schambelan M, Benson CA, Carr A, et al. Management of metabolic complications associated with antiretroviral therapy for HIV-1 infection: recommendations of an International AIDS Society-USA panel. *J Acquir Immune Defic Syndr*, 2002; 31: 257–75.
Comments: Provides recommendations for lipid and other metabolic testing and management in HIV.

MANAGEMENT

CD4 CELL COUNT

Joel E. Gallant, MD, MPH and Christopher J. Hoffmann, MD, MPH

DEFINITION
- Number of CD4 cells (T-helper lymphocytes with CD4 cell surface marker), used to assess immune status, susceptibility to OIs, need for ART and OI prophylaxis, and for defining AIDS (CD4 <200).

INDICATIONS
Facts About CD4
- Normal adult CD4 count reference ranges vary by laboratory; however, ranges are generally within 500–1500.
- Large individual variability in measurement reflecting method of determining CD4 count by calculation from 3 measured variables: WBC, % lymphocytes, and % lymphocytes that are CD4+ (CD4%). CD4% less variable than absolute count; within-subject coefficient of variation is 18% for CD4% vs 25% for CD4 count.
- Approximate corresponding values for CD4 count and CD4% are: >500 ~>29%, 200–500 ~14%–28%, <200 ~<14%.
- CD4 count usually determined by flow cytometry; specimens must be processed within 18 hrs of collection for optimal accuracy when assayed by flow cytometry.

Factors That Affect CD4 Count
- Seasonal and diurnal variation (lowest at 12:30 PM, highest at 8:30 PM), surgery, viral infections, tuberculosis.
- Decreases with some medications (e.g., corticosteroids, especially with acute use, less pronounced with chronic use; PEG-IFN, IFN; cancer chemotherapy).
- Acute changes in CD4 more often due to redistribution of CD4 in lymphatics, spleen, and bone marrow.
- Splenectomy causes abrupt, prolonged increase in CD4. In asplenic patients, CD4% provides more accurate assessment of immune status.
- HTLV-I can increase CD4 (may have low CD4% with disproportionately high CD4 count). HTLV-I common in Brazil, Caribbean, and Japan.
- Sex, race, psychologic stress, and physical stress have minimal effect on CD4. Pregnancy leads to hemodilution and a small decline in CD4 count, but no decline in CD4%.

CD4 in HIV Infection
- Abrupt decline in CD4 after acute HIV infection followed by rise. CD4 count after recovery from acute infection can return to normal range (close to preinfection baseline) or can be low.
- Without ART, annual CD4 decline correlated with viral load (VL) only on population level. VL is poor predictor of 1–2 yr CD4 decline on individual level, accounting for less then 10% of individual variation.
- On ART, biphasic increase in CD4, 50–120 in 1st 3 mos (thought to be due to redistribution of memory CD4 cells from lymphoid tissue) followed by average increase of 2–7 cells/mo via expansion of naïve CD4 cell population; CD4 increase can continue yrs after ART initiation (>6 yrs). Normalization of CD4 count more likely in patients who start therapy with higher CD4 counts.
- CD4 response generally correlates with VL suppression, but discordant results can occur; 10% have VL suppression but no CD4 rise. Lack of CD4 response is not evidence of treatment failure if VL suppressed.
- Bone marrow suppression from AZT may blunt CD4 response. Some evidence for better CD4 response with boosted PIs, integrase inhibitors, and CCR5 antagonsts than NNRTIs (specifically LPV/r vs EFV in ACTG 5142, RAL vs EFV in STARTMRK, and MVC vs EFV in MERIT).
- Abrupt decrease in CD4 often occurs after discontinuing ART (100–150 in 3–4 mos).

Idiopathic CD4 Lymphopenia (ICL)
- Idiopathic CD4 Lymphopenia (ICL) characterized by low CD4 not explained by HIV or other medical conditions.
- Defined as: (1) CD4 <300 or CD4% <20% on >2 measurements, (2) lack of HIV infection, and (3) absence of alternative explanation.
- Lower risk of OIs than with HIV infection; CD4 tends to remain stable, prognosis relatively good. PCP prophylaxis recommended for CD4 <200.

CLINICAL RECOMMENDATION

CD4 Monitoring

- Follow CD4 q3–6 mos in untreated and q3–6 mos in those on ART. Repeat when results inconsistent with prior trends. In patients on suppressive ART with CD4 above OI threshold, CD4 can be monitored q6–12 mos unless changes in clinical status, such as new HIV-related Sx or initiation of IFN, corticosteroids, or ant-neoplastic agents.
- CD4% less variable than absolute count, but less predictive of risk of OI. Can be used in cases of discrepant CD4 count results (e.g., to determine whether an apparent decline is likely to be real).
- CD4 count is most important lab result for untreated patients; VL is most important result for treated patients.

CD4 Response to ART

- If VL suppression but poor CD4 rise, assess for concomitant infections and use of drugs that suppress bone marrow. Assess concordance of CD4% trends. Consider switch from AZT to other NRTI (e.g., TDF or ABC).
- Benefit of switch to or addition of boosted PI, RAL, or MVC unknown. Studies in progress.
- IL-2 increases CD4 count, but no clinical benefit in 2 large clinical trials (SILCAAT [Levy], ESPRIT [Losso]).

SELECTED REFERENCES

Department of Health and Human Services (DHHS); Guidelines for the use of antiretroviral agents in HIV-1-infected adults and adolescents. January 10, 2011; *http://www.aidsinfo.nih.gov/ContentFiles/AdultandAdolescentGL.pdf*.
Comments: DHHS guidelines, including recommendations for CD4 count monitoring. CD4 count less important than VL in treated patients, and can be monitored every 6–12 months in stable patients with suppressed VL and high CD4 counts.

Thompson MA et al: Antiretroviral treatment of adult HIV infection: 2010 recommendations of the International AIDS Society-USA panel. *JAMA*, 2010; 304: 321.
Comments: IAS-USA guidelines for ART, including recommendations for laboratory monitoring.

Moore RD, Keruly JC. CD4+ cell count 6 years after commencement of highly active antiretroviral therapy in persons with sustained virologic suppression. *Clin Infect Dis*, 2007; 44: 441–6.
Comments: CD4 increase can continue 6 yrs after starting ART, but patients with lower nadir CD4 counts may reach a lower plateau than those with higher CD4 counts, and this is clinically relevant, with greater risk of progression or death despite undetectable VL.

HIV DIAGNOSIS

Joel E. Gallant, MD, MPH

DEFINITION

- Diagnosis of acute or chronic HIV infection.

INDICATIONS

Indications for Voluntary HIV Testing

- CDC now recommends routine, voluntary testing of all adolescents and adults without written informed consent. Annual testing recommended for those at high risk. "Opt-out" approach recommended: patient told that HIV testing will be performed, and given opportunity to refuse. Not all state laws allow implementation of these recommendations.
- When routine testing not performed, consider testing for patient request, patients at risk, conditions suggesting impaired cellular immunity (OIs, thrush, recurrent or refractory vaginal candidiasis, recurrent pneumonia, etc.), TB, shingles (especially in young adults), sexually transmitted diseases, certain laboratory abnormalities (unexplained anemia, thrombocytopenia, leukopenia/lymphopenia, or elevated total protein), pregnant women, hospitalized adults in areas of high seroprevalence.

CLINICAL RECOMMENDATION

HIV Serology

- Enzyme-linked immunoassay (EIA) plus confirmatory Western blot (WB) if EIA repeatedly reactive.
- Sensitivity 99.5% after 3 mos of infection; specificity >99.994%.

MANAGEMENT

- EIA alone: 2% false positive.
- WB: negative: "no" bands; positive: "gp120/160" + either gp41 or p24; indeterminate: any other band pattern.
- WB false-positives: rare. Causes include autoantibodies, HIV vaccines, technical/clerical error.
- WB indeterminate: causes include seroconversion (especially with p24), cross-reacting antibodies, infection with type O or HIV-2, HIV vaccines.
- False negative serology: usually due to testing window period before seroconversion. Rate = 0.3% in high-prevalence population; <0.001% in low-prevalence population. Other rare causes of false-negatives: seroreversion, atypical host response, agammaglobulinemia, infection with type N, O, or HIV-2, technical or clerical error.
- False positive serology: frequency 0.0004%–0.0007%. Causes: HIV vaccine, factitious HIV infection, influenza vaccination, technical or clerical error.
- Indeterminate serology: causes include testing in window period during seroconversion, late-stage HIV infection, cross-reacting non-specific antibodies, infection with type O or HIV-2, HIV vaccination, technical or clerical error. Perform risk assessment and measure VL. If seroconverting, VL usually high and WB positive within 1 mo.
- Acute HIV infection: expect negative or indeterminate serology with high VL.

Home Test Kits

- *Home Access Express Test*: blood test, with results by phone in 3–7 days. Double EIA with confirmatory IFA. Sensitivity and specificity >99% (800-448-8378 or *www.homeaccess.com/*).

Rapid Tests

- *OraQuick* (OraSure Technologies): HIV-1 and -2 antibody test (blood, plasma, oral fluid). Results read by provider in 20 mins. Sensitivity 100% (blood), 99.6% (oral fluid); specificity >99.5%. CLIA waived.
- *Reveal G2* (MedMira Inc.): HIV-1 antibody test (serum or plasma, centrifuge required). Sensitivity 99.8%, specificity 98.6%. Not CLIA waived.
- *Uni-Gold Recombigen* (Trinity Biotech): HIV-1 antibody test (blood, plasma, serum). Sensitivity 100%, specificity 99.7%.CLIA waived.
- *Multispot* (Bio-Rad Labs): HIV-1 and -2 antibody test (serum, centrifuge required). Sensitivity 100%, specificity 99.9%. Not CLIA waived.
- *Clearview* (Inverness Medical): HIV-1 and -2 antibody test (blood). Sensitivity 99.7%, specificity 99.9%. CLIA waived.
- *VITROS* (Ortho Clinical Diagnostics): HIV-1 and -2 antibody test (serum, centrifuge required). Sensitivity 100%, specificity 99.5%. Not CLIA waived.

Oral Fluid Tests

- *OraSure* (OraSure Technologies): Ab screen by ELISA with WB confirmation using oral mucosal collection device. Results in 3 days. Sensitivity >99.2%, specificity >99.8%.
- *OraQuick* (OraSure Technologies): see "Rapid Tests" above.

Urine Tests

- *Calypte* HIV-1 Urine EIA (Calypte Biomedical Corp). EIA only: positive results must be confirmed by serology. Sensitivity 99%, specificity 94%.

Viral Detection

- Preferred for Dx of acute retroviral syndrome (ARS). Serology preferred in asymptomatic patients, as some HIV+ patients have undetectable virus. May be helpful with indeterminate serology.
- Quantitative HIV RNA (viral load): high levels of viremia with ARS. Low-levels (<10,000) may be false-positive. Rare false-negatives in chronic infection.
- HIV DNA PCR: qualitative assay to detect cell-associated proviral DNA. May be useful for detection of HIV infection in neonates. Sensitivity >99%. Not FDA approved, and requires confirmation.
- p24 antigen: less expensive but less sensitive (90%) than HIV RNA for Dx of ARS.
- PBMC Cx: expensive and labor-intensive. Can be quantitative or qualitative. Sensitivity 95%–100%.
- *Aptima* (GenProbeInc.): qualitative HIV-1 RNA: approved for Dx of HIV infection, including acute or primary infection, and to confirm Dx in patient with repeatedly positive serology. Advantages over viral load testing unclear.
- 4th generation serology (Ag/Ab tests) shorten window period and increase likelihood of positive results in patients with ARS.

SELECTED REFERENCES

Bartlett JG, Branson BM, Fenton K, et al. Opt-out testing for human immunodeficiency virus in the United States: progress and challenges. *JAMA*, 2008; 300: 945–51.

Comments: Documents multiple barriers to widespread implementation of routine HIV screening as recommended by CDC, including state legislation. Extrapolating Maryland data to US, authors estimated late diagnosis resulted in 100,000 life-years lost.

Burke RC, Sepkowitz KA, Bernstein KT, et al. Why don't physicians test for HIV? A review of the US literature. *AIDS*, 2007; 21: 1617–24.

Comments: Documents poor uptake of 2006 CDC HIV screening recommendations in US.

Branson BM, Handsfield HH, Lampe MA, et al; Centers for Disease Control and Prevention (U.S.). Revised guidelines for testing, counseling, and referral and revised recommendations for HIV screening of pregnant women. *MMWR Recomm Rep*, 2006; 55, No. RR-14: 1–17.

Comments: Most recent CDC guidelines for HIV testing and counseling, recommending routine, voluntary testing for all adults and adolescents without written informed consent.

RESISTANCE TESTING: GENOTYPE

Lisa A. Spacek, MD, PhD

DEFINITION
- HIV gene sequencing assay to detect mutations that confer ARV drug resistance.

INDICATIONS

Acute or Chronic Infection, ART-Naïve Patients
- Genotype testing recommended for all newly Dx'd patients at time of Dx.
- High reported rates of transmitted drug resistance (8%–16%).
- Repeat testing at ART initiation may detect drug-resistant virus acquired since time of Dx.
- Choice of ART based on treatment history and drug resistance of source patient.
- Genotype testing recommended in all pregnant women prior to ART initiation.
- If transmitted integrase strand transfer inhibitor (INSTI) resistance is suspected, supplement standard resistance testing with INSTI genotypic resistance assay.

Established Infection, ART-Experienced Patients
- Treatment failure VL >1000 (genotype can sometimes be performed with VL in 500–1000 range).
- Drug resistance testing results used to select fully active drugs in cases of virologic failure.
- Suboptimal suppression of VL after ART initiation.
- Pregnancy, if VL detectable on ART.
- In setting of virologic failure on INSTI-based regimen, supplement standard resistance testing with INSTI genotypic resistance assay.

Professional Society Guidelines
- IAS-USA Recommendations.
- DHHS Guidelines.
- European AIDS Clinical Society.
- BHIVA Guidelines.

CLINICAL RECOMMENDATION

Important Considerations
- Increased transmission of resistant virus, persistence of transmitted resistant mutants, and demonstrated cost-effectiveness are reasons to perform resistance testing at time of Dx regardless of need for ART.
- Genotype preferred over phenotype in naïve patients because of ability to detect mixtures that occur during reversion to wild-type.
- Resistance detected reliably in species that make up >10%–20% of viral pool. Mixtures of susceptible and resistant virus (present at >10%–20%) can be detected with genotype.
- Minority variants not detected by standard assays. Point mutations assays, clonal sequencing, and ultra deep sequencing are methods to detect minority resistance and have unproven clinical utility.

MANAGEMENT

- May not detect mutations acquired on prior therapy: consider prior genotype results and treatment Hx.
- Not usually recommended when VL < 500 c/mL.
- Testing should be performed on ART whenever possible, or within 4 wks after discontinuation.
- *VircoTYPE* (Virco) provides a genotype resistance analysis, and uses linear regression modeling to generate predicted phenotype based on mutations and pairs of mutations in Virco's correlative genotype-phenotype database.

Genotype vs Phenotype

- Less expensive.
- Shorter turnaround time (1–2 wks).
- May detect mutations, including mixtures, before they result in phenotypic resistance.
- Consider phenotype (± genotype) in patients with more extensive resistance, where genotype interpretation can be complex, particularly in PI resistance. Phenotype may also be useful for non-subtype B virus and for assessing susceptibility to newer agents.
- When ordering phenotype, consider ordering genotype (or combined test), as phenotype alone may underestimate resistance due to mixtures.

Tools for Genotype Interpretation

- Stanford HIV Drug Resistance Database, *http://cpr.stanford.edu/cpr/.*
- Los Alamos National Laboratory HIV Drug Resistance Database, *http://resdb.lanl.gov/ Resist_DB/default.htm.*

SELECTED REFERENCES

Wittkop L, Günthard HF, de Wolf F, et al. Effect of transmitted drug resistance on virological and immunological response to initial combination antiretroviral therapy for HIV (EuroCoord-CHAIN joint project): a European multicohort study. *Lancet Infect Dis*, 2011 Feb 25. [Epub ahead of print].
Comments: Results of European collaboration found that 479 of 10,056 (4.8%) participants had at least one mutation and resistance to at least one drug. Findings support resistance testing in ART-naïve patients to determine initial ART choice.

Panel on Antiretroviral Guidelines for Adults and Adolescents. Guidelines for the use of antiretroviral agents in HIV-1-infected adults and adolescents. Department of Health and Human Services; January 1, 2011; 11–8. *http://www.aidsinfo. nih.gov/contentfiles/AdultandAdolescentGL.pdf.* Accessed March 30, 2011.
Comments: Drug resistance testing recommended at time of Dx, at ART initiation, in setting of suboptimal virologic response, virologic failure and pregnancy.

Thompson MA, Aberg JA, Cahn P, et al. Antiretroviral treatment of adult HIV infection: 2010 recommendations of the International AIDS Society-USA Panel. *JAMA*, 2010; 304: 321–333.
Comments: Baseline genotypic testing recommended in all ART-naïve patients and in cases of confirmed virologic failure.

Johnson VA, Brun-Vezinet F, Clotet B, et al. Update of the drug resistance mutations in HIV-1. *Top HIV Med*, 2010; 18: 156–163.
Note: Accessed at: *www.iasusa.org/resistance_mutations/mutations_figures.pdf.* Accessed March 30, 2011.
Comments: Nine new mutations: E138G and E138K for etravirine, E92Q for raltegravir, and M36L, M36V, H69R, L89I, L89M, and L89V for tipranavir/ritonavir.

Paredes R, Lalama CM, Ribaudo HJ, et al. Pre-existing minority drug-resistant HIV-1 variants, adherence, and risk of antiretroviral treatment failure. *J Infect Dis*, 2010; 201: 662–71.
Comments: Minority K103N or Y181C populations were determined by allele-specific polymerase chain reaction (ACTG A5095). In 183 subjects, minority K103N or Y181C mutations, or both, were detected in 8 (4.4%), 54 (29.5%), and 11 (6%), respectively. Minority Y181C mutations were associated with increased risk of virologic failure (HR, 3.5, 95%CI, 1.9-6.3) in ART-naïve, adherent patients of EFV-based regimen.

RESISTANCE TESTING: PHENOTYPE

Lisa A. Spacek, MD, PhD

DEFINITION

- HIV drug resistance assays in which RT, PR, intergrase and envelope gene sequences derived from patient plasma HIV RNA used to measure HIV replication at different concentrations of ARVs.

INDICATIONS

- Phenotype tests combined effect of all mutations, including mutational interactions. Most useful in patients with multiple mutations, especially to assess PI susceptibility.
- Quantitatively measures drug resistance and identifies ARVs with partial activity that may be useful when treatment options limited.
- Interpretation of phenotype based on two important clinical cut offs: (1) lower cut off: value where clinical response diminished (partial susceptibility), and (2) upper cut off: value above which no clinical response expected.
- Phenotype does not require understanding of genotypic correlates of resistance; therefore, may be especially useful for new drugs and non-B subtypes.
- Measures hypersusceptibility.
- Consider phenotyping when treatment history complex and/or significant resistance expected.

Professional Society Guidelines

- IAS-USA Recommendations.
- DHHS Guidelines.
- European AIDS Clinical Society.
- BHIVA Guidelines.

CLINICAL RECOMMENDATION

Important Considerations

- Genotype preferred over phenotype in ART-naive patients to detect mutations as it is cheaper and more likely to detect resistance due to wild-type/mutant mixtures; also determines HIV-1 subtype.
- Testing should be performed on ART or <4 wks of stopping ART to detect drug-resistant population that evolves under selective pressure of ART.
- Phenotype may fail to detect resistance due to wild-type/mutant mixtures, especially in patients no longer on ART.
- Simultaneous or combined genotype (e.g., *PhenoSense GT*) should generally be ordered with phenotype.

Phenotype Test Methods

- Results reported as fold change in drug susceptibility of patient's sample vs control. Susceptibility measured by inhibitory concentration (IC) or amount of drug required to inhibit viral replication by 50%.
- Biologic cut offs based on normal distribution of susceptibility to drug for wild-type strain from treatment-naïve patients.
- Clinical cut offs (CCO) based on data from cohort studies and clinical trials to determine decline in susceptibility that results in reduced virologic response.
- Detects resistance only in species that make up >10%–20% of viral population.
- VircoTYPE (Virco), a virtual phenotype, uses drug-specific linear regression modeling to predict phenotype based on genotype using Virco's genotype-phenotype correlative database.

MANAGEMENT

SELECTED REFERENCES

Panel on Antiretroviral Guidelines for Adults and Adolescents. Guidelines for the use of antiretroviral agents in HIV-1-infected adults and adolescents. Department of Health and Human Services; January 1, 2011; 11–18. http://www.aidsinfo.nih.gov/contentfiles/AdultandAdolescentGL.pdf. Accessed March 30, 2011.
Comments: Addition of phenotypic testing to genotypic testing recommended in persons with known or suspected complex drug resistance mutation patterns, particularly in PIs.

Thompson, MA, Aberg JA, Cahn P, et al. Antiretroviral treatment of adult HIV infection: 2010 recommendations of an International AIDS Society-USA panel. *JAMA*, 2010; 304: 321–323.
Comments: Drug resistance testing recommended at time of HIV diagnosis and in all cases of virologic failure.

Winters B, Van Craenenbroeck E, Van der Borght K. Clinical cut-offs for HIV-1 phenotypic resistance estimates: update based on recent pivotal clinical trial data and a revised approach to viral mixtures. *J Virol Methods*, 2009; 162: 101–8.
Comments: Updated clinical cut offs (CCO) for VircoTYPE HIV-1 drug resistance assay based on linear regression analysis used 6550 records from clinical cohorts and TITAN, POWER, and DUET clinical studies. Marginally higher CCOs seen for NRTIs.

Napravnik S, Cachafeiro A, Stewart P, Eron JJ Jr, Fiscus SA. HIV-1 viral load and phenotypic antiretroviral drug resistance assays based on reverse transcriptase activity in comparison to amplification based HIV-1 RNA and genotypic assays. *J Clin Virol*, 2010; 47: 18–22.

Comments: To evaluate test for potential use in resource-limited settings, 108 specimens were used to compare ExaVir Drug phenotype to HIV GenoSure genotype. Phenotypes were generally consistent with genotype findings for EFV, but not for NVP.

Fun A, de Jong D, Nijhuis M. Genetic barrier of DRV is decreased by *gag* polymorphisms. Presented at: 18th Conference on Retroviruses and Opportunistic Infections; February 27–March 2, 2011; Boston, MA. Available at *www.retroconference. org/2011/Abstracts/40883.htm*. Accessed March 30, 2011.

Comments: *In vitro* phenotypic resistance, 5- to 7-fold decreased susceptibility, to DRV seen as result of gag 437 mutations in subtype AG virus.

VIRAL LOAD ASSAYS

Lisa A. Spacek, MD, PhD

DEFINITION
- Quantitative plasma HIV RNA assay.
- Most important indicator of response to ART.

INDICATIONS

Commercial Viral Load Assays
- HIV RT PCR (*Amplicor HIV-1 Monitor* v1.5/Ultrasensitive, Roche Pharmaceuticals).
- Branched chain DNA (bDNA) (*Versant HIV-1 RNA* v3.0, Bayer Pharmaceuticals).
- Nucleic acid sequence-based amplification (*NucliSens HIV-1 EasyQ* v2.0, bioMérieux).
- Real-time PCR (*TaqMan HIV-1 v2.0*, Roche Pharmaceuticals).
- Real-time PCR (*RealTime HIV-1*, Abbott Laboratories).

Acute HIV Infection
- VL may be used to diagnose acute HIV infection prior to seroconversion (2%–9% without HIV infection have false + results, usually with low-level VL).
- Dx should always be confirmed by standard methods (ELISA or Western blot) 2–4 mos after acute seroconversion.

Prognosis and Risk of Opportunistic Infection
- VL decrease on ART associated with improved clinical outcome.
- VL "set point" is prognostic indicator in early stage infection, independent of CD4.
- VL predicts risk of OI independent of CD4 when CD4 <200.

Probability of Transmission
- VL directly correlated with probability of transmission in all types of exposure studied.

Therapeutic Monitoring
- Goal of ART: VL below assay's limit of detection by 24 wks.
- Repeat testing 2-8 wks after ART initiation, every 4–8 wks until suppressed, then every 3–4 mos for at least the 1st yr.
- Expected decline: 0.75–1 log at 1 wk, 1.5–2 log at 4 wks and undetectable at 16–24 wks.
- Baseline VL may affect rate of decrease, most patients with response at 24 wks had at least 1 log decrease within 4 wks of ART initiation.
- Optimal viral suppression: VL persistently below assay's limit of detection.
- May extend testing interval to 6 mos for adherent patients with suppressed VL >2–3 yrs with stable clinical and immunologic status.
- Virologic failure: confirmed VL >200. Repeat assay when VL is unexpectedly detectable.
- Sustained viremia (>500) increases risk of drug resistance and viral failure.

TABLE 3-3

Trade Name	Technique	Dynamic Range	Subtypes Amplified	Specimen Volume
Amplicor Monitor v1.5 Ultrasensitive	Real-time PCR	50–75,000 c/mL	Group M	0.5 mL
Versant v3.0	bDNA	75–500,000 c/mL	A–G	1 mL

Trade Name	Technique	Dynamic Range	Subtypes Amplified	Specimen Volume
NucliSens EasyQ v2.0	NASBA	10–10,000,000 c/mL	A, B, C, D, F, G, H, J, CRF01_AE, CRF02_AG	0.1–0.5–1 mL
TaqMan HIV-1 v2.0	Real-time PCR	20–10,000,000 c/mL	A–H, Group N	1 mL
RealTime HIV-1	Real-time PCR	40–10,000,000 c/mL	Groups M, N, and O	1 mL

CLINICAL RECOMMENDATION

Quality Assurance

- VL should be obtained when clinically stable (>4 wks after acute infection or vaccination).
- When serially monitoring VL, use same laboratory and assay technique.
- Changes >30%–50% (0.2–0.3 log) considered significant.
- Sample collection in anticoagulant EDTA avoids heparin-associated inhibition of PCR.

VL Monitoring in Untreated Patients

- Perform at baseline then every 3–4 mos in untreated patients.
- Baseline VL appears to be lower in women and blacks compared to white men, although rates of disease progression are similar.

Factors That Increase VL

- Low drug concentration: nonadherence or poor pharmacokinetics.
- Drug resistance.
- Acute infection (e.g., TB, PCP, HSV, or pneumococcal pneumonia).
- Immunizations (influenza, Pneumovax): increases are modest and transient.

Factors Not Measured by VL

- Immune function.
- CD4 regenerative reserve.
- Susceptibility to ARVs.
- Syncytial vs nonsyncytial forms; R5 vs X4 tropism.
- VL in compartments other than blood (e.g., lymph nodes, CNS, GI tract, and genital secretions).

SELECTED REFERENCES

Panel on Antiretroviral Guidelines for Adults and Adolescents. Guidelines for the use of antiretroviral agents in HIV-1-infected adults and adolescents. Department of Health and Human Services; January 1, 2011; 9–10. *http://aidsinfo.nih.gov/contentfiles/AdultandAdolescentGL.pdf*. Accessed March 30, 2011.

Comments: Viral load is the most important indicator of response to ART. Virologic failure defined as confirmed VL >200. This threshold accounts for blips and assay variability.

Thompson, MA, Aberg JA, Cahn P, et al. Antiretroviral treatment of adult HIV infection: 2010 Recommendations of the International AIDS Society-USA panel. *JAMA*, 2010; 304: 321–333.

Comments: Guidelines recognize that VL of 20-50 has unclear clinical significance. Recommendations include confirmation of viral load rebound on 2 separate tests at least 2–4 wks apart with review of regimen tolerability, drug-drug interactions, and patient adherence.

Paba P, Fabeni L, Ciccozzi M, et al. Performance evaluation of the COBAS/TaqMan HIV-1 v2.0 in HIV-1 positive patients with low viral load: a comparative study. *J Virol Methods*, 2011 Mar 23. [Epub ahead of print].

Comments: Recommendation to use same assay with longitudinal therapeutic monitoring and expected low VL.

Pas S, Rossen JW, Schoener D, et al. Performance evaluation of the new Roche Cobas AmpliPrep/Cobas TaqMan HIV-1 test version 2.0 for quantification of human immunodeficiency virus type 1 RNA. *J Clin Microbiol*, 2010; 48: 1195–200.

Comments: Version 2.0 of Roche COBAS TaqMan HIV-1 test was compared to COBAS Amplicor HIV-1 Monitor Test, v1.5; COBAS TaqMan HIV-1 v1.0; and Abbott RealTime HIV-1 assay. TaqMan v2.0 dynamic range was 20 to 10,000,000 c/mL. While a threshold of 50 c/mL was associated with virologic failure, measurements of 20 to 45 c/mL were not.

Reekie J, Mocroft A, Sambatakou H, et al. Does less frequent routine monitoring of patients on a stable, fully suppressed cART regimen lead to an increased risk of treatment failure? *AIDS*, 2008; 22: 2381–2390.

Comments: Patients who spent >80% of time fully suppressed on ART had a 38% reduced risk of virologic failure (HR, 0.6; 95% CI, 0.4-0.9). Patients with stable clinical and immunologic status may have VL monitored with extended interval of 6 mos.

MANAGEMENT

Miscellaneous

INITIAL EVALUATION

Richard D. Moore, MD, MHS

CLINICAL RECOMMENDATION

Medical History

- HPI: include date of Dx, date of infection if known, nadir CD4, peak VL, OIs and Sxs (stage HIV).
- PMH: include prior TB or exposure, PPD history, chicken pox, shingles, residence and travel, mental health (e.g., depression screening), weight change.
- Meds: ART history (if any), OTCs, dietary supplements, methadone.
- Vaccinations: tetanus, pneumococcal, hepatitis B and A, HPV, varicella, and flu (seasonal).
- Substance use: street, prescribed, recreational, needle-sharing, alcohol use (with CAGE or AUDIT), smoking.
- Sexual history: practices, barrier use, HIV status of partners, STDs.
- Social: family/partner violence, HIV status of partner and children (if any), social support, diet, exercise, education.
- Allergies: sulfonamides, penicillin, hypersensitivity to prior ARVs, and any other relevant medication allergies.
- Family history: early CVD, diabetes, hyperlipidemia.
- Women: menstrual history, contraception, infertility, pregnancy history, childbearing plans, osteoporosis Dx and treatment.

Physical Exam

- Women: include pelvic/rectal, breast exam. Evaluate for condyloma, HSV, fungal, cervical dysplasia (Pap), *Trichomonas*, *Chlamydia* and GC, HPV.
- Men: include prostate/rectal, genital exam. Evaluate for condyloma, HSV, other STIs. Consider anal Pap (HPV, dysplasia), especially in MSM.
- Skin: KS, fungal, folliculitis, prurigo nodularis.
- Body habitus: lipodystrophy, wasting, obesity.
- Oropharynx: candidiasis, OHL, KS, aphthous ulcers, periodontal disease.
- Lymphadenopathy: localized requires evaluation; generalized common with untreated HIV.
- Neurologic: cognitive dysfunction, neuropathy, focal neurologic findings.

Laboratory Assessment

- HIV serology: if lab confirmation (serology, elevated VL) not available.
- CD4 count: stage HIV. Every 3–6 mos if not on ART.
- VL (plasma HIV RNA): stage HIV. Every 3–4 mos if not on ART.
- RPR: repeat annually or more often in patients at high risk.
- Chemistries: include AST, ALT, BUN, creatinine, bilirubin, ak phos, albumin, electrolytes.
- CBC with differential.
- Fasting blood glucose ($\times$ 2): consider 2-hr OGTT or HbA1C if abnormal.
- Fasting lipid profile (TG, TC, HDL, LDL): all or prior to starting ARVs.
- Urinalysis: proteinuria may indicate HIV-related or other early renal disease (e.g., HTN, DM).
- *C. trachomatis* and *N. gonorrhea* by NAAT (all sexually active patients or w/ Sx).
- HIV genotype (if VL >1000): indicated regardless of need for ART, as mutations may disappear.
- G6PD: consider before use of dapsone, primaquine, sulfonamides, especially in patients at risk (African or Mediterranean descent).
- Hepatitis serologies: HAV (anti-HAV total or IgGAb), HBV (HBsAg, HBsAb and/or HBcAb, with HBeAg/HBeAb and HBV DNA if HBsAg+; HBV DNA if HBcAb+/HBsAb- or if elevated LFTs), and HCV (anti-HCV, with HCV PCR if anti-HCV+ or negative with risk factors or elevated LFTs).
- Anti-*Toxoplasma* IgG: evaluate for latent *Toxoplasma* infection. Counsel seronegative patients on avoiding exposure.
- Anti-CMV IgG: in non-MSM, non-IDU (MSM and IDU highly likely to be seropositive).

- Anti-varicella IgG: in patients with no history of chicken pox or shingles.
- AM testosterone level (total): if clinical indication (weight loss, fatigue, loss of libido, erectile dysfunction).
- Pregnancy test: missed menses.
- PSA: recommended for men >40 yo (AUA [Carroll]). Routine screening not recommended (ACA and USPSTF); no PSA screening after age 75 (ACS [Smith]).

Procedures

- Ophthalmologic fundoscopy: if CD4 <50 or with visual Sx.
- Chest X-ray: if PPD+ or if clinically indicated. Not routine.
- Cervical Pap: repeat at 6 mos, then annually if negative. Refer for colposcopy if abnormal.
- Anal Pap: consider, especially in MSM or women with history of anal intercourse. Repeat every 1–3 yrs. Refer for high-resolution anoscopy if abnormal.
- Anthropomorphic measures: skin-fold, extremity/neck/abdomen circumference. BIA or DEXA: not standardized; BIA can't distinguish visceral vs SQl fat. DEXA best for SQ, not visceral fat.
- Tuberculin skin test (TST) or interferon-gamma releasing assay (IGRA): repeat annually in patients at risk; repeat after immune reconstitution on ART if initially negative with low CD4.
- Vaccinations: dT or Tdap (every 10 yr), pneumococcal (one time revaccination 5 years after 1st dose; consider repeat every 5 yrs though efficacy unknown), influenza (annual), hepatitis B and A (if nonimmune). Vaccine efficacy greater with higher CD4 (>200), undetectable VL. Defer vaccination in patients about to start ART.

Other Health Maintenance

- Breast exam/mammogram in women over 40 (every 1–2 yrs; annual after age 50).
- Colonoscopy: over age 50 (repeat in 10 yrs if negative).
- PSA: high false +, not routine. Age 50–70 most likely to benefit, particularly if black or 1st degree relative with prostate cancer, but risk of false + should be first discussed.
- Bone density: women >60, or if high-risk for early osteopenia in women, or high-risk (early menopause, steroid use, hypogonadism).
- ECG: if clinically indicated. Not routine.
- PFTs: if clinically indicated. Not routine.

Counseling

- ART: preparation for life-long treatment, adherence, adverse effects, readiness before starting.
- Sexual practices, barrier and contraceptive use, pregnancy plans.
- Substance and alcohol use and treatment.
- Smoking cessation, diet, exercise, dietary supplements.
- Social support, housing, living assistance.

SELECTED REFERENCES

Smith RA, Cokkinides V, Brawley OW. Cancer screening in the United States, 2009: a review of current American Cancer Society guidelines and issues in cancer screening. *CA Cancer J Clin*, 2009; 59: 27–41.
Comments: ACS guidelines for cancer screening.

Aberg JA, Kaplan JE, Libman H, et al. Primary care guidelines for the management of persons infected with human immunodeficiency virus: 2009 update by the HIV Medicine Association of the Infectious Diseases Society of America. *Clin Infect Dis*, 2009; 49: 651–81.
Comments: Primary care guidelines of HIV-infected individuals.

Centers for Disease Control and Prevention. Recommended adult immunization schedule: United States, 2009. *MMWR*, 2009; 57: Q1–4.
Comments: Adult immunization recommendations from CDC.

Carroll P, Albertsen PC, Greene K, et al. Prostate-specific antigen best practice statement: 2009 update. American Urological Association, 2009. *www.auanet.org/content/guidelines-and-quality-care/clinical-guidelines/main-reports/psa09.pdf*. Accessed August 5, 2011.
Comments: American Urological Association recommends PSA for men >40. ACS and US Preventive Services Task Force do not agree.

Hammer SM, Eron JJ, Reiss P et al. Antiretroviral treatment of adult HIV infection: 2008 recommendations of the International AIDS Society-USA panel. *JAMA*, 2008; 300: 555–70.
Comments: IAS-USA recommendations for pretreatment evaluation of the HIV-infected adults.

MANAGEMENT

Hirsch MS, Gunthard HF, Schapiro JM, et al. Antiretroviral drug resistance testing in adult HIV-1 infection: 2008 recommendations of an International AIDS Society-USA panel. *Clinic Infect Dis*, 2008; 47: 266–85.
Comments: Up-to-date recommendations for ART resistance testing.

National Cholesterol Education Program Expert Panel on Detection, Evaluation, and Treatment of High Blood Cholesterol in Adults (Adult Treatment Panel III). Third Report of the National Cholesterol Education Program (NCEP) Expert Panel on Detection, Evaluation, and Treatment of High Blood Cholesterol in Adults (Adult Treatment Panel III) final report. *Circulation*, 2002; 106: 3143–421.
Comments: Guidelines on management of lipids.

Panel on Antiretroviral Guidelines for Adults and Adolescents. Guidelines for the use of antiretroviral agents in HIV-1-infected adults and adolescents. Department of Health and Human Services; January 1, 2011; 1–161. *http://aidsinfo.nih.gov/contentfiles/AdultandAdolescentGL.pdf*. Accessed August 5, 2011.
Comments: Guidelines for pretreatment evaluation of the HIV-infected adult and adolescent.

US Preventive Services Task Force (USPSTF). *Guide to Clinical Preventive Services*, 2010-2011. *www.ahrq.gov/clinic/pocketgd1011/*. Accessed August 5, 2011.
Comments: Guidelines to clinical preventive services for adults.

US Preventive Services Task Force (USPSTF). *Screening for Prostate Cancer: Clinical Summary of U.S. Preventive Services Task Force Recommendation*, August, 2008. *www.uspreventiveservicestaskforce.org/uspstf/uspsprca.htm*. Accessed August 5, 2011.
Comments: USPSTF recommendations: no PSA for men >75. For aged 50–75, discussion with physician, but no routine screening. Test with informed (risk/benefit) consent.

Amercian Cancer Society. Prostate cancer. Can prostate cancer be found early? *www.cancer.org/Cancer/ProstateCancer/DetailedGuide/prostate-cancer-detection*. Accessed August 5, 2011.
Comments: American Cancer Society believes evidence does not support routine screening for all men. Discussion should begin at age 50 (age 45 for men at high risk, b/o family Hx, of prostate Ca). Test with informed (risk/benefit) consent.

SECTION 4
PATHOGENS

Bacteria

CHLAMYDIA TRACHOMATIS

Noreen A. Hynes, MD, MPH

MICROBIOLOGY

- Four biovars of *C. trachomatis* cause human infection and clinical disease (trachoma, lymphogranuloma venereum, urogenital infections, etc.).
- Obligate intracellular parasite; requires eukaryotic host cell for ATP; cultivated only within cell cultured system.
- 2 distinct morphologic cycles: elementary body (metabolically inert extracellular infectious particle) and reticulate body (intracellular, replicating form).
- Most common syndromes in HIV practice involve *C. trachomatis* serovars infecting columnar or cuboidal epithelial surfaces.

CLINICAL

- Mucopurulent cervicitis.
- Nongonococcal urethritis.
- Pelvic inflammatory disease.
- Epididymitis.
- Proctocolitis.
- Bartholinitis.
- Conjunctivitis.
- Perihepatitis (Fitz-Hugh-Curtis syndrome).
- Arthritis syndromes (reactive arthritis, Reiter's syndrome).
- Lymphogranuloma venereum associated with 3 possible stages:
  - **Primary LGV:** 1 of 4 forms: papule, ulcer or erosion, herpetiform (small) lesion, or non-specific urethrtis. Manifests 3–30 days after sexual exposure; this stage missed in 50%–90% by both patient and provider; lesions heal rapidly and without scarring.
  - **Secondary LGV:** inguinal syndrome characterized by acute lymphadenitis with bubo formation and/or anogenital syndrome characterized by acute hemorrhagic proctitis. Both forms associated with fever and other constitutional symptoms with systemic infection, including inflammation and swelling of lymph nodes and surrounding tissue. In heterosexual men tender inguinal and/or femoral painful unilateral lymphadenopathy seen in 2/3 of cases; one node or entire chain may be involved with or without bubo formation. Areas overlying nodes/buboes may ulcerate, discharge pus from >1 point and create chronic fistulae. "Groove sign" noted when both inguinal and femoral chains involved simultaneously, seen in 15%–20% of cases. Complications of this stage include febrile arthritis, pneumonitis, and (rarely) perihepatitis. This stage usually occurs 2–6 wks after initial infection. Most patients do not progress beyond this stage.
  - **Tertiary LGV:** very uncommon, seen predominantly in women. Results from persistence of infection or progression into adjacent tissue leading to chronic inflammation and destruction of tissue in the involved area.

SITES OF INFECTION

- Cervix.
- Urethra.
- Conjunctiva.
- Rectum.
- Upper female reproductive tract (endometrium, Fallopian tubes).
- Oropharynx.

TREATMENT

General Principles

- Uncomplicated infection (e.g., chlamydial cervicitis, urethritis) treated with regimens of shorter duration.
- LGV: requires at least 21 days of treatment.

- Clinical syndromes involving upper genitourinary tracts (pelvic inflammatory disease, epididymitis) are often polymicrobial and treated with longer duration regimens.
- Partner therapy (sexual contacts in last 60 days) should be treated presumptively unless infection definitively ruled out.

Specific Regimens for Uncomplicated Genitourinary Infection
- Azithromycin: 1 g orally × 1 (may be given DOT; preferred if adherence questionable).
- Doxycycline: 100 mg PO twice daily × 7 days.
- Levofloxacin: 500 mg PO once daily × 7 days.
- Ofloxacin: 300 mg PO once daily × 7 days.

Complicated Chlamydial Infections
- Pelvic inflammatory disease: ceftriaxone 250 mg IM and doxycycline 100 mg PO twice daily × 14 days.
- Epididymitis: ceftriaxone 250 mg IM and doxycycline 100 mg PO twice daily × 10 days.
- LGV:
  - Doxycycline 100 mg PO twice daily × 21 days.
  - Erythromycin base 500 mg PO 4 ×day × 21 days.
  - Azithromycin 1000 mg PO once weekly × 3 wks (probably works but no clinical data; based on known antichlamydial activity).
- Erythromycin base 500 mg orally 4 times daily for 21 days.

OTHER INFORMATION
- Nucleic acid amplification tests (NAATs) are preferred method of detection as they are specific and are far more sensitive than chlamydia Cx, Ag detection tests (EIA or DFA), or unamplified nucleic acid hybridization assays.
- Currently available testing technologies include PCR, transcription-mediated amplification (*APTIMA* by Gen-Probe), and strand displacement amplification (*BDProbeTec ET* by Bectin Dickinson & Co). All can be done on urine, urethral or cervical swab samples, and are generally equivalent in sensitivity and specificity.
- CDC recommends screening of at-risk MSM at least annually for urethral and rectal GC and chlamydia and for pharyngeal GC. Standard FDA-cleared method for Dx is Cx. Although NAAT is generally more sensitive and favored by most experts to Dx extragenital infection, it may not be marketed for that purpose. Labs may offer NAAT for Dx of extragenital infection after conducting internal validation study of method. LabCorp and Quest offer NAAT for Dx of rectal and pharyngeal GC and chlamydia.
- LGV Diagnosis: clinical suspicion is key; other etiologies of presenting syndrome need to be excluded. Specimens should be collected for testing (if available). Genital or lymph node specimens (lesion swab or bubo aspirate) may be tested for *C. trachomatis* by Cx (30%–85% sensitivity), direct immunofluorescence, or nucleic acid detection. NAAT are tests of choice for all chlamydia strains including LGV; NAAT not FDA cleared for detection of *C. trachomatis* rom rectal specimens.
- Genotyping not widely available and should be requested through local state health department (CDC may assist the health department).
- Chlamydia serology (complement fixation test, single L-type immunofluorescence, or microimmunofluorescence) may support the clinical Dx but is not a definitive test; four-fold rise of IgM and IgG antibody is diagnostic of active infection. Single IgM antibody >1:64 or single IgG >1:256 considered positive for invasive disease. Interpretation of results not standardized for LGV and validity in LGV proctitis unknown. Serology has low sensitivity early in disease, but high titers alone without clinical signs/Sx does not confirm infection with LGV. Histology of collected Bx specimens not specific; the Frei test is no longer used.

SELECTED REFERENCES

Workowski KA, Berman S. Sexually transmitted diseases treatment guidelines 2010. *MMWR Recomm Rep*, 2010; 59(RR-12): 1–110.
Comments: These consensus panel guidelines provide a basis for managing most sexually acquired chlamydia infections encountered in practice.

De Vries HJ, Morre SA, White JA, Moi H. European guideline for the management of lymphogranuloma venereum, 2010. *Int J ADIS*. 2010; 8: 533–6.
Comments: European consensus guidelines for Dx and Rx of LGV. As in US, majority of cases are in MSM, and need for anal swabs is stressed.

PATHOGENS

CLOSTRIDIUM DIFFICILE

Robin McKenzie, MD

MICROBIOLOGY

- Spore-forming, anaerobic, Gram-positive rod.
- Produces toxins A and B, which bind to specific receptors in colon. Toxins attack Rho proteins, disrupting actin formation and causing cell death.
- Recent animal studies suggest that toxin B, not toxin A, is essential for virulence.
- Spores contaminate hands and hospital environment. Alcohol and other antiseptic hand rubs may be ineffective in killing spores. Handwashing physically removes spores.
- New hypervirulent strain (REA group B1/PFGE type NAP1) produces higher levels of toxins A and B, and is associated with fluoroquinolone resistance, more severe disease, and higher mortality.

CLINICAL

- Infection usually nosocomially acquired during ABx therapy or within 1–2 mos of stopping ABx. Rare infections occur in previously healthy persons not exposed to healthcare facilities or ABx, including women in peripartum period.
- Fluoroquinolones, clindamycin, cephalosporins, penicillins most commonly associated ABx; but even metronidazole, vancomycin, and some chemotherapeutic meds have been incriminated.
- Up to 1/3 of hospitalized HIV+ patients infected. High infection rates probably result from frequent ABx use and hospitalization. *C. difficile*-associated diarrhea in HIV+ patients not more severe or less responsive to treatment.
- 2/3 of infected patients are asymptomatic carriers and can spread infection to others. About 1/3 of infected patients have Sx: watery diarrhea, abdominal pain, fever, leukocytosis.
- Fulminant colitis (3% of cases) causes severe pain, distention, fever, chills. May lead to perforation, ileus, megacolon, and death.
- Gold standard for Dx is cytotoxin detection in anaerobic tissue culture of stool. Sensitive and specific but expensive and slow (24–48 hr). qPCR assays targeting the toxin B gene are as sensitive and specific, but not generally available.
- Commercial ELISA to detect toxins is quicker and easier. Specific but only 70%–80% sensitive. Detection of toxins A and B preferred since some cases caused by strains that only produce toxin B. Stool Cx is nonspecific: identifies both toxigenic and nontoxigenic strains.
- Sigmoidoscopy/colonoscopy may show normal colon in mild cases, nonspecific colitis, or pseudomembranes (raised yellow plaques). Contraindicated for perforation or toxic megacolon. (Use proctoscopy with minimal insufflation.).
- Abdominal X-ray: look for dilated colon >7 cm in diameter (toxic megacolon), free air (perforation), ileus.
- CT may show thickened bowel wall or nodules. Changes usually seen in colon only and not small bowel. Ascites may be present.

SITES OF INFECTION

- Colon: most common involved site.
- Small intestine: rarely involved.
- Extraintestinal disease: very rare—cellulitis, soft tissue infection, pericarditis, reactive arthritis.

TREATMENT

Initial Episode

- Stop ABx if possible. Consider switching PCP prophylaxis from TMP-SMX to dapsone. If Sx resolve, no further Rx needed.
- For mild cases, begin metronidazole 500 mg PO 3 ×/day or 250 mg PO 4 ×/day × 10 days. (Reserve vancomycin, which is more expensive.)
- For severe illness, increased creatinine, WBC >20,000, or metronidazole-unresponsive disease, begin vancomycin 125–500 mg PO 4 ×/day.
- If underlying ABx cannot be stopped, consider continuing metronidazole or vancomycin until 1 wk after ABx completed.

- PO therapy preferred. If PO treatment not possible, give metronidazole 500 mg IV q6h and/or vancomycin 500 mg 4 ×/day via enema or jejunal tube.
- Maintain normal volume status and electrolytes.
- Antimotility drugs (loperamide, diphenoxylate) contraindicated (increased risk of toxic megacolon).
- Monitor closely for complications: toxic megacolon, perforation, ileus. Danger signs: increasing WBC, elevated creatinine, elevated lactic acid.
- Colectomy (total) may be lifesaving for fulminant colitis and should be considered before WBC >50,000 or lactate >5.

Relapse
- 10%–30% of patients relapse, usually within 2 wks of stopping metronidazole or vancomycin.
- May be due to spores in gut or to reinfection.
- Not associated with ABx resistance. First relapse: retreat w/ metronidazole or vancomycin (equally effective).
- Multiple relapses may respond to vancomycin taper, (allows spores to germinate and then be killed): 125 mg PO 4 ×/day, twice daily, once daily, qod (1 wk at each interval), followed by 125 mg q3 days × 2 wks (6-wk total course).
- Other options: vancomycin 125 mg PO 4 ×/day for 14 days, followed by rifaximin 400 mg twice daily for 14 days; *Saccharomyces boulardii* (a yeast) or *Lactobacillus* strain GG to recolonize colon; or IV gamma globulin 400 mg/kg every 3 wks for 2 or 3 doses to provide antitoxin IgG.

FOLLOW-UP
Possible Relapse
- Do not routinely repeat toxin assay after treatment.
- Patients who relapse once are at risk for multiple relapses.
- If mild Sx recur after treatment, do not treat.
- If moderate-to-severe Sx recur, repeat toxin assay and treat as above if positive.

Complications
- If severe diarrhea, fever, leukocytosis, or abdominal distension persist, evaluate for toxic megacolon.
- Toxic megacolon can occur without diarrhea (pooling of stool in atonic bowel, isolated right-sided colitis).
- Signs of an acute abdomen (decreased bowel sounds, tenderness, rebound, guarding) suggest perforation.
- Persistent diarrhea can cause protein-losing enteropathy w/ hypoalbuminemia, ascites, and peripheral edema.

SELECTED REFERENCES

Lyras D, O'Connor JR, Howarth PM, et al. Toxin B is essential for virulence of *Clostridium difficile*. *Nature*, 2009; 458: 1176–9.

Comments: Contrary to earlier views, this study using well-established hamster model shows that toxin B, not toxin A, is main virulence factor for *C. difficile* disease.

Peterson LR, Robicsek A. Does my patient have *Clostridium difficile* infection? *Ann Intern Med*, 2009; 151: 176–9.

Comments: Recent review reports that commonly used diagnostic methods—ELISA, glutamate dehydrogenase ("common antigen") detection, direct stool cytotoxin assay via tissue Cx—all have limited sensitivity compared to qPCR assays for toxin B or its regulators in stool.

Zar FA, Bakkanagari SR, Moorthi KM, et al. A comparison of vancomycin and metronidazole for the treatment of *Clostridium difficile*-associated diarrhea, stratified by disease severity. *Clin Infect Dis*, 2007; 45: 302–7.

Comments: Randomized, double-blind, placebo-controlled trial in which 150 subjects stratified for mild or severe disease were treated with metronidazole 250 mg PO 4 ×/day or vancomycin 125 mg PO 4 ×/day. Cure rates for mild disease were 90% and 98% (P = 0.36) and for severe disease were 76% and 97% (P = 0.02). Severe disease was defined as presence of pseudomembranes, ICU admission, or 2 of the following: age >60, T >38.3, albumin <2.5, or WBC >15,000. This trial supports use of vancomycin for severe disease.

PATHOGENS

HAEMOPHILUS INFLUENZAE

Paul G. Auwaerter, MD

MICROBIOLOGY

- Small aerobic Gram-negative coccobacilli found mainly in human respiratory tract.
- Encapsulated, type b strain accounts for most bacteremic pneumonia and invasive disease, whereas nonencapsulated strains mostly cause otitis media, sinusitis, AECB, and pneumonia.
- Sensitivity of Gram stain and Cx probably ~50% in patients with *H. influenzae* pneumonia. Use of prior ABx decreases yield.

CLINICAL

- Up to 80% may be carriers of nontypeable *H. influenzae*. Colonization of type b strains (which account for most invasive disease) reduced considerably in children (<1%) w/ introduction of conjugate vaccine.
- Most infections (about 2/3) caused by nontypeable strains.
- HIV appears to be a risk factor for developing invasive disease due to *H. influenzae* type b, especially bacteremic pneumonia. However, *H. influenzae* type b remains rare, so immunization unwarranted in adults.
- Pneumonia may occasionally mimic PCP with bilateral interstitial infiltrates.
- TMP/SMX may reduce risk of community-acquired pneumonia.
- Azithromycin or clarithromycin prophylaxis may reduce infection, but no data.

SITES OF INFECTION

- Community-acquired pneumonia (CAP): *H. influenzae* responsible for 3%–40% of HIV-related bacterial pneumonia.
- Acute exacerbations of chronic bronchitis (AECB): increased colonization in smokers.
- Bacterial bronchitis.
- Acute bacterial sinusitis.
- Meningitis.
- Epiglottitis.
- Acute otitis media.
- Periorbital cellulitis: mainly children, diminished since introduction of immunization.
- Septic arthritis: rare.
- Conjunctivitis: *H. influenzae* biogroup *aegyptius* may cause severe conjunctivitis (aka Brazilian purpuric fever) mostly in children. Described in South America, but may occur elsewhere.

TREATMENT

Respiratory Infections (Mild to Moderate)

- **Preferred:** amoxicillin/clavulanate 875 mg PO q12h or oral cephalosporin (e.g., cefuroxime 250–500 mg PO twice daily or cefixime, cefpodoxime, cefaclor, loracarbef).
- **Alternative:** FQ (e.g., levofloxacin 500 mg PO once daily, moxifloxacin 400 mg PO once daily). Macrolides (azithromycin 500 mg then 250 mg once daily × 5–10 days, clarithromycin 500 mg PO twice daily × 7–10 days) cover >80% strains; beware of drug interactions with these drugs.
- Avoid ampicillin/amoxicillin for significant infections, as resistance rates can be >40% due to beta-lactamase production. Resistance to TMP-SMX may be more common in HIV+ patients.

Severe Infections (Pneumonia, Meningitis, Epiglottis)

- Life-threatening illnesses treated with parenteral therapy: ceftriaxone 1–2 g IV once daily or cefotaxime 2 g IV q4–6h or ampicillin-sulbactam or parenteral FQ (levofloxacin 750 mg IV or moxifloxacin 400 mg IV q24h).
- Dexamethasone 0.6 mg/kg/day IV in 4 divided doses for children >2 mos w/ *H. influenzae* type B (Hib) meningitis: decreases risk of deafness/neurological sequelae.

Prevention

- Children: Hib vaccines available include monovalent Hib vaccine (*ActHib*) and combination product DTaP-IPV/Hib (*Pentacel*). These are recommended at ages 2 mos, 4 mos, 6 mos, and 12–15 mos. HIV+ children are viewed as being at high risk of infection, and should not skip booster doses in case of vaccine shortages. Booster doses can be made up with wany product.
- **Note:** the monovalent Hib vaccine (*PedvaxHib*), may be available for providers serving American Indian/Alaska Native children through states' immunization programs from the VFC Pediatric Vaccine Stockpile. The vaccine schedule is the same as above.

- Adults: Hib vaccine not recommended because most infections are with nonencapsulated strains not covered by vaccine.
- With invasive Hib disease, unimmunized contacts (adults and children <48 mos) should receive rifampin prophylaxis 20 mg/kg/day (600 mg max) × 4 days to eradicate carrier state and reduce secondary cases. Contact defined as spending >4 h/ day for at least 5/7 days preceding hospitalization of index case.
- Chemoprophylaxis not recommended if all household contacts <48 mos have completed immunization series.
- Effectiveness of rifampin only if taken within 7 days of index case hospitalization.

OTHER INFORMATION
- With introduction of infant immunization program w/ Hib vaccine, childhood meningitis, epiglottitis, bacteremia, and arthritis now all uncommon.

SELECTED REFERENCES

Centers for Disease Control, 2011. Recommended adult immunization schedule 2011. June 7, 2011. *www.cdc.gov/vaccines/recs/schedules/adult-schedule.htm*. Accessed August 10, 2011.
Comments: *H. influenza* type b is not a routine vaccination for adults. For child recommendations, see *www.cdc.gov/vaccines/recs/schedules/child-schedule.htm*.

LISTERIA MONOCYTOGENES

Khalil G. Ghanem, MD, PhD

MICROBIOLOGY
- A small nonsporulating, catalase positive, Gram-positive bacillus.
- In clinical specimens, it may appear as a Gram-variable coccus, diplococcus, or diphtheroid.
- 7 spp. identified; in general, only *L. monocytogenes* pathogenic in humans.
- Grows well at 4–10°C (i.e., routine temperatures in refrigerators).
- Widespread in nature; recovered from raw vegetables, unpasteurized milk, meats, fish, and poultry. Person-to-person transmission unlikely (except vertically from mother to infant).

CLINICAL
- HIV+ patients have 60 to >150-fold increased risk of infection, especially w/ advanced immunosuppression (CD4 <50–100).
- Routine TMP-SMX prophylaxis may prevent infections in those at highest risk, which may explain relatively low incidence.
- Up to 60% of systemic infections (bacteremia, endocarditis, and CNS infections) may be preceded by gastroenteritis with fever.
- Seizures (~25%) and movement disorders (15%–20%) not uncommon w/ CNS infections; may also mimic basilar meningitis seen w/ TB.
- Dx: blood and CSF Cx; CSF shows PMN predominance; in 30% of cases, monos may predominate. CSF Gram stain may show no organisms (~70%), or may show small Gram-positive to Gram-variable bacilli/coccobacilli/diphtheroids.

SITES OF INFECTION
- CNS: meningitis, meningoencephalitis, rhombencephalitis (cranial nerve palsies, cerebellar signs, and hemiparesis), cerebritis and abscesses (unlike other bacteria, subcortical abscesses occur, but rarely).
- Cardiovascular: bacteremia, endocarditis, myocarditis (rare), arteritis (rare).
- Skin: skin infections.
- GI: gastroenteritis, hepatic abscesses and cholecystitis (rare).
- Eyes: conjunctivitis and endophthalmitis.
- Bone: osteomyelitis and septic arthritis.
- Lung: pleuropulmonary infections.
- GU: involvement of placenta leading to neonatal death; chorioamnionitis.

TREATMENT
Prevention
- Adapted from Lorber B; Listeriosis; *Clin Infect Dis*; 1997;24:1–9.

PATHOGENS

- Thoroughly cook all meat and poultry.
- Wash all raw vegetables.
- Avoid unpasteurized milk products.
- Avoid soft cheeses (cream cheese, yogurt, and cottage cheese are safe).
- Avoid deli meats, or heat thoroughly before consuming.

Treatment

- No randomized controlled trials comparing treatment regimens.
- Ampicillin is drug of choice; TMP-SMX is alternative.
- Meningitis: ampicillin 2 g IV q4h + gentamicin 1.7 mg/kg q8h × 3 wks OR TMP-SMX 15–20 mg/kg/day divided q8h. If abscess, treat until abscess disappears (~6 wks).
- No data on once-daily aminoglycoside dosing.
- Endocarditis: ampicillin + gentamicin × 4–6 wks (same dose as above).
- Bacteremia without CNS involvement or endocarditis: ampicillin × 2 wks.

FOLLOW-UP

- ART w/ immune reconstitution may decrease risk of infection.
- In 1 study, mortality in HIV+ patients (~29%) higher than in HIV-negative patients (~17%).

OTHER INFORMATION

- Immunity to *Listeria* has been shown to be cell-mediated.
- Other at-risk groups include infants, the elderly, and pregnant women in addition to immunocompromised patients.
- Cephalosporins and older generation fluoroquinolones have inadequate activity against *L. monocytogenes* and should not be used. Limited data on newer fluoroquinolones *in vivo*.

SELECTED REFERENCES

Drevets DA, Bronze MS. *Listeria monocytogenes*: epidemiology, human disease, and mechanisms of brain invasion. *FEMS Immunol Med Microbiol*, 2008; 53: 151–65.
Comments: Comprehensive article reviews salient epidemiologic and clinical manifestations of *L. monocytogenes* infections, and summarizes molecular mechanisms involved in human disease.

Goulet V, Hedberg C, Le Monnier A, et al. Increasing incidence of listeriosis in France and other European countries. *Emerg Infect Dis*, 2008; 14: 734–40.
Comments: Authors report that incidence of listeriosis in France and 8 other European countries has been increasing, most evident among adults >60 and not associated with foodborne outbreaks or pregnancy.

MYCOBACTERIUM KANSASII

Christopher J. Hoffmann, MD, MPH

MICROBIOLOGY

- Slow-growing mycobacterium (2–6 wks in Cx).
- Acid-fast rod on Kinyoun or Ziehl-Neelsen staining.
- Water is major environmental reservoir, infection probably through aerosol route.

CLINICAL

- 2nd most common cause of nontuberculous mycobacterial disease in HIV/AIDS patients in USA (after MAC). Usually causes lung disease, but disseminated disease also occurs.
- In HIV+ patients, single + Cx may indicate disease.
- Dx: mycobacterial Cx from infected site. 2007 ATS criteria for non-HIV: (1) compatible Sx or parenchymal lung abnormalities on imaging; (2) 2+ positive sputa or 1+ from BAL; and (3) exclusion of other diseases. (these criteria may be too strict for HIV+ patients).
- On AFB microscopy may appear longer and wider than *M. tuberculosis*, but this feature not reliable enough for Dx.
- No FDA approved rapid tests for species-specific Dx from primary clinical specimen.
- Disease typically with CD4 <200 (most often <50). Typical clinical presentation: fever, cough, pulmonary infiltrates, and/or cavities. CXR: >50% bilateral disease with consolidation of nodules or effusion. Cavitation <10%. Normal <10%.
- Clinical features similar to TB. Primarily pulmonary disease, but can also disseminate.

- DDx: TB, other nontuberculous mycobacterial diseases, lymphoma, nocardiosis, histoplasmosis, coccidiodomycosis, bacterial pneumonia.

SITES OF INFECTION

- Lung: most common site. Cavitary disease with higher CD4, alveolar or interstitial infiltrates with lower CD4. CXR normal in about 10%.
- Disseminated disease: can occur with CD4 <100; usually with concomitant pulmonary disease.
- Bone: osteomyelitis can occur.
- CNS: CNS disease can occur.

TREATMENT

Standard Treatment Regimen (Am J Respir Crit Care Med, 2007; 175: 367–416)

- Rifampin (10 mg/kg/day or 600 mg max PO once daily) + isoniazid (5 mg/kg/day or 300 mg max PO once daily + pyridoxine 50 mg PO once daily) + ethambutol (15 mg/kg/day) + pyridoxine (50 mg/day). 2 mos of initial ethambutol 25 mg/kg/day no longer recommended. Treatment endpoint: 12 m of negative sputa.
- Consider adding clarithromycin (500 mg twice daily) for severe disease and very low CD4.
- Rifampin resistant disease: 3-drug regimen including clarithromycin or azithromycin, moxifloxacin, ethambutol, sulfamethoxozole, or streptomycin (based on susceptibility testing). Cure less likely than with rifampin-based regimen.

DRUG-DRUG INTERACTIONS

- RIF not recommended with DLV, APV, FPV, ATV, IDV, NFV, SQV, TPV, NVP, ETR. Use with caution and monitor liver enzymes if used with LPV/r + RTV 300 mg twice daily. RIF + NVP not recommended, but some may consider using in resource-limited setting based on a small case series showing success. Interaction between DRV and RIF not well characterized, however not recommended combination.
- RIF + EFV: RIF standard dose, EFV 800 mg once daily.
- Rifabutin is alternative to RIF with APV, FPV, ATV, IDV, NFV, RTV, TPV, DRV or LPV/r but must adjust rifabutin dose (see specific drug modules for dose recommendations).
- No significant drug-drug interactions between RIF and NRTIs or ENF.

Other Considerations

- Treat >18 mos (>12 mos after Cx converts to negative).
- Immune reconstitution inflammatory syndrome (IRIS) can occur after starting either mycobacterial or ART.

FOLLOW-UP

- For pulmonary disease, obtain sputum AFB smear and Cx monthly until 3 consecutive negative Cx.
- Monitor LFTs in patients on INH and/or RIF; monitor for retinal toxicity (Snellen and Ishihara tests) monthly while on EMB.
- May take 2–4 mos for Cx to convert to negative. If still positive after 4 mos, obtain repeat susceptibility testing.

OTHER INFORMATION

- Acquired drug resistance associated with treatment failure or relapse. Avoid addition of a single drug to a failing regimen.

SELECTED REFERENCES

Cattamanchi A, Nahid P, Marras TK, et al. Detailed analysis of the radiographic presentation of *Mycobacterium kansasii* lung disease in patients with HIV infection. *Chest*, 2008; 133: 875–80.
Comments: Description of CXR findings with *M. kansasii* among HIV+ patients in San Francisco.

Griffith DE, Aksamit T, Brown-Elliott BA, et al. An official ATS/IDSA statement: diagnosis, treatment, and prevention of nontuberculous mycobacterial diseases. *Am J Respir Crit Care Med*, 2007; 175: 367–416.
Comments: ATS guidelines for diagnosing and managing NTM disease.

Levine B, Chaisson RE. *Mycobacterium kansasii*: a cause of treatable pulmonary disease associated with advanced human immunodeficiency virus (HIV) infection. *Ann Intern Med*, 1991; 114: 861–8.
Comments: Retrospective case series: among 19 HIV+ patients w/ *M. kansasii* disease, 14 had only pulmonary disease, 2 had only extrapulmonary disease, and 3 had both. Median CD4 49. Ten patients treated with anti-TB drugs; all improved. Among 9 untreated patients, 2 developed progressive cavitary pulmonary disease and died from *M. kansasii*.

PATHOGENS

MYCOBACTERIUM SPP.

Christopher J. Hoffmann, MD, MPH

MICROBIOLOGY

- *Mycobacteria* spp. divided into rapid growers (<7 days) and slow growers (>7 days) based on time to mature growth on agar plates.
- Rapid growing: *M. fortuitum* (3–7 days) and *M. chelonae.*
- Slow growing: *M. gordonae* (7–10 days), *M. malmoense, M. marinum* (7–10 days), *M. ulcerans* and *M. xenopi* (3–8 wks in Cx), *M. terrae, M. nonchromogenicum.*
- Very slow growing: *M. genavense.* Alert lab: requires incubation in broth media for >8 wks.
- *M. haemophilum:* "blood-loving," slow growing. Alert lab: requires ferric iron supplementation and temperature 30°C.
- Risk for nontuberculous mycobacterial (NTM) disease in HIV+ patients is directly proportional to CD4 count. Invasive non-TB disease rare with CD4 count >50 (except for *M. marinum*) and Sx usually chronic (>30 days) prior to Dx. High CD4 and short duration of Sx make NTM unlikely cause of illness; in this setting positive sputum isolates more likely to be colonizers or contaminants.

CLINICAL

- *M. abscessus:* causes skin and soft tissue disease, lymphadenitis, and pulmonary disease.
- *M. chelonae:* causes skin and soft tissue disease and lymphadenitis.
- *M. fortuitum:* cutaneous disease (cellulitis, abscesses, ulcers) most common and can have contiguous spread to bones/joints; catheter-related infections, disseminated disease, lymphadenitis less common; pulmonary disease rare. Institutional/nosocomial disease outbreaks due to contaminated water have been reported.
- *M. genovense:* typically CD4 <50. Similar manifestations to MAC—fever, weight loss, abdominal pain, anemia, lymphadenopathy, diarrhea, splenomegaly. Abdominal lymphadenopathy and splenomegaly often more pronounced than MAC. Also causes cutaneous infections. Can be associated with IRIS. Cx of liver or bone marrow more sensitive than blood Cx.
- *M. gordonae:* rare cause of human disease—isolation from clinical specimen usually represents environmental contamination from water.
- *M. haemophilum:* cutaneous disease with multiple papules, nodules, or ulcerations, often overlying joints. Also causes arthritis, osteomyelitis, pulmonary disease, and disseminated infection. Suspect if prior clinical specimens AFB smear positive but Cx-negative (requires iron enriched culture media).
- *M. marinum:* cutaneous plaques, any CD4 count.
- *M. malmoense:* rare cause of pulmonary, lymphadenitis, disseminated infection. Most reports of disease in northern and western European Union.
- *M. ulcerans:* causes Buruli ulcer, cause of subcutaneous nodules which progress to indurated plaques and eventually undermined ulcerations, and rarely, osteomyelitis. Mostly occurs in tropical Africa. No difference in presentation noted between HIV-uninfected and HIV-infected individuals. Not transmitted person-to-person.
- *M. xenopi:* occurs at low CD4, pulmonary most common usually with pulmonary nodules or diffuse reticulonodular disease; may resemble TB. Disseminated disease can occur. However, is often a contaminant. Outbreaks associated with hot water taps, bronchoscopes in institutions. Significance of positive respiratory Cxs should be carefully considered. In symptomatic patients with abnormal CXR, repeated isolation from respiratory specimens usually indicates disease if no alternative etiology.

TREATMENT

M. abscessus, M. chelonae

- No consensus. Clarithromycin 500 mg PO twice daily for 6 mos. For serious infections, add tobramycin + imipenum for 1st 2–6 wks.

M. fortuitum

- Localized, limited skin disease: monotherapy with clarithromycin 500 mg PO twice daily, trimethoprim/sulfamethoxazole DS 1 tab PO twice daily, or doxycycline 100 mg PO twice daily; duration typically 3–4 mos.

- Severe disease: amikacin (15 mg/kg q day) plus either beta-lactam (cefoxitin 2 g q6h or imipenem 1 g q6h) or fluoroquinolone (moxifloxacin 400 mg PO once daily) until clinical improvement, then oral therapy with at least 2 drugs; duration typically 6–12 mos.
- Use *in vitro* susceptibility tests to guide ABx selection.

M. haemophilum
- Clarithromycin: 500 mg PO twice daily + rifampin (RIF) 600 mg PO once daily + moxifloxacin 400 mg PO once daily ± amikacin 15–20 mg/kg IV once daily.
- Cycloserine: (250 mg PO twice daily) active *in vitro*.

M. genavense
- Clarithromycin: 500 mg PO twice daily + RIF 600 mg PO once daily + ethambutol (EMB) 15 mg/kg PO once daily.
- Duration: indefinite if no immune reconstitution. If immune reconstitution, consider stopping if treated >1 yr + CD4 >100 for 3–6 mos + asymptomatic.
- *M. genavense* associated with IRIS: treat as for IRIS with MAC (see 6–7). Typically can continue ART and antimycobacterial treatment; treat Sx with NSAIDS. Some patients require steroids.

M. gordonae
- No consensus. Isoniazid (INH) 300 mg PO once daily + RIF 600 mg PO once daily + EMB 15 mg/kg PO once daily + streptomycin (SM) 15 mg/kg once daily (*Clin Infect Dis* 1992;14:1229).
- Clarithromycin: active *in vitro*.

M. marinum
- Clarithromycin: 500 mg PO twice daily or RIF 600 mg PO once daily + EMB 15 mg/kg PO once daily. All therapy for at least 3 mos.

M. malmoense
- Clarithromycin: 500 mg PO twice daily + RIF 600 mg PO once daily + EMB 15 mg/kg PO once daily.
- Alternatives: SM 15 mg/kg once daily; INH 300 mg PO once daily (+ vitamin B6 50 mg PO once daily).
- Duration: prolonged (at least 18–24 mos), and indefinite if no immune reconstitution.

M. ulcerans
- Surgical excision. Antimicrobial therapy not successful.

M. xenopi
- Clarithromycin 500 mg PO twice daily + RIF 600 mg PO once daily + EMB 25 mg/kg q day for 2 mos then 15 mg/kg once daily ± SM 15 mg/kg 3 ×/wk (*Am J Respir Crit Care Med* 1997;156:S1).
- Duration: prolonged (2 yrs or more). High rates of failure and relapse.
- Moxifloxacin: active *in vitro*.

FOLLOW-UP
- *M. genavense*: follow for improvement in symptoms, and conversion of blood cultures to negative. Monitor LFTs on rifampin; monitor visual acuity and color vision monthly on ethambutol.
- *M. gordonae*: monitor LFTs on isoniazid, rifampin; visual acuity and color vision monthly on ethambutol; vestibular and renal function on streptomycin.
- *M. haemophilum*: monitor LFTs on rifampin, renal function on amikacin.
- *M. malmoense*: monitor LFTs on rifampin and isoniazid; monitor visual acuity and color vision monthly on ethambutol.
- *M. xenopi*: monitor sputum cultures monthly until 3 consecutive negatives. Monitor LFTs on rifampin; visual acuity and color vision monthly on ethambutol; vestibular and renal function on streptomycin.

SELECTED REFERENCES

Alvarez-Uria G, Falcó V, Martín-Casabona N, et al. Non-tuberculous mycobacteria in the sputum of HIV-infected patients: infection or colonization? *Int J STD AIDS*, 2009; 20: 193–5.

Comments: Study of colonization vs invasive disease among hospitalized patients with mycobacterial sputum Cx.

Thomsen VO, Dragsted UB, Bauer J, et al. Disseminated infection with *Mycobacterium genavense*: a challenge to physicians and mycobacteriologists. *J Clin Microbiol*, 1999; 37: 3901–5.

PATHOGENS

Comments: For Dx of *M. genavense* disease, shortest Cx detection times and highest Cx recovery rates were from liver and bone marrow specimens (vs blood). Liver: 75% of specimens Cx positive, median time 6 days to positive Cx. Bone marrow: 70% of specimens Cx positive, median time 15 days. Blood: 25% Cx positive, median time 46 days.

el-Helou P, Rachlis A, Fong I, et al. *Mycobacterium xenopi* infection in patients with human immunodeficiency virus infection. *Clin Infect Dis*, 1997; 25: 206–10.
Comments: Description of clinical spectrum of *M. xenopi* infection among HIV+ patients in a region where *M. xenopi* relatively common. Among 24 patients with 1 or more positive respiratory Cx, 75% felt to have colonization, 25% (all with advanced AIDS) deemed to have disease.

Saubolle MA, Kiehn TE, White MH, et al. *Mycobacterium haemophilum*: microbiology and expanding clinical and geographic spectra of disease in humans. *Clin Microbiol Rev*, 1996; 9: 435–47.
Comments: Good review of microbiology and clinical manifestations of *M. haemophilum*.

Bessesen MT, Shlay J, Stone-Venohr B, et al. Disseminated *Mycobacterium genavense* infection: clinical and microbiological features and response to therapy. *AIDS*, 1993; 7: 1357–61.
Comments: For treatment of *M. genavense* disease, clarithromycin-containing regimens associated with clinical improvement and clearance of mycobacteremia.

NEISSERIA GONORRHOEAE

Khalil G. Ghanem, MD, PhD

MICROBIOLOGY
- Nonmotile, nonspore-forming, Gram-negative diplococcus.
- Infects cuboidal and columnar epithelium leading to a vigorous inflammatory response.
- Selective growth media (Thayer-Martin and New York City) most common; Cx routinely available in Dx of GC infection in settings that can process specimens appropriately. Swabs from urethral, cervical, rectal, pharyngeal, and ocular sites can be Cx'd.
- Nonamplified molecular testing, including EIA and DNA hybridization probes, may be used. Cervical and urethral swabs can be tested.
- Nucleic acid amplification tests (NAATs) are the gold standard and may be performed on urethral swabs, cervical swabs, urine, and self-collected vaginal swabs; CDC recommends their use on rectal and pharyngeal swabs even though they are not FDA cleared for that indication.

CLINICAL
- Sx in men: acute urethritis (purulent urethral discharge, dysuria) is predominant manifestation; incubation 2–7 days; 10% of epididymitis in young men due to GC; asymptomatic infection less common than in women (up to 30%).
- Sx in women: asymptomatic (up to 90% in some studies); vaginal discharge, dysuria, spotting. PID is serious complication of ascending infection.
- Anorectal: may be only site of infection in up to 40% of MSM and 5% of women. Sx may include tenesmus, purulent discharge, and rectal bleeding, though most asymptomatic.
- Disseminated GC infection (DGI): asymmetrical migratory polyarthritis (knees, elbows), tenosynovitis, and dermatitis (hemorrhagic papules/pustules); blood Cx positive in 50%; >80% of mucosal Cx are positive; joint fluid findings: >50,000 PMNs and Cx usually positive.
- Gram stain (urethra) >90% sensitive in symptomatic men, less sensitive (40%–60%) in women (endocervical site) and asymptomatic men (~50%–70% sensitivity); NAATs have >95% sensitivity and ~99% specificity in both symptomatic and asymptomatic patients.
- NAATs from oropharyngeal or rectal sites not currently FDA licensed; but CDC considers them the test of choice for detecting extragenital infections; most commercial labs provide these tests.

SITES OF INFECTION
- GU: urethritis, epididymitis, cervicitis, Skene's and Bartholin's gland infections, endometritis, salpingitis, pelvic peritonitis, and tubo-ovarian abscess.
- CV: DGI; endocarditis (rare).
- GI: gingivitis (rare), pharyngitis, proctitis, and perihepatitis (Fitz-Hugh-Curtis syndrome).

- Musculoskeletal: osteomyelitis (rare) and septic arthritis.
- Eyes: conjunctivitis.
- CNS: meningitis (very rare).

TREATMENT

Drug Resistance

- ~18% of strains in the US resistant to PCN, TCN, or both.
- Fluoroquinolone-resistant *N. gonorrhoeae* (FQRNG) strains are now widespread in US, Asia, and Europe.
- Increase in azithromycin resistance in the past several years; cases reported in California and Hawaii.
- Cephalosporin (ceftriaxone and cefixime) resistance in Japan and Europe has been reported; no resistance reported in US in 2009, but MICs to cephalosporins are increasing.

General Principles

- Prevention: condoms highly effective at preventing transmission.
- Treatment recommendations for HIV-infected patients similar to uninfected patients.
- Dual therapy using a cephalosporin (preferably ceftriaxone) and a macrolide is now recommended by the CDC for the treatment of GC (even if concomitant *Chlamydia trachomatis* infection is ruled out).
- PCN, FQ, and TCN should not be used.
- Spectinomycin is no longer available in the US.
- Azithromycin (2 g orally in a single dose) is the only alternate agent that may be used in cephalosporin-allergic patients.

Antimicrobial Therapy

- From: CDC. Sexually transmitted diseases treatment guidelines 2010. *MMWR* 2010:59 (No. RR-12).
- Uncomplicated urethral, cervical, anorectal, and oropharyngeal infections: ceftriaxone 250 mg IM × 1 (preferred) OR cefixime 400 mg PO × 1 (alternate) PLUS Azithromycin 1g PO × 1.
- DGI: ceftriaxone 1 g IV q12h until clinical response, then switch to PO cefixime 400 mg twice-daily to complete a 7 day course.
- GC conjunctivitis: ceftriaxone 1 g IM × 1.
- PID outpatient: ceftriaxone 250 mg IM × 1 + doxycycline 100 mg PO twice-daily +/− metronidazole 500 mg PO twice-daily × 14 days.
- PID inpatient: clindamycin 900 mg IV q8h + gentamicin 2 mg/kg IV × 1 loading, then 1.7mg/kg IV q8h (monitor levels) once daily gentamicin (5 mg/kg) OR cefotetan 2 g IV q12h + doxycycline 100 mg IV/PO q12h. Can switch to PO doxycycline 24–48 hrs after clinical improvement to complete a 14 day course.

FOLLOW-UP

- No test of cure necessary after Rx.
- Repeat NAATs should not be performed within 2 wks after Rx as persistent nucleic acid can give false-positive results.
- All sex partners in past 60 days should be tested and treated presumptively if follow-up uncertain.
- Persistent Sx despite adequate therapy and no reexposure warrants Cx with susceptibility testing.
- Outpatient Rx of PID warrants F/U within 72 hrs to ensure clinical improvement.

OTHER INFORMATION

- Updated information on gonorrhea can be found at: *www.cdc.gov/std/Gonorrhea/*.

SELECTED REFERENCES

Centers for Disease Control and Prevention (CDC): Cephalosporin susceptibility among Neisseria gonorrhoeae isolates—United States, 2000–2010. *MMWR* 60:873, 2011.
Comments: This paper demonstrates the increasing MICs of N. gonorrhoeae strains in the U.S. to cephalosporins. Of note, no cases of cephalosporin resistant GC were documented.

Centers for Disease Control and Prevention (CDC): Neisseria gonorrhoeae with reduced susceptibility to azithromycin—San Diego County, California, 2009. *MMWR* 60:579, 2011.
Comments: This report from the CDC highlights the emerging problem of azithromycin-resistant strains in California.

PATHOGENS

Centers for Disease Control and Prevention (CDC). Update to CDC's sexually transmitted diseases treatment guidelines, 2006: fluoroquinolones no longer recommended for treatment of gonococcal infections. *MMWR*, 2007; 56: 332–6.
Comments: The CDC no longer recommends FQ as first-line agents for treating gonorrhea in the US.

Gunn RA, O'Brien CJ, Lee MA, et al. Gonorrhea screening among men who have sex with men: value of multiple anatomic site testing, San Diego, California, 1997–2003. *Sex Transm Dis*, 2008; 35: 845–8.
Comments: 33% of total gonorrhea cases among gay men would have been missed if urethra had been the only site tested for GC. Rectal and pharyngeal sites significantly increased the yield.

PSEUDOMONAS AERUGINOSA

Khalil G. Ghanem, MD, PhD

MICROBIOLOGY

- Aerobic, motile, oxidase-positive, Gram-negative rod, 0.5–0.8 mcm × 1.5–3 mcm.
- Isolated from soil, water, plants, and animals—including humans (especially moist sites such as perineum, axillae, and ears).
- Thrives in moist environments of the hospital (respiratory equipment, clean solutions, disinfectants, sinks, mops, food) and the community (swimming pools, whirlpools, hot tubs, contact lens solutions).
- Defects in humoral and cellular immunity, loss of mucosal integrity, and leukocyte abnormalities, especially w/ advanced HIV disease, may predispose to infection.
- Drug resistance is common and based on permeability changes of the outer membrane, efflux pumps, and beta-lactamases. Multidrug-resistant strains becoming more common.

CLINICAL

- Infections, both nosocomial and community acquired, are associated w/ HIV infection, leukopenia, and especially advanced immunosuppression.
- Both bacteremic (central lines, pneumonia, skin, UTI) and nonbacteremic (sinusitis, pneumonia and skin) forms of *P. aeruginosa* infection occur.
- Risk factors: antibiotic use, indwelling vascular catheters, hospitalization, leukopenia, immunosuppression.
- Dx: Cx (blood, urine, sputum) mandatory before therapy; assess ABx susceptibility in view of increasing resistance.

SITES OF INFECTION

- Respiratory: bronchitis; pneumonia (often recurrent and/or chronic); similar to patients w/ CF; lobar, cavitary, diffuse interstial, bronchiectatic, and empyemas all reported.
- Skin: papules, nodules, folliculitis, abscesses, and ecthyma gangrenosum (usually as a result of systemic infection).
- ENT: orbital cellulitis; sinusitis (recurrent and/or chronic); parapharyngeal abscesses, and malignant otitis externa, particularly in diabetic patients.
- GU: complicated UTI, pyelonephritis.
- Bone: osteomyelitis.
- CV: endocarditis mostly in IDU.

TREATMENT

General Principles

- Combination therapy usually preferred, especially w/ serious infections, and as initial therapy for all infections while awaiting susceptibility testing. However, prospective data on combination therapy lacking (*Clin Infect Dis* 16:404, 1993).
- Combination therapy, if used, should include synergistic drugs such as beta-lactams + aminoglycosides. Surgical intervention should supplement ABx therapy in cases of infected fluid collections.
- Duration of therapy depends on extent of infection and host-related factors. (immunosuppression status). HIV-infected patients w/ advanced immunosuppression may require longer courses (3–4 wks).

- Consider hospital and community resistance patterns when choosing initial Rx for suspected *P. aeruginosa* infections. Modify Rx based on susceptibility testing.

Antimicrobials

- Antipseudomonal penicillins: piperacillin (200–300 mg/kg/day divided q4h up to 500 mg/kg /day, usually 3 g q4h); ticarcillin (3 g q4h).
- Cephalosporins: ceftazidime (2 g q8h), cefepime (2 g q8h).
- Carbapenems: imipenem (0.5 g q6h), meropenem (1 g q8h); ertapenem should not be used.
- Monobactams: aztreonam (up to 2 g q6h). Note: High resistance.
- Aminoglycosides: should be used at therapeutic once-daily dosing (gentamicin and tobramycin 5.1 mg/kg/day).
- Fluoroquinolones: based on susceptibility pattern. Ciprofloxacin tends to have better antipseudomonal activity.
- Dose adjustments should be made based on creatinine clearance and liver function, as appropriate.
- When extensive resistance precludes use of above drugs, colistin (2.5–5 mg/kd/d given q12h) is an option (*Clin Infect Dis* 14:403, 1992).

Follow-up

- Expect recurrences in HIV-infected patients w/ persistent immunosuppression (20%–40% recurrence rates documented).
- No formal recommendations for secondary prophylaxis; decisions should be tailored based on clinical setting.

Selected References

Falagas ME, Kasiakou SK Colistin: the revival of polymyxins for the management of multidrug-resistant gram-negative bacterial infections. *Clin Infect Dis*, 2005; 40: 1333–41.
Comments: Polymyxins active against selected Gram-negative bacteria, including *Acinetobacter* spp., *Pseudomonas aeruginosa*, *Klebsiella* spp., and *Enterobacter* spp. These drugs have been used extensively worldwide for decades. However, parenteral use of these drugs associated w/ nephrotoxicity and neurotoxicity.

Hidron AI, Edwards JR, Patel J, et al. NHSN annual update: antimicrobial-resistant pathogens associated with healthcare-associated infections: annual summary of data reported to the National Healthcare Safety Network at the Centers for Disease Control and Prevention, 2006–2007. *Infect Control Hosp Epidemiol*, 2008; 29: 996–1011.
Comments: Recent surveillance study of pathogens causing device-associated and procedure-associated healthcare-associated infections (HAIs) reported by hospitals in the National Healthcare Safety Network (NHSN) that highlights the emergence of carbapenem-resistant *P. aeruginosa* (2%).

Klibanov OM, Raasch RH, Rublein JC. Single versus combined antibiotic therapy for gram-negative infections. *Ann Pharmacother*, 2004; 38: 332–7.
Comments: Recent review suggests that although most studies were not randomized, double-blind, or controlled, monotherapy with agents active against isolated organisms, including *P. aeruginosa*, may be appropriate for most patients. Efficacy outcomes did not significantly differ in most studies comparing single and combination therapies. Some trials suggest that combination therapy may be preferred in neutropenic patients and those with pseudomonal infections.

RHODOCOCCUS EQUI

Eric Nuermberger, MD

Microbiology

- Pleomorphic Gram-positive bacillus, weakly acid-fast.
- Grows well on ordinary media, but may be mistaken as diphtheroid contaminant.
- Rarely isolated from healthy persons, suspect immunosuppressive condition.
- Soil inhabitant; infection typically via inhalation, but may be via inoculation or ingestion.
- Recognized equine pathogen, but only 20%–30% of infected humans have contact with horses.

Clinical

- CXR: unilobar nodular infiltrate or consolidation, often upper lobe, frequently cavitates, TB mimic; may see multilobar involvement or pleural effusion.

PATHOGENS

- High-resolution chest CT also may show ground-glass opacities, centrilobular nodules, or tree-in-bud appearance.
- Dx may require invasive procedure, but blood Cx positive in up to 2/3 of HIV+ patients.
- Histopathology: dense histiocytic infiltrate with necrosis, intracellular bacteria; may see PAS+ macrophages or malakoplakia (histiocytic aggregates with basophilic cytoplasmic inclusions laminated with calcium, iron).
- 2/3 of *R. equi* infections are in HIV+ patients; CD4 typically <100.
- Mortality 55% in pre-HAART era.
- Rare OI, incidence: 3/1000 in hospitalized AIDS patients.

SITES OF INFECTION

- Lung: most common site (approximately 80%); often insidious fever, cough, fatigue, weight loss.
- Cutaneous: nodule, abscess, ulcer at inoculation site or with disseminated disease.
- Musculoskeletal: osteomyelitis, septic arthritis, psoas abscess.
- Adenitis: cervical, mesenteric.
- Less common: nodule or abscess in brain, liver, spleen, kidney, prostate after dissemination.
- DDx: TB, other mycobacterial infections, fungal infections, actinomycosis, nocardiosis, lung abscess, lung cancer, lymphoma, metastatic neoplasm.

TREATMENT

General Principles

- No treatment standard established.
- Susceptibility testing recommended to guide therapy and to investigate treatment failures.
- Combination therapy strongly recommended to prevent emergence of resistance.
- Begin with 2–3 parenteral agents for 2–4 wks, then change to 2-drug oral regimen for at least 6 mos and 1–2 mos beyond resolution of disease.
- In largest series (*Diagn Microbiol Infect Dis* 47:441, 2003), mostly pre-HAART era, 43% died of the disease or progressed despite treatment, only 15% cured.
- For patients with AIDS, relapse occurs frequently enough that lifelong suppressive therapy with 1–2 oral agents is recommended beyond treatment of active disease unless immune reconstitution achieved.
- ART confers survival benefit.
- Consider surgical drainage or resection of large cavities or abscesses in those who fail to respond to ABx.

Parenteral Agents

- Most commonly reported: vancomycin + 1–2 of the following: carbapenem, aminoglycoside, or rifampin.
- Vancomycin: 15 mg/kg IV twice daily.
- Amikacin: 15 mg/kg IV once daily or gentamicin 5–7 mg/kg IV once daily.
- Imipenem 500 mg IV q6h or meropenem 1 g IV q8h or ertapenem 1 g IV once daily.
- Rifampin (RIF): 600 mg IV once daily (not for monotherapy).
- Consider fluoroquinolone for patients intolerant to 2 or more of above agents: moxifloxacin 400 mg IV once daily or levofloxacin 750 mg IV once daily, or levofloxacin 500 mg IV once daily.

ORAL AGENTS

- Most commonly reported: RIF + macrolide, tetracycline or fluoroquinolone.
- RIF: 600 mg PO once daily (not for monotherapy).
- Clarithromycin: 500 mg PO twice daily, erythromycin 500 mg PO 4 ×/day or azithromycin 500 mg PO once daily.
- Minocycline: 100 mg PO twice daily or doxycycline 100 mg PO twice daily.
- Moxifloxacin: 400 mg PO once daily or levofloxacin 500–750 mg PO once daily.
- Other drugs commonly active: TMP/SMX, clindamycin, linezolid.

FOLLOW-UP

- As with TB, failure to respond to Rx (improved symptoms and CXR) after 2 mos should prompt sputum Cx and susceptibility testing.
- Recommended treatment duration is at least 6 mos and 1–2 mos after all disease manifestations resolve.
- Lifelong suppressive therapy recommended for patients w/ AIDS unless immune reconstitution achieved.

OTHER INFORMATION

- Simultaneous OIs are common.
- 2 cases of apparent person-to-person transmission suggest that other immunocompromised patients should not share room with patients with cavitary or sputum Cx-positive disease. Need for airborne isolation unclear.

SELECTED REFERENCES

Torres-Tortosa M, Arrizabalaga J, Villanueva JL, et al. Prognosis and clinical evaluation of infection caused by *Rhodococcus equi* in HIV-infected patients: a multicenter study of 67 cases. *Chest*, 2003; 123: 1970–6.

Comments: Multicenter retrospective study from Spain is largest series in HIV+ patients (N = 67). Cure or regression achieved in 57%, but mortality attributable to *Rhodococcus* in 34%. Despite time period studied (1990–1998), absence of ART was the only independent predictor of mortality.

Weinstock DM, Brown AE. *Rhodococcus equi*: an emerging pathogen. *Clin Infect Dis*, 2002; 34: 1379–85.

Comments: Comprehensive review. HIV+ patients (2/3 of all cases) more likely to have disseminated disease, simultaneous OIs, and worse outcomes than immunocompetent or organ transplant patients, although most cases reported from pre-HAART era.

SALMONELLA SPP.

Amita Gupta, MD, MHS

MICROBIOLOGY

- Facultatively anaerobic, Gram-negative bacillus, foodborne (95% cases: outbreaks linked to multiple vehicles including eggs, poultry, meats, dairy or vegetables) or zoonotic pathogen, except *S. typhi* (typhoid fever) and *S. paratyphi* (paratyphoid fever), which colonize/infect humans only.
- Nontyphoidal strains classified by agglutination reactions to O antigens identifying serogroups A–E; approximately 2500 serovars/serotypes exist. Most common in US are *S. typhimurium*, *S. enteriditis*, *S. newport*, *S. enterica*, or *S. choleraesuis* sometimes used as single name for clinically familiar serovars (e.g., *S. enterica typhimurium*).
- Typhoidal species *S. typhi* (serogroup D) and *S. paratyphi* more difficult to Cx. Increased yield when blood, bone marrow, and intestinal secretions Cx'd before or soon after ABx initiated.
- Recovery of organism possible from almost any site, but most commonly stool followed by blood.
- Grows on standard media for stool; fresh stool specimen preferred; rectal swabs inferior.

CLINICAL

- Nontyphoidal *Salmonella* gastroenteritis: nausea, vomiting, diarrhea ± fever, bloody stools (only ~50% of the time) usually occur within 6–72 hrs of ingestion of contaminated food or water; usually self-limited lasting 3–7 days. Occasionally more prolonged illness with fever, bloody diarrhea, weight loss. Mean carriage after resolution of Sx up to 4–5 wks and varies by serotype. *Salmonella* cannot be reliably be distinguished from other common enteric pathogens on a clinical basis.
- Extraintestinal salmonellosis: almost any site can be involved; clinical disease depends on site (see Sites of Infection section below). Bacteremia usually occurs with advanced immunosuppression. Approximately 5%–10% develop localized infection after bacteremia.
- HIV+ patients at 20–100-fold increased risk of salmonellosis than general population, and more likely to have invasive disease, including recurrent bacteremia (which is AIDS-defining).
- Patients with AIDS and *Salmonella* bacteremia at risk for relapse, recurrence when not on ART.
- Typhoid fever (*S. typhi*) rarely reported with HIV even in developing world; rare in US but consider in returning traveler, particularly from India, other Asian countries, South America, and Africa. Sx initially nonspecific but then may develop fever, abdominal pain ± diarrhea, neuropsychiatric 10%–15%, rose spots 15%–30%, hepatomegaly 50%. Lasts up to 4 wks without ABx and complications can occur. Paratyphoid illness similar but usually less severe.

PATHOGENS

- Acquisition might be facilitated by HIV-associated achlorhydria, agents that decrease acid secretion, HIV-associated changes in gut immunity.

SITES OF INFECTION
- GI tract: gastroenteritis, enteric fever (acute fever, abdominal tenderness ± diarrhea, and nonspecific Sx mostly due to *S. typhi* and *S. paratyphi*); rectal ulcers.
- Bacteremia: AIDS increases risk; recurrent nontyphoidal bacteremia is AIDS-defining illness.
- Extraintestinal sites (rare): endocarditis, aortitis/arteritis, lung abscess, osteomyelitis, meningitis and brain abscess, parotitis, liver abscess, UTI, septic and reactive arthritis, genital abscess, soft tissue infections.
- Carriage: transient, asymptomatic carrier state can occur with median duration of excretion in stool of 3–4 wks. Chronic carrier state: persistence of *Salmonella* in stool or urine for >1 yr. Biliary tree (gallbladder) major nidus. Occurs in <1% with nontyphoid and 1%–4% with typhoid strains. Antimicrobials can increase persistence of transient carriage but often used to treat chronic carriage.

TREATMENT
Mild-to-Moderate Illness
- HIV-infected persons at increased risk for invasive, recurrent, and most notably, drug-resistance.
- If deciding to treat, choice usually empiric, so choice often guided by desire to cover common enteric pathogens.
- Immunocompetent patients without HIV often do not require treatment; condition self-limited and ABx may prolong carrier state (IDSA Guidelines CID 2001;32:331). Most experts recommend treatment in HIV population, though no data from clinical trials support this recommendation.
- Treatment duration not well defined: 7–14 days for mild, nonbacteremic cases with CD4 >200; >4–6 wks for AIDS, CD4 <200, or bacteremic cases.
- Fluid and electrolyte replacement important.
- If susceptibilities unknown, use PO fluoroquinolone (preferred ciprofloxacin), azithromycin, or TMP-SMX initially, then modify Rx according to susceptibilities when available. Ampicillin and TMP-SMX resistance now more common (see Treatment Regimens and Doses below).
- Fluoroquinolones, 3rd-generation cephalosporins and azithromycin effective for *S. typhi* and *S. paratyphi*.

Severe Illness
- Hospitalized patients or patients with severe diarrhea (>5 stools/day and/or T >101°F, tenesemus, blood, or fecal leukocytes), bacteremia, or extraintestinal infections such as meningitis, lung abscess, osteomyelitis should be empirically treated with PO or IV fluoroquinolones (preferred ciprofloxacin as most data with this FQ). Alternatives include azithromycin or IV/IM 3rd-generation cephalosporin such as ceftriaxone. Narrow treatment once susceptibilities known.
- Fluid and electrolyte replacement important.
- Possible or confirmed *S. typhi* infection: ciprofloxacin or ceftriaxone × 10–14 days. Alternatively azithromycin 1 g PO × 1 then 500 mg PO once daily × 6 days. If associated with shock, consider dexamethasone a few minutes before antibiotic: 3 mg/kg then 1 mg/kg q6h × 8 doses (NEJM 310:82,1984: Mortality benefit but study did not include HIV+ patients). Consider ID consultation.

Treatment
- **Preferred agent:** ciprofloxacin: 500 mg PO twice daily for gastroenteritis; 750 mg PO twice daily if bacteremia; 400 mg IV twice daily if unable to take oral medications or concern about poor absorption. Can also use ofloxacin 400 mg PO twice daily or norfloxacin 400 mg PO twice daily (norfloxacin not recommended for bacteremia).
- Little to no data for other fluoroquinolones but likely to be effective. Levofloxacin 500 mg PO or IV once daily; moxifloxacin 400 mg PO or IV once daily.
- TMP/SMX: effective, but resistance reported. 1 DS PO twice daily.
- Ceftriaxone: effective for both nontyphoidal and typhoidal salmonellosis. 1–2 g IV or IM once daily. Cefotaxime 1–2 g IV q8h also effective.

- Azithromycin: effective alternative for both nontyphoidal and typhoidal salmonellosis, particularly in patients with multiple allergies or pregnant patients. 500 mg PO once daily.
- Aztreonam: alternative in patients with multiple allergies based on *in vitro* data. 1–2 g IV q8h.

FOLLOW-UP
Relapse or Chronic Carriage
- Causes of treatment failure: resistance, malabsorption of PO ABx, sequestered focus of infection, or drug interactions.
- Monitor response to Rx, especially in patients w/ advanced HIV+ infection. F/U stool Cx to demonstrate cure not required except with clinical failure or for public health reasons (e.g., food service or healthcare worker).
- Transient, asymptomatic carrier state can occur with median duration of excretion in stool of 3–4 wks. Chronic carrier state refers to persistence in stool or urine for >1 yr. Biliary tree (gallbladder) is major nidus. Occurs in <1% with nontyphoid and 1%–4% with typhoid strains.
- ABx can increase persistence of transient carriage but often used to treat chronic carrier state. Ceftriaxone or fluoroquinolones preferred. If biliary disease present, best results with cholecystectomy and 10–14-days ABx course initiated before surgery.
- Recurrent septicemia: some experts consider prolonged course of antimicrobials (>6 mos) but not well studied; benefits must be weighed against risks of prolonged antimicrobial exposure.

OTHER INFORMATION
- AZT has documented anti-*Salmonella* activity *in vitro*, and appears to be clinically useful in prevention of relapse.
- Prevention: (1) handwashing with soap/hand sanitizers after potential contact with human feces, handling of raw meats, eggs, poultry, handling pets or other animals, before and after sex; (2) cook meats, poultry thoroughly; (3) wash fresh produce; (4) avoid unprotected sex practices that may result in oral exposure to feces; (5) avoid eating raw or undercooked eggs, unpasteurized dairy products or fruit juices, and raw seed sprouts.
- Useful websites: *www.cdc.gov/foodnet/* and *www.cdc.gov/narms/* (CDC's foodborne diseases websites); *www.idsociety.org/* (select practice guidelines for HIV/AIDS).
- Report salmonellosis to local and/or state public health authorities.
- Pregnant women can be treated in similar fashion as nonpregnant women. Fluoroquinolone-induced arthropathy seen in animal model but nearly 400 cases of quinolone use in pregnancy did not show association with arthropathy or birth defects. Alternate agents such as azithromycin, expanded spectrum cephalosporins, or TMP-SMX can also be considered based on Cx susceptibility results.

SELECTED REFERENCES
Kaplan JE, Benson C, Holmes KH, et al. Guidelines for prevention and treatment of opportunistic infections in HIV-infected adults and adolescents: recommendations from CDC, the National Institutes of Health, and the HIV Medicine Association of the Infectious Diseases Society of America. *MMWR Recomm Rep*, 2009; 58: 1–207.
Comments: Latest guidelines from CDC/NIH/IDSA. Specific recommendations for *Salmonella* in HIV+ patients on S152–153.

CDC. *National Antimicrobial Resistance Monitoring System for Enteric Bacteria (NARMS): Human Isolates Final Report, 2005.* Atlanta, GA: US Department of Health and Human Services, CDC, 2008. *www.cdc.gov/NARMS/annual/2005/NARMSAnnualReport2005.pdf.* Accessed June 18, 2009. Atlanta, Georgia: U.S. Department of Health and Human Services, CDC, 2008.
Comments: Report and figures on national trends in antimicrobial resistance among *Salmonella*.

Hohmann EL. Nontyphoidal salmonellosis. *Clin Infect Dis*, 2001; 32: 263–9.
Comments: Good clinical review of salmonellosis.

Guerrant RL, Van Gilder T, Steiner TS, et al. Practice guideliens for the management of infectious diarrhea. *Clin Infect Dis*, 2001; 32(3): 331–51.

Hoffman SL, Punjabi NH, Kumala S, et al. Reduction of mortality in chloramphenicol-treated severe typhoid fever by high-dose dexamethasone. *N Engl J Med*, 1984; 310: 82–8.

PATHOGENS

STAPHYLOCOCCUS SPP.

Khalil G. Ghanem, MD, PhD

MICROBIOLOGY

- *Staphylococci* (*Staph*): clustered Gram-positive beta-hemolytic bacteria. *S. aureus* (SA) is coagulase positive.
- Coagulase-negative *Staph* (CoNS): >30 species, 15 of which are human pathogens. *S. epidermidis*, *S. saprophyticus* (novobiocin resistant), *S. haemolyticus*, *S. lugdunensis*, and *S. schleiferi* are most commonly isolated.
- SA produces several toxins, including enterotoxins, epidermolytic toxins, and toxic shock syndrome toxins (TSST).
- Staph grow rapidly on blood agar and other nonselective media. They can survive harsh environmental conditions, high salt media, and are relatively heat-resistant.
- Methicillin resistance: >80% of CoNS, and an increasing number of both hospital-acquired and community-acquired SA (MRSA) encompasses all β-lactam antibiotics, including cephalosporins. Vancomycin-intermediate resistance (VISA) and vancomycin-resistant strains have emerged.

CLINICAL

- Both MRSA and MSSA infections occur more frequently in HIV+ patients. Advanced immunosuppression increases risk.
- Increased prevalence of IDU among HIV+ patients, frequent hospitalization, frequent use of antimicrobials, and need for long-term venous access have further increased risk of SA infections, especially MRSA.
- Signs and Sx depend on degree of immunosuppression and site of infection (see Sites of Infection section, following).
- Dx: SA and CoNS grow easily in Cx; blood, urine, CSF, sputum, skin, and bone Cx, as indicated, should be obtained. Further investigation depends on site of infection.
- Community-acquired (CA-) MRSA strains now account for >75% of soft tissue infections.
- CA-MRSA vs hospital-acquired MRSA: (1) more susceptible to ABx other than beta-lactams; (2) genotypes not the same as isolates from local hospitals; (3) mainly harbor different methicillin-resistance cassettes; (4) CA-MRSA isolates more likely to encode a putative virulence factor called Panton-Valentine leukocidin.
- Currently, 1 strain of CA-MRSA predominates (staphylococcal chromosomal cassette type IV, sequence type 8, Panton-Valentine leukocidin gene positive).

SITES OF INFECTION

- Skin and soft tissue: cellulitis, folliculitis (SA), furuncles and carbuncles (SA), impetigo (SA), post-operative wound infections.
- Musculoskeletal: pyomyositis (SA), abscesses (mostly SA), osteomyelitis, septic arthritis, prosthetic joint infections.
- Cardiovascular: bacteremia, endocarditis, pericarditis (SA).
- Pulmonary: necrotizing pneumonia (SA), empyema (SA).
- Neurological: abscesses, meningitis (mostly SA), and shunt infections (both SA and CoNS).
- GI: epidemic acute food poisoning (SA).
- Systemic: toxic shock syndrome.
- Urinary tract: isolation of SA from urine should prompt immediate evaluation for an endovascular source.

TREATMENT

General Principles

- Penicillin not effective to treat SA or CoNS infections due to widespread resistance.
- >80% of CoNS and a growing number of hospital-acquired and community acquired SA are methicillin-resistant.
- Vancomycin should not be used to treat MSSA as a convenience; efficacy inferior to beta-lactams.
- Short courses of parenteral therapy (2 wks) for endovascular infections should be discouraged in HIV-infected patients.

- CA-MRSA may be sensitive to >1 of following: clindamycin, TMP-SMX, fluoroquinolones, or macrolides. Once resistance profile known, they may be used for non-life threatening infections (usually skin, soft tissue, and bone infections).
- Regimen and duration depends on site of infection and sensitivity of organisms; in general skin, soft tissue infections, and uncomplicated pulmonary infections require 10–14 days of Rx, endovascular and bone infections at least 4–6 wks of therapy.
- When infected collections of fluid are found (empyema, abscesses), surgical drainage must accompany antimicrobial Rx.
- Any indwelling vascular lines should be removed; success of eradicating endovascular Staph infections (especially SA) without foreign body removal is low (<30%).
- Isolation of SA from blood requires therapy. Unlike CoNS, SA should not be viewed as a contaminant.

Decolonization

- MRSA decolonization has not led to reduction in infection in all patient populations; effect of any decolonization strategy seems to last only about 90 days.
- Mupirocin: eradication of nasal colonization after initial (5–7 days) use is 88% for HIV + patients, but resistance develops quickly.
- Chlorhexidine baths used in combination with intranasal mupirocin in uncontrolled trials and during outbreaks.

Antimicrobials

- PO: cephalexin (500 mg PO 4 ×/day), dicloxacillin (500 mg PO 4 ×/day), clindamycin (300 mg PO 4 ×/day), fluoroquinolones (advanced generation FQ tend to have better gram + coverage, e.g., levofloxacin, moxifloxacin), TMP-SMX, and minocycline.
- IV: antistaphylococcal PCN (nafcillin [1–2 g IV q4h] or oxacillin [1–2 g IV q4h]); if MRSA, vancomycin (15 mg/kg IV q12h); linezolid (600 mg IV q12h).
- Synergy: gentamicin 1 mg/kg IV q8h; rifampin 300 mg IV/PO q12h. Limit to 1st 5 days of Rx. No benefit has been shown in extending the course.
- Endocarditis: MSSA: nafcillin or oxacillin ± gentamicin or rifampin; MRSA: vancomycin ± gentamicin or rifampin × 4–6 wks. Short courses for right-sided endocarditis not recommended in HIV-infected patients; new data for daptomycin (6 mg/kg IV q24h) (Fowler) in MSSA and MRSA endocarditis.
- CoNS: vancomycin ± rifampin; occasionally may be sensitive to FQ or TMP-SMX; tigecycline, linezolid, and daptomycin are alternate choices.
- Intermediate resistance and full resistance to vancomycin in SA have been reported. Case reports suggest that the use of linezolid in combination with rifampin may be successful.
- Susceptibility to fluoroquinolones, aminoglycosides, clindamycin, TMP-SMX, and rifampin must be ascertained prior to the use of these agents.

FOLLOW-UP

- Adjust ABx doses based or renal and hepatic function. Redose vancomycin when trough level <10–15; in general, no need to measure peak/trough levels of aminoglycosides when used at synergistic doses.
- Incomplete Rx may lead to hematogenous dissemination of SA and complications days to years after discontinuation of Rx.
- Resistance to erythromycin in CA-MRSA may suggest inducible resistance to clindamycin; ensure that a D-test is performed before clindamycin is prescribed.

SELECTED REFERENCES

Cenizal MJ, Hardy RD, Anderson M, et al. Prevalence of and risk factors for methicillin-resistant *Staphylococcus aureus* (MRSA) nasal colonization in HIV-infected ambulatory patients. *J Acquir Immune Defic Syndr*, 2008; 48: 567–71.

Comments: Study of 146 HIV+ patients: the prevalence of MRSA nasal colonization was relatively high compared with prior studies; axillary colonization was rare. Prior MRSA/MSSA infection, not receiving antibiotics, and lower CD4 count associated with MRSA nasal colonization. TMP-SMX seemed to be protective of colonization.

Diep BA, Chambers HF, Graber CJ, et al. Emergence of multidrug-resistant, community-associated, methicillin-resistant *Staphylococcus aureus* clone USA300 in men who have sex with men. *Ann Intern Med*, 2008; 148: 249–57.

Comments: Infection with multidrug-resistant USA300 MRSA was common among MSM, and multidrug-resistant MRSA infection might be sexually transmitted in this population of 9 hospitals in San Francisco and 2 outpatient clinics in San Francisco and Boston.

PATHOGENS

Moran GJ, Krishnadasan A, Gorwitz RJ, et al. Methicillin-resistant *S. aureus* infections among patients in the emergency department. *N Engl J Med*, 2006; 355: 666–74.
Comments: SA isolated from 320 of 422 patients with skin and soft-tissue infections (76%). Prevalence of MRSA was 59% overall and ranged from 15%–74%. Among MRSA isolates, 95% susceptible to clindamycin, 6% to erythromycin, 60% to fluoroquinolones, 100% to rifampin and TMP-SMX, and 92% to tetracycline.

STREPTOCOCCUS PNEUMONIAE

Lisa A. Spacek, MD, PhD and Eric Nuermberger, MD

MICROBIOLOGY

- *Streptococcus pneumoniae* (pneumococcus): Gram-positive diplococcus with polysaccharide capsule, demonstrated by Quellung reaction or capsular swelling when antibodies bind to capsular polysaccharide antigen.
- Grows well on standard media, but prior antibiotics may preclude growth.
- Ecologic niche is nasopharynx, colonizes 5%–10% of adults, 20%–40% of children. Definite pathogen when isolated from sterile site (blood, CSF, joint fluid, etc.). Probable pathogen in respiratory specimens (Gram stain or Cx) or when urinary antigen positive in patient w/ pneumonia.
- Dx: sputum Gram stain and Cx, blood Cx, and urine antigen. Blood Cx more sensitive in HIV+ patients due to greater likelihood of bacteremia. Cx data important due to increased risk of TMP/SMX and macrolide resistance in patients on ABx for OI prophylaxis.
- Rapid urinary antigen test (*Binax*): 70%–90% sensitive, 90% specific for bacteremic pneumonia; lower yield in nonbacteremic pneumonia; data show test results are independent of HIV status.

CLINICAL

- Pneumonia, classic presentation: abrupt onset of fever, rigors, productive cough, pleurisy; exam: tachycardia, tachypnea, hypoxia, findings consistent with lung consolidation, maybe pleural rub; CXR: typically lobar pneumonia ± effusion, but multilobar, even diffuse infiltrates possible. HIV infected patients more frequently present with bacteremia, multilobar involvement, and parapneumonic effusions.
- Incidence of invasive disease 100 × higher in patients with AIDS; lower incidence in those on ART.
- Risk factors include low CD4, older age, asthma, cigarette smoking, IV drugs, and alcohol use.
- HIV does not clearly affect treatment response or increase mortality, but pneumonia recurs in 8%–25% within 6 mos (usually reinfection).
- Due to increased incidence of TB (see p. 32) in HIV+ patients, consider *M. tuberculosis* as etiology. If TB likely, avoid fluoroquinolone monotherapy, as respiratory quinolones are active against *M. tuberculosis*.
- Common cause of meningitis in adults and children > 6 mos. May be due to direct extension from sinuses or middle ear or associated with head trauma, CSF leak, or disruption of dura.

SITES OF INFECTION

- Lung: pneumonia, pleural effusion, empyema, acute exacerbation of chronic bronchitis (AECB).
- Sinuses: sinusitis.
- Middle ear: otitis media.
- CNS: meningitis.
- Joints: septic arthritis.
- Peritoneum: spontaneous bacterial peritonitis.
- Heart: purulent pericarditis, endocarditis.
- Skin: cellulitis.
- Eye: conjunctivitis.

TREATMENT
Respiratory Tract Infections

- For empiric therapy of pneumonia, see Pneumonia, Bacterial (p. 28). In non-ICU patients, beta-lactam + macrolide OR respiratory fluoroquinolone. In ICU patients, IV beta-lactam +

either IV azithromycin or an IV respiratory fluoroquinolone. In PCN-allergic, aztreonam + IV respiratory fluoroquinolone. In all regimens, avoid empiric use of macrolide monotherapy in those on macrolide for MAC prophylaxis.

- Pneumonia (PCN-sensitive, MIC <2), ICU patient, parenteral: penicillin G 2–4 MU q4h or ampicillin 1–2 g q6h (preferred) OR ceftriaxone 1 g IV once daily or twice daily or cefotaxime 1–2 g IV q6–8h (alternatives). Addition of a macrolide or fluoroquinolone (levofloxacin, moxifloxacin) may be beneficial in severe pneumonia until improvement noted.
- Pneumonia (PCN-sensitive, MIC <2), ward patient: preferred Rx is IV beta-lactam + a macrolide. If PCN allergy or Hx (past 3 mos) of Rx with beta-lactam, IV respiratory fluoroquinolone recommended. Penicillin G 2–4 MU q4h or ampicillin 1–2 g q6h (preferred) OR ceftriaxone 1 g IV once or twice daily or cefotaxime 1–2 g IV q6–8h (alternatives). Moxifloxacin 400 mg IV/PO once daily, levofloxacin 500–750 mg IV/PO once daily or clindamycin 600 mg IV q8h (IgE-mediated beta-lactam allergy).
- Pneumonia (PCN-sensitive, MIC <2), outpatient: preferred Rx is oral beta-lactam + oral macrolide. If PCN allergy or Hx of Rx with beta-lactam, respiratory fluoroquinolone recommended. Amoxicillin 2–3 g/day (preferred), cefpodoxime 200 mg twice daily, cefprozil 500 mg twice daily, cefuroxime 500 mg twice daily, cefdinir 300 mg twice daily, clarithromycin 1 g once daily (XL) or 500 mg twice daily, azithromycin 500 mg × 1, then 250–500 mg once daily, doxycycline 100 mg twice daily.
- Pneumonia (PCN-resistant, MIC >2): ceftriaxone or cefotaxime (as above) if MIC to either agent is <2 OR fluoroquinolone IV/PO once daily (levofloxacin 500–750 mg, moxifloxacin 400 mg). Also vancomycin, linezolid, or high-dose amoxicillin (3 g/day with PCN MIC <4 μg/mL).
- Sinusitis, empiric: amoxicillin 500 mg 3 ×/day or 750 mg twice daily, doxycycline 100 mg twice daily (ACP guidelines, *Ann Intern Med*; 2001; 134(7): 595–9).
- Acute exacerbation of chronic bronchitis: same as for sinusitis above (ACP guidelines, *Ann Intern Med*; 2001; 134(7): 595–9).

Meningitis

- For empiric therapy of presumed bacterial meningitis, see Bacterial Meningitis, Acute, Community-Acquired: vancomycin + a 3rd-generation cephalosporin; add ampicillin to cover *Listeria monocytogenes* in those >50 yrs. In those at risk for Gram-negative bacilli, consider using meropenem rather than cephalosporin.
- PCN-sensitive (MIC <0.1): penicillin G 4 million units IV q4h or ampicillin 2 g IV q4h (preferred); ceftriaxone 2 g IV q12h or cefotaxime 2–3 g IV q4–6h (alternatives).
- PCN nonsusceptible (MIC 0.1–1): ceftriaxone or cefotaxime (as earlier) (preferred); cefepime 2 g IV q8h or meropenem 2 g IV q8h (alternatives).
- PCN-resistant (MIC >2): vancomycin 15 mg/kg q8–12h + ceftriaxone or cefotaxime (as earlier) (preferred); moxifloxacin 400 mg IV q24h (alternative).

Prevention

- ART decreases risk of pneumonia; TMP/SMX and azithromycin prophylaxis do not, but may increase risk of pneumococcal drug resistance.
- Pneumovax, a 23-valent polysaccharide vaccine, reduces risk of meningitis and bacteremic pneumonia in adults. Unlike conjugate vaccine, Pneumovax includes 19A serotype, most prevalent cause of invasive disease in children and 2nd most common in adults.
- Pneumovax recommended for patients with CD4 >200, optional if CD4 <200.
- Revaccinate every 5 yrs and when CD4 >200 if initial vaccination was given when <200.
- Annual influenza vaccination may decrease risk of pneumococcal superinfection of influenza.

SELECTED REFERENCES

Kaplan JE, Benson C, Holmes KH, et al. Guidelines for prevention and treatment of opportunistic infections in HIV-infected adults and adolescents: recommendations from CDC, the National Institutes of Health, and the HIV Medicine Association of the Infectious Diseases Society of America. *MMWR Recomm Rep*, 2009; 58: 31–36. **Comments:** Discussion specific to bacterial respiratory disease highlights role of *S. pneumoniae* due to high incidence of pneumococcal pneumonia and accompanying bacteremia in those with HIV/AIDS.

[No authors listed]. Pneumococcal vaccination of adults: polysaccharide or conjugate? *Med Lett Drugs Ther*, 2009; 51: 47–8. **Comments:** This brief comparative review of polysaccharide vs conjugate pneumococcal vaccine argues for use of polysaccharide as preferred choice due to wider spectrum (includes serotype 19A) and proven reduced risk of meningitis and bacteremic pneumonia.

PATHOGENS

Mandell LA, Wunderink RG, Anzueto A, et al. Infectious Diseases Society of America/American Thoracic Society consensus guidelines on the management of community-acquired pneumonia in adults. *Clin Infect Dis*, 2007; 44 suppl 2: S27–72.
Comments: New comprehensive consensus guidelines for management of immunocompetent persons are largely applicable to HIV+ patients with respect to pneumococcal pneumonia.

Tunkel AR, Hartman BJ, Kaplan SL, et al. Practice guidelines for the management of bacterial meningitis. *Clin Infect Dis*, 2004; 39: 1267–84.
Comments: IDSA meningitis guidelines discuss impact of beta-lactam resistance in *S. pneumoniae* and include empiric and pathogen-directed treatment recommendations.

Richter SS, Heilmann KP, Dohrn CL, et al. Changing epidemiology of antimicrobial-resistant *Streptococcus pneumoniae* in the United States, 2004–2005. *Clin Infect Dis*, 2009; 48: e23–33.
Comments: Epidemiology of drug resistance: intermediate PCN, MIC 0.1–1 µg/mL, increased from 13% to 18%; PNC-resistant, MIC >2, decreased from 22% to 15%; increase in serotypes 19A (2% to 35%) and 35B (1% to 13%).

Domingo P, Suarez-Lozano I, Torres F, et al. Bacterial meningitis in HIV-1-infected patients in the era of highly active antiretroviral therapy. *J Acquir Immune Defic Syndr*, 2009; 51: 582–7.
Comments: Prospective study of 32 episodes of spontaneous bacterial meningitis in HIV+ vs 267 episodes in HIV-negative persons, matched by age and yr of infection. *S. pneumoniae* was most frequent etiologic agent among HIV+ patients. Neurologic complications more common (P = 0.02), case fatality rate greater (P = 0.004), and more frequent incidence of neurologic sequelae (P = 0.001) in HIV+.

Madeddu G, Fois AG, Pirina P, et al. Pneumococcal pneumonia: clinical features, diagnosis and management in HIV-infected and HIV noninfected patients. *Curr Opin Pulm Med*, 2009; 15: 236–42.
Comments: Comparative review of pneumococcal pneumonia in HIV+ vs HIV-negative patients endorses sputum and blood Cx as well as urinary antigen for Dx evaluation of pneumonia in HIV+ patients.

Hung CC, Chang SY, Su CT, et al. A 5-year longitudinal follow-up study of serological responses to 23-valent pneumococcal polysaccharide vaccination among patients with HIV infection who received highly active antiretroviral therapy. *HIV Med*, 2010; 11(1): 54–63.
Comments: This 5-yr study evaluated serologic response to 23-valent pneumococcal polysaccharide vaccine in 169 HIV-infected patients on ART. Participants were stratified by CD4 at vaccination: ,100 (N = 35); 100–199 (N = 36); 200–349 (N = 34); and $350 (N = 64). Antibody response to vaccination declined during follow-up in those with CD4 ,100 and those who did not achieve viral suppression.

Snow V, Lascher S, Mottur-Pilson C. Evidence base for management of acute exacerbations of chronic obstructive pulmonary disease. *Ann Intern Med*; 2001; 134(7): 595–9.
Comments: ACP/ASIM recommendations for treatment of AECB. Although *S. pneumoniae* and *H. influenzae* commonly implicated, most exacerbations likely due to viral infections. There is marginal support for treating severe exacerbations in pts with most severe underlying obstructive disease with antibacterials. Recommended agents are amoxicillin, doxycycline and TMP-SMX.

Fungi

ASPERGILLUS SPP.

Dionissios Neofytos, MD, MPH and Paul G. Auwaerter, MD

MICROBIOLOGY

- Ubiquitous filamentous mold, hyphae (2–5 μm) usually septated with 45° angle branching.
- Diagnosis mainly based on colony morphology on solid media and specific microscopic features.
- Noninvasive diagnostic tests now available: galactomannan antigen in serum and BAL (good sensitivity/specificity in the right patient population), PCR (not well studied), beta-D-glucan (not specific).
- *A. fumigatus* most common cause of human disease. *A. flavus* next most common, followed by *A. terreus*, *A. niger* (usually a contaminant), *A. versicolor*, and *A. nidulans*. Recently, new *Aspergillus* spp. (*A. lentulus*) described.
- *A. terreus* may be resistant to amphotericin products. *A. fumigatus*: azole-resistance reported. *A. lentulus*: may be resistant to itraconazole, voriconazole, caspofungin.

CLINICAL

- Portal of entry: respiratory tract >skin. *Aspergillus* conidia inhaled and migrate to bronchi/ lung parenchyma, germinate into hyphae, which can invade tissue. Alveolar macrophages and neutrophils important host defences.
- Broad spectrum of disease from noninvasive: colonization, allergic bronchopulmonary aspergillosis (ABPA), aspergilloma (lung nodule), to more invasive: chronic pulmonary necrotizing aspergillosis, invasive or disseminated aspergillosis.
- Invasive disease generally seen with immune suppression: transplant (bone marrow and organ) recipients, hematologic malignancy, neutropenia, corticosteroids, HIV/AIDS, chronic granulomatous disease.
- HIV: common risk factors include advanced HIV (CD4 <50), steroid use, prior OI, and neutropenia. May present as sinusitis, tracheobronchitis, otitis, or pneumonia, but colonization of respiratory tract common.
- Frequent bronchial colonizer in patients w/ structural lung disease (e.g., bronchiectasis, carcinoma, sarcoid, prior TB).
- Invasive lung disease w/ pleuritic chest pain, cough, hemoptysis, dyspnea. Lung imaging w/ nodular/ cavitary lesions, patchy infiltrates, "halo-sign" (hemorrhage), and "crescent-sign" (necrosis).
- Dx of invasive disease: proven: histopathological/Cx evidence; probable: host factors, clinical criteria and mycological criteria (microscopy/Cx/galactomannan antigen); possible (absence of mycological support).

SITES OF INFECTION

- Lung: allergic bronchopulmonary aspergillosis (ABPA), tracheobronchitis w/ white plaques, aspergilloma, chronic necrotizing aspergillosis, invasive aspergillosis.
- Sinuses: allergic, fungus ball, invasive disease.
- CNS: abscess (contiguously through sinuses or hematogenously), mycotic infarction.
- Skin: primary (inoculation, armboard-related, catheter-related) or secondary (disseminated) in heavily immunosuppressed patients.
- Heart: endocarditis (risk factors: prosthetic heart valve surgery, IV drug abuse, central line infection).
- Eye: endophthalmitis (hematogenous or direct inoculation), keratitis from trauma.
- Disseminated to kidney, liver, spleen, and CNS; blood Cx rarely positive.

TREATMENT

Invasive or Disseminated Infection

- **Preferred:** voriconazole 6 mg/kg IV q12h × 2 then 4 mg/kg IV q12h.
- **Alternative:** amphotericin B 1.0–1.5 mg/kg/day IV or lipid formulation amphotericin 5.0 mg/kg/day IV.
- **Salvage:** caspofungin 70 mg IV × 1 dose, then 50 mg IV q24h.
- **Salvage:** posaconazole 200 mg PO q6h × 7 days, then 400 mg PO q8–12h with food.

PATHOGENS

- Combination therapy often employed (e.g., voriconazole + caspofungin, amphotericin + voriconazole) but limited data to support practice and cost high.
- If neutropenic, use G-CSF. Decrease/stop corticosteroids/other immunosuppression if possible.
- Avoid IV voriconazole if CrCl <50 because cyclodextrin accumulates, although no good data.

Aspergilloma

- Often requires no intervention. Must be distinguished from necrotic mass in cavity due to invasive pulmonary aspergillosis.
- Significant hemoptysis: consider pulmonary artery embolization, partial lung resection (if adequate PFTs).
- Medical treatment of unclear benefit. Main conundrum: is there invasive/progressive disease? Some data suggest itraconazole may be helpful, but rate of invasive disease low, despite risk factors.

Local Disease (Sinus/HEENT, Cutaneous, and Other)

- Medical therapy as in invasive disease.
- Surgery to remove necrotic tissue, active infection, e.g., brain, bone, heart valve, skin, sinuses.

Allergic Bronchopulmonary Aspergillosis

- Prednisone: 0.5 mg/kg/day × 1 wk then 0.5 mg/kg every other day × 5 wks with taper.
- Itraconazole: 200 mg PO twice daily × 16 wks leads to quicker steroid taper and improved pulmonary parameters. Role of voriconazole not studied.

FOLLOW-UP

Aspergillus Infections

- Voriconazole: 4 mg/kg PO twice daily once clinically stable.
- Duration uncertain, but usually until no clinical evidence of active disease and reduced immunosuppression.
- Treatment failure: some define as no response within 96 hrs or persistent fever. Beware of "transient" worsening of chest CT findings upon resolution of neutropenia and possibly immune reconstitution. Consider adding caspofungin (70 mg IV × 1 dose, then 50 mg IV once daily) or voriconazole. Limited data available for combination therapy.
- Very limited data to correlate galactomannan assay titers with response.

OTHER INFORMATION

- Serious disease remains difficult to treat. However, outcomes have improved due to a number of factors (risk factor identification, high clinical suspicion, noninvasive diagnostic tests, effective/safe antifungal agents).

SELECTED REFERENCES

Walsh T, Anaissie E, Denning D, et al. Treatment of aspergillosis: clinical practice guidelines of the Infectious Diseases Society of America. *Clin Infect Dis*, 2008; 46: 327–60.
Comments: Revised treatment guidelines for treatment of aspergillosis.

De Pauw B, Walsh TJ, Donnelly JP, et al. Revised definitions of invasive fungal disease from the European Organization for Research and Treatment of Cancer/Invasive Fungal Infections Cooperative Group and the National Institute of Allergy and Infectious Diseases Mycoses Study Group (EORTC/MSG) Consensus Group. *Clin Infect Dis*, 2008; 46(12): 1813–21.
Comments: Revised definitions of invasive fungal infections, including invasive aspergillosis. Important assitions: galactomannan assay in serum/BAL.

Herbrecht R, Denning DW, Patterson TF, et al. Voriconazole versus amphotericin B for primary therapy of invasive aspergillosis. *New Engl J Med*, 2002; 347: 408–15.
Comments: Important paper that has made voriconazole preferred treatment for aspergillosis based on randomized trial of 277 patients w/ invasive aspergillosis (most had hematological malignancies). Voriconazole response rate 53% vs 32% for amphotericin B. Survival also superior: 71 vs 58%.

BLASTOMYCES DERMATITIDIS

Amita Gupta, MD, MHS

MICROBIOLOGY

- Dimorphic fungus found along Mississippi, Missouri, St. Lawrence, and Ohio rivers and regions that border Great Lakes in US and Canada. Occurs in Africa, and a few cases have been reported in Europe, Middle East, and India.

- Grows as a broad-based budding yeast at 37°C. At 25°C, produces mycelia and can produce conidia.
- Grows in moist soil with acidic pH and high organic content (decaying vegetation, close to water, areas of high humidity).
- Commercially available molecular probe offers rapid identification of culture.

CLINICAL

- Almost any organ can be involved (see Sites of Infection below). Disease ranges from asymptomatic to rapidly fatal. Most primary infections asymptomatic or mild. Human infection most commonly results from inhalation of conidia. Rare reports of sexual transmission or accidental infection of lab personnel.
- Acute pulmonary infection (<3 wks of Sx duration) often asymptomatic or mis-Dx'd as viral syndrome due to nonspecific Sx of fever, myalgias, cough. Most cases Dx'd after chronic (>3 wks) manifestations appear.
- In immunocompetent individuals incubation period 30–45 days. Relatively uncommon OI in HIV. CD4 usually <200. Similar clinical manifestations but disease can progress more rapidly with advanced HIV. Reactivation disease may play role in up to 25% of cases with advanced HIV.
- Mortality rate in HIV-infected patients <54% in pre-HAART era. Insufficient data in HAART era, but outcome expected to be improved.
- Cx is gold standard for Dx: sensitivity ~90%. Fungal Cx of sputum, skin, CSF, urine, infected tissue, and/or bone lesions. Brain-heart infusion or Sabouraud's glucose agar typically used. Detection from any sterile site diagnostic. Important to notify lab and pathology personnel about possibility of blastomycosis, as accidental autoinoculation (i.e., lab exposures) have been reported.
- In many cases, Dx can be made by visualization of characteristic broad-based budding yeast from body fluid or aspirated skin lesions; wet mount (with 10% KOH or fungal stain) under light microscopy. Centrifugation of CSF, BAL, urine, pleural fluid recommended to optimize detection. Histopathology specimens best seen with fungal stains (e.g., Gimori methanamine staining); PAS stain can also be helpful (thick-walled broad-based yeast cells seen). Pyogranulomatous tissue response (noncaseating) or pseudoepitheliomatous hyperplasia can be seen on pathology.
- *Blastomyces* antigen test (EIA-MiraVista Diagnostics). Positive EIA of blood or urine found in 72% of cases of disseminated and 100% of pulmonary cases. Specificity limited by cross-reactive antigens with other fungi, e.g., *Histoplasma*, *Paracoccidioides*, and *Penicillium marneffei*.
- False-positive *Histoplasma* antigen tests possible due to cross-reactive antigens.
- Skin testing and sero-Dx using complement fixation antibodies or immunodiffusion precipitin bands not recommended due to poor sensitivity and specificity.
- (1-3)-beta-D-glucan test (Fungitell®): *Blastomyces* usually not detected due to little (1,3)-beta-D-glucan produced in the yeast phase. Enzyme immunoassay with A antigen of *B. dermatitidis* cross reacts with *Histoplasma*. Newer serology test based on BAD1 protein (no cross-reaction) or chemiluminescent DNA probes may be useful (more sensitive) but not commercially available.

SITES OF INFECTION

- Disseminated disease: usually presents as indolent, progressive illness with significant weight loss and pulmonary complaints but may progress to an acute sepsis syndrome. Dissemination occurs in ~63% of HIV+ patients with blastomycosis.
- CNS: in 1 review, cerebral abscess or meningitis in 11/24 HIV+ patients (46%). Consider CNS evaluation to assure appropriate therapy.
- Skin: lesions can be papulopustular, ulcerative, subcutaneous nodules. Central crusting with "black dots" can occur. If purulent drainage, can often see yeast forms on microscopic examination. Less common in patients with AIDS (~20%).
- Lung: most common site of infection. Fever, cough, dyspnea, and pleuritic chest pain. Chest X-ray abnormal in up to 2/3 of cases. Infiltrates on CXR can be lobar, interstitial, miliary, interstitial, nodular, masslike, or rarely cavitary. Pleural effusions can also occur. Patients may develop ARDS.
- Osteolytic bone lesions, often with cold abscess (predilection for ribs, vertebrae, long bones, skull, face).
- Prostatitis, epididymitis, or renal disease.

PATHOGENS

TREATMENT

Initial Therapy: Nonmeningeal Disease

- Lipid formulation amphotericin 3–5 mg/kg or amphotericin B 0.7–1 mg/kg/day for 1–2 wks or until improvement noted. Switch to oral therapy with itraconazole as preferred azole, 200 mg 3 ×/day for 3 days then twice daily. Treat for at least 12 mos.
- IDSA recommends measuring serum itraconazole levels after 2 wks of itraconazole to ensure adequate levels of drug exposure.
- Surgery for refractory focal disease such as cavitary lung lesions and CNS abscesses.
- If no CNS disease, mild or localized disease and CD4 >200, can consider initial treatment with itraconazole but limited data.
- Discontinuation: azole can be safely discontinued in persons who have received at least 1 yr of appropriate azole, have CD4 >150 × >6 mos, and are receiving ART.

Suppressive Therapy: Nonmeningeal Disease and Discontinuation

- Long-term suppressive therapy should be given to prevent relapse until good immune response to ART can be achieved.
- 1st line: itraconazole 200 mg PO once daily (liquid formulation preferred).
- 2nd line: fluconazole 200–400 mg PO twice daily; less effective but can be used in patients with meningeal disease or patients who experience toxicity on itraconazole.

Initial Therapy: Brain Abscess or Meningitis

- Amphotericin lipid formulation 5 mg/kg/day IV × 4–6 wks then switch to oral azole.
- Most appropriate azole to use is unclear. Possible options for oral azole: fluconazole (800 mg/day), itraconazole (200 mg 2–3 ×/day), or voriconazole (200–400 mg twice daily) × >12 mos and until resolution of CSF abnormalities.
- Azoles should not be used as initial therapy for CNS blastomycosis; should be used only after initial response to amphotericin.

Suppressive Therapy: Meningeal Disease and Discontinuation

- Long-term suppressive therapy should be given to prevent relapse of disease until good immune response to ART can be achieved.
- 1st line: fluconazole 400 mg PO twice daily may be useful but data scant.
- 2nd line: itraconazole 100–200 mg PO twice daily (liquid formulation preferred).
- Discontinuation: limited data, but likely that azole can be safely discontinued in patients who have received at least 1 yr of appropriate azole, have CD4 >150 for >6 mos, and are receiving ART.

FOLLOW-UP

- Azoles should not be given during pregnancy.
- Follow for drug toxicities, clinical response, and counsel patient regarding drug with azoles.
- Consider discontinuation of antifungal maintenance therapy after >12 mos of antifungal therapy completed, CD4 count >150 for >6 mos and full resolution of clinical disease due to blastomycosis.
- Data from pediatric study suggest follow-up of urine antigen titers may be useful to gauge treatment response.

SELECTED REFERENCES

McKinnel JA, Pappas PG. Blastomycosis: new insights into diagnosis, prevention, and treatment. *Clin Chest Med*, 2009; 30: 227–239.
Comments: Comprehensive review of blastomycosis.

Chapman SW, Dismukes WE, Proia LA, et al. Clinical practice guidelines for the management of blastomycosis: 2008 update by the Infectious Diseases Society of America. *Clin Infect Dis*, 2008; 46: 1801–12.
Comments: Guidelines published by IDSA for treatment of blastomycosis.

CANDIDA SPP.

Dionissis Neofytos, MD, MPH

MICROBIOLOGY

- Thin walled, ovoid yeast cells typically 4–6 mcm in size (*C. glabrata* smaller).
- >150 spp., but ~9 are frequent pathogens in humans, including *C. albicans*, *C. krusei*, *C. glabrata*, *C. parapsilosis*, *C. tropicalis*, *C. dubliniensis*, and *C. lusitaniae*.

- Microscopy of clinical specimens reveals yeast forms and pseudohyphae w/ some true hyphae. Gram stain: large Gram + cocci.
- Grow well in routine blood Cx bottles and on agar plates. Blood cultures positive in 50%–70% of candidemia cases. Antigen (e.g., beta-D-glucan) and PCR assays may be of some help for diagnosis of candidemia. *C. albicans* and *C. dubliniensis* germ-tube positive (early hyphal-like extensions at 24 hrs of culture). All other *Candida* spp. germ-tube negative. PNA-FISH testing on a positive blood Cx: rapid detection of *C. albicans* and *C. glabrata*.
- *C. albicans* found as part of normal flora of mouth, vagina, GI tract. *C. parapsilosis* associated with central line infections and outbreaks from transmission from healthcare workers. *C. tropicalis* associated with poor outcomes in severely immunocompromised (i.e., neutropenic) hosts. *C. glabrata* and *C. krusei* associated with prior exposure to azoles.

CLINICAL

- *C. albicans* is most common spp. causing disease in humans, but non-*albicans Candida* spp. such as *C. glabrata* and *C. krusei* becoming more common. Distribution and epidemiology of *Candida* spp. varies around the world.
- **Oropharyngeal candidiasis (OPC):** white pseudomembranous plaques coating tongue and palate (thrush); removable by scraping the plaques leaving a raw, painful, and bleeding mucosa. Also includes erythematous candidiasis and angular cheilitis.
- **Esophagitis:** odynophagia and dysphagia; endoscopy reveals ulcers and pseudomembranes; OPC often present but not required. If empiric Rx fails, consider endoscopy to r/o CMV, herpes, aphthous, or azole-resistant *Candida* esophagitis.
- **Vaginitis:** itching, burning, cheesy white discharge (although scant discharge not uncommon); not more refractory to therapy than in HIV-negative patients.
- Growth of *Candida* from BAL or sputum usually due to contamination from upper respiratory source; lung Bx demonstrating yeast and inflammation is gold standard, but pneumonia extremely uncommon.
- **Candidemia:** associated with multiple risk factors, including abdominal surgery, administration of broad-spectrum antibiotics, central lines, TPN, hemodialysis, mechanical ventilation. Mortality remains high (35%–47%) (*Mayo Clin Proc.* 2008; 83: 1011–21).

SITES OF INFECTION

- GI: OPC; acute and chronic atrophic candidiasis; esophagitis; gastric, small bowel and colonic ulcers (uncommon); hepatic and splenic abscesses, peritonitis (associated w/ surgery/trauma or peritoneal dialysis catheter).
- CV: candidemia (often associated w/ central venous catheters); endocarditis; myocardial abscesses.
- CNS: meningitis.
- GU: vulvovaginal candidiasis; UTI; perinephric abscesses.
- Skin: folliculitis; balanitis; intertrigo; paronychia and onychomycosis.
- Respiratory: pneumonia (rare).
- Eyes: endophthalmitis.
- Bone and joints: septic arthritis; osteomyelitis.

TREATMENT

General Principles

- *In vitro* susceptibility testing best established for fluconazole, but available for multiple agents; recommended for candidemia isolates; most useful when disease refractory to Rx, with *C. glabrata* and *C. krusei*, which may be fluconazole-resistant, and in cases where switch from parenteral Rx to oral fluconazole being considered.
- Risk factors for azole resistance: CD4 <50, TMP-SMX use for PCP prophylaxis, and previous exposure to azoles.
- Reduced susceptibility or resistance to azoles may occur in *C. albicans* w/ prolonged exposure to fluconazole. Increasing dose (up to 800 mg/day) may overcome resistance.
- Higher MICs to echinocandins reported among isolates of *C. parapsilosis*; of unclear clinical significance.
- Resistance to echinocandins emerging in high-risk patients (i.e., with hematologic malignancies, transplant).

PATHOGENS

- *C. krusei* intrinsically resistant to fluconazole; it may still be susceptible to broad-spectrum azoles (i.e., voriconazole, posaconazole). Increasing resistance to fluconazole w/ *C. glabrata* and *C. dubliniensis.*
- *C. lusitaniae* tends to be resistant to amphotericin B.
- For candidemia, removal of central venous lines (if feasible) recommended to promote clearance of organism.
- For candidemia, ophthalmology evaluation should be obtained to R/O endophthalmitis.

Chemotherapy
- See guidelines: *Clin Infect Dis* 2004; 38: 165–89.
- **OPC(1):** clotrimazole troches 10 mg 5 times daily or nystatin 200,000–400,000 U 5 ×/day. Alternates are fluconazole 100–200 mg PO once daily; itraconazole solution 200 mg PO once daily, amphotericin B 1–5 mL 4 times daily (can be prepared w/ 100 mg/mL solution). Duration: 7–14 days after clinical improvement.
- **OPC(2):** start with topical formulations; if no response, switch to fluconazole; if no response, consider higher doses of fluconazole (up to 800 mg/day); if no response can switch to PO itraconazole, IV caspofungin, or amphotericin B.
- **Esophagitis:** fluconazole 100–200 mg PO/IV once daily (up to 800 mg once daily); itraconazole 200 mg PO once daily; alternatives include voriconazole 6 mg/kg mg PO/IV twice daily; amphotericin B 0.3–0.7 mg/kg/day IV; caspofungin 50 mg IV once daily. Duration: 14–21 days after clinical improvement.
- **Vaginitis** (*MMWR* 2006;55[RR-11]:45): topical creams (e.g., clotrimazole 1% 5 g/day × 7–14 days); vaginal tablets (e.g., clotrimazole 100 mg twice daily × 3 days); PO tablets (fluconazole 150 mg PO × 1 dose—not in pregnancy).
- **Candidemia and disseminated/deep-seated infection:** consider an echinocandin (caspofungin 70 mg IV load then 50 mg q24h, micafungin 100–150 mg IV q24h, anidulafungin 200 mg IV load then 100 mg IV q24h) or amphotericin B (0.6–1.0 mg/kg/day IV) or 1 of its lipid formulations or fluconazole 800 mg load then 400 mg q24h. Duration: 14 days after last + blood Cx and Sx resolution; longer in cases of endophthalmitis, endocarditis, osteomyelitis, septic arthritis, or other complications.
- **Candidemia in nonneutropenic hosts:** fluconazole 800 mg IV/PO load then 400 mg q24h, caspofungin 70 mg IV load then 50 mg q24h, micafungin 100–150 mg IV q24h, anidulafungin 200 mg IV load then 100 mg IV q24h, amphotericin B 0.6–1.0 mg/kg/day IV or lipid formulation.
- **Candidemia in neutropenic hosts:** limited data available. Amphotericin B 0.7–1.0 mg/kg/day or lipid formulations 3–5 mg/kg/day IV, caspofungin 70 mg IV load then 50 mg q24h, micafungin 100–150 mg IV q24h, anidulafungin 200 mg IV load then 100 mg IV q24h. Alternative: fluconazole 6–12 mg/kg IV/PO q24h: only for stable patients without prior azole exposure.

FOLLOW-UP
- Sx of OPC, esophagitis, and vaginitis typically respond within 3–5 days.
- If no response, consider endoscopy for esophagitis; consider modifying therapy for OPC (switch to fluconazole, increase dose, or switch to another agent); if still no response, consider Cx and sensitivity testing.
- Immune reconstitution with ART decreases recurrences; even incomplete viral suppression helpful.
- Maintenance therapy, OPC: clotrimazole or nystatin preferred; alternates include fluconazole 100 mg PO once daily or itraconazole 200 mg PO once daily.
- Maintenance therapy, esophagitis: consider for frequent recurrence; fluconazole 200 mg PO once daily preferred; alternatives include itraconazole 200 mg PO once daily.
- For complicated vaginitis, consider topical creams administered for > 7 days or fluconazole 150 mg PO × 2 doses separated by 72 h. Vaginitis due to non-*C. albicans* spp. may respond to topical boric acid (600 mg/day × 14 days) or to topical 5-FC (*Clin Infect Dis*, 2004; 38: 161–89).

OTHER INFORMATION
- Itraconazole available in 2 formulations: (1) capsules taken with meals and acidic drinks (e.g., cola) to increase absorption; (2) liquid formulation taken on empty stomach.

- Azoles are potent inhibitors of P450 cytochrome; drug-drug interactions with PIs, EFV, PPIs, CCBs, nafcillin, carbamazepine, phenytoin, calcineurin inhibitors, St. John's wort, etc. Review prior to administration.
- Echinocandins associated with minimal adverse events. Please note possible interaction of caspofungin with cyclosporine. Caspofungin and micafungin should be dose-adjusted in cases of hepatic dysfunction.

SELECTED REFERENCES

Reboli AC et al: Anidulafungin versus fluconazole for invasive candidiasis. *N Engl J Med* 356:2472, 2007; June 14.
Comments: Noninferiority trial showing equivalency of these compounds for IC (superiority of anidulafungin was observed). Treatment successful in 75.6% of pts treated with anidulafungin vs. 60.2% for fluconazole (difference, 15.4%; 95% CI, 3.9 to 27.0).

Kuse ER et al: Micafungin versus liposomal amphotericin B for candidaemia and invasive candidosis: a phase III randomised double-blind trial. *Lancet* 369:1519, 2007 May 5.
Comments: Nearly equivalent efficacy (90%) in both arms but micafungin better tolerated than liposomal amphotericin.

Spanakis EK, Aperis G, Mylonakis E. New agents for the treatment of fungal infections: clinical efficacy and gaps in coverage. *Clin Infect Dis*, 2006; 43: 1060–8.
Comments: Excellent review of the latest FDA approved antifungals and those expected to be approved (e.g., posaconazole).

Pappas PG, Rex JH, Sobel JD, et al. Guidelines for treatment of candidiasis. *Clin Infect Dis*, 2004; 38: 161–89.
Comments: Updated guidelines for the management of candidiasis.

Gafter-Gvili A, Vidal L, Goldberg E, Leibovici L, Paul M. Treatment of invasive candida infections: systematic review and meta-analysis. *Mayo Clin Proc*, 2008; 83(9): 1011–21.

PENICILLIUM MARNEFFEI

Khalil G. Ghanem, MD, PhD

MICROBIOLOGY

- Dimorphic fungus: mold at 25°C with short, hyaline, septate, and branched hyphae; yeast at 37°C with cerebriform, smooth, light tan colonies; reverse side on agar appears pink due to pigment production.
- Yeast form 3–6 × 1.5–2 m, round/ellipsoidal, with round central septum, and mixed with hyphae.
- Reservoir host: bamboo rats; isolated from these animals (liver, lungs, spleen, and feces) in various parts of Southeast Asia; organism also isolated from soil of bamboo rats' burrows.
- Divides by fission (manifested by the central septum in the yeast form); transmitted primarily via inhalation; also direct inoculation, possibly ingestion.

CLINICAL

- Endemic in Southeast Asia (Thailand, Vietnam, Hong Kong) and southern China.
- 80% of cases occur in immunocompromised hosts. HIV: 3rd leading OI in endemic areas after *M. TB* and *C. neoformans*. Risk increases with advanced immunosuppression (CD4 <200).
- Signs and Sx: fever, weight loss, anemia, skin lesions, dry cough, chest pain, lymphadenopathy, hepatosplenomegaly.
- Dx (1): appropriate travel history. CXR: infiltrates and cavitation. Bx: bone marrow, skin lesions, or lymph nodes; stains: Wright's, Giemsa, H and E, GMS, or PAS (see Microbiology second bullet above); immunohistochemistry.
- Dx (2): Cx: blood has variable yield (sensitivity up to 76%); bone marrow Cx.
- Dx (3): serology and PCR available.
- Clinical DDx: TB, histoplasmosis.
- Laboratory DDx: *H. capsulatum*, which divides by budding, unlike *Penicillium*.

SITES OF INFECTION

- Pulmonary: infiltrates and cavitation.
- GI: diarrhea and hepatosplenomegaly (especially in children with AIDS).
- Skin: lesions, especially in face, upper trunk and arms; umbilicated papules typical; oral and genital ulcers.

PATHOGENS

- Cardiovascular: pericarditis (rare).
- Heme: lymphadenopathy, anemia, and cytopenias.
- Bone: osteomyelitis, osteolytic lesions.

TREATMENT
Primary Therapy
- Amphotericin B: (0.6 mg/day IV × 2 wks) followed by itraconazole (400 mg PO once daily × 10 wks) appears most effective (*Clin Infect Dis*, 1998; 26: 1107–10). Consider itraconazole levels.

FOLLOW-UP
Secondary Prophylaxis
- High relapse rate of therapy (>50%) if immunosuppression persists and secondary prophylaxis not instituted.
- Consider itraconazole suppressive therapy (200 mg/day) unless immunosuppression reversed (Sun).
- Limited data suggest that discontinuation of 2° prophylaxis in patients with immune reconstitution may be feasible (*J Antimicrob Chemother* 63: 340, 2009).

SELECTED REFERENCES
Sirisanthana T, Supparatpinyo K, Perriens J, et al. Amphotericin B and itraconazole for treatment of disseminated *Penicillium marneffei* infection in human immunodeficiency virus-infected patients. *Clin Infect Dis*, 1998; 26: 1107–10.
Comments: Open-label, nonrandomized study of amphotericin B 0.6 mg/kg/day IV × 2 wks, followed by itraconazole 400-mg PO once daily × 10 wks. Of 74 HIV-infected patients studied who had disseminated *P. marneffei* infection, 72 (97.3%) responded to treatment.

Supparatpinyo K, Perriens J, Nelson KE, et al. A controlled trial of itraconazole to prevent relapse of *Penicillium marneffei* infection in patients infected with the human immunodeficiency virus. *New Engl J Med*, 1998; 339: 1739–43.
Comments: Double-blinded trial of 72 patients with AIDS in complete remission after treatment for *P. marneffei* infection. Patients randomly assigned to receive either itraconazole (200 mg PO once daily) or placebo as maintenance therapy. None of 36 patients assigned to itraconazole had relapse within 1 yr, whereas 20 of 35 patients assigned to placebo had relapses.

Wu TC, Chan JW, Ng CK, et al. Clinical presentations and outcomes of *Penicillium marneffei* infections: a series from 1994 to 2004. *Hong Kong Med J*, 2008; 14: 103–9.
Comments: Retrospective study of 47 cases of penicilliosis. Fever, malaise, and anemia were the commonest presentations. Most diagnoses were obtained from blood cultures (83%) and lymph node biopsies (34%). 5 (11%) died. Most patients received induction amphotericin B, followed by oral itraconazole; a smaller proportion (21%) received oral itraconazole only.

Sun HY, Chen MY, Hsiao CF, et al. Endemic fungal infections caused by *Cryptococcus neoformans* and *Penicillium marneffei* in patients infected with human immunodeficiency virus and treated with highly active anti-retroviral therapy. *Clin Microbiol Infect*, 2006; 12: 381–8.
Comments: Study reports that discontinuation of secondary prophylaxis after initiation of ART in patients with penicilliosis is feasible. Only 1 episode of penicillosis recurred (relapse rate of 1.72/100 person-years; 95% CI, 1.44–2.10/100 PY) after median follow-up of 35.3 mos.

Parasites

ACANTHAMOEBA SPP.

Lisa A. Spacek, MD, PhD and Khalil G. Ghanem, MD, PhD

MICROBIOLOGY

- 1 of 4 genera of free-living amebas associated with disease in humans; >20 spp. described.
- Life cycle w/ 2 stages: actively dividing trophozoite and dormant cysts (double-walled 10–15 mcm in diameter); cysts resistant to chlorine, low temperature, antibiotics.
- Encystation occurs under environmental stress: food deprivation, desiccation, change in temperature, pH.
- Ubiquitous in nature: isolated from air, soil, freshwater, salt water, chlorinated swimming pools, sewage, fish, reptiles, birds, mammals.
- Transmission: inhalation most common route; direct inoculation of skin can occur.

CLINICAL

- Cause of granulomatous amebic encephalitis (GAE), chronic sinusitis, otitis, cutaneous lesions in AIDS patients.
- Disseminated disease more common with advanced immunosuppression; immunity is predominantly T-cell mediated.
- Infrequently diagnosed before death due to low level of suspicion or pathological misdiagnosis.
- Sx of GAE: subacute onset of headache, confusion, stiff neck; CT and MRI show nonspecific enhancing lesions (usually in midbrain, brainstem, and cerebellum); may be cyst-like.
- Dx of GAE: CSF with pleocytosis; wet mount of CSF (trophozoites resemble macrophages); H and E staining; calcofluor white fluorescently stains cysts and trophozoites in tissue section; special growth medium and cell Cx can be used.
- Dx of skin lesions: Bx; staining/Cx as above.
- Real-time PCR assays validated for diagnosis of keratitis.

SITES OF INFECTION

- Skin: most common manifestation in AIDS; painful ulcerated nodules on trunk or extremeties; may be due either to direct inoculation or hematogenous spread; 73% mortality. Leukocytoclastic vasculitis reported.
- CNS: GAE; CD4 usually <200; fulminant course; mortality high; CSF may show lymphocytic pleocytosis, low glucose and high protein but may be normal.
- ENT: chronic sinusitis and otitis.
- Eyes: painful, chronic corneal ulcers associated with use of contact lenses; this form occurs in immunocompetent patients.
- Bone: osteomyelitis.
- Lungs: may be primary portal of entry; pneumonia may occur.

TREATMENT

General Points

- Early Dx yields best chance of cure.
- Combination therapy is the rule for treating infections; diamidine derivatives (propamidine, pentamidine, dibromopropamidine) have greatest activity. Other active drugs: ketoconazole, fluconazole, sulfadiazine, TMP-SMX, 5-flucytosine, rifampin.
- Test for drug sensitivity. Drugs must be cysticidal to prevent recurrence from dormant cysts.
- Prognosis may be improved with immune restoration due to ART.

CNS Disease

- Fluconazole 800 mg/day + sulfadiazine 1–2 g PO q6h + surgery effective in AIDS patient with localized CNS involvement (± 5-FC 25 mg/kg q6h).
- ART.

Cutaneous Disease

- IV pentamidine 4 mg/kg/day + topical chlorhexidine + topical ketoconazole successful for cutaneous disease without CNS involvement.
- ART.

PATHOGENS

459

Ocular Disease
- Refer to ophthalmologist immediately.
- Successful regimen for AK: polyhexamethylene biguanide 0.02% ± chlorhexidine 0.02% ± propamidine isethionate and dipropamidine (Brolene) 0.1% ± hemamidine 0.1% (Perez-Santonja).
- ART.

SELECTED REFERENCES

Hammersmith KM. Diagnosis and management of *Acanthamoeba* keratitis. *Curr Opin Ophthalmol*, 2006; 17: 327–31.
Comments: Recent review highlighting increased frequency of infections, associated with frequent replacement soft contact lenses. Good outcome with early Dx; providers should consider Dx especially in contact lens wearer with suspected herpes keratitis.

Visvesvara GS, Moura H, Schuster FL. Pathogenic and opportunistic free-living amoebae: *Acanthamoeba* spp., *Balamuthia mandrillaris, Naegleria fowleri*, and *Sappinia diploidea*. *FEMS Immunol Med Microbiol*, 2007; 50: 1–26.
Comments: Recent summary of free-living amoebae-associated infection; reviews types of disease and diagnostic methods.

Marciano-Cabral F, Cabral G. *Acanthamoeba* spp. as agents of disease in humans. *Clin Microbiol Rev*, 2003; 16: 273–307.
Comments: Review on *Acanthamoeba* in both immunocompromised and competent hosts. Authors detail latest diagnostic techniques, including PCR.

CYCLOSPORA CAYETANENSIS

Lisa A. Spacek, MD, PhD and Khalil G. Ghanem, MD, PhD

MICROBIOLOGY
- Obligate intracellular coccidian parasite; infects epithelial cells of small intestine.
- Excreted in stool as oocysts (spherical, 8–10 mcm in diameter), which may be shed intermittantly and at low levels. Sporulation (maturation of oocysts) occurs outside host and takes 7–12 days.
- Transmitted by fecal-contaminated soil, food, and water. Humans only known host and reservoir. Human-to-human transmission unlikely as excreted oocysts must sporulate before becoming infectious.
- Both sporadic infections and outbreaks occur. Infections tend to be seasonal with spring and summer being peak seasons in the US, associated with imported raspberries, mixed salad greens, and basil.
- Found in travelers to endemic areas, i.e., Peru, Nepal, Haiti, Guatemala, Indonesia.

CLINICAL
- Infects both immunocompetent/compromised patients. Increased risk of disease with advanced immunosuppression.
- Incubation period 7–11 days; onset of Sx usually sudden.
- Sx: prolonged, relapsing watery diarrhea, crampy abdominal pain, fatigue, anorexia, myalgias, and fever; vomiting uncommon.
- More asymptomatic carriage and shorter duration of illness in residents of endemic areas compared to travelers.
- Dx: concentrate by centrifugation in formalin-ethyl acetate, organisms stain variably acid-fast using modified Ziehl-Neelsen or Kinyoun method (light pink to deep red); blue autofluorescence under UV microscopy; "hot" modified safranin method stains oocysts a brilliant reddish orange; PCR available.
- Mixed infections with other parasites such as *Cryptosporidium* have been reported.

SITES OF INFECTION
- Small intestine: found in cytoplasm of jejunal epithelial cells.
- Gallbladder: cases of acalculous cholecystitis have been reported in AIDS patients.

TREATMENT
Chemotherapy
- TMP-SMX DS 1 tab twice daily × 7–10 days.
- With relapse some patients may require secondary prophylaxis: TMP-SMX DS 1 tab/3 × wk.
- Nitazoxanide may be effective, 500 mg PO twice daily × 3 days; not FDA approved for this indication.

SELECTED REFERENCES

Centers for Disease Control and Prevention (CDC). Preliminary FoodNet data on the incidence of infection with pathogens transmitted commonly through food—10 States, 2008. *MMWR Morb Mortal Wkly Rep*, 2009; 58: 333–7.
Comments: This report describes preliminary surveillance data on incidence of food-transmitted pathogens for 2008 and trends since 1996. Incidence of *Cyclospora* infections was 0.04 per 100,000 population in 2008.

Chacin-Bonilla L. Transmission of *Cyclospora cayetanensis* infection: a review focusing on soil-borne cyclosporiasis. *Trans R Soc Trop Med Hyg*, 2008; 102: 215–6.
Comments: This review focuses on transmission of *C. cayetanensis* via fecal-contaminated soil. Risk factors for infection include extreme poverty, lack of toilet or latrine, defecation practices, and soil contact.

Lalonde LF, Gajadhar AA. Highly sensitive and specific PCR assay for reliable detection of *Cyclospora cayetanensis* oocysts. *Appl Environ Microbiol*, 2008; 74: 4354–8.
Comments: This study describes a preliminary validation of DNA extraction for *C. cayetanensis* oocysts and a sensitive and specific novel PCR assay.

Herwaldt BL. *Cyclospora cayetanensis*: a review, focusing on the outbreaks of cyclosporiasis in the 1990s. *Clin Infect Dis*, 2000; 31: 1040–57.
Comments: Author focuses on foodborne and waterborne outbreaks of cyclosporiasis documented from 1990–1999. These highlight need for healthcare personnel to consider that seemingly isolated cases of infection could be part of widespread outbreaks and should be reported to public health officials.

ENTAMOEBA HISTOLYTICA

Joseph M. Vinetz, MD

MICROBIOLOGY
- Protozoan parasite, cause of diarrhea, dysentery, liver abscess, and other syndromes.
- Quadrinucleate cyst passed in feces initiates infection, excystation occurs in intestinal umen.
- Galactose/N-acetyl-D-galactosamine (Gal/GalNAc)-specific lectin mediates parasite adhesion to colonic mucins, allowing colonization, and later invasion.
- Invasion related to penetration of mucous layer, killing of epithelial cells by amoebapore (5kDa protein).
- Immunity mediated by mucosal IgA recognition of Gal/GalNAc lectin.

CLINICAL
- Occurs primarily in developing countries, but immigrants and travelers diagnosed with infection in US.
- Onset of colitis usually gradual with Sxs >1 wk, distinguishing it from bacterial dysentery.
- Dx (1) of amebic colitis: observation of red cell-containing motile trophozoites on fresh stool smear (insensitive); always heme + stool.
- On O and P, visualized ameba must be distinguished clinically from *Entamoeba dispar*, a morphologically identical parasite that is noninvasive and does not cause disease.
- Dx (2) Colonoscopy: biopsy or scraping at margin of colonic mucosal ulcer—parasite may be seen; H and E shows necrosis, classic flask-shaped ulcer.
- Dx (3) Antigen test: distinguishes *E. histolytica* from *E. dispar* is available; more sensitive than microscopy of stool.
- Dx (4) Serology: 99% sensitive for amebic liver abscess; 88% sensitive for colitis, but Ab may be present yrs later so that serology may not be useful in immigrants from *E. histolytica*-endemic regions.
- Dx (5) Ultrasound of liver: cannot distinguish amebic from pyogenic abscess, but can guide aspiration if necessary.
- Dx (6) Liver abscess aspiration: yields anchovy paste-like material; lack of WBCs (due to lysis by parasite) clue to diagnosis, parasites usually not seen.

SITES OF INFECTION
- Colon: dysentery, ameboma (tumor-like lesion of colonic lumen), toxic megacolon.
- Liver: abscess; can rupture causing peritonitis.
- Lung: empyema (right-sided; direct extension from liver).
- Heart: pericarditis (direct extension from liver).
- Brain: abscess (hematogenous spread, rare).

PATHOGENS

- Skin: usually perineal, genital.
- GU: rectovaginal fistula.

TREATMENT

Intestinal Colonization

- *E. dispar* does not require Rx.
- Lumenal agents alone should be used (not absorbed).
- Iodoquinol: 650 mg PO 3 times daily × 20 days.
- Paromomycin: 25–35 mg/kg/day in 3 divided doses × 7 days.

Invasive

- Metronidazole: 500–750 mg PO 3 times daily × 7–10 days.
- Tinidazole: 2 g PO × 3–5 days.
- Liver abscess aspiration not usually necessary, does not speed recovery.
- Consider adding luminal agent, otherwise relapse of extraintestinal disease may occur months later.

OTHER INFORMATION

- Amebic colitis should be ruled out prior to treatment of Crohn's disease; corticosteroids will worsen amebiasis.
- Clinical and laboratory findings: colitis: fever 10% of the time; 1/2 of patients have weight loss; abdominal pain frequent; no WBCs in stool (lysed by organism), invariably heme + parasites detected <50% of the time with stool microscopy; peripheral WBC higher with progressively severe Sx. Liver abscess: fever in 90%, 1/2 of patients have Sx >4 wks, abscess in right lobe of liver in 80% (similar to pyogenic abscesses so this is not distinguishing feature); most patients have elevated WBC count, transaminases and alk phos, may have elevated bilirubin with jaundice.

SELECTED REFERENCES

Petri WA, Singh U. Diagnosis and management of amebiasis. *Clin Infect Dis*, 1999; 29: 1117–25.
Comments: Useful summary of treatment approaches including antiparasitic drugs and role of aspiration of liver abscess.

Haque R, Huston CD, Hughes M, et al. Amebiasis. *New Engl J Med*, 2003; 348: 1565–73.
Comments: State of the art article on amebiasis that remains topical and useful.

GIARDIA LAMBLIA

Joseph M. Vinetz, MD

MICROBIOLOGY

- Protozoan parasite, reservoir primarily human, potentially domestic and sylvatic animals; fecal-oral or waterborne transmission.
- Most commonly identified fecal parasite in North America; common in mountainous areas of Northeast, Rocky Mountain states, Northwest; pockets of high prevalence in urban areas.
- Fecal-oral transmission, including oral-anal transmission during sexual activities.

CLINICAL

- At presentation, most patients have had >7 days of diarrhea; weight loss >10 lbs in >50%.
- Treatment-refractory, or relapsing cases seen in immunocompromised, including HIV/AIDS.
- Risk factors: children in home who attend daycare centers; travel to endemic area; ingestion of unfiltered water while camping/hiking or well water on farm; fecal-oral sexual contact.
- Dx: stool exam for cysts/trophozoites; stool *Giardia* antigen test (slightly more sensitive than microscopy, 100% specific).
- Stools profuse and watery; become greasy and foul smelling over time; blood, pus and mucus absent.
- Typical presentation: acute onset diarrhea, bloating, flatulence, cramps, accompanied by malaise, nausea, anorexia, and classically with "sulfuric belching".
- Clinical manifestations not different in HIV+ vs HIV-negative; incidence and prevalence unclear, range from very low to ~5% in developed countries to as high as 15% in developing countries.
- Treatment failures occur with all therapies; need to investigate sexual partners to ensure that transmission/reinfection not occuring.
- Treatment may be difficult in immunocompromised patients, with higher risk for relapse.

SITES OF INFECTION
- GI: upper small bowel, adherent to enterocytes; biliary tract involvement (rare).
- No extraintestinal disease.

TREATMENT

Metronidazole
- 250 mg 3 times daily × 5–7 days (not FDA approved, but clinical standard with widespread experience).
- Refractory cases: use in combination with quinacrine has been reported effective.
- Efficacy 80%–95%.
- When taken w/ alcohol, can produce disulfiram-like effect.
- In pregnancy, no standard recommendations because of theoretical risk of metronidazole-induced teratogenicity (not yet observed).
- Has been used in pregnancy for trichomoniasis; teratogenic potential appears minimal; use restricted to last 2 trimesters.
- Clinical resistance has been seen with metronidazole.

Tinidazole
- 2 g PO as single dose.
- FDA approved 2004.
- >90% efficacy rate, appears to have better side effect profile than metronidazole.

Furazolidone
- 100 mg PO four times daily × 7–10 days.
- Efficacy ~80%, lower than metronidazole.
- Side effects: GI, turns urine brown, mild hemolysis with G6PD deficiency, not approved for use in pregnancy.

Quinacrine
- 100 mg PO 3 times daily × 5–7 days.
- Not commercially available in the US or Canada. Available only from Panorama Pharmacy, 8215 Van Nuys Blvd., Panorama City, CA 91402. Tel: (818) 988-7979.
- Has been used in combination with metronidazole in refractory cases; use full doses of both drugs.

Paromomycin
- 25–30 mg/kg/day in 3 divided doses, × 5–10 days.
- Efficacy low, ~60%–70%.
- Can be used in pregnancy, if treatment cannot be delayed beyond delivery.

Nitazoxanide
- 500 mg twice daily × 10 days, then 1 g twice daily × 15 days.
- Anecdotal evidence for use in treatment-refractory cases (*Clin Microbiol Rev* 14:114, 2001).

Albendazole
- 400 mg q day × 3 days.
- Has *in vitro* anti-*Giardia* activity but clinical efficacy not demonstrated in clinical trials.

FOLLOW-UP

Refractory/Relapsing Giardiasis
- Refractory/relapsing cases in HIV/AIDS: if 2 courses of metronidazole do not eradicate infection (as documented by ELISA), alternatives include quinacrine + metronidazole (*Am J Trop Med Hyg* 68:384, 2003), tinidazole, or possibly nitazoxanide (*Clin Microbiol Rev* 14:114, 2001).

OTHER INFORMATION
- Commonly transmitted to family members of infected child, who is likely to be in daycare setting.
- Sexual partners should be screened for infection, as they could be reservoir for reinfection, especially among MSM.

SELECTED REFERENCES

Abboud P, Lemée V, Gargala G, et al. Successful treatment of metronidazole- and albendazole-resistant giardiasis with nitazoxanide in a patient with acquired immunodeficiency syndrome. *Clin Infect Dis*, 2001; 32: 1792–4.
Comments: This case report describes efficacy of nitazoxanide, an FDA approved agent, in metronidazole and albendazole-resistant giardiasis in a patient with AIDS.

Yoder JS, Beach MJ, Centers for Disease Control and Prevention (CDC). Giardiasis surveillance—United States, 2003–2005. *MMWR Surveill Summ*, 2007; 56: 11–8.

PATHOGENS

Comments: Epidemiological information about giardiasis in the United States.

Nash TE, Ohl CA, Thomas E, et al. Treatment of patients with refractory giardiasis. *Clin Infect Dis*, 2001; 33: 22–8.
Comments: Clinical discussion from Ted Nash, the major investigative leader in the field.

Gardner TB, Hill DR. Treatment of giardiasis. *Clin Microbiol Rev*, 2001; 14: 114–28.
Comments: A comprehensive discussion of treatment options in giardiasis, including some options not readily available in the US.

ISOSPORA BELLI

Khalil G. Ghanem, MD, PhD

MICROBIOLOGY

- Coccidian protozoal parasite; mature oocyst 22–33 × 12–15 mcm contains 2 sporocysts, which contain 4 trophozoites each.
- Sporulated oocysts are ingested; sporozoites penetrate epithelial cells of small intestine and develop into trophozoites.
- Transmission occurs by ingestion of fecally contaminated water and food.
- Epidemiology: endemic in Central and South America, Africa, and Southeast Asia; in US, usually associated with HIV infection and institutional living.

CLINICAL

- Sx: profuse, watery, noninflammatory diarrhea (with cases of hemorrhagic diarrhea reported); malaise; crampy abdominal pain; fever uncommon; malabsorption syndrome. Incubation period ~7 days.
- Dx: wet mount or iodine stains of fecal smears are adequate; multiple samples improve sensitivity, as shedding is intermittent; autofluorescence microscopy more sensitive than iodine stain (*Arch Pathol Lab Med* 120:1023, 1996); PCR available; can be seen in duodenal aspirates and intestinal Bx.
- Extraintestinal spread to gallbladder, liver, and spleen has been reported.
- Cases in the US are relatively rare due to routine use of TMP-SMX for PCP prophylaxis in all HIV+ patients w/ CD4 <200.

SITES OF INFECTION

- Small intestine: diarrhea, malabsorption.
- Gallbladder: acalculous cholecystitis.
- Liver and spleen: dissemination reported (rare).
- Rheumatological: reactive arthritis may occur.

TREATMENT

Chemotherapy

- TMP-SMX DS 1 tab PO twice daily × 7 days. Higher doses and longer duration of therapy for acute infection have also been used.
- Sulfa allergic: pyrimethamine 75 mg/day × 14 days + folinic acid × 14 days (*Ann Intern Med* 109:474, 1988 Sep. 15).
- Sulfa allergic: ciprofloxacin 500 mg PO twice daily × 1 wk. Less effective than TMP-SMX.

Secondary Prophylaxis

- Up to 50% of immunosuppressed patients relapse following primary therapy.
- TMP/SMX DS 1 tab PO 3 ×/wk (Verdier) for secondary prophylaxis.
- Sulfa allergic: pyrimethamine 25 mg PO once daily + folinic acid (*Ann Intern Med* 109:474, 1988 Sep. 15).
- Ciprofloxacin 500 mg PO 3 ×/wk can also be used, but is less effective than TMP-SMX.
- Duration indefinite unless immune recovery; no published recommendations on discontinuation of secondary prophylaxis with immune reconstitution, but presumably safe.

FOLLOW-UP

- Shedding may persist even after adequate therapy; follow patients symptomatically.

SELECTED REFERENCES

Verdier RI, Fitzgerald DW, Johnson WD, et al. Trimethoprim-sulfamethoxazole compared with ciprofloxacin for treatment and prophylaxis of *Isospora belli* and *Cyclospora cayetanensis* infection in HIV-infected patients. A randomized, controlled trial. *Ann Intern Med*, 2000; 132: 885–8.

Comments: 22 patients with with chronic diarrhea due to *I. belli* randomly assigned to receive PO TMP-SMX DS 1 tab twice daily or ciprofloxacin (500 mg) twice daily * 7 days. Patients who responded received prophylaxis for 10 wks (1 tab 3 times weekly). Diarrhea resolved more rapidly with TMP-SMX than with ciprofloxacin. All patients receiving secondary prophylaxis with TMP-SMX remained disease-free, and 15 of 16 receiving secondary prophylaxis with ciprofloxacin remained disease-free.

Franzen C, Müller A, Salzberger B, et al. Uvitex 2B stain for the diagnosis of Isospora belli infections in patients with the acquired immunodeficiency syndrome. *Arch Pathol Lab Med*; 1996; 120(11): 1023–5.

Comments: Wet-mounts examined by phase-contrast and bright-field microscopy; smears stained with modified acid-fast stain compared to fluorescent stain with Uvitex 2B. Using fluorescent stain, the oocysts of *I. belli* stained bright white/blue fluorescent and showed a structure similar to that of oocysts in acid fast stains.

Weiss LM, Perlman DC, Sherman J, et al. Isospora belli infection: treatment with pyrimethamine. *Ann Intern Med*; 1988 Sep 15; 109(6): 474–5.

Comments: 2 pts with AIDS, sulfonamide allergy, and *I. belli* infection are reported. They were treated successfully with pyrimethamine 75 mg/day alone; recurrence prevented with pyrimethamine 25 mg/day.

LEISHMANIA SPP.

Paul G. Auwaerter, MD and Joseph M. Vinetz, MD

MICROBIOLOGY

- Protozoan parasite; HIV increases risk of visceral (hepatosplenic and bone marrow) disease; not opportunistic cutaneous or mucocutaneous disease. 2nd most common OI tissue protozoan in HIV after *Toxoplasma gondii* worldwide.
- Transmitted by sandfly vectors. Also shared needles among IDUs, primarily in endemic urban settings.
- Forms: visceral leishmaniasis: *L. donovani* (Asia), *L. infantum* (southern Europe, Mediterranean), *L. chagasi* (Brazil).
- Cutaneous leishmaniasis: *L. major* and *L. tropica* (Old World), *L. mexicana, L. amazonensis, L. peruviana, L. guyanensis* (New World), *L. (viania) braziliensis* (cutaneous and mucocutaneous).
- Amastigote forms seen within macrophages; flagellated promastigote forms seen in cultures, transmitted from insect vector.

CLINICAL

- Visceral leishmaniasis (VL) as an OI in HIV/AIDS occurs due to decreased T-cell immunity associated with progressive HIV infection; 75% with CD4 <200, only 5% with CD4 >500. Particular risk groups include IDUs in southern Europe (needle sharing); residents of or from endemic areas of India, Brazil, Sudan, where agents of visceral leishmaniasis present.
- Syndrome of hepatosplenomegaly, pancytopenia, skin hyperpigmentation (variable); nutritional wasting, bacterial superinfections may be cause of death. Cutaneous lesions more common in HIV-related disease.
- Relapse after treatment common in AIDS and other severe immunocompromising conditions (corticosteroids, organ transplantation); may occur mos to yrs after leaving endemic region where initial infection occurred.
- Cutaneous leishmaniasis not generally considered to be an HIV-related OI.
- Dx (1): Giemsa or DFA stain of splenic or bone marrow aspirate with demonstration of parasites (amastigotes) within macrophages (method of choice). Cx is gold standard but limited to reference/research labs (use diphasic NNN media); also PCR (experimental) or isoenzyme analysis in specialized labs, serology (less helpful in endemic regions; note, crossreactivity with *T. cruzi* for patients in Central/South America).

PATHOGENS

- Dx (2): patients with suspected VL, examine peripheral or buffy coat sample prior to invasive procedure in advanced AIDS patients, as up to 50% have evidence of visible amastigotes seen within monocytes.
- Dx (3): serologic testing of HIV-related visceral leishmaniasis less sensitive than in non-AIDS.
- Need to distinguish from *Histoplasma capsulatum* (similar sized intramacrophage organism but has a pseudocapsule surrounding it), visualize rod-shaped kinetoplast in *Leishmania*.
- Up to 10% of HIV+ patients with amastigotes seen on peripheral smear may be asymptomatic.
- Mortality 10%–20% of AIDS patients with VL in 1st episode; 60% alive at 1 yr.

SITES OF INFECTION
- Liver/spleen: hepatosplenomegaly (may be profound).
- Bone marrow: pancytopenia.
- Dissemination: seen in fulminant or unsuspected cases (organisms seen in lung, skin, GI mucosa, pancreas, myocardium, larynx, adrenals).
- Cutaneous: rare reports of disseminated cutaneous infection in patients with advanced HIV or arising in setting of immune reconstitution.

TREATMENT
General Considerations
- Response may vary depending on infecting organism, host, and locale of acquisition. Recommend consulting with expert knowledgeable in management of leishmaniasis.
- Treatment of VL in HIV/AIDS limited to above agents, different than Rx for cutaneous disease, which has more possibilities.
- Lifelong maintenance therapy likely necessary; no studies demonstrate whether maintenance can be stopped even if after immunologic response to ART.
- Most experts regard liposomal amphotericin as treatment of choice in patients with VL and HIV. Antimonials used widely in developing world due to cost and infusion difficulties with amphotericin products.
- Many treatment studies done in Spain; efficacy of above regimens in VL in New World not demonstrated adequately.
- Role of miltefosine (oral agent effective in VL due to *L. donovani* in India) not well known in treatment or maintenance therapy in HIV/AIDS or in New World.
- For cutaneous recommendations, see Leishmania spp. module in the Johns Hopkins ABX Guide.
- In *L. infantum* VL in Spain, comparison of amphotericin B lipid complex (ABLC) to glucantime shows somewhat greater efficacy when given at 3 mg/kg/day IV × 10 days with fewer side effects. Much more expensive.
- ART should be initiated or optimized following standard practice for HIV + patients.

Liposomal Amphotericin (Preferred)
- Use 4 mg/kg/day IV on days 1–5, 10, 17, 24, 31, and 38.
- Total cumulative dose of 20–60 mg/kg body weight recommended.
- Maintenance therapy for secondary prevention usually indicated, but no consensus on dose or duration. See Follow-up section on next page.
- The optimal amphotericin dosage is unclear. Reports with efficacy include conventional amphotericin B 0.5–1.0 mg/kg/day IV to achieve a total dose of 1.5–2.0 grams (BII), or liposomal or lipid complex preparations of 2–4 mg/kg body weight administered on consecutive days or in an interrupted schedule (e.g., 4 mg/kg on days 1–5, 10, 17, 24, 31, and 38) to achieve total cumulative dose of 20–60 mg/kg body weight (BII).

(SbV IV, Pentostam, Pentavalent Antimony, Preferred)
- 20 mg *SbV IV* daily × 28 days.
- Call CDC Drug Service for assistance in obtaining *Pentostam*: (404) 639-3670.
- Meglumine antimoniate (*Glucantime*): same dosing, not available in US.
- With pentavalent antimony, ~50%–60% of cases show initial improvement.
- Relapse rate without reversal of immunosuppression or antirelapse/suppressive therapy: 40% at 6–9 mos, 90% at 12 mos.
- Do not use in pregnancy due to teratogenicity.

Miltefosine (Alternative)
- Miltefosine (not FDA approved): oral, appears effective: 2.5 mg/kg/day × 28 days (max daily dose, 150 mg).

- For women, need negative pregnancy test before starting therapy and use of effective contraception.
- Relapse rates may be higher than with antimonials.

Conventional Amphotericin B (Alternative)
- Liposomal preparations preferred due to toxicity concerns.
- Amphotericin B 0.7–1 mg/kg once daily or alternate days, total dose unclear in HIV/AIDS.
- Reports with efficacy include conventional amphotericin B 0.5–1.0 mg/kg/day IV to achieve a total dose of 1.5–2.0 g.

Meglumine Antimonate (Alternative)
- Alternative antimonial.
- 20 mg Sb/kg/day IV or IM × 28 days.
- May be available in US through compounding pharmacies, e.g., Medical Center Pharmacy, New Haven, CT (203-688-6816) or others (see *www.pccarx.com/*).

Paromomycin
- 15 mg/kg/day IM × 21 days.
- Use only in regions without disease that could include mucosal involvement.

FOLLOW-UP

Treatment Failure
- For patients who fail to respond to initial therapy or experience relapse after initial treatment, repeat course of initial regimen, or use one of the recommended alternatives for initial therapy as outlined previously.
- Subsequent response rates appear similar to initial therapies.

Maintenance therapy
- If not receiving ART, risk of relapse at 6 and 12 mos, in the absence of maintenance therapy, is 60% and 90%, respectively.
- Post-induction therapy, recommended secondary prophylaxis using antileishmanial drug q2–4 wks.
- Maintenance is especially important if CD4 <200.
- No specific regimen favored regarding amphotericin products or antimonials.
- Abelcet 3 mg/kg IV q21 days × 1 yr (*J Antimicrob Chemother*; 2004 Mar; 53(3): 540–3.) but appears to be suboptimal with a 50% relapse rate at 1 yr.
- 1 small study (*Scand J Infect Dis*; 2008; 40(6–7): 523–6) used miltefosine 50 mg 3 ×/wk after induction until immune reconstitution.
- Allopurinol not recommended due to high relapse rates.
- Unclear when to stop, perhaps with strongly positive response to ART (i.e., CD4 >200) but clinical studies lacking.

OTHER INFORMATION
- For visceral disease, lipid formulations of amphotericin B as effective as antimonials or conventional amphotericin B, with less toxicity but higher cost.
- Failure of liposomal amphotericin not due to resistance, so retreatment with lipsomal amphotericin should be considered rather than switching.

SELECTED REFERENCES

Kaplan JE, Benson C, Holmes KH, et al. Guidelines for prevention and treatment of opportunistic infections in HIV-infected adults and adolescents: recommendations from CDC, the National Institutes of Health, and the HIV Medicine Association of the Infectious Diseases Society of America. *MMWR Recomm Rep*, 2009; 58: 1–207.
Comments: Recommendations specific to HIV+ patients. Data for maintenance therapy is limited.

Drugs for parasitic infections. *The Medical Letter*, 2007; 5: e1–14. *www.dpd.cdc.gov/dpdx/HTML/PDF_Files/MedLetter/Leishmania.pdf*. Accessed August 11, 2011.
Comments: Recommendations for treatment of VL based upon this module.

Lachaud L, Bourgeois N, Plourde M, et al. Parasite susceptibility to amphotericin B in failures of treatment for visceral leishmaniasis in patients coinfected with HIV type 1 and *Leishmania infantum*. *Clin Infect Dis*, 2009; 48: e16–22.
Comments: Treatment failure in setting of HIV does not appear to be due to the development of *in vitro* resistance to amphotericin B. Authors suggest continued consideration of this drug in patients who relapse.

Sinha S, Fernández G, Kapila R, et al. Diffuse cutaneous leishmaniasis associated with the immune reconstitution inflammatory syndrome. *Int J Dermatol*, 2008; 47: 1263–70.

PATHOGENS

Comments: Report of IRIS causing extensive cutaneous disease following institution of ART.

Bartlett JG, Auwaerter PG, Pham PA. Johns Hopkins ABX Guide; Diagnosis and Treatment of Infectious Diseases. Burlington, MA: Jones and Bartlett Learning; 2012.

López-Vélez R, Videla S, Márquez M, et al. Amphotericin B lipid complex versus no treatment in the secondary prophylaxis of visceral leishmaniasis in HIV-infected patients. *J Antimicrob Chemother*; 2004 Mar; 53(3): 540–3.
Comments: A secondary prophylaxis study treating *L. infantum* visceral leishmaniasis in Spain; placebo vs. *Abelcet*. Small pt numbers (N=17); endpoint was non-relapse of VL at 1 yr. 50% of pts receiving ABLC relapsed by 1 yr; 78% of pts with no Rx relapsed. This dosage regimen appears suboptimal.

Marques N, Sá R, Coelho F, et al. Miltefosine for visceral leishmaniasis relapse treatment and secondary prophylaxis in HIV-infected patients. *Scand J Infect Dis*; 2008; 40(6–7): 523–6.
Comments: Report of 5 pts treated with 50mg 3times/week, and cessation after immune reconstitution.

TRICHOMONAS VAGINALIS

Barbara E. Wilgus, MSN, CRNP

MICROBIOLOGY
- *Trichomonas vaginalis:* sexually transmitted protozoan flagellate.

CLINICAL
- Humans are only natural host of *T. vaginalis.*
- WHO estimates that trichomoniasis accounts for almost 1/2 of all curable vaginal infections worldwide.
- ~50% asymptomatic.
- Sx: vaginal discharge (42%), odor (50%), vulvar edema or erythema (22%–37%).
- Though discharge classically described as frothy, this is present in only ~10% of patients.
- Strawberry cervix: red punctate lesions on the cervix most easily seen with colposcopy.
- Urethritis most frequent clinical syndrome in males, though often asymptomatic.
- Most common Dx for women is demonstration of motile trichomonads on saline wet prep. Sensitivity 60%–70%; specificity 100%. Wet prep is insensitive for Dx in men.
- Dx: point-of-care antigen detection tests have been licensed. Sensitivity >83%; specificity 98.6%.
- Cx specific for *T. vaginalis* may be useful in some settings.

SITES OF INFECTION
- Cervix: cervicitis.
- Vagina: vaginitis.
- Male urethra: nongonocccal urethritis.
- Prostate: chronic prostatitis.

TREATMENT
Antimicrobial Therapy
- Metronidazole: 2 g PO (single dose) curative in 97%.
- Alternative metronidazole 500 mg PO twice daily × 7 days has been shown in randomized controlled trial to be more effective for HIV+women; CDC recommends consideration for seven-day treatment first-line in HIV+ women.
- Tinidazole: 2 g PO (single dose) is standard; however, studies have shown that 1.5–4.5 g/day × 7–14 days more effective with cure of 80%–100% in cases of metronidazole resistance.
- Metronidazole intravaginal gel: limited efficacy (<50%); should not be used. Metronidazole resistance in 2%–5%, high-level resistance is rare. Consultation and susceptibility testing is available from CDC if treatment failure to both metronidazole and tinidazole.
- Alcohol avoidance with oral metronidazole and tinidazole recommended (disulfuram-like reaction).
- Alcohol content in LPV/r and RTV liquid may result in disulfuram-like reaction with metronidazole or tinidazole coadministration.

Treatment of Sexual Partners
- Sexual partners should be treated with same medication as index case.
- Patient should be counseled to abstain from sex until treatment of self and partner complete.

FOLLOW-UP

- Patient should return for reevaluation if Sx persist.
- 3-mo post-Rx rescreening now suggested in CDC guidelines.
- Men/women asymptomatic after treatment: follow-up is unnecessary.

OTHER INFORMATION

- *Trichomonas* infection associated with increased risk of post-operative infection, tubal infertility, atypical PID, increased HIV transmission and infectivity, as well as increased risk of preterm birth.
- Incidence, persistence, recurrence in HIV infected women not correlated with immune status.

SELECTED REFERENCES

Workowski KA, Berman SM; Centers for Disease Control and Prevention. Sexually transmitted diseases treatment guidelines, 2010. *MMWR Recomm Rep*, 2010; 59 (RR-12): 58–61.
Comments: Comprehensive review, STD clinical standards of practice, most recent practice guideline from CDC.

Schwebke JR, Burgess D. Trichomoniasis. *Clin Microbiol Rev*, 2004; 17: 794–803.
Comments: Comprehensive, excellent resource.

Swygard H, Seña AC, Hobbs MM, et al. Trichomoniasis: clinical manifestations, diagnosis and management. *Sex Transm Infect*, 2004; 80: 91–5.
Comments: Offers overview of diagnostic and treatment guidelines for trichomoniasis, including metronidazole-resistant strains.

Kissinger P, Mena L, Levison J, et al. A randomized treatment trial: single versus 7-day dose of metronidazole for the treatment of *Trichomonas vaginalis* among HIV-infected women. *J Acquir Immune Defic Syndr*, 2010; 55: 565–71.
Comments: RCT of single dose versus prolonged therapy for treatment of trichomonas in HIV+ women, compelling enough results to suggest treatment changes in most recent CDC guidelines.

Nye MB, Schwebke JR, Body BA. Comparison of APTIMA *Trichomonas vaginalis* transcription-mediated amplification to wet mount microscopy, culture, and polymerase chain reaction for diagnosis of trichomoniasis in men and women. *Am J Obstet Gynecol*, 2009; 200: 188–97.
Comments: Good comparison study of diagnostic modalities for detection of trichomonas.

PATHOGENS

Viruses

CYTOMEGALOVIRUS

Lisa A. Spacek, MD, PhD and Khalil G. Ghanem, MD, PhD

MICROBIOLOGY

- Member of human herpesvirus beta subfamily w/ envelope and dsDNA; viral DNA polymerase is target for drugs. Latency established after infection. Transmission via saliva, blood, genital secretions, breast milk, urine, or feces. Reactivation (increasing w/ advancing immune suppression) responsible for most HIV-related disease.
- **CMV retinitis:** full-thickness necrotizing retinitis, most common manifestation of CMV in patients w/ AIDS.
- **CMV, gastrointestinal:** EGD w/ Bx for esophagitis; colonoscopy with Bx for colonic disease; Dx defined by clinical Sx, macroscopic mucosal lesions on endoscopy, and CMV by Cx, histopathology, immunohistochemical analysis, or *in situ* hybridization. Histology reveals large basophilic intranuclear "owl's eye" and intracytoplasmic inclusion bodies.
- **CMV, neurologic:** CSF WNL for encephalitis, but in polyradiculomyelitis often w/ PMNs, mildly increased protein levels and low glucose. Most sensitive is PCR of CSF for CMV; Cx usually +; MRI may show characteristic periventricular white matter changes (encephalitis).
- **CMV pneumonitis:** uncommon condition. Positive Cx from BAL does not establish Dx. Both clinical Sx (see below) and Bx results demonstrating viral inclusions must be used together for Dx.

CLINICAL

- Up to 50% of patients w/ AIDS developed CMV disease in pre-HAART era; ~32% developed CMV retinitis.
- **Retinitis:** painless loss of vision, decreased acuity, floaters, flashing lights, leading to retinal detachment. Lesions yellow-white fluffy (peripheral lesions sometimes granular) retinal infiltrates w/ areas of hemorrhage. Progression leads to atrophic gliotic scar. Immediate ophtho consult if CD4 <100 and ocular symptoms or other CMV-related disease.
- **GI:** fever, nausea, odynophagia, dysphagia, and substernal chest pain w/ esophagitis; diarrhea, abdominal cramps, weight loss w/ colitis; hepatitis also occurs. Colonic mucosal hemorrhage with perforation can be life-threatening complication.
- **Neurological:** dementia, ventriculoencephalitis, or ascending polyradiculomyelopathy; progressive bilateral leg weakness, areflexia, and urinary retention w/ radiculomyelitis; lethargy, confusion, fever, ataxia, and cranial nerve abnormalities w/ encephalitis.
- **Pulmonary:** uncommon. Fever, SOB, diffuse pulmonary infiltrates, and no other infection that could account for these Sx (up to 50% of patients w/ PCP will have positive CMV Cx from bronchial specimens: requires Rx only for PCP).

SITES OF INFECTION

- Primary infection: mononucleosis-like syndrome w/ fever, lymphadenopathy, and hepatitis.
- Eyes: retinitis.
- GI tract: esophagitis; colitis; gastritis; pancreatitis (less common); cholecystitis (less common); hepatitis.
- Nervous system: encephalitis; radiculomyelitis; mononeuritis multiplex; myelitis.
- Lungs: pneumonitis.
- CV: myocarditis.
- Hematologic: thrombocytopenia and hemolytic anemia.

TREATMENT

Prevention

- Most cases of CMV disease due to reactivation of latent infection (up to 70% of adults seropositive; up to 90% of MSM seropositive).
- Best approach for prevention is initiating ART before CD4 <200.
- If CD4 count <100, yearly ophthalmological exams mandatory.

- Any ophthalmological complaint in patients w/ advanced immunosuppression requires immediate ophthalmologic consultation.
- Preemptive therapy in patients w/ advanced immunosuppression in absence of organ system involvement not recommended.
- Preemptive diagnostics on urine, stool, and BAL fluid (i.e., CMV antigenemia or quantitative PCR) do not correlate with future disease course.

Antiviral Therapy: Induction

- See individual sections (CMV Retinitis, p. 60; CMV, Gastrointestinal, p. 57; and CMV, Neurologic, p. 58) for specific details and alternate therapies.
- Choice of therapy should be guided by side effect profile of each drug.
- Retinitis: Painless loss of vision, decreased acuity, floaters, flashing lights, leading to retinal detachment. Lesions yellow-white fluffy (peripheral lesions sometimes granular) retinal infiltrates w/ areas of hemorrhage. Progression leads to atrophic gliotic scar. Immediate ophtho consult if CD4 <100 and ocular symptoms or other CMV-related disease.
- **GI:** ganciclovir 5 mg/kg IV twice daily × 3–4 wks OR foscarnet 60 mg/kg IV q12h OR valganciclovir 900 mg PO twice daily × 3–4 wks w/ food if Sx not interfering w/ oral intake.
- **Neurological:** in general, poor response to Rx. Ganciclovir 5 mg/kg IV twice daily + foscarnet 90 mg/kg IV q12h × 3–6 wks, followed by maintenance combination Rx. ART is most effective.
- **Pneumonitis:** ganciclovir 5 mg/kg IV twice daily × 3–4 wks OR foscarnet 90 mg/kg IV q12h OR valganciclovir 900 mg PO twice daily × 3 wks.
- In retinitis, GI disease and pneumonitis, no data demonstrate adverse effect from ART initiation, and immediate treatment with ART recommended. In neurologic disease, delay of ART may be prudent but not data-based.

Antiviral Therapy: Maintenance Phase

- Maintenance therapy with PO valganciclovir in patients with AIDS only studied for CMV retinitis.
- Retinitis: valganciclovir 900 mg PO once daily + change of ganciclovir implant q6mos.
- GI: maintenance may be necessary w/ relapse.
- Pneumonitis: unclear if maintenance Rx necessary or beneficial.

Treatment-Related Side Effects

- Ganciclovir: neutropenia, thrombocytopenia, and catheter-related toxicities.
- Valganciclovir: neutropenia and thrombocytopenia.
- Foscarnet: nephrotoxicity, neurotoxicity, nausea, genital ulceration, and catheter-related complications.
- Cidofovir: nephrotoxicity, neutropenia, uveitis, hypotony.
- Immune recovery vitritis associated w/ ART has been reported and can be treated w/ systemic or periocular steroids (Kempen).

Resistance

- Resistance most likely to develop w/ prolonged underdosing of antivirals.
- Mutations in the CMV UL97 phosphotransferase gene confer variable ganciclovir resistance. Mutations in UL97 and UL54 genes confer high-level resistance to ganciclovir and cross-resistance to cidofovir.
- Cross-resistance less likely between ganciclovir and foscarnet (although cases have been reported).
- If no response to therapy, resistance testing can be performed by specialized labs; turn around time usually 10–14 days.

FOLLOW-UP

Monitoring

- Clinical response to therapy most useful indicator.
- Limited data on utility of serum markers (CMV antigenemia or quantitative PCR) in monitoring response to therapy or predicting recurrent disease.

OTHER INFORMATION

- ART is necessary adjunct to CMV-specific therapy. Short-term mortality for patients without immune reconstitution is very high.

SELECTED REFERENCES

Centers for Disease Control and Prevention. Guidelines for prevention and treatment of opportunistic infections in HIV-infected adolescents and adults. *MMWR Recomm Rep*, 2009; 58: 55–60.
Comments: OI guidelines from CDC, NIH, and HIVMA of the IDSA released March 24, 2009.

PATHOGENS

Kedhar SR, Jabs DA. Cytomegalovirus retinitis in the era of highly active antiretroviral therapy. *Herpes*, 2007; 14: 66–71.
Comments: Relapse of CMV retinitis can occur at CD4 of 1250 cells. CMV retinitis and uveitis associated with immune recovery remain causes of vision loss in this population.

Kempen JH, Min YI, Freeman WR, et al. Risk of immune recovery uveitis in patients with AIDS and cytomegalovirus retinitis. *Ophthalmology*, 2006; 113: 684–94.
Comments: 374 patients (539 eyes) w/ AIDS and CMV retinitis. 36 patients (9.6%) (50 eyes) Dx'd with immune recovery uveitis (IRU). Factors associated with IRU were >25% retinal area (OR, 2.72) or treatment with intravitreous injection of cidofovir (OR, 10.6). Eyes with IRU more commonly had cystoid macular edema (45.5% vs 3.7%, P <0.001) and epiretinal membrane (48.9% vs 13.3%, P <0.001).

EPSTEIN-BARR VIRUS

Paul G. Auwaerter, MD

MICROBIOLOGY

- Member of human gamma herpesvirus family. 90%–95% in US infected by adult years. Most HIV+ individuals also harbor EBV.
- Establishes latent infection. Spread mostly by asymptomatic shedding of virus into salivary secretions.
- Primary infection = subclinical or infectious mononucleosis (IM); peak incidence of IM in teens and early 20s.
- Presence of EBV may be considered as a tumor marker in proper clinical context.

CLINICAL

- EBV infection established in most individuals prior to HIV infection.
- EBV+ and HIV: >60 × risk of non-Hodgkin lymphoma (NHL) over general population, though overall risk remains small.
- In HIV, EBV most highly associated with Lymphoma, Primary CNS (PCNSL) (see p. 18). EBV CSF PCR + in ~100%. Studies suggest CSF PCR equivalent to brain Bx (sensitivity 83%–100%, specificity 93%–100%).
- Significance of EBV PCR in other tissues and fluids less certain, though described with smooth muscle tumors in HIV+ patients (Suankraty). Clinical reliability depends on assay used.
- Serum Monospot (heterophile antibodies) used to Dx IM (~90%), although additional 10% may require Dx through EBV-specific serology, e.g., EBV capsid IgM, IgG, and EBNA antibodies.
- False positive Monospot may be caused by acute HIV infection, and Sx can be similar. If risk factors exist, consider testing IM suspects with HIV viral load assay (acute retroviral syndrome).
- Role of EBV PCR (quantitative) of blood uncertain: conflicting data regarding correlation with risk of NHL.
- Since EBV establishes latency within cells, eradication impossible.

SITES OF INFECTION

- HIV-related lymphomas: B-cell lymphoma (~100% CNS, ~50% peripheral lymphomas associated w/ EBV), T/NK-cell lymphoma (10%–100% depending on histological grade), sporadic Burkitt Lymphoma (~25%), primary effusion lymphoma (70%–80%, but 100% also contain HHV-8). See Lymphoma, Non-Hodgkin (NHL) p. 16, Lymphoma, Hodgkin p. 15, Lymphoma, Primary CNS (PCNSL) p. 18.
- Nasopharyngeal carcinoma.
- Leiomyosarcoma: mainly in children.
- Oral hairy leukoplakia (OHL): white/gray patches on lateral margins of tongue caused by intense lytic-phase replication of EBV. Patches may spread to other parts of tongue. DDx = thrush, squamous cell CA, leukoplakia. Dx by appearance and location, cannot scrape off, unlike *Candida*.
- Infectious mononucleosis: cardinal triad of fever, lymphadenopathy, and pharyngitis. Unclear if presentation of primary EBV infection different in setting of HIV. More details about IM found in the Epstein-Barr section of the *Johns Hopkins ABX Guide* (Bartlett JG, Auwaerter PG, Pham PA. *Johns Hopkins ABX Guide: Diagnosis and Treatment of Infectious Diseases.* Burlington, MA: Jones and Bartlett Learning; 2012.).

TREATMENT

Oral Hairy Leukoplakia

- Treatment usually unnecessary. ART preferred as means to improve immune system and control lytic-phase EBV replication.
- Other options include cryotherapy, surgical removal, and topical podophyllin with variable results.
- Acyclovir: 800 mg PO 5 ×/day for 2–3 wks can limit EBV replication and may improve appearances; however, lesions recur with stopping therapy. Other drugs likely to work include valacyclovir, valganciclovir and famciclovir.

Infectious Mononucleosis

- IM usually self-limited <3 wks average, rest and supportive care.
- Corticosteroids (prednisone 40–60 mg/day) indicated for airway obstruction, severe thrombocytopenia, or hemolytic anemia. Some give for severe pharyngitis or constitutional Sx (controversial).
- Acyclovir/ganciclovir: no role in IM. Reduces viral shedding in mouth, but no clinical benefit.
- Ganciclovir employed by some for EBV CNS disease, but little data backing this practice.

SELECTED REFERENCES

Carbone A, Cesarman E, Spina M, et al. HIV-associated lymphomas and gamma-herpesviruses. *Blood*, 2009; 113: 1213–24.
Comments: Thorough overview from an oncologic perspective points out that EBV-driven lymphomas often present with plasmablastic differentiation in HIV+ patients, and that ART appears to improve outcomes with combined chemotherapy protocols.

Tsibris AM, Paredes R, Chadburn A, et al. Lymphoma diagnosis and plasma Epstein-Barr virus load during vicriviroc therapy: results of the AIDS Clinical Trials Group A5211. *Clin Infect Dis*, 2009; 48: 642–9.
Comments: Because 4 lymphomas developed during a phase II trial of vicriviroc (a CCR5 antagonist), plasma EBV DNA was monitored in 116 patients who did not experience increases in detectable levels, suggesting that CCR5 antagonism by this drug did not lead to EBV reactivation.

Corcoran C, Rebe K, van der Plas H, et al. The predictive value of cerebrospinal fluid Epstein-Barr viral load as a marker of primary central nervous system lymphoma in HIV-infected persons. *J Clin Virol*, 2008; 42: 433–6.
Comments: Some have questioned specificity of CSF EBV PCR in Dx of CNS lymphoma in HIV+ patients. This study suggests that addition of quantitative aspect (namely >10,000 c/mL) improves specificity and positive predictive value compared to qualitative result for Dx of PCNSL (96% vs 66% and 50% vs 10%, respectively).

Reznik DA. Oral manifestations of HIV disease. *Top HIV Med*, 2005; 13: 143–8.
Comments: Excellent photos of many oral lesions common to HIV.

Triantos D, Porter SR, Scully C, et al. Oral hairy leukoplakia: clinicopathologic features, pathogenesis, diagnosis, and clinical significance. *Clin Infect Dis*, 1997; 25: 1392–6.
Comments: OHL generally only seen in later HIV infection, and its presence predicts AIDS. Why OHL develops and whether EBV reactivates from latency or superinfection remains uncertain. Despite appearance of the tongue, OHL does not appear to be a premalignant lesion.

Suankratay C, Shuangshoti S, Mutirangura A, et al. Epstein-Barr virus infection-associated smooth-muscle tumors in patients with AIDS. *Clin Infect Dis*; 2005; 40: 1521, 2005 May 15; 40(10): 1521–8.
Comments: Case series describing an association.

HUMAN HERPESVIRUS 8

Joel N. Blankson, MD, PhD

MICROBIOLOGY

- Human herpesvirus 8 (HHV-8): human gammaherpes virus, also known as Kaposi sarcoma-associated herpesvirus (KSHV).
- 20%–30% of gay men are HHV-8 seropositive vs 1% of HIV-negative blood donors. Associated with receptive anal intercourse and number of partners. An unknown cofactor may be involved in transmission.
- HHV-8 gene products promote spindle cell proliferation and angiogenesis and therefore may eventually lead to tumor formation.
- For diagnostic and specific information see Kaposi sarcoma, p. 14; and Castleman Disease, p. 13.

PATHOGENS

CLINICAL
- Cause of HIV-associated Kaposi sarcoma (KS); typically characterized by violaceous vascular lesions on skin, mucous membranes, and/or viscera (e.g., GI tract, lungs).
- HIV-associated KS seen mostly in MSM. HHV-8 found in saliva and semen. An unknown cofactor may also be involved.
- Associated with multicentric Castleman Disease, lymphoproliferative disorder mostly seen in HIV+ patients, characterized by B-type symptoms, lymphadenopathy, hypergammaglobulinemia.
- Associated with primary effusion lymphoma; a non-Hodgkin disease B-cell lymphoma mostly seen in HIV+ patients. Presents with body cavity based effusions in the absence of a solid tumor. Poor prognosis with survival usually less than 6 mos. Dx made by cytology of cells in effusion.
- Probable cause of classical KS (non-HIV associated). Typically affects elderly Mediterranean and eastern European men.
- Probable cause of endemic African KS.
- Can be transmitted via blood transfusions, less likely to occur in regions of low seroprevelence.
- In a recent study of AIDS-associated KS, having KS as AIDS-defining illness and having improving CD4 counts on ART were good prognostic signs whereas age >50 and the presence of another AIDS-associated illness associated with poor prognosis.

SITES OF INFECTION
- HHV-8 DNA has been detected in saliva and semen.
- HHV-8 DNA has been detected in endothelial cells and spindle cells in KS lesions.
- HHV-8 DNA has been detected in B cells in Castleman Disease and primary effusion lymphoma.

TREATMENT

HHV-8 Infection
- Treatment not indicated for asymptomatic HHV-8 seropositive patients. Foscarnet and cidofovir have *in vitro* anti-HHV-8 activity.
- Initiation of ART should be strongly considered, as immune reconstitution may reverse some of the manifestations of HHV-8 infection.
- PIs may have direct antiangiogenic effects. Rebound of KS seen when PIs replaced with NNRTIs in 2 small case series.

Kaposi Sarcoma (Local Disease <25 Lesions)
- ART, cryotherapy, topical alitretinoin, intralesional vinblastine, radiation therapy, surgery (see Kaposi sarcoma, p. 14).

Kaposi Sarcoma (Systemic Disease)
- ART, combination chemotherapy (see Kaposi sarcoma, p. 14).
- KS probably a late consequence of HHV-8 infection, as foscarnet and cidofovir, drugs with *in vitro* anti-HHV-8 activity, have little effect on established disease.

Multicentric Castleman Disease
- ART, combination chemotherapy, anti-IL-6 antibody, ganciclovir, valganciclovir (see Castleman disease, p. 13).

SELECTED REFERENCES

Nguyen HQ, Magaret AS, Kitahata MM, et al. Persistent Kaposi sarcoma in the era of highly active antiretroviral therapy: characterizing the predictors of clinical response. *AIDS*, 2008; 22: 937–945.
Comments: Retrospective analysis showed that chemotherapy and ART were the 2 factors associated with positive outcomes in 114 patients with KS. No difference in outcome seen in PI-based vs NNRTI-based ART.

Stebbing J, Sanitt A, Nelson M, et al. A prognostic index for AIDS-associated Kaposi's sarcoma in the era of highly active antiretroviral therapy. *Lancet*, 2006; 367: 1495–502.
Comments: Study defining positive and negative prognostic factors in AIDS associated KS.

Grabar S, Abraham B, Mahamat A. Differential impact of combination antiretroviral therapy in preventing Kaposi's sarcoma with and without visceral involvement. *J Clin Oncol*, 2006; 24: 3408–14.
Comments: Large retrospective study showing dramatic decrease in incidence of KS related to ART. No difference in incidence seen in patients on PI- vs NNRTI-based regimens.

Chang Y, Cesarman E, Pessin MS, et al. Identification of herpesvirus-like DNA sequences in AIDS-associated Kaposi's sarcoma. *Science*, 1994; 266: 1865–9.
Comments: First identification of HHV-8 sequences in KS lesions.

HUMAN T-LYMPHOTROPIC VIRUS-TYPES I/II

Joel N. Blankson, MD, PhD

MICROBIOLOGY

- Human T-cell leukemia virus I and II (HTLV I and II): members of human type C retroviruses.
- Dx by HTLV-I or HTLV-II ELISA; greater sensitivity than Western blot and PCR.

CLINICAL

- Most infections asymptomatic in general population. Not known if HIV+ patients more likely to develop disease.
- HTLV-I endemic in Caribbean, southern Japan, parts of Africa, South America. Transmitted by breastfeeding, contaminated blood products, IDU, sexual contact.
- HTLV-II endemic in IDUs; seroprevalence approximately 20%.
- HTLV-I infection: 5% lifetime risk of adult T-cell leukemia (ATL) in general population. Presents with type B Sx, lymphadenopathy. Skin involvement (plaques, nodules) common.
- HTLV-I infection: 0.5%–2.0% lifetime risk of HTLV-I-associated myelopathy/tropical spastic paraparesis (HAM/TSP) in general population. Progressive disease with leg stiffness, weakness, low back pain, bladder dysfunction.
- HTLV-I coinfected patients have higher CD4 counts than HTLV-I-negative/HIV+ patients. OIs occur at higher CD4 counts than seen in HTLV-I-negative patients.
- HTLV-I can cause immunosuppression; associated with *Strongyloides* hyperinfection, and decreased reactivity to PPD.
- Effect of HTLV-I/II on HIV disease progression controversial, with different studies reaching opposite conclusions.
- Vast majority of patients with HTLV-I infection will not develop disease.
- HTLV-II not definitively shown to cause human disease, but a few reports suggest that it can cause HAM/TSP-like syndrome.

SITES OF INFECTION

- CD4 cells are main target of infection of HTLV-I.
- HTLV-I-infected CD4 cells found in CSF of patients with HAM/TSP.
- In ATL, circulation of monoclonal transformed cells bearing HTLV-I provirus.
- HTLV-II infects peripheral blood mononuclear cells.

TREATMENT

Asymptomatic Infection

- No evidence for benefit of antiviral therapy. HTLV genome integrated into host DNA; therefore, eradication probably not possible.

ATL

- Conventional chemotherapy.
- Small prospective phase II trial showed encouraging results with AZT 1 g/day PO and alfa interferon (9 MU/day SQ).

HAM/TSP

- Corticosteroids, cyclophosphamides, alfa interferon, IVIG, plasmapheresis, and danazol have been used with inconsistent results.
- NRTIs have been tried based on *in vitro* activity against HTLV-I. AZT (1–2 g/day) or 3TC (150 mg twice daily) alone or AZT (250 mg twice daily) and 3TC (150 mg twice daily) used in 3 small studies. While decreased proviral HTLV-I load seen, Sx did not improve in most patients. TDF recently shown to have good *in vitro* activity against HTLV-I. In recent small randomized study of HIV-negative patients, 6 mos of AZT (300 mg twice daily) and 3TC (150 mg twice daily) had no effect on HTLV proviral load or clinical Sx.
- If ART to be initiated in coinfected patients, include AZT, TDF, and/or 3TC in patients with HAM/TSP or ATL if possible.
- If NRTIs to be started for coinfected patients with HAM/TSP, should be used as component of ART to prevent NRTI resistance.

Prevention

- CDC recommends that patients with asymptomatic infection not breastfeed, donate blood, or share needles. Latex condoms should be used.

PATHOGENS

SELECTED REFERENCES

Centers for Disease Control and the USPHS Working Group. Guidelines for counseling persons infected with human T-lymphotropic virus type I (HTLV-I) and type II (HTLV-II). Centers for Disease Control and Prevention and the USPHS Working Group. Ann Intern Med, 1993; 118: 448–54.
Comments: A practical set of guidelines from the CDC.

Turci M, Pilotti E, Ronzi P, et al. Coinfection with HIV-1 and human T-cell lymphotropic virus type II in intravenous drug users is associated with delayed progression to AIDS. *J Acquir Immune Defic Syndr*, 2006; 41: 100–6.
Comments: Study showing protective effective of HTLV-II coinfection in HIV-1 positive IDUs. Interestingly, in 5 treated coinfected patients there was increase in HTLV-II proviral load, while HIV viral load dropped, suggesting that ART does not treat HTLV-II.

Beilke MA, Theall KP, O'Brien M, et al. Clinical outcomes and disease progression among patients coinfected with HIV and human T-lymphotropic virus types 1 and 2. *Clin Infect Dis*, 2004; 39: 256–63.
Comments: Study showed improved survival and decreased progression to AIDS in HTLV-II-coinfected patients. These patients more likely to have other clinical complications, however. Trend towards improved survival in HTLV-I-coinfected patients. While higher CD4 counts seen in coinfected patients, no difference in frequency of OIs.

Araujo A, Hall WW. Human T-lymphotropic virus type II and neurological disease. *Ann Neurol*, 2004; 56: 10–9.
Comments: Critical review of literature linking HTLV-II to neurological disease.

HUMAN PAPILLOMAVIRUS

Khalil G. Ghanem, MD, PhD

MICROBIOLOGY

- Nonenveloped DNA virus; over 35 types cause anogenital infection.
- Exposure to HPV virtually universal in sexually active adults; majority of infections subclinical and asymptomatic.
- Prevalence of oral and genital HPV infections increase in HIV+ patients with lower CD4 counts.
- HIV+ women have 7-fold higher risk of anal and cervical cancer than HIV-negative women; HIV+ men have 37-fold higher risk of anal cancer than HIV-negative men.

CLINICAL

- 90% of genital warts associated with types 6 and 11.
- Cervical, anal intraepithelial lesions, vaginal, and vulvar dysplasia associated with oncogenic types (16, 18, 31, 33, 35 and others).
- Some studies suggest that HPV type-specific prevalence may differ between HIV+ and HIV-negative patients.
- HIV: clinical manifestations occur at any CD4 count; more advanced disease associated with persistence of oncogenic types, increasing risk of squamous intraepithelial lesions, and manifestations that may be more refractory to standard therapy.
- Dx: anogenital warts usually by visual inspection, though Bx may be required to rule out malignancy or to confirm HPV-related epithelial changes if Dx unclear visually. Intraepithelial lesions (cervical, anal, etc.) indicated by cytologic screening tests (Pap smear) followed by colposcopy or high-resolution anoscopy with Bx.
- Cervical Pap smear in HIV+ women has utility similar to that in HIV-negative women for identification of high-grade cervical lesions.
- In HIV+ women, cervical Pap recommended at baseline evaluation and 6 mos; then annually after 2 sequential normal tests. Abnormal result (atypical squamous cells cannot exclude HSIL [ASC-H], low-grade squamous intraepithelial lesion [LSIL], high-grade squamous intraepithelial lesion [HSIL], and atypical glandular cells [AGC]) should lead to colposcopy with Bx.
- 2006 Bethesda Guidelines suggest that ASCUS may be managed as in HIV-negative women: reflex HPV testing or repeat Pap every 6 mos until 2 sequential normal results. No need for immediate colposcopy.
- High rates of anal dysplasia in MSM; cytologic screening (anal Pap) may be useful for cancer prevention, though best screening intervals and management of abnormal cytology not

established. In some centers, screening at 6–12 mo intervals is practice standard; abnormal Pap results managed with high-resolution anoscopy and Bx of suspicious lesions performed with any grade of abnormal result.

SITES OF INFECTION
- Cervix.
- Vagina/perineum.
- Anus (especially among MSM and women).
- Penis/scrotum.
- Respiratory tract: recurrent respiratory papillomatosis (rare; occurs in infants perinatally exposed).
- Oral.

TREATMENT
Principles of Therapy
- Effect of ART on HPV-related cancer unclear. Some studies have suggested increased regression of high-grade dysplastic lesions, while others have not.
- Goal of therapy for genital warts: remove clinically evident lesions and relieve Sx (if present); unclear impact on HPV transmission.

Topical Treatment
- Podophyllotoxin/podofilox (0.5% gel, solution, or cream): topical application qwk × 6 wks (patient-applied).
- Imiquimod: topical administration 3 ×/wk to the wart (patient-applied; leave on for 6–10 hrs). Continue until complete resolution.
- Cryotherapy: liquid nitrogen (applied by clinician).
- Bichloroacetic acid or trichloroacetic acid (applied by clinician).
- Wart clearance and recurrence rates similar for treatments cited, though patient-applied therapies less costly overall.

Prevention
- Condoms effective at decreasing risk of HPV transmission.
- Vaccines for prevention of HPV infection (a quadrivalent vaccine currently marketed targeting HPV 6, 11, 16, and 18 and a bivalent vaccine awaiting FDA approval targeting 16 and 18) are not currently recommended in HIV+ patients because of lack of efficacy data; there are ongoing studies to determine immunogenicity in this population.

OTHER INFORMATION
- Cesarean section not protective against perinatal transmission, though clinically important disease in infant very rare.
- Specialized surgical methods may be required for removal of extensive anogenital warts: choice of tangential scissor excision, shave excision, curettage, electrosurgery, carbon dioxide laser techniques dependent upon location and experience of clinician.

SELECTED REFERENCES
Wright TC Jr, Massad LS, Dunton CJ, et al. 2006 consensus guidelines for the management of women with abnormal cervical cancer screening tests. *Am J Obstet Gynecol*, 2007; 197: 337–9.
Comments: The latest consensus guidelines are summarized in the "Clinical Relevance" section above; recommendations for HIV+ women now more closely approximate those of HIV-negative women.

Cutts FT, Franceschi S, Goldie S, et al. Human papillomavirus and HPV vaccines: a review. *Bull World Health Organ*, 2007; 85: 719–26.
Comments: This comprehensive review article summarizes the efficacy data for both the bivalent and quadrivalent HPV vaccines. Please note that, to date, there are no data on HPV vaccine efficacy in HIV+ women. An ongoing ACTG trial should answer that question.

Clifford GM, Gonçalves MA, Franceschi S, et al. Human papillomavirus types among women infected with HIV: a meta-analysis. *AIDS*, 2006; 20: 2337–44.
Comments: This study suggests that although HPV-16 is still an important cause of disease in HIV+ women, other high-risk types as well as infections with multiple HPV types are important to consider in this population.

PATHOGENS

PARVOVIRUS B19

Richard D. Moore, MD, MHS

MICROBIOLOGY

- Viral agent of Fifth disease, a childhood exanthem.
- Exposure leads to antibody response with subsequent resistance to further infection.
- 80% of all adults have antibodies to the organism; 65% of HIV-infected adults have antibodies (possibly unable to maintain humoral response).
- Virus has tropism for erythroid precursors in marrow, with pure red blood cell (RBC) aplasia.

CLINICAL

- In HIV+ persons, reactivation of latent infection or newly-acquired infection may cause clinical disease.
- Despite high seroprevalence of IgG to B19, incidence as clinical cause of anemia probably <1% of HIV+ patients.
- Anemia can be profound with Hgb <8.0 mg/dL.
- Manifestations: pure RBC aplasia, typically minimal to no neutropenia or thrombocytopenia. Anemia typically normocytic, normochromic; low reticulocyte count a hallmark.
- Dx (1): bone marrow shows giant pronormoblasts with clumped basophilic chromatin, and clear cytoplasmic vacuoles.
- Dx (2): B19 DNA positive by PCR or dot-blot hybridization using sequence-specific DNA probes for parvovirus B19. IgG and IgM antibodies often absent (absence of neutralizing antibody = chronic infection) and unreliable for Dx.
- Many clinicians will treat based on PCR/dot-blot results in appropriate clinical setting without proceeding to bone marrow Bx.

SITES OF INFECTION

- Infection of pronormoblast, earliest RBC precursor in bone marrow.

TREATMENT

Treatment

- IV immune globulin (IVIG) infusion 0.4 g/kg/day for 5 days.
- Reports of B19 anemia improvement from ART, but may persist even with effective ART.
- Routine IVIG maintenance probably not indicated with CD4 >300, but repeated infusions more likely for CD4 <80. Can persist for many months.

FOLLOW-UP

RELAPSE

- Relapse can occur, particularly in those with CD4 <100. Requires IVIG at dose of 1–2 g/kg for 2 days, with possible monthly maintenance dose of 0.4 g/kg.

SELECTED REFERENCES

Morelli P, Bestetti G, Longhi E, et al. Persistent parvovirus B19-induced anemia in an HIV-infected patient under HAART. Case report and review of literature. *Eur J Clin Microbiol Infect Dis*, 2007; 26: 833–7.
Comments: Persistent B19 anemia over 17 mos with effective ART.

Mouthon L, Guillevin L, Tellier Z. Intravenous immunoglobulins in autoimmune- or parvovirus B19-mediated pure red-cell aplasia. *Autoimmun Rev*, 2005; 4: 264–9.
Comments: Routine maintenance therapy probably not indicated in HIV-infected patients with CD4 >300, whereas repeated infusions might be necessary if CD4 <80.

Young NS, Brown KE. Parvovirus B19. *New Engl J Med*, 2004; 350: 586–97.
Comments: Good review of clinical presentation and mechanism of disease associated with parvovirus B19 (not specific to HIV).

APPENDIX I
DRUG-DRUG INTERACTION TABLES

DRUG-DRUG INTERACTION – ABACAVIR (ABC)

Drug	Effect of Interaction	Recommendations/Comments
Alcohol	ABC AUC increased by 41%.	Clinical significance unknown. No dose adjustment recommended.
Food	ABC AUC was decreased by 5% (NS).	Administer ABC with or without food.
Lamivudine (3TC)	3TC AUC decreased by 15%.	Not clinically significant. Use standard dose.
Methadone	Methadone clearance increased by 23%; ABC: 34% decrease in Cmax.	Monitor for methadone withdrawal, but dose adjustment unlikely to be necessary.
Ribavirin	Decreased EVR to Hepatitis C virus treatment.	Avoid coadministration.
Tenofovir (TDF)	Suboptimal virologic suppression when ABC/TDF/3TC once daily was used as a triple nucleoside regimen without PIs or nonnucleoside reverse transcriptase inhibitors (NNRTIs). However, preliminary analysis of ABC/AZT/3TC with TDF as nucleoside regimen did not show similar suboptimal results, and no evidence of drug interaction.	Do not coadminister ABC/TDF/3TC once daily as a triple nucleoside regimen. Minimal data on use of this combination with a 4th agent.
Tipranavir (TPV)	Decreased ABC AUC by 40%.	Clinical significance unknown. Active intracellular carbovir triphosphate not measured. Use standard dose.
Zidovudine (AZT)	No significant interaction.	Use standard dose.

DRUG-DRUG INTERACTION – ATAZANAVIR (ATV)

Drug	Effect of Interaction	Recommendations/Comments
Abacavir (ABC)	ABC plasma concentration decreased by 17%.	Unknown mechanisms and clinical implications.
Alfuzosin	May significantly increase alfuzolin serum concentrations resulting in hypotension.	Avoid coadministration.
Alprazolam	May increase serum level of alprazolam.	Applies to all PIs: consider alternative benzodiazepines (i.e., lorazepam, oxazepam, or temazepam).
Amiodarone	May significantly increase amiodarone serum level.	Applies to all PIs: data limited to case report of increased amiodarone levels with indinavir (IDV) coadministration. ATV not recommended to be coadministered with amiodarone. If coadministration cannot be avoided, monitor for amiodarone ADR (PFTs, TSH). Consider monitoring serum level of amiodarone, but its long half-life may make titration difficult.

Drug	Effect of Interaction	Recommendations/Comments
Amlodipine	May increase serum level of amlodipine.	Applies to all PIs: data limited to an interaction study conducted with atazanavir (ATV) and diltiazem, which resulted in doubling of diltiazem serum level (this led to PR interval prolongation). All PIs have the potential for prolonging the PR interval with calcium channel blocker coadministration. Calcium channel blockers should be started with a low dose and slowly titrated with close monitoring of BP and pulse.
Antacids	May significantly decrease in ATV serum levels.	Avoid coadministration. Separate administration time, ATV 400 mg 2 hrs before AC or 1 hr after buffered didanosine (ddI) or antacid administration.
Artemether (artemisinin)	May increase serum level of artemether.	Applies to All PIs: close monitoring for artemether toxicity (bone marrow suppression, bradycardia and seizure).
Astemizole	May significantly increase astemizole serum level.	Contraindicated due to potential for cardiac arrhythmias. Recommended alternative antihistamine: loratadine, fexofenadine, desloratidine, or cetirizine.
Atenolol	Atenolol AUC increased by 25%; Cmin: no significant change. ATV not affected.	No effect on PR or QTc interval with coadministration. Start with low-dose atenolol with slow-dose titration.
Atorvastatin	May increase atorvastatin serum concentrations.	Start with atorvastatin 10 mg/day, then titrate to therapeutic effect.
Azathioprine	Interaction unlikely.	Applies to all PIs and NNRTI: use standard dose.
Bepridil	May significantly increase bepridil serum level.	The manufacturer of ATV does not recommend bepridil coadministration; this contraindication should extend to all PIs since a significant increase in bepridil serum level can result in pro-arrhythmic events such as VT, PVC, and VFib.
Bosentan	May significantly increase bosentan serum concentrations.	Coadminister bosentan only after ritonavir (RTV) dosing has reached steady-state. In patients on RTV >10 days: start bosentan at 62.5 mg once daily or every other day. In patients already on bosentan: d/c bosentan for at least 36 hrs prior to initiation of RTV-boosted PIs and restart bosentan at 62.5 mg once daily or every other day after RTV has reached steady-state (after 10 days).
Carbamazepine	May decrease serum levels of ATV.	Consider alternative anticonvulsants (i.e., valproic acid, lamotrigine, levetiracetam, or topiramate). With coadministration, monitor anticonvulsants level and consider TDM of ATV.

ATAZANAVIR *(cont.)*

Drug	Effect of Interaction	Recommendations/Comments
Chlordiazepoxide	May increase serum level of chlordiazepoxide.	Applies to all PIs: consider alternative benzodiazepines (i.e., lorazepam, temazepam, or oxazepam).
Cisapride	May significantly increase cisapride serum level.	Contraindicated due to potential for cardiac arrhythmias. Recommended alternative: metoclopramide.
Clarithromycin	ATV AUC increased by 28%. Clarithromycin AUC increased by 94%. 14-hydroxyclarithromycin metabolite AUC decreased by 70%.	QTc prolongation observed with coadministration. 50% of clarithromycin dose recommended. Consider azithromycin.
Clorazepate	May increase serum level of clorazepate.	Applies to all PIs: consider alternative benzodiazepines (i.e., lorazepam, temazepam, or oxazepam).
Cyclophosphamide	May increase serum level of cyclophosphamide.	Applies to all PIs: data limited to an interaction study conducted with IDV resulting in a 50% increase in cyclophosphamide serum level. Since all PIs have potential of increasing cyclophosphamide levels, close monitoring of cyclophosphamide-induced toxicity recommended.
Cyclosporine	May significantly increase serum level of cyclosporine.	Applies to all PIs: monitor serum level of cyclosporine closely with coadministration. Cyclosporine dose may need to be decreased.
Darunavir (DRV)	No significant interaction.	Dose: DRV 600/100 mg twice daily plus ATV 300 mg once daily.
Didanosine (ddI) (buffered)	No effect on ddI serum level. ATV AUC decreased by 87%, Cmin decreased by 84% (single dose study ATV 400 mg × 1 with ddI buffered 200 mg × 1).	Administer ATV 400 mg 1 hr after ddI (buffered) administration. Consider ddI EC. The combination of ddI, FTC, and unboosted ATV did not perform well in a randomized ACTG trial.
Disopyramide	May increase disopyramide serum levels.	Applies to all PIs: no data. Monitor disopyramide serum level (target: 2 to 7.5 mcg/mL).
Docetaxel	May increase serum level of docetaxel.	Applies to all PIs: no data. Close monitoring of chemotherapy induced toxicity recommended.
Dofetilide	May significantly increase serum level of dofetilide.	Applies to all PIs: no data. Use with caution. Monitor QTc closely and adjust dofetilide dosing based on QTc prolongation and renal function. Consider an alternative class III antiarrhythmic such as bretylium or ibutilide.

Drug	Effect of Interaction	Recommendations/Comments
Echinacea	May decrease ATV serum level. Echinacea (400 mg 4 × days) decreased CYP3A4 substrate (midazolam) by 23%.	Applies to all PIs and NNRTIs. Clinical significance unknown but should avoided until the safety of this combination is further evaluated.
Efavirenz (EFV)	ATV AUC decreased by 74%, Cmax decreased by 59%, Cmin decreased by 93%.	Coadministration of ATV as a sole PI with EFV not recommended. Boosting ATV 400 mg + RTV 100 mg daily recommended with coadministration of standard dose of EFV. Avoid coadministration in patients with PI resistance.
Ergot Alkaloid	May significantly increase serum level of ergotamine resulting in acute ergot toxicity.	Contraindicated. Consider alternative agent for migraine such as sumatriptan (but not eletriptan since it is a CYP3A4 substrate and significant drug-drug interaction occurred with a CYP3A4 inhibitor).
Estazolam	May increase serum level of estazolam.	Applies to all PIs: consider alternative benzodiazepines (i.e., lorazepam, temazepam, or oxazepam).
Ethinyl Estradiol and Norethindrone	Norethindrone Cmax: increased 67%; AUC: increased 110%; Cmin: increased 262%; Ethinyl estradiol AUC: increased 48%; Cmax: no significant change; Cmin: increased 91% (with unboosted ATV).	Clinical significance unknown. Dose: with unboosted ATV coadministration, do not exceed EE 30 mcg/day. Monitor for OC adverse drug reaction. With ATV/r coadministration, use at least EE 35 mcg/day. Consider an additional barrier form of contraception.
Ethosuximide	May increase serum levels of ethosuximide.	Applies to all PIs: consider switching to valproic acid for the treatment of absence seizure.
Etoposide	May increase serum level of etoposide.	Applies to all PIs: no data. Close monitoring of chemotherapy induced toxicity recommended.
Etravirine (ETR)	With unboosted ATV: ETR AUC increased by 50%, but ATV Cmin decreased by 47%. With ATV/r: ETR AUC increased by 30% and ATV AUC and Cmin decreased by 14% and 38%, respectively.	Avoid with unboosted ATV with ETR coadministration. Unclear clinical significance with ATV/r, but the manufacturer recommends avoiding coadministration. Consider ATV/r 300/100 mg once daily + ETR 200 mg twice daily with TDM.
Felodipine	May increase serum level of felodipine.	Applies to all PIs: data limited to an interaction study conducted with ATV and diltiazem, which resulted in doubling of diltiazem serum level (this led PR interval prolongation). All PIs have potential of prolonging PR interval with calcium channel blocker coadministration. Calcium channel blockers should be started with low dose and slowly titrated with close monitoring of BP and pulse.

ATAZANAVIR *(cont.)*

Drug	Effect of Interaction	Recommendations/Comments
Fentanyl	May significantly increase fentanyl serum level.	Use with caution. Consider morphine.
Flecainide	May increase antiarrhythmic serum level.	Applies to all PIs: avoid coadministration; if necessary, monitor flecainide trough level with coadministration. Target: 200–1000 ng/mL. Toxicity frequent with trough serum levels above 1000 ng/mL.
Fluconazole	No significant interaction.	Use standard dose.
Flurazepam	May increase serum level of flurazepam.	Applies to all PIs: consider alternative benzodiazepines (i.e., lorazepam, temazepam, or oxazepam).
Fluticasone	May significantly increase systemic corticosteroid exposure.	Avoid long-term coadministration. Consider beclomethasone.
Food (light meal)	ATV AUC increased by 70%.	ATV should be administered with food.
Fosamprenavir (FPV)	ATV AUC decreased by 33%. APV AUC increased by 78%. (Dose studied: FPV 1400 mg daily + ATV 400 mg daily).	Insufficient data; clinical significance unknown. Avoid or consider TDM in PI-experienced patients.
Garlic Supplement	No data.	Studies only done with saquinavir (SQV) resulting in SQV serum level reduction. No data with other PIs or NNRTIs. Avoid coadministration.
Granisetron	May increase serum level of granisetron.	Applies to all PIs: due to the large therapeutic index of granisetron, potential interaction unlikely to be clinically significant.
H2 Blocker	ATV/r + famotidine: Cmin decreased by 28% (but comparable to ATV/r Cmin when coadministered with TDF).	Avoid coadministration if possible. If ATV/r (300/100 mg) is coadministered with famotidine, the max recommended dose for ARV-naive patients is famotidine 40 mg twice daily. Max dose for ARV-experienced patients is famotidine 20 mg twice daily with ATV/r coadministration. Administer ATV 2 hrs before or 10 hrs after H2 blocker is preferred. If coadministered with TDF + famotidine 20 mg twice daily, increase ATV/r to 400/100 mg once daily (consider TDM).
Heroin (diamorphine)	Drug interactions unlikely.	Applies to PIs and NNRTIs: interaction unlikely but illicit drug use should be avoided for obvious reasons.
Ifosfamide	May increase serum level of ifosfamide.	Applies to all PIs: no data. Close monitoring of chemotherapy-induced toxicity recommended.
Irinotecan	May increase irinotecan serum level.	Applies to all PIs: coadministration of ATV is contraindicated by manufacturer.

Drug	Effect of Interaction	Recommendations/Comments
Itraconazole	CYP3A4 inhibitor and substrate: potential for bidirectional inhibition with increase levels of PIs and itraconazole.	Except for IDV, there are no recommendations for dose adjustment for other PIs or NNRTIs. Reduce IDV dose to 600 mg q8h and do not exceed 400 mg/day of itraconazole. No data with IDV/ RTV coadministration. Consider IDV 800 mg twice daily + RTV 100 mg twice daily with aggressive hydration due to the potential increased risk of nephrolithiasis.
Ketoconazole	ATV unaffected. Ketoconazole not studied.	Standard dose ATV with ketoconazole coadministration.
Lidocaine	May increase antiarrhythmic serum levels.	Applies to all PIs: no data. Use with caution, monitor lidocaine serum level (target: 1.5 to 6 mcg/mL) with coadministration.
Lopinavir/ritonavir (LPV/r)	ATV geometric mean Cmin increased by 45% with LPV/r 400/100 mg twice daily coadministration (compared to ATV/r 300/100 mg daily). LPV PK comparable to historical data.	Dose: ATV 300 mg daily + LPV/r 400/100 mg twice daily.
Lovastatin	Serum levels of lovastatin may be significantly increased.	Contraindicated. Recommended alternatives include pravastatin, rosuvastatin, and fluvastatin (and possibly atorvastatin- start with 10 mg/day). Monitor for adverse effect due to limited clinical data.
Maraviroc (MVC)	MVC AUC increased 388%.	Dose: ATV/r 300/100 mg once daily + MVC 150 mg twice daily. In PI-naive patients, unboosted ATV can also be considered with MVC.
Mefloquine	May increase serum levels of mefloquine.	Applies to all PIs: if available, consider mefloquine serum level monitoring. Monitor for mefloquine toxicity (i.e., dizziness, LFTs, and periodic ophthalmic examination).
Methadone	No data.	Interaction unlikely but should monitor for sedation with coadministration.
Mexiletine	May increase antiarrhythmic serum levels.	Applies to all PIs: no data. Use with caution. Monitor EKG and serum level. Serum levels exceeding 1.5 to 2 mcg/mL have been associated with an increased risk of toxicity.

ATAZANAVIR *(cont.)*

Drug	Effect of Interaction	Recommendations/Comments
Midazolam	May significantly increase midazolam concentrations.	Concurrent administration of oral midazolam is contraindicated. IV midazolam may be considered with close monitoring. Consider alternative benzodiazepines (temazepam, oxazepam, or lorazepam).
Milk Thistle	No data.	Data limited to an interaction study with milk thistle and IDV. IDV AUC: unchanged; IDV Cmin: decreased by 47%. Clinical significance unknown. Unknown effect of the metabolism of other PIs or NNRTIs. Avoid coadministration with PIs and NNRTIs until it can be further evaluated.
Mirtazapine	May increase serum level of mirtazapine.	Applies to all PIs: use with caution. Consider an alternative antidepressant (i.e., SSRI: escitalopram, citalopram, sertraline, or fluoxetine).
Mycophenolate	Interaction unlikely. No significant interaction observed with NVP.	Applies to all PIs and NNRTIs: no significant interaction observed with NVP. Use standard dose.
Nefazodone	May increase serum level of nefazodone.	Applies to all PIs: use with caution. Consider an alternative antidepressant (i.e., SSRI: escitalopram, citalopram, sertraline, or fluoxetine).
Nevirapine (NVP)	Unboosted ATV Cmin was significantly lower with NVP coadministration.	NVP Cmin increased 46% and ATV Cmin decreased 41%. Avoid coadministration.
Nifedipine	May increase serum level of nifedipine.	Applies to all PIs: data limited to an interaction study conducted with ATV and diltiazem, which resulted in doubling of diltiazem serum level (this led to PR interval prolongation). All PIs have potential of prolonging the PR interval with calcium channel blocker coadministration. Calcium channel blockers should be started at low dose and slowly titrated with close monitoring of BP and pulse.
Nisoldipine	May increase serum level of nisoldipine.	Applies to all PIs: data limited to an interaction study conducted with ATV and diltiazem, which resulted in doubling of diltiazem serum level (this led to PR interval prolongation). All PIs have potential of prolonging the PR interval with calcium channel blockers coadministration. Calcium channel blockers should be started at low dose and slowly titrated with close monitoring of BP and pulse.

Drug	Effect of Interaction	Recommendations/Comments
Paclitaxel	ATV may increase paclitaxel serum concentrations.	Monitor for paclitaxel toxicity with coadministration.
Phencyclidine (PCP)	May significantly increase serum level of PCP.	Applies to all PIs: avoid PCP use with PIs (and all illicit drug use for obvious reasons).
Phenobarbital	May decrease serum levels of ATV.	Consider alternative anticonvulsants (i.e., valproic acid, lamotrigine, levetiracetam, or topiramate). With coadministration, monitor anticonvulsants level and consider TDM of ATV.
Phenytoin	May decrease serum levels of ATV.	Consider alternative anticonvulsants (i.e., valproic acid, lamotrigine, levetiracetam, or topiramate). With coadministration, monitor anticonvulsants level and consider TDM of ATV.
Pimozide	May significantly increase pimozide serum level resulting in QTc prolongation.	Contraindicated. Consider alternative: olanzapine.
Posaconazole	ATV AUC increased 2.5-fold. Posaconazole AUC increased 3.7-fold.	Monitor for potential increase in adverse drug reactions.
Propafenone	May increase antiarrhythmic serum levels.	Applies to all PIs: no data. Coadministration should be avoided. Serum levels are not routinely recommended due to the poor correlation with efficacy and toxicity.
Proton Pump Inhibitors (PPIs: omeprazole, rabeprazole, esomeprazole, lansoprazole, and pantoprazole)	ATV Cmin decreased by 78%. Cmin decreased by 46% if separated by 12 hrs.	Coadministration of PPI and ATV is contraindicated in ARV-experienced patients. In ARV-naïve patients, ATV/r (300/100 mg) + omeprazole (20 mg (max)separated by 12 hrs) may be considered, but not recommended by author. PPI equivalence: omeprazole (*Prilosec*) 20 mg = rabeprazole (*Aciphex*) 20 mg ~ esomeprazole (*Nexium*) 20 mg lansoprazole (*Prevacid*) 30 mg = pantoprazole (*Protonix*) 40 mg.
Quinidine	May increase antiarrhythmic serum levels.	Applies to all PIs: no data. Contraindicated with RTV. With all PIs and NNRTIs coadministration, monitor EKG (QTc) and serum level: target: 2 to 5 mcg/mL.
Raltegravir (RAL)	RAL AUC increased 41%.	Dose: ATV/r 300/100 mg once daily + RAL 400 mg twice daily.
Ranolazine	May significantly increase ranolazine serum concentrations.	Contraindicated. May increase risk of QTc prolongation.
Repaglinide	ATV may increase repaglinide serum concentrations.	Monitor blood glucose closely with coadministration.

ATAZANAVIR (cont.)

Drug	Effect of Interaction	Recommendations/Comments
Rifabutin (RFB)	RFB AUC increased by 110%, Cmin increased by 243% (with RFB 150 mg once daily) ATV AUC increased by 191%.	Recommended dosing with coadministration: ATV 400 mg once daily with RFB 150 mg 3 ×/wk. Or ATV/r 300/100 mg daily with RFB 150 mg 3 ×/wk.
Rifampin	ATV may be significantly decreased.	Coadministration with rifampin not recommended. RFB may be safer alternative. Dose: ATV 400 mg daily + RFB 150 mg 3 ×/wk.
Rifapentine	ATV serum levels may be significantly decreased.	Avoid coadministration. Consider using RFB.
Ritonavir (RTV)	ATV AUC increased by 238%, Cmin increased by 1089% (dose: ATV/r 300/100 mg once daily).	Boosting ATV 300 mg with 100 mg RTV results in better PK profile (doubles total ATV exposure and increases ATV trough by 10-fold), which may be preferred in PI-experienced patients.
Rosuvastatin	Rosuvastatin AUC increased 213%.	Start with rosuvastatin 5 mg/day. Close monitoring recommended due to limited clinical data.
Salmeterol	May increase salmeterol serum concentrations.	Avoid coadministration with boosted ATV. Consider formoterol.
Saquinavir (SQV)	SQV AUC increased by 449% (SQV dosed at 1200 mg once daily with ATV 400 mg once daily.) ATV not measured.	Beneficial PK interactions, which allows daily administration of SQV, but combination was inferior to LPV/r. ATV 400 mg + SQV 1200 mg once daily (did not perform well in trials). Consider ATV 300 mg + RTV 100 mg + SQV 1500–2000 mg once daily (limited data).
Sildenafil	May increase sildenafil serum level.	Applies to all PIs: use with close monitoring. Do not exceed 25 mg in a 48-hr period.
Simvastatin	May significantly increase simvastatin levels.	Contraindicated. Alternative that may be used include atorvastatin, pravastatin, rosuvastatin, fluvastatin. Monitor for adverse effect due to limited clinical data.
Sirolimus	May significantly increase serum level of sirolimus.	Applies to all PIs: dose sirolimus based on serum level. A significantly reduction of sirolimus dose with coadministration of all PIs is highly likely.
St. John's wort	May significantly decrease ATV serum level.	Contraindicated. Studies only done with IDV but St. John's wort may affect the metabolism of other PIs and NNRTIs. Use an alternative (more effective) antidepressant.

Drug	Effect of Interaction	Recommendations/Comments
Tacrolimus	May significantly increase serum level of tacrolimus.	Applies to all PIs: dose tacrolimus based on serum level. A significantly reduction of tacrolimus dose with all PIs coadministration is recommended.
Tadalafil	May increase serum level of tadalafil.	Applies to all PIs: start with 5 mg. Do not exceed 10 mg in 72 hrs. Consider sildenafil due to more clinical data and shorter half-life allowing for easier titration.
Tamoxifen	May increase serum level of tamoxifen.	Applies to all PIs: no data. Close monitoring of tamoxifen induced toxicity recommended.
Teniposide	May increase serum level of teniposide.	Applies to all PIs: no data. Close monitoring of teniposide-induced toxicity recommended.
Tenofovir (TDF)	ATV AUC decreased by 28% (compared to boosted ATV/r 300/100 mg), but still significantly (200%) higher than unboosted ATV. TDF not measured.	Interaction unlikely to be significant when ATV is boosted due to high ATV concentrations achieved with additional RTV (100 mg). Avoid use of TDF with unboosted ATV. If coadministered with TDF + famotidine 20 mg twice daily, increase ATV/r to 400/100 mg once daily.
Terfenadine	May significantly increase terfenadine serum level.	Contraindicated due to the potential for cardiac arrhythmias. Recommended alternative antihistamine: loratadine, fexofenadine, desloratidine, or cetirizine.
Tetrahydrocannabinol (THC)	Based on data with nelfinavir (NFV) and IDV interactions are unlikely.	Applies to PIs and NNRTIs: interactions are unlikely.
Tipranavir (TPV)	ATV may be significantly decreased.	Avoid coadministration.
Trazodone	May increase serum level of trazodone.	Applies to all PIs: use with caution. Consider alternative antidepressant (i.e., SSRI: escitalopram, citalopram, sertraline, or fluoxetine).
Triazolam	May significantly increase serum level of triazolam.	Contraindicated. Consider alternative benzodiazepines (temazepam, oxazepam, or lorazepam).
Vardenafil	May significantly increase serum level of vardenafil.	Applies to all PIs: do not exceed vardenafil 2.5 mg in 72 hrs (with RTV) or 2.5 mg in 24 hrs (with other PIs). Consider sildenafil due to more clinical data and less pronounced interaction.

ATAZANAVIR *(cont.)*

Drug	Effect of Interaction	Recommendations/Comments
Verapamil	May increase serum level of verapamil.	Applies to all PIs: data limited to an interaction study conducted with ATV and diltiazem, which resulted in doubling of diltiazem serum level (this led to PR interval prolongation). All PIs have the potential of prolonging the PR interval with calcium channel blocker coadministration. Calcium channel blockers should be started with 50% of the dose and slowly titrated with close monitoring of BP and pulse.
Vinblastine	May increase serum level of vinblastine.	Applies to all PIs: no data. Close monitoring of vinblastine-induced toxicity recommended.
Vincristine	May increase serum level of vincristine.	Applies to all PIs: no data. Close monitoring of vincristine-induced toxicity recommended.
Vitamin C	No data.	Data limited to interaction study with IDV and vitamin C (1 g/day) resulting in IDV AUC decreased by 14% and Cmin by 32%. Avoid coadministration until more data available.
Voriconazole	May decrease voriconazole AUC. Voriconazole may increase coadministered ATV.	Significant interaction with EFV and RTV (400 mg twice daily). Low-dose RTV boosting (200 mg/day) decreased voriconazole AUC by 39%; coadministration should be avoided or should be used with caution. In severe cases of invasive aspergillosis, the addition or substitution of voriconazole with *AmBisome* or caspofungin should be considered. Monitor voriconazole serum concentrations (target Cmin >2mcg/mL).
Zidovudine/ lamivudine (AZT/3TC)	AZT and 3TC AUC unaffected, but AZT trough decreased 30% (intracellular concentrations not measured). ATV not studied.	Standard dose AZT/3TC with ATV.

DRUG-DRUG INTERACTION – BUPROPION

Drug	Effect of Interaction	Recommendations/Comments
Alcohol	May increase risk of seizures.	Avoid coadministration.
Cimetidine	May increase effect of bupropion.	Start with low-dose buproprion and titrate slowly.
Fluoroquinolones	May decrease seizure threshold with high-dose buproprion.	Monitor for seizure with coadministration.

Drug	Effect of Interaction	Recommendations/Comments
Imipenem	May decrease seizure threshold with high-dose buproprion.	Monitor for seizure with coadministration.
Levodopa	May increase buproprion side effects.	Toxicity enhanced with coadministration. Monitor for nausea, vomiting, excitation, restlessness, and postural tremor. Start with low dose and titrate slowly.
Lopinavir/ritonavir (LPV/r)	LPV/r decreased bupropion AUC 57%.	Titrate bupropion to effect.
MAO Inhibitors	May increase the risk of hypertension.	Contraindicated; do not coadminister.
Nicotine Patch	May increase the risk of hypertension.	Monitor BP closely.
Ritonavir (RTV)	RTV did not significantly increase bupropion concentrations.	No seizure reported with PI coadministration; use standard doses.
Theophylline	May decrease seizure threshold with high-dose buproprion.	Monitor for seizure with coadministration.
Tricyclic Antidepressants	May decrease seizure threshold with high-dose buproprion.	Monitor for seizure with coadministration.
Warfarin	May increase or decrease INR.	Monitor INR closely.

DRUG-DRUG INTERACTION – CIPROFLOXACIN

Drug	Effect of Interaction	Recommendations/Comments
Antacids (magnesium, aluminum, calcium, Al-Mg contained in buffered ddI), vitamins, and minerals	Cations bind to ciprofloxacin resulting in decreased absorption and loss therapeutic efficacy.	Avoid coadministration. Administer ciprfloxacin at least 2 hrs before cations.
Didanosine (ddI) (buffered suspension)	Antacid buffer binds to ciprofloxacin resulting in decreased absorption and loss therapeutic efficacy.	Avoid coadministration. Administer ciprfloxacin at least 2 hrs before cations. No interaction with ddI EC.
Glyburide	May cause hyper or hypoglycemia.	Monitor glucose levels closely.
Methotrexate	May increase methotrexate serum concentrations.	Monitor for methotrexate toxicity.
Mexiletine	Ciprofloxacin may inhibit CYP1A2 resulting in increased mexiletine concentrations.	Monitor mexiletine serum concentrations with coadministration.

CIPROFLOXACIN *(cont.)*

Drug	Effect of Interaction	Recommendations/Comments
Nonsteroidal anti-inflammatory drugs (NSAIDs)	May increase risk of seizure.	Avoid coadministration in patients with seizure history.
Probenecid	Probenecid interferes with renal tubular secretion of ciprofloxacin, this may result in 50% increase in serum levels of ciprofloxacin.	No dose adjustment.
Sevelamer	Ciprofloxacin absorption significantly decreased.	Avoid coadministration. Administer ciprofloxacin 2 hrs before sevelamer.
Sucralfate	Decreased absorption of ciprofloxacin.	Do not coadminister. Administer ciprofloxacin at least 2 hrs before sucralfate.
Theophylline	Increases theophylline concentrations by 17%–257%.	Monitor theophylline serum concentrations with coadministration.
Warfarin	Ciprofloxacin inhibit R-warfarin metabolism. Case reports of ciprofloxacin enhancing anti-coagulation effect of warfarin.	Monitor INR closely.

DRUG-DRUG INTERACTION – CLARITHROMYCIN

Drug	Effect of Interaction	Recommendations/Comments
Alfuzosin	Risk of QTc prolongation increased.	Contraindicated.
Alprazolam	Alprazolam serum levels may be increased.	Consider lorazepam, oxazepam, or temazepam.
Amiodarone	Amiodarone serum levels may be increased.	Monitor.
Astemizole	Risk of QTc prolongation increased.	Contraindicated.
Atazanavir (ATV)	ATV AUC increased by 28%. Clarithromycin AUC increased by 94%. QTc prolongation has been observed with coadministration.	Consider azithromycin or reduce clarithromycin dose by 50%. Further renal dose adjustment is required but not outlined by specific guidelines. Suggestion: CrCl 30–60 mL/min, 250 mg q24h; CrCl < 30 mL/min, 250 mg q48h.
Carbamazepine	Carbamazepine serum levels increased by 60%.	Avoid coadministration or monitor serum level.
Cisapride	Risk of QTc prolongation increased.	Contraindicated.

Drug	Effect of Interaction	Recommendations/Comments
Colchicine	May increase the risk of colchicine toxicity.	Avoid coadministration.
Cyclosporine	Cyclosporine serum levels may be increased.	Monitor.
Diazepam	Diazepam serum levels may be increased.	Consider lorazepam, oxazepam, or temazepam.
Digoxin	Digoxin serum levels may be increased. Increased digoxin toxicity has been reported with coadministration.	Monitor serum level.
Darunavir/ ritonavir (DRV/r)	Clarithromycin AUC increased by 57%.	Consider azithromycin.
Efavirenz (EFV)	Clarithromycin AUC decreased by 39%. Clinical significance unknown although high incidence of rash was observed in healthy volunteers with coadministration.	Consider azithromycin.
Ergot Alkaloids	Risk of ergotism increased.	Avoid coadministration.
Etravirine (ETR)	ETR AUC increased 42%. Clarithromycin AUC decreased 39%. 14-hydroxyclarithromycin (active metabolite, though not as effective against MAC) AUC increased 21%.	Consider azithromycin.
Fentanyl	Fentanyl serum levels may be increased.	Consider morphine.
Fosamprenavir (FPV)	FPV AUC increased by 18% (studied with APV). Clarithromycin AUC not affected.	No dose adjustment necessary.
Indinavir (IDV)	IDV AUC increased 295%. Clarithromycin AUC increased 53%.	No dose adjustment necessary.
Lopinavir (LPV)	Lovastatin serum levels may be increased.	No dose adjustment necessary. See RTV for LPV/r.
Lovastatin	Clarithromycin AUC may be increased.	Consider pravastatin.
Maraviroc (MVC)	MVC serum levels may be increased.	MVC 150 mg twice daily.
Midazolam	Midazolam serum levels may be increased.	Consider lorazepam, oxazepam, or temazepam.

CLARITHROMYCIN *(cont.)*

Drug	Effect of Interaction	Recommendations/Comments
Nevirapine (NVP)	NVP AUC increased by 26%. Clarithromycin AUC decreased by 29%. 14-hydroxyclarithromycin (active metabolite, though not as effective against MAC) AUC increased by 27%.	No dose adjustment necessary.
Pimozide	Risk of QTc prolongation increased.	Contraindicated.
Raltegravir (RAL)	No data but an interaction is unlikely.	No dose adjustment necessary.
Ranolazine	Risk of QTc prolongation increased.	Contraindicated.
Rifabutin (RFB)	RFB AUC increased by 56%. Clarithromycin AUC decreased by 44%. 14-hydroxyclarithromycin (active metabolite, though not as effective against MAC) AUC increased by 57%.	Consider azithromycin.
Rifampin	Rifampin AUC increased 99% and Cmax increased 69%. Clarithromycin AUC decreased 44% and Cmax decreased 41%. Increased rifampin toxicity has been observed with coadministration.	Avoid coadministration.
Ritonavir (RTV)	Clarithromycin AUC increased by 77% and Cmin increased by 182%.	Consider azithromycin or reduce clarithromycin dose by 50%. Further renal dose adjustment is required but not outlined by specific guidelines.
Saquinavir (SQV)	SQV AUC increased by 177%. Clarithromycin AUC increased by 45%.	No dose adjustment necessary. See RTV for SQV/r.
Simvastatin	Simvastatin serum levels may be increased.	Consider pravastatin.
Sirolimus	Sirolimus serum levels may be increased.	Monitor serum level.
Tacrolimus	Tacrolimus serum levels may be increased.	Monitor serum level.
Terfenadine	Risk of QTc prolongation increased.	Contraindicated.
Theophylline	Theophylline serum levels may be increased.	Monitor serum level.

Drug	Effect of Interaction	Recommendations/Comments
Tipranavir/ ritonavir (TPV/r)	TPV AUC increased by 66%. Clarithromycin AUC increased by 19%.	Consider azithromycin.
Triazolam	Triazolam serum levels may be increased.	Consider lorazepam, oxazepam, or temazepam.
Warfarin	Anticoagulation may be increased.	Monitor INR.

DRUG-DRUG INTERACTION – DAPSONE

Drug	Effect of Interaction	Recommendations/Comments
Bismuth	Dapsone absorption may be decreased.	Avoid coadministration. Administer dapsone 2 hrs before bismuth.
Cimetidine	Dapsone absorption may be decreased.	Avoid coadministration. Administer dapsone 2 hrs before H-2 blockers.
Didanosine (ddI) (buffered suspension)	Dapsone solubility may decreased and result in decreased absorption.	Clinical significance unknown (a PK study did not find interaction). Used enteric coated ddI.
Esomeprazole	Dapsone absorption may be decreased.	Avoid coadministration.
Famotidine	Dapsone absorption may be decreased.	Avoid coadministration. Administer dapsone 2 hrs before H-2 blockers.
Lansoprazole	Dapsone absorption may be decreased.	Avoid coadministration.
Nizatidine	Dapsone absorption may be decreased.	Avoid coadministration. Administer dapsone 2 hrs before H-2 blockers.
Omeprazole	Dapsone absorption may be decreased.	Avoid coadministration.
Pantoprazole	Dapsone absorption may be decreased.	Avoid coadministration.
Primaquine	Risk of hemolysis may be increased, particularly in G6PD deficiency.	Avoid or monitor closely with coadministration.
Probenecid	Dapsone serum concentrations may be increased.	Monitor for anemia with coadministration.
Pyrimethamine	Risk of anemia may be increased.	Monitor.
Rabeprazole	Dapsone absorption may be decreased.	Avoid coadministration.
Ranitidine	Dapsone absorption may be decreased.	Avoid coadministration. Administer dapsone 2 hrs before H-2 blockers.

DAPSONE *(cont.)*

Drug	Effect of Interaction	Recommendations/Comments
Ribavirin	Risk of hemolysis may be increased.	Avoid or monitor closely with coadministration.
Rifampin	Dapsone serum levels decreased by 85%–90%.	Avoid coadministration.
Sucralfate	Dapsone absorption may be decreased.	Avoid coadministration. Administer dapsone 2 hrs before sucralfate.
Trimethoprim (TMP)	TMP serum levels increased by 48%. Dapsone serum levels increased by 40%. Methemoglobinemia has been reported with coadministration.	Clinical significance unknown, but cases of methemoglobinemia reported with TMP + dapsone in patients who tolerated dapsone alone.
Zidovudine (AZT)	Risk of anemia may be increased.	Monitor.

DRUG-DRUG INTERACTION – DARUNAVIR (DRV)

Drug	Effect of Interaction	Recommendations/Comments
Acid-Reducing Agents (PPIs, H-2 blocker)	No change in DRV AUC. Omeprazole AUC decreased by 42%.	Use standard dose.
Alfuzosin	May increase alfuzosin serum concentrations.	Contraindicated. Consider doxazosin and terazosin for BPH (with close monitoring).
Amiodarone	DRV/r may increase serum concentration of amiodarone.	Avoid or use with dose adjustment and close monitoring.
Astemizole	DRV/r may significantly increase serum concentration of astemizole.	Contraindicated due to the potential for cardiac arrhythmia.
Atazanavir (ATV)	No interaction.	Dose: ATV 300 mg once daily + DRV/r 600/100 mg twice daily.
Atorvastatin	Increased atorvastatin exposure by approximately 4-fold.	Dose: start with atorvastatin 10 mg once daily and titrate slowly. Avoid doses >40 mg/day. Rare events of hypersensitivity including facial edema and rhabomyolysis associated with DRV coadministration.
Bepridil	DRV/r may increase serum concentration of bepridil.	Avoid or use with dose adjustment and close monitoring.

Drug	Effect of Interaction	Recommendations/Comments
Bosentan	May significantly increase bosentan serum concentrations.	Coadminister bosentan only after RTV dosing has reached steady-state. In patients on RTV >10 days: start bosentan at 62.5 mg once daily or every other day. In patients already on bosentan: d/c bosentan for >36 hrs prior to initiation of RTV-boosted PIs and restart bosentan at 62.5 mg once daily or every other day after RTV has reached steady-state (after 10 days).
Buprenorphine	Buprenorphine serum concentrations not significantly affected, but norbuprenorphine active metabolite AUC was increased 46%.	Subjects did not require buprenorphine dose adjustment, but clinicians should monitor for possible increased sedation.
Calcium Channel Blockers (e.g., amlodipine, diltiazem, felodipine, nifedipine, and nicardipine)	DRV/r may increase serum concentration of amlodipine, diltiazem, felodipine, nifedipine, and nicardipine.	May need to decrease calcium channel blockers dose by 50%. Use with close monitoring.
Carbamazepine	No significant decrease in DRV/r AUC. Carbamazepine serum concentrations increased 45%.	Monitor carbamazepine serum concentrations with coadministration.
Cisapride	DRV/r may significantly increase serum concentration of cisapride.	Contraindicated due to the potential for cardiac arrhythmia.
Clarithromycin	DRV: no change. Clarithromycin AUC increased 57%.	Dose: adjust clarithromycin dose according to renal function. CrCl 30–60 mL/min = 250 mg twice daily, CrCl<30 mLmin = 250 mg once daily. Avoid with QTc prolongation. Consider using azithromycin.
Cyclosporine	DRV/r may significantly increase serum concentration of cyclosporine.	Avoid or use with dose adjustment and close monitoring of cyclosporine serum concentration.
Efavirenz (EFV)	DRV Cmin decreased by 31%. EFV AUC and Cmin increased 21% and 17%, respectively.	Dose not established since initial PK study used only DRV 300/100 mg twice daily. Consider: DRV/r 600/100 mg twice daily plus EFV 600 mg once daily.
Enfuvirtide (ENF)	No interaction.	Use standard dose.
Ergot Alkaloid	DRV/r may significantly increase serum concentration of ergot alkaloid.	Contraindicated due to the potential for acute ergotism.

DARUNAVIR *(cont.)*

Drug	Effect of Interaction	Recommendations/Comments
Ethinyl Estradiol/ Norethindrone	DRV/r decreased ethinyl estradiol AUC 44%.	Use with caution. Use an alternative form of contraception.
Etravirine (ETR)	ETR AUC decreased by 37%.	Despite drug-drug interaction, good clinical efficacy with DRV/r plus ETR coadministration. No dosage adjustments necessary. ETR 200 mg twice daily plus DRV/r 600/100 mg twice daily.
Fluticasone	DRV/r may increase serum concentration of fluticasone.	Concurrent use of fluticasone and RTV might lead in increased fluticasone plasma concentrations and decreased cortisol, resulting in Cushing's syndrome. Avoid long-term coadministration or use with dose adjustment and close monitoring. Consider beclomethasone.
Fosamprenavir (FPV)	No data.	Avoid coadministration.
Indinavir (IDV)	IDV AUC and Cmin increased 23% and 125%, respectively. DRV AUC and Cmin increased 24% and 44%, respectively.	Dose not established. May increase risk of nephrolithiasis.
Itraconazole	DRV/r may increase serum concentration of itraconazole.	Monitor itraconazole serum concentrations.
Ketoconazole	DRV AUC increased 42%. Ketoconazole AUC increased 212%.	Do not exceed ketoconazole 200 mg once daily or use alternative agent.
Lidocaine	DRV/r may increase serum concentration of lidocaine.	Avoid or use with dose adjustment and close monitoring.
Lopinavir (LPV)	DRV AUC and Cmin decreased 53% and 65%, respectively. LPV AUC and Cmin increased 37% and 72%, respectively.	Avoid coadministration.
Lovastatin	DRV/r may significantly increase simvastatin serum concentration.	Contraindicated. Consider alternative statin (pravastatin, atorvastatin, and possibly rosuvastatin).
Maraviroc (MVC)	MVC AUC increased 4-fold.	Dose: DRV/r 600/100 mg twice daily plus MVC 150 mg twice daily.
Methadone	DRV/r decreased R-methadone AUC by 16%.	Monitor for sign and Sx of withdrawal. Titratemethadone dose as needed.
Midazolam	DRV/r may significantly increase serum concentration of midazolam.	Contraindicated due to potential for increased sedation. Consider lorazepam.
Nelfinavir (NFV)	No data.	Avoid coadministration.

Drug	Effect of Interaction	Recommendations/Comments
Nevirapine (NVP)	No significant change in DRV AUC and Cmin. NVP AUC and Cmin increased 27% and 47%, respectively.	Limited data (historical control comparison). Consider: DRV/r 600/100 mg twice daily plus NVP 200 mg twice daily.
Paroxetine	Paroxetine AUC decreased by 39%. DRV: no change.	Titrate paroxetine to therapeutic effect.
Phenobarbital	May significantly decrease DRV serum concentration.	Avoid coadministration. Consider valproic acid or levitaracetam.
Phenytoin	May significantly decrease DRV serum concentration.	Avoid coadministration. Consider valproic acid or levitaracetam.
Pimozide	DRV/r may significantly increase serum concentration of pimozide.	Contraindicated due to potential for QTc prolongation.
Pravastatin	Pravastatin AUC increased 81%, but highly variable.	Dose: start with 10 mg once daily and titrate slowly. Rare events of hypersensitivity including facial edema and rhabomyolysis associated with DRV coadministration.
Prednisone	DRV/r may increase serum concentration of prednisone.	Concurrent use of prednisone and RTV might lead in increased prednisone plasma concentrations and decreased cortisol, resulting in Cushing's syndrome. Avoid long-term coadministration or use with dose adjustment and close monitoring.
Propafenone	DRV/r may increase serum concentration of propafenone.	Avoid or use with dose adjustment and close monitoring.
Quinidine	DRV/r may increase serum concentration of quinidine.	Avoid or use with dose adjustment and close monitoring.
Raltegravir (RAL)	Interaction unlikely.	Use standard dose of both drugs.
Ranolazine	May significantly increase ranolazine serum concentrations.	Contraindicated. May increase risk of QTc prolongation.
Rifabutin (RFB)	DRV/r may increase serum concentration of RFB. No data on DRV PK with coadministration.	Dose: consider RFB 150 mg every other day with DRV/r coadministration.
Rifampin	May significantly decrease DRV serum concentration.	Avoid coadministration. Consider RFB.
Rifapentine	May significantly decrease DRV serum concentrations.	Avoid coadministration. Consider dose adjusted RFB (150 mg every other day) with DRV/r.
Rosuvastatin	May increase rosuvastatin serum concentration.	No data. Initiate with low dose rosuvastatin (5 mg) with coadministration.
Salmeterol	May increase salmeterol serum concentrations.	Avoid coadministration. Consider formoterol.

DARUNAVIR *(cont.)*

Drug	Effect of Interaction	Recommendations/Comments
Saquinavir (SQV)	DRV AUC and Cmin decreased 25% and 42%, respectively. No change in SQV serum concentration.	Avoid coadministration.
Sertraline	Sertraline AUC decreased by 49%. DRV: no change.	Titrate sertraline to therapeutic effect.
Sildenafil	No significant change in sildenafil AUC between 25 mg (with DRV/r) and 100 mg (without DRV/r).	Use with caution. Do not exceed 25 mg in 48h.
Simvastatin	DRV/r may significantly increase simvastatin serum concentration.	Contraindicated. Consider alternative statin (pravastatin, atorvastatin, and possibly rosuvastatin).
Sirolimus	DRV/r may significantly increase serum concentration of sirolimus.	Avoid or use with dose adjustment and close monitoring of sirolimus serum concentration.
St. John's wort	May significantly decrease DRV serum concentration.	Avoid coadministration.
Tacrolimus	DRV/r may significantly increase serum concentration of tacrolimus.	Avoid or use with dose adjustment and close monitoring of tacrolimus serum concentration.
Tadalafil	DRV/r may significantly increase serum concentration of tadalafil.	Avoid or use with dose adjustment and close monitoring. Dose adjustment: tadalafil 10 mg q72h.
Tenofovir (TDF)	DRV: no change. TDF AUC and Cmin increased 22% and 37% respectively.	Use standard dose.
Terfenadine	DRV/r may significantly increase serum concentration of terfenadine.	Contraindicated due to potential for cardiac arrhythmia.
Tipranavir (TPV)	May significantly decrease DRV serum concentrations.	Avoid coadministration.
Trazodone	DRV/r may increase serum concentration of trazodone.	Use with dose adjustment and close monitoring.
Triazolam	DRV/r may significantly increase serum concentration of triazolam.	Contraindicated due to potential for increased sedation. Consider lorazepam.
Vardenafil	DRV/r may significantly increase serum concentration of vardenafil.	Avoid or use with dose adjustment and close monitoring. Use with caution. Dose adjustment: vardenafil 2.5 mg q 72h.

Drug	Effect of Interaction	Recommendations/Comments
Voriconazole	DRV/r may decrease voriconazole serum concentration.	Use with caution. Monitor voriconazole serum concentration (target Cmin > 2 mcg/mL).
Warfarin	S-warfarin AUC decreased 21%.	Use with close INR monitoring.

DRUG-DRUG INTERACTION – DELAVIRDINE (DLV)

Drug	Effect of Interaction	Recommendations/Comments
Alfuzosin	May increase alfuzosin serum concentrations.	Avoid coadministration.
Alprazolam	May increase alprazolam serum levels.	Contraindicated. Consider lorazepam, oxazepam, or temazepam with DLV coadministration.
Amiodarone	May significantly increase amiodarone serum levels.	Use with caution. Data limited to case report of increased amiodarone levels with IDV coadministration. Monitor for amiodarone ADR (PFTs and TSH). Consider monitoring serum levels of amiodarone. Long half-life may make titration difficult (consider alternative antiarrhythmics with cardiology consult).
Amlodipine	May increase serum level of amlodipine.	Applies to all PIs and DLV: data limited to an interaction study conducted with ATV and diltiazem, which resulted in doubling of diltiazem serum levels (this led to PR interval prolongation). All PIs and DLV has the potential of prolonging the PR interval with calcium channel blocker coadministration. Calcium channel blockers should be started with 50% of the dose and slowly titrated with close monitoring of BP and pulse.
Amphetamine	May increase amphetamine serum levels.	Clinical significance unknown. Use with caution.
Antacids	DLV AUC: decreased by 41%; decreased absorption of DLV.	Clinically significant. Separate antacid dose by at least 1 hr before or 2 hrs after DLV.
Artemether (artemisinin)	May increase serum levels of artemether.	Applies to all PIs and DLV: close monitoring for artemether toxicity (bone marrow suppression, bradycardia and seizure).

DELAVIRDINE (cont.)

Drug	Effect of Interaction	Recommendations/Comments
Astemizole	May significantly increase astemizole serum levels.	Contraindicated due to the potential for cardiac arrhythmias. Recommended alternative antihistamine: loratadine, fexofenadine, desloratidine, or cetirizine.
Azathioprine	Interaction unlikely.	Applies to all PIs and NNRTIs: use standard dose.
Bepridil	May significantly increase bepridil serum levels.	Applies to all PIs and DLV: no data. The manufacturer of ATV, RTV, and APV does not recommend bepridil coadministration, this contraindication should extend to all PIs and DLV since a significant increase in bepridil serum levels can result in pro-arrhythmic events such as VT, PVC, and VFib.
Carbamazepine	DLV levels may be decreased and carbamazepine levels may be increased.	Coadministration not recommended. Monitor carbamazepine levels and consider TDM of PIs and NNRTI. Consider alternative agents: valproic acid, lamotrigine, levetiracetam, or topiramate.
Chlordiazepoxide	May increase serum levels of chlordiazepoxide.	Applies to all PIs and DLV: consider alternative benzodiazepines (lorazepam, temazepam, or oxazepam).
Cisapride	May significantly increase cisapride serum levels.	Contraindicated due to potential for cardiac arrhythmias. Recommended alternative: metoclopramide.
Clarithromycin	Clarithromycin AUC: increased by 100%; 14-hydroxyclarithromycin AUC: decreased by 75%; DLV AUC: increased by 44%.	Dose adjustment recommended with impaired renal function. Cr clearance 30–60 mL/min: 50% of clarithromycin dose. Cr clearance <30 mL/min: 25% of clarithromycin dose. Consider azithromycin.
Clorazepate	May increase serum levels of clorazepate.	Applies to all PIs and DLV: consider alternative benzodiazepines (lorazepam, temazepam, or oxazepam).
Cyclophosphamide	May increase serum levels of cyclophosphamide.	Applies to all PIs and DLV: data limited to an interaction study conducted with IDV resulting in a 50% increase in cyclophosphamide serum levels. Since all PIs and DLV have the potential of increasing cyclophosphamide levels, close monitoring of cyclophosphamide-induced toxicity is recommended.
Cyclosporine	May increases serum levels cyclosporine.	Monitor serum levels of cyclosporine closely with coadministration. Cyclosporine dose may need to be decreased.

Drug	Effect of Interaction	Recommendations/Comments
Didanosine (ddI) (buffered)	DLV AUC: decreased by 20%.	Consider ddI EC or administer DLV at least 1 hr prior to buffered ddI tabs/suspension.
Diltiazem	May increase serum levels of diltiazem.	Applies to all PIs and DLV: data limited to an interaction study conducted with ATV which resulted in doubling of diltiazem serum levels (this led to PR interval prolongation). All PIs and DLV have the potential of prolonging the PR interval with diltiazem coadministration. Diltiazem should be started with 50% of the dose and slowly titrated with close monitoring of BP and pulse.
Disopyramide	May increase disopyramide serum levels.	Applies to all PIs and DLV: no data. Monitor disopyramide serum level (target: 2 to 7.5 mcg/mL).
Docetaxel	May increase serum levels of docetaxel.	Applies to all PIs and DLV: no data. Close monitoring of chemotherapy-induced toxicity recommended.
Dofetilide	May significantly increase serum levels of dofetilide.	Applies to all PIs and DLV: no data. Use with caution. Monitor QTc closely and adjust dofetilide dosing based on QTc prolongation and renal function. Consider an alternative class III antiarrhythmic such as bretylium or ibutilide.
Echinacea	May decrease DLV serum levels. Echinacea (400 mg 4 × days) decreased CYP3A4 substrate (midazolam) by 23%.	Applies to all PIs and NNRTIs. Clinical significance unknown but should avoided until the safety of this combination is further evaluated.
Ergot Alkaloids	May significantly increase serum levels of ergotamine resulting in acute ergot toxicity.	Contraindicated. Consider alternative agent for migraine such as sumatriptan (but not eletriptan since it is a CYP3A4 substrate and significant drug interaction occurred with a CYP3A4 inhibitor).
Estazolam	May increase serum levels of estazolam.	Applies to all PIs and DLV: consider an alternative benzodiazepines (lorazepam, oxazepam, or temazepam).
Ethinyl Estradiol	Ethinyl estradiol levels decreased by 20%.	Clinical significance unknown. Patients should be aware of potential interaction. Alternative birth control methods should be recommended.
Ethosuximide	May increase serum levels of ethosuximide.	Applies to all PIs and DLV: consider switching to valproic acid for the treatment of absence seizure.
Etoposide	May increase serum levels of etoposide.	Applies to all PIs and DLV: no data. Close monitoring of chemotherapy-induced toxicity recommended.

DELAVIRDINE *(cont.)*

Drug	Effect of Interaction	Recommendations/Comments
Etravirine (ETR)	May increase ETR serum concentrations.	Avoid coadministration.
Felodipine	May increase serum levels of felodipine.	Applies to all PIs and DLV: data limited to an interaction study conducted with ATV and diltiazem, which resulted in doubling of diltiazem serum levels (this led PR interval prolongation). All PIs and DLV have the potential of prolonging PR interval with calcium channel blockers coadministration. Calcium channel blockers should be started with 50% of the dose and slowly titrated with close monitoring of BP and pulse.
Fentanyl	May significantly increase serum levels of fentanyl.	Use with caution. Consider morphine.
Flecainide	May increase antiarrhythmic serum levels.	Applies to all PIs and DLV: avoid coadministration; if necessary, monitor flecainide trough level with coadministration. Target: 200–1000 ng/mL. Toxicity is frequent with trough serum levels above 1000 ng/mL.
Fluconazole	No interaction.	Use standard doses of both drugs.
Fluoxetine	DLV Cmin increased by 50%.	Not significant. Use standard dose.
Flurazepam	May increase serum levels of flurazepam.	Applies to all PIs and DLV: consider an alternative benzodiazepines (lorazepam, oxazepam, or temazepam).
Food	DLV AUC was not affected by food.	Administer DLV with or without food.
Garlic Supplement	No data.	Studies only done with SQV resulting in SQV serum level reduction. No data with DLV. Avoid coadministration.
Granisetron	May increase serum levels of granisetron.	Applies to all PIs and DLV: consider an alternative benzodiazepines (lorazepam, oxazepam, or temazepam).
H2-Blocker	May decrease DLV absorption.	Contraindicated.
Heroin (diamorphine)	Drug interaction unlikely.	Interaction unlikely but illicit drug use should be avoided for obvious reasons.
Ifosphamide	May increase serum levels of ifosphamide.	Applies to all PIs and DLV: no data. Close monitoring of chemotherapy-induced toxicity recommended.
Indinavir (IDV)	IDV AUC: increased by 44% (compared to 800 mg q8h dose).	With coadministration, decrease IDV to 600 mg q8h and use standard dose of DLV.

Drug	Effect of Interaction	Recommendations/Comments
Irinotecan	May increase irinotecan serum levels.	Applies to all PIs and DLV: Coadministration of ATV is contraindicated by manufacturer. All PIs and DLV also have the potential for significant interaction with irinotecan, therefore the coadministration should be done with extreme caution.
Ketoconazole	DLV Cmin: increased by 50%.	No clinical data; consider dose adjustment: DLV 200–400 mg 3×/day.
Lidocaine (systemic)	May increase lidocaine serum levels.	No data. Use with caution, monitor lidocaine serum levels (target: 1.5 to 6 mcg/mL) with coadministration.
Lopinavir/ritonavir LPV/r	May increase LPV serum levels.	Unlikely to be significant. Use standard dose for both drugs.
Lovastatin	May significantly increase lovastatin levels.	Contraindicated. Recommended alternatives include pravastatin, rosuvastatin, or fluvastatin (and possibly atorvastatin— start at 10 mg/day). Monitor for adverse effect due to limited clinical data.
Maraviroc (MVC)	DLV may increase MVC serum concentrations.	Dose: DLV 400 mg 3 times daily + MVC 150 mg twice daily.
Mefloquine	May increase serum levels of mefloquine.	Applies to all PIs and DLV: monitor mefloquine levels. Monitor for mefloquine toxicity (dizziness, LFTs, and periodic ophthalmic examination).
Methadone	DLV AUC not affected by methadone. Methadone PK was not evaluated but DLV may have the potential for increasing methadone serum levels.	Use standard DLV dose. Monitor for sedation; methadone dose may need to be decreased.
Mexiletine	May increase antiarrhythmic serum levels.	Applies to all PIs and DLV: no data. Use with caution. Monitor EKG and serum levels. Serum levels exceeding 1.5 to 2 mcg/mL have been associated with an increased risk of toxicity.
Midazolam	May significantly increase midazolam levels.	Single dose IV midazolam may be used; chronic midazolam administration (oral or intravenous) should be avoided. Consider alternative benzodiazepines (lorazepam, temazepam, or oxazepam).
Milk Thistle	No data.	Data limited to an interaction study with milk thistle and IDV. IDV AUC unchanged; IDV Cmin decreased by 47%. Clinical significance unknown. Avoid coadministration with DLV.

DELAVIRDINE *(cont.)*

Drug	Effect of Interaction	Recommendations/Comments
Mirtazapine	May increase serum levels of mirtazapine.	Applies to all PIs and DLV: use with caution. Consider an alternative antidepressant (i.e., SSRI: escitalopram, citalopram, sertraline, or fluoxetine).
Mycophenolate	Interaction unlikely. No significant interaction observed with NVP.	Applies to all PIs and NNRTIs: no significant interaction observed with NVP. Use standard dose.
Nefazodone	May increase serum levels of nefazodone.	Applies to all PIs and DLV: use with caution. Consider an alternative antidepressant (i.e., SSRI: escitalopram, citalopram, sertraline, or fluoxetine).
Nelfinavir (NFV)	NFV AUC: increased by 72%; DLV AUC: decreased by 42%; Cmin: decreased by 52%.	Clinical significance unknown. Alternative PI should be considered.
Nifedipine	May increase serum levels of nifedipine.	Applies to all PIs and DLV: data limited to an interaction study conducted with ATV and diltiazem, which resulted in doubling of diltiazem serum levels (this led to PR interval prolongation). All PIs and DLV have the potential of prolonging the PR interval with calcium channel blockers coadministration. Calcium channel blockers should be started with 50% of the dose and slowly titrated with close monitoring of BP and pulse.
Nisoldipine	May increase serum levels of nisoldipine.	Applies to all PIs and DLV: data limited to an interaction study conducted with ATV and diltiazem, which resulted in doubling of diltiazem serum levels (this led to PR interval prolongation). All PIs and DLV have the potential of prolonging the PR interval with calcium channel blockers coadministration. Calcium channel blockers should be started with 50% of the dose and slowly titrated with close monitoring of BP and pulse.
Paclitaxel	Case reports of increased paclitaxel serum levels.	Data limited to case reports of severe toxicity associated with DLV coadministration with paclitaxel. Close monitoring of paclitaxel-induced toxicity is recommended.
Phencyclidine (PCP)	May significantly increase serum levels of PCP.	Avoid PCP with DLV coadministration. Avoid all illicit drug use for obvious reasons.

Drug	Effect of Interaction	Recommendations/Comments
Phenobarbital	May decrease serum level of PIs and NNRTIs. PIs and NNRTIs may increase or decrease phenobarbital serum level.	Consider alternative anticonvulsants (i.e., valproic acid, lamotrigine, levetiracetam, or topiramate). With coadministration, monitor anticonvulsants level and consider TDM of PIs and NNRTIs.
Phenytoin	DLV AUC: decreased by approx 90% (population PK).	Coadministration not recommended. Monitor phenytoin levels and adjust as indicated. Consider alternative agents: (i.e., valproic acid, lamotrigine, levetiracetam, or topiramate).
Pimozide	May significantly increase pimozide serum levels resulting in QTc prolongation.	Contraindicated. Consider alternative: olanzapine.
Propafenone	May increase propafenone serum level.	Use with caution. Serum levels are not routinely recommended due to the poor correlation with efficacy and toxicity.
Proton Pump Inhibitors (PPI) (omeprazole or pantoprazole)	May decrease DLV absorption.	Coadministration is not recommended.
Quinidine	May increase quinidine levels.	No data. Use with caution with close monitoring of EKG (QTc) and serum levels: target: 2 to 5 mcg/mL.
Ranolazine	May increase ranolazine serum concentrations.	Avoid coadministration.
Rifabutin (RFB)	RFB AUC: increased by 100%; DLV AUC: decreased by 80%.	Contraindicated.
Rifampin	DLV AUC: decreased by 96%.	Do not coadminister.
Rifapentine	DLV serum levels may be significantly decreased.	Avoid coadministration.
Ritonavir (RTV)	RTV AUC: increased by 61%; Cmin: increased by 55%. No difference in DLV PK parameters.	No dose adjustment necessary.
Rosuvastatin	Other CYP3A4 inhibitor (i.e., erythromycin) did not affect rosuvastatin serum levels.	Interaction unlikely, but close monitoring recommended due to limited clinical data.
Saquinavir (SQV)	SQV AUC: increased by 500%; DLV AUC: decreased by 15%.	A beneficial interaction. No adjustment necessary. Use SQV 800 mg 3×/day + DLV 400 mg 3×/day.
Sildenafil	May increase sildenafil serum levels.	Use with caution. Do not exceed 25 mg in 48 hrs.
Simvastatin	May significantly increase simvastatin levels.	Contraindicated. Consider: pravastatin, rosuvastatin or low dose atorvastatin (start with 10 mg/day).

DELAVIRDINE *(cont.)*

Drug	Effect of Interaction	Recommendations/Comments
Sirolimus	May increase serum levels of sirolimus.	Dose sirolimus based on serum levels. A significantly reduction of sirolimus dose with DLV coadministration is highly likely.
St. John's wort	DLV clearance may be increased significantly.	Studies only done with IDV, but St. John's wort likely to affect the metabolism of DLV. Do not coadminister.
Tacrolimus	May increase serum levels of tacrolimus.	Dose tacrolimus based on serum levels. A significantly reduction of tacrolimus dose with DLV coadministration is highly likely.
Tadalafil	May increase serum levels of tadalafil.	Applies to all PIs and DLV: start with 5 mg. Do not exceed 10 mg in 72 hrs. Consider sildenafil due to more clinical data and shorter half-life allowing for easier titration.
Tamoxifen	May increase serum levels of tamoxifen.	Applies to All PIs and DLV: no data. Close monitoring of tamoxifen-induced toxicity recommended.
Teniposide	May increase serum levels of teniposide.	Applies to all PIs and DLV: no data. Close monitoring of teniposide-induced toxicity recommended.
Terfenadine	May increase terfenadine levels.	Contraindicated due to the potential for cardiac arrhythmias. Recommended alternative antihistamine: loratadine, fexofenadine, desloratidine, or cetirizine.
Tetrahydrocannabinol (THC)	Based on data with NFV and IDV interactions are unlikely.	Applies to PIs and NNRTIs: interactions are unlikely but illicit drug use should be avoided for obvious reasons.
Trazodone	May increase serum level of trazodone.	Applies to all PIs and DLV: use with caution. Consider an alternative antidepressant (i.e., SSRI: escitalopram, citalopram, sertraline, or fluoxetine).
Triazolam	May significantly increase triazolam serum levels.	Contraindicated. Consider alternative benzodiazepines (temazepam, oxazepam, or lorazepam).
Vardenafil	May significantly increase serum levels of vardenafil.	Applies to all PIs and DLV: do not exceed vardenafil 2.5 mg in 72 hrs (with RTV) or 2.5 mg in 24 hrs (with other PIs and DLV). Consider sildenafil due to more clinical data and less pronounced interaction. Avoid coadministration with IDV.

Drug	Effect of Interaction	Recommendations/Comments
Verapamil	May increase serum levels of verapamil.	Applies to all PIs and DLV: data limited to an interaction study conducted with ATV and diltiazem, which resulted in doubling of diltiazem serum levels (this led PR interval prolongation). All PIs and DLV have the potential of prolonging PR interval with calcium channel blockers coadministration. Calcium channel blockers should be started with 50% of the dose and slowly titrated with close monitoring of BP and pulse.
Vinblastine	May increase serum levels of vinblastine.	Applies to all PIs and DLV: no data. Close monitoring of vinblastine induced toxicity recommended.
Vincristine	May increase serum levels of vincristine.	Applies to all PIs and DLV: no data. Close monitoring of vincristine-induced toxicity recommended.
Voriconazole	May increase voriconazole AUC. Voriconazole may increase DLV AUC.	No data with DLV. Use with close monitoring.
Warfarin	May increase warfarin effects.	Other NNRTIs and PIs may also affect warfarin requirements. Monitor INR closely and adjust warfarin as indicated.

DRUG-DRUG INTERACTION – DIDANOSINE (DDI)

Drug	Effect of Interaction	Recommendations/Comments
Allopurinol	May significantly increase ddI serum levels. ddI (buffered formulation) AUC increased by 120%.	PK studies conducted with ddI (buffered), but interaction also applies to ddI EC. Do not coadminister.
Atazanavir (ATV)	ATV AUC: decreased by 87%; Cmin: decreased by 84% with ddI (buffered). ddI EC: ddI AUC increased by 26% and ATV AUC decreased by 11%.	Administer ddI (pediatric solution) on empty stomach 2 hrs before or 1 hr after food or ATV. Use ddI EC if possible, since interaction unlikely to be significant, especially when ATV is boosted with RTV (ATV/r 300/100 mg).
Cidofovir	3 mg/kg IV (with probenecid) on days 1 and 8 ddI AUC: increased by 60%. Possible inhibition of renal tubular secretion by probenecid and/or cidofovir.	Applies to pediatric solution. Monitor for ddI toxicity, but unlikely to be significant since cidofovir is only administered qow with probenecid.
Cisplatin	May increase risk of peripheral neuropathy.	Monitor for peripheral neuropathy. Irreversible neuropathy with continued use. Avoid long-term coadministration.

DIDANOSINE *(cont.)*

Drug	Effect of Interaction	Recommendations/Comments
Dapsone	Dapsone: no change. Early single dose PK study found a decrease in dapsone serum levels, however multiple dose studies did not find a significant change in dapsone serum levels with ddI (buffer) coadministration.	No significant interaction. Use standard dose. ddI EC not studied but interaction unlikely.
Delavirdine (DLV)	DLV AUC decreased by 32%.	Applies to ddI buffered formulation only. Separate administration time by at least 2 hrs or use ddI EC formulation (not studied but interaction unlikely).
Disulfiram	May increase risk of peripheral neuropathy.	Monitor for peripheral neuropathy. Irreversible neuropathy with continued use. Avoid long-term coadministration.
Fluoroquinolone (ciprofloxacin)	Ciprofloxacin: AUC decreased by 26% with ddI (buffered). ddI: not affected. Ciprofloxacin not affected by ddI EC.	Consider ddI EC (ciprofloxacin not affected) or administer ddI suspension 6 hrs prior to or 2 hrs after ciprofloxacin administration. Study performed with ciprofloxacin, but all other fluoroquinolones may also be significantly affected by buffered ddI.
Food	ddI AUC decreased by 18%–27% w/ EC formulation; AUC decreased by 47% with buffered formulation.	Administer all forms of ddI on empty stomach (1 hr before or 2 hrs after meals).
Ganciclovir (IV and PO)	Coadministration with ddI (buffered formulation) resulted in a 111% increased in ddI AUC. Ganciclovir AUC decreased by 21%.	Clinical significance unknown, but monitor closely for ddI toxicity. No data with ddI EC.
Gold Compounds	May increase risk of peripheral neuropathy.	Monitor for peripheral neuropathy. Irreversible neuropathy with continued use. Avoid long-term coadministration.
Hydralazine	May increase risk of peripheral neuropathy.	Monitor for peripheral neuropathy. Irreversible neuropathy with continued use. Avoid long-term coadministration.
Hydroxyurea	Increased risk of pancreatitis and peripheral neuropathy.	Do not coadminister.
Indinavir (IDV)	IDV: no change (with ddI EC). IDV AUC decreased by 84% (with ddI buffered).	No significant interaction with ddI EC (use standard dose). Administer IDV 1 hr before or after ddI (pediatric solution).

Drug	Effect of Interaction	Recommendations/Comments
Isoniazid	May increase risk of peripheral neuropathy.	Give isoniazid with pyridoxine to decrease the risk of neuropathy. Monitor for peripheral neuropathy. Irreversible neuropathy with continued use. Avoid long-term coadministration.
Itraconazole	Itraconazole Cmax: undetectable.	Applies to ddI (pediatric solution). Administer itraconazole caps at least 2 hrs after ddI suspension. No interaction with ddI EC (preferred).
Ketoconazole	Ketoconazole: No change (with ddI EC). Decreased in ketoconazole absorption (with ddI buffered).	No significant interaction with ddI EC (use standard dose). Administer itraconazole caps at least 2 hrs after ddI suspension.
Methadone	ddI (buffered) AUC decreased by 60%. Methadone serum levels not affected. No interaction with ddI EC formulation.	Do not coadminister ddI (pediatric powder) with methadone. Use ddI EC with methadone.
Metronidazole	May increase risk of peripheral neuropathy (rare).	Monitor for peripheral neuropathy. Irreversible neuropathy with continued use. Avoid long-term coadministration.
Pentamidine (IV)	May increase risk of pancreatitis.	Caution when administering to patients with history of alcoholism. Avoid in patients currently abusing alcohol.
Pyridoxine (vitamin B6), high dose	May increase risk of peripheral neuropathy.	Monitor for peripheral neuropathy. Irreversible neuropathy with continued use. Avoid long-term coadministration.
Ribavirin	Increased risk of mitochondrial toxicity FDA case reports: 21 out of 27 cases associated with pancreatitis, 5 deaths due to lactic acidosis (all 5 taking ddI + ribavirin).	Contraindicated. Do not coadminister. Use an alternative nucleoside reverse transcriptase inhibitor (NRTI).
Ritonavir (RTV)	ddI AUC: decreased by 15%.	Applies to pediatric solution. Clinical significance unknown. Separate ddI and RTV administration by at least 2 hrs. No data with ddI EC but interaction unlikely.
Stavudine (d4T)	Increased risk of peripheral neuropathy, pancreatitis, and lactic acidosis.	Do not coadminister.
Tenofovir (TDF)	ddI EC AUC: increased by 48% (fasted); ddI EC AUC: increased by 60% (fed) TDF: no change. Suboptimal response in 91% of patients with ddI/TDF/3TC.	Dose adjust ddI to 250 mg PO once daily (>60 kg) with TDF coadministration. Combination with unadjusted ddI dose may lead to CD4 decline. Do not use ddI/TDF/3TC as sole triple nucleoside regimen or NNRTI/ddI/TDF due to high rates of virologic failure.

DIDANOSINE *(cont.)*

Drug	Effect of Interaction	Recommendations/Comments
Tetracyclines	Not studied. May decrease tetracyclines serum levels due to chelation by the divalent cation of the ddI buffer.	Applies to pediatric solution. Consider ddI EC or administer ddI suspension 6 hrs prior to or 2 hrs after tetracycline administration. No data with ddI EC but interaction unlikely.
Thalidomide	May increase risk of peripheral neuropathy.	Monitor for peripheral neuropathy. Irreversible neuropathy with continued use. Avoid long-term coadministration.
Valganciclovir	Not studied. ddI AUC may be significantly increased.	Clinical significance unknown. Monitor for ddI toxicity (neuropathy, pancreatitis, and lactic acidosis).
Vincristine	May increase risk of peripheral neuropathy.	Monitor for peripheral neuropathy. Irreversible neuropathy with continued use. Avoid long-term coadministration.

DRUG-DRUG INTERACTION – DOXYCYCLINE

Drug	Effect of Interaction	Recommendations/Comments
Acitretin	May increase intracranial pressure.	Contraindicated.
Bismuth Salts	Bismuth salts chelate tetracyclines resulting in a decreased absorption of tetracycline.	Administer bismuth 2 hrs after tetracycline.
Carbamazepine	Coadministration may decrease tetracyclines serum concentrations.	Avoid carbamazepine coadministration. Monitor closely for tetracycline therapy failure.
Cholestyramine	Coadminstration may significantly reduce tetracyclines absorption.	Avoid coadministration.
Colestipol	Coadminstration significantly reduce tetracyclines absorption.	Avoid coadministration.
Didanosine (ddI) (buffer in peds formulation) contains cations:	Polyvalent metal cations form an insoluble chelate with tetracyclines resulting in decreased absorption and serum levels of tetracyclines.	Separate administration by 4 hrs.
Digoxin	Coadministration may result in increased digoxin concentration (in about 10% of patients).	Monitor serum level with sign and symptoms of digoxin toxicity.

Drug	Effect of Interaction	Recommendations/Comments
Methoxyflurane	Case reports of renal failure with coadministration with tetracycline.	Avoid coadministration.
Non-depolarizing Neuromuscular Blocker (e.g., vecuronium, pancuronium, rocuronium)	May potentiate non-depolarizing neuromuscular blocker.	Use with close monitoring.
Oral Contraceptives	Tetracyclines may decrease the efficacy of oral contraceptives.	Consider an additional form of contraception.
Penicillins	*In vitro* antagonism when coadministered. Bacteriocidal effect of penicillins may be diminished *in vivo*.	Avoid coadministration.
Phenobarbital	Coadministration may decrease tetracyclines serum concentrations.	Avoid phenobarbital coadministration. Monitor closely tetracycline for therapy failure.
Phenytoin	Coadministration may decrease tetracyclines serum concentrations.	Avoid phenytoin coadministration. Monitor closely for tetracycline therapy failure.
Polyvalent Metal Cations (aluminum, zinc, magnesium, iron, calcium [milk])	Polyvalent metal cations form an insoluble chelate with tetracyclines resulting in decreased absorption.	Separate administration by 4 hrs.
Quinapril	Magnesium excipient may reduce tetracyclines absorption.	Avoid coadministration.
Rifabutin (RFB)	Coadministration may decrease tetracyclines serum concentrations.	Avoid RFB coadministration. Monitor closely for tetracycline therapy failure.
Rifampin	Coadministration may decrease tetracyclines serum concentrations.	Avoid rifampin coadministration. Monitor closely for tetracycline therapy failure.
Urinary Alkalinizers (sodium lactate, sodium bicarbonate)	Coadministration results in increased urinary excretion of tetracyclines by 24%–65%.	Avoid coadministration.
Warfarin	Coadministration may increase INR.	Monitor INR closely.

DRUG-DRUG INTERACTION – EFAVIRENZ (EFV)

Drug	Effect of Interaction	Recommendations/Comments
Alprazolam	May decrease alprazolam concentrations.	Titrate to effect or consider lorazepam.
Amodiaquine	Amodiaquine AUC increased with coadministration.	Coadministration of EFV with artesunate plus amodiaquine may result in significant LFT elevations. With EFV coadministration, significant increase in amodiaquine AUC (114% and 302%) reported in 2 patients.
Artemether (artemisinin)	May decrease serum level of artemether.	Close monitoring of artemether therapeutic efficacy (i.e., parasite count on blood smear and clinical signs and symptoms of clinical improvement). Coadministration of EFV with artesunate plus amodiaquine may result in significant LFT elevations.
Astemizole	May significantly increase astemizole serum level.	Contraindicated due to the potential for cardiac arrhythmias. Recommended alternative antihistamine: loratadine, fexofenadine, desloratidine, or cetirizine.
Atazanavir (ATV)	ATV AUC: decreased 74%; Cmin: decreased 93% (without RTV coadministration) ATV AUC: increased 241%; Cmin: increased 671% (with RTV coadministration).	Recommended dosing: ATV 400 mg + RTV 100 mg once daily + EFV 600 mg qhs (consider ATV TDM especially in PI-experienced patients). Unboosted ATV not recommended with EFV.
Atorvastatin	Atorvastatin: AUC decreased by 43%.	May require atorvastatin dose increase with close monitoring of LFTs and CPK.
Azathioprine	Interaction unlikely.	Applies to all PIs and NNRTIs: use standard dose.
Azithromycin	Azithromycin AUC unchanged.	No significant interaction. Use standard dose.
Bepridil	May increase bepridil serum concentrations.	May increase risk of QTc prolongation. Contraindicated.
Buprenorphine	Buprenorphine AUC and Cmin decreased by 50%. EFV not affected.	No withdrawal symptoms noted when buprenorphine Cmin decreased from 0.85 ng/mL to 0.42 ng/mL. It should be noted that withdrawal symptoms may not be seen until a decrease to 0.23 ng/mL. Use standard dose buprenorphine with titration to therapeutic effect.
Bupropion	Bupropion AUC decreased 55%.	Titrate to therapeutic effect.

Drug	Effect of Interaction	Recommendations/Comments
Carbamazepine	EFV AUC decreased by 34% and carbamazepine AUC decreased by 27%.	Avoid coadministration. Consider alternative anticonvulsant (e.g., valproic acid, lamotrigine, levetiracetam, or topiramate). With coadministration, monitor carbamazepine levels and consider EFV TDM.
Caspofungin	May decrease caspofungin serum level.	Monitor for caspofungin therapeutic failure, may need to increase dose to 70 mg/day.
Cetirizine	EFV: no significant change, cetirizine: no change.	No significant interaction. Use standard dose of both drugs.
Cisapride	May increase cisapride serum level.	Contraindicated due to potential for cardiac arrhythmias. Recommended alternative: metoclopramide.
Clarithromycin	Clarithromycin AUC: decreased 39%; 14-hydroxyclarithromycin AUC: increased 34%.	Clinical significance unknown. High incidence of rash seen in healthy volunteer receiving this combination. Consider alternative macrolide (azithromycin).
Clarithromycin	Clarithromycin AUC decreased 39%.	High incidence of rash with coadministration. Consider azithromycin.
Cocaine	May theoretically increase serum level of hepatotoxic metabolite.	Avoid illicit drugs for obvious reasons.
Cyclophosphamide	May decrease serum level of cyclophosphamide.	No data. Monitor for chemotherapeutic response. Cyclophosphamide dose may need to be increased.
Cyclosporine	May significantly decrease serum level of cyclosporine.	Monitor serum level of cyclosporine closely with coadministration. Cyclosporin dose may need to be increased.
Darunavir (DRV)	DRV Cmin decreased by 31%. EFV AUC and Cmin increased 21% and 17%, respectively (studied with DRV/r 300/100 mg twice daily).	Dose not established. Consider DRV 600/100 mg twice daily with EFV 600 mg qhs. With once daily DRV/r, only 900/100-mg dose has been tested with EFV. Based on PK data, either DRV/r 800/100 mg or 950/100 mg once daily plus EFV 600 mg qhs can be considered in PI-naive patients.
Diltiazem (and other dihydro-pyridines calcium channel blockers: nifedipine, amlodipine)	Diltiazem AUC decreased by 69% with coadministration. EFV AUC increased by 11%.	Titrate diltiazem dose to effect. Higher diltiazem and other calcium channel blocker doses may be needed.
Docetaxel	May decrease serum level of docetaxel.	No data. Docetaxel dose may need to be increased.

EFAVIRENZ (cont.)

Drug	Effect of Interaction	Recommendations/Comments
Echinacea	May decrease EFV serum level. Echinacea decreased CYP3A4 substrate (midazolam) by 23%.	Clinical significance unknown but should avoided until the safety of this combination is further evaluated.
Ergot Derivatives	May significantly increase serum level of ergotamine resulting in acute ergot toxicity.	Contraindicated. Consider alternative agent for migraine such as sumatriptan but not eletriptan, since it is a CYP3A4 substrate and significant drug-drug interaction occurred with CYP3A4 inhibitor.
Ethinyl Estradiol	Ethinyl estradiol AUC increased 37%.	Clinical significance unknown. No data on progesterone component of oral contraceptive available. Alternative form of birth control should be recommended. Contraceptive failures have been reported with implantable hormonal contraceptive.
Etoposide	May decrease serum level of etoposide.	No data. Etoposide dose may need to be increased.
Famotidine	No significant interaction.	Use standard dose.
Fatty Meal (54% fat) or Low-Fat Meal (4%)	EFV AUC increased by 50% and 22% with high-fat and low fat-meal, respectively. Fatty meal increased EFV tabs Cmax by 79% and EFV caps Cmax by 51%.	Manufacturer recommends taking EFV on an empty stomach due to the potential for increased CNS side effect from high EFV Cmax. May not be necessary after initial side effects have resolved.
Fluconazole	Fluconazole AUC increased 16%.	No significant interaction. Use standard dose.
Fluoxetine	EFV AUC not significantly affected by SSRI (population PK).	No significant interaction. Use standard dose.
Fosamprenavir (FPV)	APV Cmin decreased by 36% (dose used FPV/r 1400 /200 mg once daily). APV Cmin decreased by 17% (dose used FPV 700/100 mg twice daily).	Recommended dosing: FPV/r 1400/300 mg once daily (in PI-naive patients only) or FPV/r 700/100 mg twice daily + EFV 600 mg qhs.
Garlic Supplement	No data.	Reduction on SQV serum level. No data with EFV. Avoid coadministration.
Heroin (diamorphine)	Drug interactions unlikely.	Interaction unlikely but illicit drug use should be avoided for obvious reasons.
Ifosphamide	May decrease serum level of ifosphamide.	Applies to EFV and NVP: no data. Ifosphamide dose may need to be increased.

Drug	Effect of Interaction	Recommendations/Comments
Indinavir (IDV)	IDV AUC: decreased 19%; Cmin: decreased 48%.	Clinically significant: recommended dose: IDV 1000 mg q8h + EFV 600 mg qhs or IDV/r 800/200 mg twice daily + EFV 600 mg qhs.
Itraconazole	Itraconazole AUC decreased by 39%. EFV AUC not affected.	For invasive fungal infections, monitor itraconazole serum levels with coadministration. Consider alternative antifungal (i.e., fluconazole: no significant interaction).
Ketoconazole	May decrease ketoconazole serum levels.	May need to increase ketoconazole dose (i.e., fluconazole: no significant interaction).
Levonorgestrel	Levonorgestrel AUC decreased 56%.	Use a second form of contraception with EFV coadministration.
Lopinavir/ritonavir (LPV/r)	LPV AUC decreased (non-significant); Cmin decreased 39%.	Clinically significant: consider LPV/r 600/150 mg (3 tabs) twice daily + EFV 600 mg qhs, especially in PI-experienced patients. Standard dose of 400/100 mg twice daily may be adequate in PI-naive patients.
Lorazepam	No significant change.	Use standard dose.
Lovastatin	May decrease lovastatin serum concentrations.	No data. Consider atorvastatin.
Maraviroc (MVC)	MVC AUC decreased by 45%.	MVC 600 mg twice daily + EFV 600 mg qhs. If PIs (i.e., LPV/r or SQV/r) are included in regimen, MVC 150 mg twice daily recommended.
Medroxyprogesterone (DMPA)	No significant drug interaction. EFV AUC was not significantly affected. DMPA concentrations were not reported.	Efficacy of DMPA was not affected by EFV coadministration. Use standard dose of both drugs. Counsel patient on the potential for teratogenicity of EFV.
Mefloquine	May decrease serum level of mefloquine.	If available, consider mefloquine serum level monitoring. Close monitoring of mefloquine therapeutic efficacy (i.e., parasite count on blood smear and clinical signs and XX of clinical improvement).
Methadone	Methadone AUC: decreased 57%.	Monitor for opiate withdrawal. May need to increase the maintenance dose of methadone.
Midazolam	May increase midazolam level.	Do not coadminister. Consider lorazepam (not significantly affected by EFV), oxazepam, or temazepam.

EFAVIRENZ *(cont.)*

Drug	Effect of Interaction	Recommendations/Comments
Milk Thistle	No data.	Data limited to interaction study with milk thistle and IDV. IDV AUC unchanged; IDV Cmin decreased by 47%. Clinical significance unknown. Avoid coadministration.
Mycophenolate	Interaction unlikely. No significant interaction observed with NVP.	No significant interaction observed with NVP. Use standard dose.
Nelfinavir (NFV)	NFV AUC: increased 20%. M8 AUC: decreased 37%.	No significant interaction. Use standard dose: NFV 1250 mg twice daily + EFV 600 mg qhs.
Nevirapine (NVP)	EFV AUC: decreased 22%; Cmin: decreased 36%.	Coadministration not recommended due to overlapping resistance profile. With coadministration consider increasing EFV to 800 mg once daily.
Paclitaxel	May decrease serum level of paclitaxel.	Applies to EFV and NVP: no data. Monitor for chemotherapeutic response. Paclitaxel dose may need to be increased.
Paroxetine	Paroxetine AUC not affected.	No significant interaction. Use standard dose.
Phenobarbital	EFV and anticonvulsants levels may be decreased.	Consider alternative anticonvulsants (i.e., valproic acid, lamotrigine, levetiracetam, or topiramate). With coadministration, monitor anticonvulsants level and consider EFV TDM.
Phenytoin	EFV and anticonvulsants levels may be decreased.	Consider alternative anticonvulsants (i.e., valproic acid, lamotrigine, levetiracetam, or topiramate). With coadministration, monitor anticonvulsants level and consider EFV TDM.
Pimozide	May increase risk of cardiac arrhythmias.	Contraindicated.
Posaconazole	Posaconazole AUC decreased 50%.	Avoid coadministration if possible; consider alternative antifungal. With coadministration TDM recommended. For invasive fungal disease, consider posaconazole 400 mg q8h.
Pravastatin	Pravastatin AUC decreased 44%.	Clinical significance unknown. May need to increase dose of pravastatin.
Raltegravir (RAL)	RAL AUC decreased by 36%, but Cmin not significantly affected.	Dose: RAL 400 mg twice daily + EFV 600 mg qhs.
Rifabutin (RFB)	RFB AUC: decreased 38% No change in EFV AUC.	Recommended dosing: increase RFB to 450 mg/day or 600 mg 3 ×/wk with EFV 600 mg qhs.

Drug	Effect of Interaction	Recommendations/Comments
Rifampin	EFV AUC: decreased 26%; no change in rifampin AUC.	Recommended dosing: EFV 800 mg/day with rifampin 600 mg once daily in patients >50 kg (monitor for EFV CNS side effects). May decrease to EFV 600 mg/day if 800 mg dose not easily tolerated. Consider TDM.
Rifapentine	EFV serum levels may be significantly decreased.	Avoid coadministration. Consider using RFB with dose adjustment.
Ritonavir (RTV)	RTV AUC: increased 18% EFV AUC: increased 21%.	No significant interaction. Use standard dose of RTV and EFV.
Rosiglitazone	EFV Cmin decreased by 6% (non-significant) (n = 10).	Use standard dose.
Rosuvastatin	Other CYP3A4 inhibitor (i.e., erythromycin) did not affect rosuvastatin serum level.	Rosuvastatin AUC and Cmax unexpectedly increased 2.1 and 4.7-fold at steady state with LPV/r coadministration. Despite increased rosuvastatin exposure, the LDL-lowering effects were attenuated with LPV/r coadministration. Close monitoring recommended due to limited clinical data.
Saquinavir (SQV)	SQV/r AUC: decreased 62% (with unboosted SQV); SQV Cmin: decreased 10% (w/ boosted SQV 400 mg/ RTV 400 mg); RTV Cmin: no significant change; EFV: no significant change.	Do not coadminister unboosted SQV with EFV. Recommended dose: SQV/r 1000/100 mg + EFV 600 mg qhs.
Sertraline	Sertraline AUC decreased 39%.	Titrate sertraline to effect.
Simvastatin	Simvastatin: AUC decreased by 68%.	May require simvastatin dose increase with close monitoring of LFTs and CPK.
Sirolimus	May significantly decrease serum level of sirolimus.	Applies to EFV and NVP: dose sirolimus based on serum level. May need to increase sirolimus dose.
St. John's wort	Not studied, may decrease EFV levels.	Contraindicated. Use an alternative (more effective) antidepressant.
Tacrolimus	May significantly decrease serum level of tacrolimus.	Dose tacrolimus based on serum level. May need to increase tacrolimus dose.
Tamoxifen	May decrease serum level of tamoxifen.	No data. Monitor for chemotherapeutic response. Tamoxifen dose may need to be increased.
Teniposide	May decrease serum level of teniposide.	No data. Monitor for chemotherapeutic response. Teniposide dose may need to be increased.
Terfenadine	May significantly increase terfenadine serum level.	Contraindicated due to the potential for cardiac arrhythmias. Recommended alternative antihistamine: loratadine, fexofenadine, desloratidine, or cetirizine.

EFAVIRENZ *(cont.)*

Drug	Effect of Interaction	Recommendations/Comments
Tetrahydrocan-nabinol (THC)	Based on data with NFV and IDV interactions are unlikely.	Applies to PIs and NNRTIs: interactions are unlikely but illicit drug use should be avoided for obvious reasons.
Tipranavir (TPV)	No significant change in TPV and EFV PK parameters with higher TPV/r dose (750/200 mg twice daily).	Consider TPV/r 500/200 mg twice daily + EFV 600 mg once daily.
Triazolam	May increase triazolam serum level.	Contraindicated. Consider lorazepam (not significantly affected by EFV), oxazepam, or temazepam.
Vinblastine	May decrease serum level of vinblastine.	Applies to EFV and NVP: no data. Monitor for chemotherapeutic response. Vinblastine dose may need to be increased.
Vincristine	May decrease serum level of vincristine.	Applies to EFV and NVP: no data. Monitor for chemotherapeutic response. Vincristine dose may need to be increased.
Voriconazole	EFV (400 mg PO once daily) decreased steady state voriconazole (200 mg q12h) AUC by 77%. EFV AUC was increased by 44%. No significant change in voriconazole and EFV AUC with voriconazole 400 mg q12h plus EFV 300 mg qhs.	EFV should not be coadministered with voriconazole at the standard doses. Dose: EFV 300 mg qhs plus voriconazole 400 mg twice daily. Monitor voriconazole Cmin (target Cmin >2 mcg/mL). Consider EFV TDM.
Warfarin	Not studied; may increase or decrease warfarin effects; monitor INR and adjust warfarin as indicated.	Monitor INR and adjust warfarin as indicated.

DRUG-DRUG INTERACTION – EMTRICITABINE (FTC)

Drug	Effect of Interaction	Recommendations/Comments
Food	FTC AUC was not affected by food.	Administer FTC with or without food.
Tenofovir (TDF)	TDF Cmin was increased by 20%; AUC was unchanged.	Interaction not significant. Use standard dose.
Zidovudine (AZT)	No significant drug interaction.	Use standard dose.

Drug-Drug Interaction – Etravirine (ETR)

Drug	Effect of Interaction	Recommendations/Comments
Antiarrhythmics (amiodarone, bepridil, disopyramide, flecainide, lidocaine, mexiletine, propafenone, and quinidine)	Antiarrhythmics serum concentrations may be decreased with ETR coadministration.	Use with caution. Monitor antiarrhythmics serum concentrations.
Anticonvulsants (carbamazepine, phenobarbital, and phenytoin)	ETR serum concentrations may be significantly decreased.	Avoid coadministration.
Antifungals	All azole antifungals may increase ETRs serum concentrations. Itraconazole and ketoconazole's serum concentrations may be decreased with ETR coadministration. On the other hand, posaconazole is unlikely to be affected by ETR.	With ETR coadministration, monitor itraconazole serum concentrations. Dose adjustment may be needed.
Atazanavir (ATV)	With unboosted ATV coadministration ETR AUC increased by 50%, but ATV Cmin decreased by 47%.	Avoid unboosted ATV coadministration.
Atazanavir/ ritonavir (ATV/r)	With ATV/r coadministration ETR AUC increased by 30% and ATV AUC and Cmin decreased by 14% and 38%, respectively.	Unclear clinical significance, but manufacturer recommends avoiding coadministration. With coadministration, consider TDM.
Atorvastatin	Atorvastatin AUC decreased by 37%. No change in ETR AUC.	The dose of atorvastatin may need to be increased.
Clarithromycin	ETR AUC increased by 42%. Clarithromycin AUC decreased by 39%, but 14-OH-clarithromycin increased by 21%.	Consider azithromycin for MAC treatment. Clinical significance unclear for infections involving *S. pneumoniae* and *H. influenzae* since 14-OH-clarithromycin metabolite is active.
Clopidogrel	May decrease the efficacy of clopidogrel.	Avoid coadministration.
Darunavir/ ritonavir (DRV/r)	DRV AUC increased by 15%. ETR AUC and Cmin decreased by 37% and 49%, respectively.	Despite significant reduction in ETR serum concentrations, good virologic response observed in clinical trials. No dose adjustment necessary.
Dexamethasone	ETR serum concentrations may be decreased.	Use with caution. Consider an alternative corticosteroid.

ETRAVIRINE *(cont.)*

Drug	Effect of Interaction	Recommendations/Comments
Didanosine (ddI)	ETR AUC increased 11% (NS). No significant change in ddI AUC.	No dosage adjustments necessary.
Digoxin	Digoxin AUC increased by 18%.	Limited data. Consider monitoring digoxin serum concentrations.
Ethinyl Estradiol and Norethindrone	Ethinyl estradiol AUC increased by 22%. Norethindrone AUC decreased by 5%.	Clinical significance unknown. Consider the use of an additional barrier form of contraception.
Fluconazole	Fluconazole increased ETR AUC 86%. Fluconazole not affected by ETR.	Use standard doses.
Fosamprenavir/ ritonavir (FPV/r)	APV AUC 12h, increased by 69%. ETR comparable to historical control.	Unclear clinical significance with FPV/r, but manufacturer recommends avoiding coadministration. With coadministration, consider TDM.
HMG-CoA Reductase Inhibitors (lovastatin, simvastatin, rosuvastatin, and pravastatin)	Lovastatin and simvastatin serum concentrations may be decreased. Rosuvastatin and pravastatin are unlikely to be affected with ETR coadministration.	Rosuvastatin and pravastatin may be considered.
Immunosuppressants (cyclosporine, sirolimus, and tacrolimus)	ETR may decrease immunosuppressant serum concentrations.	Monitor serum concentrations of immunosuppressants closely with coadministration.
Indinavir (IDV)	IDV AUC decreased 46%, ETR AUC increased 51%.	Unboosted PIs should be avoided with ETR.
Lopinavir/ ritonavir (LPV/r)	LPV AUC decreased 18%. ETR Cmin decreased by 45%.	No dosage adjustments necessary. No dosage adjustments necessary. ETR Cmin reduction with LPV/r was comparable to the observed reduction with DRV/r coadministration.
Maraviroc (MVC)	MVC AUC decreased by 53%. ETR not affected.	Increase MVC to 600 mg twice daily. If a CYP3A4 inhibitor, such as DRV/r, is coadministered with MVC plus ETR, decrease MVC to 150 mg twice daily.
Methadone	No change in active R (-) methadone.	No dosage adjustments necessary.
Midazolam	Midazolam AUC decreased by 37%.	Limited data. Titrate midazolam to effect. May also decrease triazolam serum concentrations.
Nelfinavir (NFV)	May decrease NFV serum concentrations.	Unboosted PIs should be avoided with ETR.

Drug	Effect of Interaction	Recommendations/Comments
Omeprazole	ETR AUC increased 41%. Omeprazole AUC increased 332% (limited data).	No dosage adjustments necessary.
Raltegravir (RAL)	ETR AUC increased by 10%. No significant change in RAL AUC.	No dosage adjustments necessary.
Ranitidine	ETR AUC decreased 14%.	No dosage adjustments necessary.
Rifabutin (RFB)	ETR AUC and Cmin decreased 37% and 35%, respectively. RFB AUC decreased 17%.	Use standard dose RFB 300 mg daily, but avoid coadministration with DRV/r or SQV/r plus ETR due to potential additive decrease in ETR exposure.
Rifampin	ETR serum concentrations may be significantly decreased.	Avoid coadministration.
Rifapentine	ETR serum concentrations may be significantly decreased.	Avoid coadministration.
Ritonavir RTV (600 mg twice daily)	ETR AUC decreased 46%.	Avoid coadministration with high-dose RTV.
Saquinavir+ Lopinavir/ritonavir (SQV+LPV/r)	Minor AUC changes in PIs.	No dosage adjustments.
Saquinavir/ ritonavir (SQV/r)	ETR AUC and Cmin decreased 33% and 29%, respectively. No significant change in SQV AUC.	No dosage adjustments necessary.
Sildenafil	Sildenafil AUC decreased 57%.	Titrate sildenafil to effect.
St. John's wort	ETR serum concentrations may be decreased.	Avoid coadministration.
Tenofovir (TDF)	ETR AUC decreased by 19%, TDF AUC increased by 15%.	No dosage adjustments necessary.
Tipranavir/ ritonavir (TPV/r)	ETR AUC decreased by 76%. TPV and RTV AUC increased by 18% and 23%, respectively.	Avoid coadministration.
Voriconazole	Voriconazole increased ETR AUC 36%. Voriconazole AUC was slightly increased by 14% (not clinically significant).	Use standard dose, but consider monitoring of voriconazole serum concentrations when treating invasive fungal infections due to high PK variability.
Warfarin	Warfarin AUC increased by 82%.	Limited data. Use with close INR monitoring.

DRUG-DRUG INTERACTION – FLUCONAZOLE

Drug	Effect of Interaction	Recommendations/Comments
Astemizole	May increase astemizole serum concentrations.	Contraindicated.
Benzodiazepines (alprazolam, diazepam, midazolam, triazolam)	May increase benzodiazepine serum concentrations.	Use with caution. Benzodiazepine dose may need to be decreased.
Cisapride	May increase cisapride serum concentrations.	Contraindicated.
Clopidogrel	May decrease the efficacy of clopidogrel.	Avoid coadministration.
Cyclosporine	Cyclosporine concentrations may be significantly increased.	Monitor cyclosporine concentrations closely. Cyclosporine dose may need to be decreased.
Efavirenz (EFV)	No significant interaction.	Usual dose.
Etravirine (ETR)	May increase ETR serum concentrations.	No data. Monitor for LFTs and rash with coadministration.
Fentanyl	Fentanyl serum concentrations may be significantly increased.	Use with caution. Fentanyl dose may need to be decreased.
Lovastatin	May increase lovastatin serum concentrations.	Consider pravastatin or rosuvastatin.
Maraviroc (MVC)	May increase MVC serum concentrations.	No data. Use standard dose.
Nevirapine (NVP)	NVP clearance decreased by 2-fold.	Monitor LFTs closely with coadministration.
Oral Hypoglycemics	Risk of hypoglycemia may be increased.	Monitor closely.
Phenytoin	Phenytoin AUC was increased by 88%.	Monitor phenytoin concentrations closely with coadministration.
Raltegravir (RAL)	Interaction unlikely.	Use standard dose.
Rifabutin (RFB)	No effect on fluconazole, but RFB serum concentrations increased by 80%.	Monitor for RFB-associated toxicity (i.e., uveitis). RFB dose may need to be decreased.
Rifampin	May significantly decrease fluconazole serum concentrations.	Avoid coadministration. Consider RFB.
Simvastatin	May increase simvastatin serum concentrations.	Consider pravastatin or rosuvastatin.
Sirolimus	Sirolimus concentrations may be significantly increased.	Monitor sirolimus concentrations closely. Sirolimus dose may need to be significantly decreased.

Drug	Effect of Interaction	Recommendations/Comments
Tacrolimus	Tacrolimus levels may be significantly increased (monitor tacrolimus levels closely).	Monitor tacrolimus concentrations closely. Tacrolimus dose may need to be significantly decreased.
Terfenadine	May increase terfenadine serum concentrations.	Contraindicated.
Warfarin	INR may be significantly increased.	Monitor INR closely with coadministration.
Zidovudine (AZT)	AZT AUC increased by 74%.	Monitor for AZT-associated toxicity.

DRUG-DRUG INTERACTION – FOSAMPRENAVIR (FPV)

Drug	Effect of Interaction	Recommendations/Comments
Alfuzosin	May significantly increase alfuzosin serum concentrations.	Avoid coadministration.
Alprazolam	May increase serum levels of alprazolam.	Applies to all PIs: consider alternative benzodiazepine (lorazepam, temazepam, or oxazepam).
Amilodipine	May increase serum levels of amlodipine.	Applies to all PIs: data limited to an interaction study conducted with ATV and diltiazem, which resulted in doubling of diltiazem serum levels (this led to PR interval prolongation). All PIs have the potential of prolonging the PR interval with calcium channel blocker coadministration. Calcium channel blockers should be started with 50% of the dose and slowly titrated with close monitoring of BP and pulse.
Amiodarone	May significantly increase amiodarone serum levels.	Applies to all PIs: data limited to case report of increased amiodarone levels with IDV coadministration. The manufacturer of RTV, APV, and ATV recommends against use of amiodarone, but all PIs have the same potential of significantly increasing amiodarone serum levels. If coadministration cannot be avoided, monitor for amiodarone ADRs (PFTs and TSH). Consider monitoring serum levels of amiodarone, but its long half-life may make titration difficult.
Antacids	APV AUC decreased 18%, but trough not affected.	Consider administration of FPV 2 hrs before or 1 hr after antacids OR use FPV/r with antacid coadministration.
Artemether (artemisinin)	May increase serum levels of artemether.	Applies to all PIs: close monitoring for artemether toxicity (bone marrow suppression, bradycardia, and seizure).

FOSAMPRENAVIR *(cont.)*

Drug	Effect of Interaction	Recommendations/Comments
Astemizole	May significantly increase astemizole serum levels.	Contraindicated due to the potential for cardiac arrhythmias. Recommended alternative antihistamine: loratadine, fexofenadine, desloratidine, or cetirizine.
Atazanavir (ATV)	ATV AUC decreased 22%. FPV AUC increased 78%.	Clinical significance of a 22% decrease in ATV AUC unknown. Consider FPV/r 700/100 mg twice daily + ATV 300 mg once daily.
Atorvastatin	Atorvastatin AUC increased by 130% (w/o RTV) and 150% (w/ RTV). No change in APV AUC.	Start with low doses (10–20 mg/day) and avoid doses > 40 mg/day or consider alternative agents (pravastatin, fluvastatin, or possibly rosuvastatin).
Azathioprine	Interaction unlikely.	Applies to all PIs and NNRTI: use standard dose.
Bepridil	May significantly increase bepridil serum levels.	Applies to all PIs: no data. The manufacturer of ATV, RTV, and APV does not recommend bepridil coadministration, this contraindication should extend to all PIs since a significant increase in bepridil serum levels can result in pro-arrhythmic events such as VT, PVC, and VFib.
Bosentan	Bosentan serum concentrations may be significantly increased.	Coadminister bosentan only after RTV has reached steady-state. In patients on RTV >10 days: start bosentan at 62.5 mg once daily or every other day. In patients already on bosentan: d/c bosentan for >36 hrs prior to initiation of RTV-boosted PIs and restart bosentan at 62.5 mg once daily or every other day after RTV has reached steady-state (after 10 days).
Carbamazepine	May decrease levels of PIs and NNRTI. PIs and NNRTI may increase or decrease carbamazepine levels.	Applies to all PIs and NNRTIs: consider alternative anticonvulsants (valproic acid, lamotrigine, levetiracetam, or topiramate). Monitor carbamazepine levels and consider TDM of PIs and NNRTIs.
Chlordiazepoxide	May increase serum levels of chlordiazepoxide.	Applies to all PIs: consider alternative benzodiazepines (lorazepam, temazepam, or oxazepam).
Cisapride	May significantly increase cisapride serum levels.	Contraindicated due to potential for cardiac arrhythmias. Recommended alternative: metoclopramide.
Clarithromycin	May increase clarithromycin AUC with FPV/r.	No data with FPV, but APV increased 18% with clarithromycin coadministration. Consider dose adjustment renal insufficiency. CrCl 30–60 mL/min: 50% of dose. <30 mL/min: 25% of the dose.

Drug	Effect of Interaction	Recommendations/Comments
Clorazepate	May increase serum levels of clorazepate.	Applies to all PIs: consider alternative benzodiazepines (lorazepam, temazepam, or oxazepam).
Cyclophosphamide	May increase serum levels of cyclophosphamide.	Applies to all PIs: data limited to an interaction study conducted with IDV resulting in a 50% increase in cyclophosphamide serum levels. Since all PIs have the potential of increasing cyclophosphamide levels, close monitoring of cyclophosphamide-induced toxicity is recommended.
Cyclosporine	May significantly increase serum levels of cyclosporine.	Applies to all PIs: monitor serum levels of cyclosporine closely with coadministration. Cyclosporine dose may need to be decreased.
Darunavir (DRV)	No data.	Avoid coadministration.
Dexamethasone	May decrease APV serum levels.	Use with caution. Consider boosting (FPV/r 700/100 mg).
Digoxin	Digoxin serum concentration may be increased with FPV/r coadministration.	Monitor digoxin serum concentrations closely with coadministration.
Diltiazem	May increase serum levels of diltiazem.	Applies to all PIs: data limited to an interaction study conducted with ATV which resulted in doubling of diltiazem serum levels (this led to PR interval prolongation). All PIs have the potential of prolonging the PR interval with diltiazem coadministration. Diltiazem should be started with 50% of the dose and slowly titrated with close monitoring of BP and pulse.
Disopyramide	May increase disopyramide serum levels.	Applies to all PIs: no data. Monitor disopyramide serum levels (target: 2–7.5 mcg/mL).
Docetaxel	May increase serum levels of docetaxel.	Applies to all PIs: no data. Close monitoring of chemotherapy-induced toxicity recommended.
Dofetilide	May significantly increase serum levels of dofetilide.	Applies to all PIs: no data. Use with caution. Monitor QTc closely and adjust dofetilide dosing based on QTc prolongation and renal function. Consider an alternative class III antiarrhythmic such as bretylium or ibutilide.

FOSAMPRENAVIR *(cont.)*

Drug	Effect of Interaction	Recommendations/Comments
Efavirenz (EFV)	FPV/r 700/100 mg twice daily + EFV 600 mg qhs × 2 wks: APV Cmin decreased by 17% compared to twice daily boosted FPV. FPV/r 1400/200 mg once daily + EFV 600 mg qhs × 2 wks: APV Cmin decreased by 36% with EFV coadministration compared to once daily boosted FPV.	Recommended dose: FPV/r 700/100 mg twice daily + EFV 600 mg once daily OR FPV/r 1400/300 mg once daily + EFV 600 mg qhs.
Ergot Alkaloid	May significantly increase serum levels of ergotamine resulting in acute ergot toxicity.	Contraindicated. Consider alternative agent for migraine such as sumatriptan (but not eletriptan since it is a CYP3A4 substrate and significant drug interaction occurred with CYP3A4 inhibitor).
Estazolam	May increase serum levels of estazolam.	Applies to all PIs: consider alternative benzodiazepines (lorazepam, temazepam, or oxazepam).
Ethinyl Estradiol/ Norethindrone	May increase ethinyl estradiol serum concentrations. APV serum concentrations may decrease.	Avoid coadministration. Ethinyl estradiol Cmin increased 32%. Norethindrone AUC increased 18%, and Cmin increased 45%. APV AUC decreased 22%, and Cmin decreased 20% (studied using old formulation of APV).
Ethosuximide	May increase serum levels of ethosuximide.	Applies to All PIs: consider switching to valproic acid for the treatment of absence seizure.
Etoposide	May increase serum levels of etoposide.	Applies to all PIs: no data. Close monitoring of chemotherapy-induced toxicity recommended.
Etravirine (ETR)	APV AUC increased by 69%.	Manufacturer recommends avoiding coadministration, but clinical significance unclear. Consider FPV/r 700/100 mg twice daily with standard dose ETR.
Felodipine	May increase serum levels of felodipine.	Applies to all PIs: data limited to an interaction study conducted with ATV and diltiazem, which resulted in doubling of diltiazem serum levels (this led to PR interval prolongation). All PIs have the potential of prolonging the PR interval with calcium channel blockers coadministration. Calcium channel blockers should be started with 50% of the dose and slowly titrated with close monitoring of BP and pulse.

Drug	Effect of Interaction	Recommendations/Comments
Flecainide	May increase serum levels of flecainide.	Applies to all PIs: avoid coadministration; if necessary, monitor flecainide trough levels with coadministration. Target: 200–1000 ng/mL. Toxicity is frequent with trough serum levels above 1000 ng/mL.
Fluconazole	Interaction unlikely.	Use standard doses of both drugs.
Flurazepam	May increase serum levels of flurazepam.	Applies to all PIs: consider alternative benzodiazepines (lorazepam, temazepam, or oxazepam).
Fluticasone	Fluticasone AUC increased 350-fold (studied with RTV 100 mg q12h).	Avoid long-term coadministration. Consider beclomethasone.
Garlic Supplement	49% and 51% reduction in SQV AUC and Cmin, respectively.	Studies only done with SQV, but garlic may affect the serum levels of other PIs and NNRTIs. Avoid coadministration of garlic with other PIs and NNRTIs.
Granisetron	May increase serum levels of granisetron.	Applies to all PIs: due to the large therapeutic index of granisetron, potential interaction is unlikely to be clinically significant.
Heroin (diamorphine)	Drug interactions unlikely.	Applies to PIs and NNRTIs: interaction unlikely but illicit drug use should be avoided for obvious reasons.
Ifosphamide	May increase serum levels of ifosphamide.	Applies to all PIs: no data. Close monitoring of chemotherapy-induced toxicity recommended.
Indinavir (IDV)	APV AUC increased 33%.	Dose regimens not established. Avoid.
Irinotecan	May increase irinotecan serum levels.	Applies to all PIs: Coadministration of ATV is contraindicated by manufacturer. All PIs also have the potential for significant interaction with irinotecan, therefore coadministration should be done with extreme caution.
Itraconazole	May increase itraconazole serum concentrations.	Monitor for itraconazole serum concentrations.
Ketoconazole	May increase APV and ketoconazole serum concentrations.	With old APV formulation, APV AUC increased 32% and ketoconazole AUC increased 44%. Use standard dose of both drugs, but do not exceed ketoconazole 200 mg/day.
Lidocaine	May increase antiarrhythmic serum levels.	Applies to all PIs: no data. Use with caution, monitor lidocaine serum levels (target: 1.5–6 mcg/mL) with coadministration.

FOSAMPRENAVIR *(cont.)*

Drug	Effect of Interaction	Recommendations/Comments
Lopinavir/ ritonavir LPV/r	FPV 1400 mg twice daily + LPV/r 533/133 mg twice daily: APV Cmin decreased by 42% (compared to FPV/r 700/100 mg twice daily) but 3-fold higher Cmin (compared to FPV 1400 mg twice daily historical control); no significant change in LPV serum levels (compared to LPV/r 400/100 mg twice daily).	Coadministration generally not recommended. Consider FPV 1400 mg twice daily + LPV/r 600/150 mg twice daily. Consider TDM with coadministration.
Lovastatin	Serum levels of lovastatin may be significantly increased.	Contraindicated. Recommended alternatives include pravastatin, rosuvastatin, or fluvastatin (and atorvastatin–start with 10 mg/day). Monitor for ADRs due to limited clinical data.
Maalox	APV AUC decreased by 18%.	No significant interaction.
Maraviroc (MVC)	FPV/r may increase serum concentrations of MVC.	No data. Consider FPV/r 700/100 mg twice daily + MVC 150 mg twice daily.
Mefloquine	May increase serum levels of mefloquine.	Applies to all PIs: monitor mefloquine serum levels and mefloquine-induced toxicity (i.e., dizziness, LFTs, and periodic ophthalmic examination).
Methadone	S-methadone serum concentrations may be decreased. May decrease R-methadone AUC by 13% (studied with APV).	Studied with APV. S-methadone (active) was decreased 13% and APV AUC was decreased 25%; no withdrawal symptom observed. Coadminister with close monitoring.
Midazolam	May significantly increase midazolam levels.	Chronic use of midazolam should be avoided; single use IV midazolam may be used. Consider alternative benzodiazepines (temazepam, oxazepam, orlorazepam).
Milk Thistle	Data limited to a drug interaction study with milk thistle and IDV. IDV AUC unchanged but Cmin decreased by 47%.	Clinical significance unknown. May affect the serum levels of other PIs and NNRTIs.
Mirtazapine	May increase serum levels of mirtazapine.	Applies to all PIs: use with caution. Consider an alternative antidepressant (i.e., SSRI: escitalopram, citalopram, sertraline, or fluoxetine.).
Mycophenolate	Interaction unlikely. No significant interaction observed with NVP.	Applies to all PIs and NNRTI: no significant interaction observed with NVP. Use standard dose.

Drug	Effect of Interaction	Recommendations/Comments
Nefazodone	May increase serum levels of nefazodone.	Applies to all PIs: use with caution. Consider an alternative antidepressant (i.e., SSRI: escitalopram, citalopram, sertraline, or fluoxetine).
Nelfinavir (NFV)	APV AUC increased 150%.	Inadequate data; avoid coadministration.
Nevirapine (NVP)	APV serum concentration increased by 29% (compared to historical control). NVP increased 13%.	FPV/r 700/100 mg twice daily + NVP 200 mg twice daily.
Nifedipine	May increase serum levels of nifedipine.	Applies to all PIs: data limited to an interaction study conducted with ATV and diltiazem, which resulted in doubling of diltiazem serum levels (this led to PR interval prolongation). All PIs have the potential of prolonging the PR interval with calcium channel blockers coadministration. Calcium channel blockers should be started with 50% of the dose and slowly titrated with close monitoring of BP and pulse.
Nisoldipine	May increase serum levels of nisoldipine.	Applies to all PIs: data limited to an interaction study conducted with ATV and diltiazem, which resulted in doubling of diltiazem serum levels (this led to PR interval prolongation). All PIs and DLV have the potential of prolonging the PR interval with calcium channel blockers coadministration. Calcium channel blockers should be started with 50% of the dose and slowly titrated with close monitoring of BP and pulse.
Paclitaxel	May significantly increase serum levels of paclitaxel.	Applies to all PIs: since all PIs have the potential of significantly increasing paclitaxel serum levels, close monitoring of paclitaxel-induced toxicity is recommended.
Paroxetine	Paroxetine AUC decreased by 55% with FPV/r.	Titrate to therapeutic effect.
Phencyclidine (PCP)	May significantly increase serum levels of PCP.	Applies to all PIs: illicit drug use should be avoided for obvious reasons.
Phenobarbital	May decrease serum levels of PIs and NNRTIs. PIs and NNRTIs may increase or decrease phenobarbital serum level.	Applies to all PIs and NNRTI: consider alternative anticonvulsants (valproic acid, lamotrigine, levetiracetam, or topiramate). With coadministration, monitor anticonvulsants levels and consider TDM of PIs and NNRTIs.

FOSAMPRENAVIR (cont.)

Drug	Effect of Interaction	Recommendations/Comments
Phenytoin	May decrease serum levels of PIs and NNRTIs. PIs and NNRTIs may increase or decrease phenytoin serum levels.	Applies to all PIs and NNRTIs: consider alternative anticonvulsants (valproic acid, lamotrigine, levetiracetam, or topiramate). With coadministration, monitor anticonvulsants levels and consider TDM of PIs and NNRTIs.
Pimozide	May significantly increase pimozide serum levels resulting in QTc prolongation.	Contraindicated. Consider alternative: olanzapine.
Propafenone	May significantly increase serum levels of propafenone.	Applies to all PIs: no data. Coadministration should be avoided. Serum levels are not routinely recommended due to the poor correlation with efficacy and toxicity.
Proton Pump Inhibitors (PPI)	No significant interaction.	FPV may be coadministered with PPI.
Quinidine	May increase antiarrhythmic serum levels.	Applies to all PIs: no data. Contraindicated with RTV. With all Ps and NNRTIs coadministration, monitor EKG (QTc) and serum levels: target: 2–5 mcg/mL.
Raltegravir (RAL)	RAL and APV AUC decreased 37% and 36%, respectively (with unboosted FPV). RAL AUC decreased 55% (with FPV/r 700/100 mg twice daily).	Clinical significance unknown. Avoid unboosted FPV with RAL coadministration. Use FPV/r with close monitoring or consider alternative boosted PI with RAL coadministration.
Ranitidine (and other H-2 blockers)	APV AUC decreased by 30%.	Interaction not significant with boosted FPV (FPV/r 700/100 mg twice daily).
Ranolazine	May significantly increase ranolazine serum concentrations.	Contraindicated. May increase risk of QTc prolongation.
Rifabutin (RFB)	Based on APV data, an increase in RFB levels is expected.	CDC recommendation: FPV 1400 mg twice daily + RFB 150 mg once daily OR 300 g 3 ×/wk OR FPV 700 mg + RTV 100 mg twice daily + 150 mg every other day OR 150 mg 3 ×/wk.
Rifapentine	FPV serum levels may be significantly decreased.	Avoid coadministration. Consider using RFB.
Rifampin	No data, but significant decrease in APV serum levels expected.	Coadministration not recommended.

Drug	Effect of Interaction	Recommendations/Comments
Ritonavir (RTV)	When coadministered with RTV, APV AUC increased by over 2-fold, Cmin increased by 4-fold w/ once daily administration and 6-fold w/ twice daily administration (compared to FPV 1400 mg twice daily).	Dose for PI experienced patients: FPV/r 700/100 mg twice daily. Daily administration (FPV/r 1400/200 mg once daily) can be used in PI-naive patients.
Rosuvastatin	No interaction.	Usual dose. Close monitoring recommended due to limited clinical data.
Salmeterol	May increase salmeterol serum concentrations.	Avoid coadministration with boosted FPV. Consider formoterol.
Saquinavir (SQV)	SQV AUC decreased 14% (NS).	Limited data. Avoid or consider SQV/r 1000/100–200 mg twice daily + FPV 700 mg twice daily.
Sildenafil	May increase sildenafil serum levels.	Applies to all PIs: start with 25 mg, and avoid dosing on consecutive days.
Simvastatin	May significantly increase simvastatin levels.	Contraindicated. Alternatives include atorvastatin (start with 10–20 mg/day), pravastatin, rosuvastatin, or fluvastatin. Monitor for adverse effect due to limited clinical data.
Sirolimus	May significantly increase serum levels of sirolimus.	Applies to all PIs: dose sirolimus based on serum levels. A significantly reduction of sirolimus dose with all PIs coadministration is highly likely.
St. John's wort	May significantly decrease FPV levels.	Contraindicated. Use an alternative (more effective) antidepressant.
Tacrolimus	May significantly increase serum level of tacrolimus.	Applies to all PIs: dose tacrolimus based on serum level. A significantly reduction of tacrolimus dose with all PIs coadministration is recommended.
Tadalafil	May increase serum level of tadalafil.	Applies to all PIs: start with 5 mg. Do not exceed 10 mg in 72 hrs. Consider sildenafil due to more clinical data and shorter half-life allowing for easier titration.
Tamoxifen	May increase serum level of tamoxifen.	Applies to all PIs: no data. Close monitoring of tamoxifen-induced toxicity recommended.
Teniposide	May increase serum level of teniposide.	Applies to all PIs: no data. Close monitoring of teniposide-induced toxicity recommended.

FOSAMPRENAVIR *(cont.)*

Drug	Effect of Interaction	Recommendations/Comments
Terfenadine	May significantly increase terfenadine serum level.	Contraindicated due to the potential for cardiac arrhythmias. Recommended alternative antihistamine (loratadine, fexofenadine, desloratidine, or cetirizine).
Tetrahydrocannabinol (THC)	Based on data with NFV and IDV interactions are unlikely.	Applies to PIs and NNRTIs: interactions are unlikely but illicit drug use should be avoided for obvious reasons.
Tipranavir (TPV)	APV AUC decreased 44%.	Avoid coadministration.
Trazodone	May increase serum level of trazodone.	Applies to all PIs: use with caution. Consider an alternative antidepressant (i.e., SSRI: escitalopram, citalopram, sertraline, or fluoxetine).
Triazolam	May significantly increase triazolam serum level.	Contraindicated. Consider alternative benzodiazepines (temazepam, oxazepam, and lorazepam).
Vardenafil	May significantly increase serum level of vardenafil.	Applies to all PIs: do not exceed vardenafil 2.5 mg in 72 hrs (with RTV) OR 2.5 mg in 24 hrs (with other PIs). Consider sildenafil due to more clinical data and less pronounced interaction. Avoid coadministration with IDV.
Verapamil	May increase serum level of verapamil.	Applies to all PIs: data limited to an interaction study conducted with ATV and diltiazem, which resulted in doubling of diltiazem serum level (this led PR interval prolongation). All PIs have the potential of prolonging PR interval with calcium channel blocker coadministration. Calcium channel blockers should be started with 50% of the dose and slowly titrated with close monitoring of BP and pulse.
Vinblastine	May increase serum level of vinblastine.	Applies to all PIs: no data. Close monitoring of vinblastine-induced toxicity recommended.
Vincristine	May increase serum level of vincristine.	Applies to all PIs: no data. Close monitoring of vincristine-induced toxicity recommended.
Voriconazole	May decrease voriconazole AUC with FPV/r. Voriconazole may increase coadministered ART.	Significant interaction with RTV (400 mg twice daily); contraindicated. Voriconazole AUC decreased 39% with RTV 200 mg/day coadministration; avoid coadministration with boosted PI. Consider another antifungal for aspergillosis (i.e., *AmBisome* or caspofungin) or use with TDM.

Drug	Effect of Interaction	Recommendations/Comments
Warfarin	Case report of increased warfarin requirements after RTV initiation.	Other PIs and NNRTIs may also affect warfarin requirements. Monitor INR closely with coadministration.

DRUG-DRUG INTERACTION – INDINAVIR (IDV)

Drug	Effect of Interaction	Recommendations/Comments
Alprazolam	May increase serum levels of alprazolam.	Consider an alternative benzodiazepine (lorazepam, temazepam, or oxazepam).
Amiodarone	In a case report amiodarone levels increased by 44%.	Contraindicated. Monitor for amiodarone toxicity. Consider alternative antiarrhythmic with cardiology consult.
Amlodipine	Amlodipine serum concentrations increased 90%.	All PIs have the potential of prolonging the PR interval with calcium channel blocker coadministration. Calcium channel blockers should be started with 50% of the dose and slowly titrated with close monitoring of BP and pulse.
Artemether (artemisinin)	May increase serum levels of artemether.	Applies to all PIs: close monitoring for artemether toxicity (bone marrow suppression, bradycardia, and seizure).
Astemizole	May significantly increase astemizole serum levels.	Contraindicated due to the potential for cardiac arrhythmias. Recommended alternative antihistamine: loratadine, fexofenadine, desloratidine, or cetirizine.
Atorvastatin	May increase atorvastatin levels.	Avoid combination. Consider alternative agents: pravastatin, fluvastatin, or rosuvastatin. With coadministration, use low-dose atorvastatin and monitor for ADRs due to limited clinical data.
Atovaquone	No significant interaction.	Use standard dose of both drugs.
Azathioprine	Interaction unlikely.	Use standard doses.
Bepridil	May significantly increase bepridil serum levels.	No data. Manufacturers of ATV, RTV, and APV do not recommend bepridil coadministration; this contraindication should extend to all PIs since significant increase in bepridil serum levels can result in pro-arrhythmic events such as VT, PVC, and VF.

INDINAVIR *(cont.)*

Drug	Effect of Interaction	Recommendations/Comments
Bosentan	Bosentan serum concentrations may be significantly increased with IDV/r.	Coadminister bosentan only after RTV dosing has reached steady-state. In patients on RTV >10 days: start bosentan at 62.5 mg once daily or every other day. In patients already on bosentan: d/c bosentan for >36 hrs prior to initiation of RTV-boosted PIs and restart bosentan at 62.5 mg once daily or every other day after RTV has reached steady-state (after 10 days).
Carbamazepine	IDV levels: decreased 4%–25% of mean population values.	Consider alternative anticonvulsants (i.e., valproic acid, lamotrigine, levetiracetam, or topiramate). With coadministration, monitor anticonvulsants levels and consider TDM of IDV.
Chlordiazepoxide	May increase serum levels of chlordiazepoxide.	Applies to all PIs: consider an alternative benzodiazepine (lorazepam, temazepam, oroxazepam).
Cisapride	May significantly increase cisapride serum levels.	Contraindicated due to potential for cardiac arrhythmias. Recommended alternative: metoclopramide.
Clarithromycin	Clarithromycin AUC increased 53%.	Reduce clarithromycin dose by 50% in patients with CrCL 30–60 mL/min. Reduce clarithromycin dose by 75% in patients with CrCL <30 mL/min.
Clorazepate	May increase serum levels of clorazepate.	Applies to all PIs: consider an alternative benzodiazepine (lorazepam, oxazepam, or temazepam).
Cyclophosphamide	Cyclophosphamide: clearance decreased by 1.5 fold; IDV: no change.	Clinical significance unknown. May require cyclophosphamide dose adjustment.
Cyclosporine	May significantly increase serum levels of cyclosporine.	Applies to all PIs: monitor serum levels of cyclosporine closely with coadministration. Cyclosporine dose may need to be decreased.
Darunavir (DRV)	IDV AUC and Cmin increased 23% and 125%, respectively. DRV AUC and Cmin increased 24% and 44%, respectively.	Dose not established. May increase risk of nephrolithiasis.
Dexamethasone	May decrease IDV serum concentrations at steady-state.	Avoid unboosted IDV. Use IDV/r with dexamethasone with close monitoring for virologic efficacy.
Didanosine (ddI) (buffered suspension)	IDV AUC decreased by 84%.	Administer IDV 1hr before or after ddI (buffered). Consider using ddI EC since there are no interactions with IDV.

Drug	Effect of Interaction	Recommendations/Comments
Digoxin	Digoxin serum concentration may be increased with IDV/r coadministration.	Monitor digoxin serum concentration closely with coadministration.
Diltiazem	May increase serum levels of diltiazem.	Data limited to an interaction study conducted with ATV which resulted in doubling of diltiazem serum levels (this led to PR interval prolongation). All PIs have the potential of prolonging PR interval with diltiazem coadministration. Diltiazem should be started with 50% of the dose and slowly titrated with close monitoring of BP and pulse.
Disopyramide	May increase disopyramide serum levels.	Applies to all PIs: no data. Monitor disopyramide serum levels (target: 2 to 7.5 mcg/mL).
Docetaxel	May increase serum levels of docetaxel.	Applies to all PIs: no data. Close monitoring of chemotherapy-induced toxicity recommended.
Dofetilide	May significantly increase dofetilide levels.	No data. Use with caution. Monitor QTc closely and adjust dofetilide dosing based on QTc prolongation and renal function. Consider an alternative class III antiarrhythmic such as bretylium or ibutilide.
Doxorubicin	Doxorubicin: no change in clearance; IDV: no change.	Use standard dose. Close monitoring recommended due to limited clinical data.
Dronabinol	No significant interaction.	Use standard doses of both drugs.
Echinacea	May decrease IDV serum level. Echinacea (400 mg 4 ×/day) decreased CYP3A4 substrate (midazolam) by 23%.	Applies to all PIs and NNRTIs. Clinical significance unknown but should avoided until the safety of this combination is further evaluated.
Efavirenz (EFV)	IDV AUC: decreased by 31%–35%; EFV: no effect.	Recommended dosing: IDV 1000 mg q8H + EFV 600 mg qhs or IDV/r 800/200 mg twice daily + EFV 600 mg qhs.
Ergot Alkaloids	May significantly increase ergotamine levels. Case report of ergotism has been reported.	Contraindicated. Consider alternative agent for migraine such as sumatriptan (but not eletriptan since it is a CYP3A4 substrate and significant drug-drug interaction occurred with CYP3A4 inhibitor).
Estazolam	May increase serum levels of estazolam.	Applies to all PIs: consider an alternative benzodiazepine (lorazepam, oxazepam, or temazepam).
Ethosuximide	May increase serum levels of ethosuximide.	Applies to all PIs: consider switching to valproic acid for the treatment of absence seizure.

INDINAVIR *(cont.)*

Drug	Effect of Interaction	Recommendations/Comments
Etoposide	May increase serum levels of etoposide.	Applies to all PIs: no data. Close monitoring of chemotherapy-induced toxicity recommended.
Etravirine (ETR)	IDV AUC decreased 46% (studied with unboosted IDV).	No data with IDV/r. Avoid coadministration.
Etravirine (ETV)	IDV Cmin increased by 10-fold (dose: IDV/r 800/100 mg twice daily compared to IDV 800 mg q8h).	Dose: IDV/r 800/100 mg twice daily (high rate of nephrotoxicity) or IDV/RTV 400/400 mg twice daily (high rate of GI toxicity).
Felodipine	May increase serum levels of felodipine.	Applies to all PIs: data limited to an interaction study conducted with ATV and diltiazem, which resulted in doubling of diltiazem serum levels (this led PR interval prolongation). All PIs have the potential of prolonging PR interval with calcium channel blocker coadministration. Calcium channel blockers should be started with 50% of the dose and slowly titrated with close monitoring of BP and pulse.
Fentanyl	May significantly increase serum levels of fentanyl.	Use with caution. Consider morphine.
Flecainide	May increase antiarrhythmic serum levels.	Applies to all PIs: avoid coadministration; if necessary, monitor flecainide trough levels with coadministration. Target: 200–1000 ng/mL. Toxicity is frequent with trough serum levels above 1000 ng/mL.
Fluconazole	No significant interaction.	Use standard dose of both drugs.
Flurazepam	May increase serum levels of flurazepam.	Applies to all PIs: consider an alternative benzodiazepine (lorazepam, oxazepam, or temazepam).
Fluticasone	Fluticasone serum concentration may be increased with IDV/r coadministration.	Avoid long term coadministration. Consider beclomethasone.
Food	IDV AUC decreased by 77% with a 784 kcal meal (48.6 g fat, 31.3 g protein). IDV not significantly affected by a light meal (toast and jelly, apple juice, coffee with skim milk and sugar, or a meal of corn flakes).	Take on an empty stomach or with light snack >1 hr ac and >2 hrs pc when IDV given as the sole PI. IDV coadministered with RTV (IDV 800 mg twice daily + RTV 100 mg twice daily) removes food effect and is preferred.

Drug	Effect of Interaction	Recommendations/Comments
Garlic Supplements	Studies only done with SQV and revealed 49% and 51% reduction of SQVC min and AUC, respectively when coadministered with garlic supplement (3.5 grams twice daily).	Unknown interaction with other PIs. Studies only done with SQV but garlic supplement may affect serum levels of other PIs and NNRTIs. Avoid coadministration with PIs and NNRTIs.
Granisetron	May increase serum levels of granisetron.	Applies to all PIs: due to the large therapeutic index of granisetron, potential interaction is unlikely to be clinically significant.
Grapefruit or Seville Orange Juice	No significant interaction. IDV AUC decreased by 26%.	Clinically significant interaction unlikely. Studies conducted with unboosted IDV. Clinical significance unknown but boosting IDV with RTV (IDV/r 800/100 mg twice daily) will likely overcome any potential interaction.
Heroin (diamorphine)	Drug interactions unlikely.	Applies to PIs and NNRTIs: interaction unlikely but illicit drug use should be avoided for obvious reasons.
Ifosfamide	May increase serum levels of ifosfamide.	Applies to all PIs: no data. Close monitoring of chemotherapy-induced toxicity recommended.
Irinotecan	May increase irinotecan serum levels.	Applies to all PIs: Coadministration of ATV is contraindicated by manufacturer. All PIs also have the potential for significant interaction with irinotecan, therefore the coadministration should be done with extreme caution.
Itraconazole	IDV serum levels may be increased by itraconazole.	Dose: IDV 600 mg q8h. When coadministered with itraconazole, IDV 600 mg q8h has equivalent PK compared to IDV 800 mg q8h. Do not exceed itraconazole 200 mg twice daily. No data with IDV/r coadministration. Consider IDV/r 800/100 mg twice daily with aggressive hydration due to potential increased risk of nephrolithiasis.
Ketoconazole	IDV AUC: increased by 68%.	Dose: IDV to 600 mg q8h. Consider IDV/r 800/100 mg twice daily (do not exceed ketoconazole 200 mg/day) with aggressive hydration due to potential increased risk of nephrolithiasis.
Lidocaine	May increase antiarrhythmic serum levels.	Applies to all PIs: no data. Use with caution, monitor lidocaine serum levels (target: 1.5 to 6 mcg/mL) with coadministration.

INDINAVIR *(cont.)*

Drug	Effect of Interaction	Recommendations/Comments
Lopinavir/ritanavir (LPV/r)	IDV AUC increased by 20%, Cmin increased by 46%; IDV Cmin increased by 247%; LPV no change.	Dose: IDV 600 mg or 666 mg twice daily + LPV/r 400/100 mg twice daily.
Lovastatin	May significantly increase lovastatin levels.	Contraindicated. Recommended alternatives include pravastatin, rosuvastatin, or fluvastatin. Monitor for ADRs due to limited clinical data.
Maraviroc (MVC)	MVC serum concentrations may be increased.	Decrease MVC to 150 mg twice daily.
Mefloquine	May increase serum levels of mefloquine.	Applies to all PIs: monitor mefloquine serum levels and for mefloquine toxicity (i.e., dizziness, LFTs, and periodic ophthalmic examination).
Methadone	No change in methadone or IDV serum levels.	No interaction. Use standard dose of both drugs.
Mexiletine	May increase antiarrhythmic serum levels.	Applies to all PIs: no data. Use with caution. Monitor EKG and serum levels. Serum levels exceeding 1.5 to 2 mcg/mL have been associated with an increased risk of toxicity.
Midazolam	May significantly increase midazolam levels.	Concurrent administration contraindicated due to potential for prolonged sedation. Consider alternative benzodiazepines (lorazepam, oxazepam, or temazepam). Single-dose midazolam may be used (chronic use not recommended).
Milk Thistle (silymarin)	IDV AUC: unchanged IDV Cmin: decreased by 25%.	Clinical significance unknown. Since milk thistle has not shown clinical benefit for the treatment of viral hepatitis, avoid coadministration with IDV until it can be further evaluated.
Mirtazapine	May increase serum levels of mirtazapine.	Applies to all PIs: use with caution. Consider an alternative antidepressant (i.e., SSRI: escitalopram, citalopram, sertraline, or fluoxetine).
Mycophenolate	Interaction unlikely. No significant interaction observed with NVP.	Applies to all PIs and NNRTIs: no significant interaction observed with NVP. Use standard dose.
Nefazodone	May increase serum levels of nefazodone.	Applies to all PIs: use with caution. Consider an alternative antidepressant (i.e., SSRI: escitalopram, citalopram, sertraline, or fluoxetine).

Drug	Effect of Interaction	Recommendations/Comments
Nelfinavir (NFV)	NFV AUC: increased by 83%.	Dose: IDV 1200 mg twice daily + NFV 1250 twice daily (limited clinical data).
Nevirapine (NVP)	No effect on NVP; decrease IDV AUC by 28%.	IDV 1000 mg q8h + NVP 200 mg twice daily or IDV/r 800/200 mg twice daily + NVP standard dose.
Nifedipine	May increase serum levels of nifedipine.	Applies to all PIs: data limited to an interaction study conducted with ATV and diltiazem, which resulted in doubling of diltiazem serum levels (this led to PR interval prolongation). All PIs have the potential of prolonging the PR interval with calcium channel blocker coadministration. Calcium channel blockers should be started with 50% of the dose and slowly titrated with close monitoring of BP and pulse.
Nisoldipine	May increase serum levels of nisoldipine.	Applies to all PIs: data limited to an interaction study conducted with ATV and diltiazem, which resulted in doubling of diltiazem serum levels (this led to PR interval prolongation). All PIs have the potential of prolonging the PR interval with calcium channel blocker coadministration. Calcium channel blockers should be started with 50% of the dose and slowly titrated with close monitoring of BP and pulse.
Norethindrone and Ethinyl Estradiol	Norethindrone levels increased by 26% and Ethinyl estradiol by 24%.	Use of barrier method of contraception is recommended to prevent pregnancy.
Omeprazole	No significant interaction.	Use standard dose.
Paclitaxel	May increase paclitaxel serum levels.	Applies to all PIs: since all PIs have the potential of significantly increasing paclitaxel serum levels, close monitoring of paclitaxel-induced toxicity is recommended.
Phencyclidine (PCP)	May significantly increase serum levels of PCP.	Applies to all PIs. Avoid all illicit drug use with PIs and NNRTIs.
Phenobarbital	May decrease IDV serum levels. PIs and NNRTIs may increase or decrease phenobarbital serum levels.	Applies to All PIs and NNRTIs: consider alternative anticonvulsants (i.e., valproic acid, lamotrigine, levetiracetam, or topiramate). With coadministration, monitor anticonvulsants levels and consider TDM of PIs and NNRTIs.

INDINAVIR *(cont.)*

Drug	Effect of Interaction	Recommendations/Comments
Phenytoin	May significantly decrease IDV serum levels.	Applies to all PIs and NNRTIs: consider alternative anticonvulsants (i.e., valproic acid, lamotrigine, levetiracetam, or topiramate). Monitor anticonvulsant levels and consider TDM of PIs and NNRTIs.
Pimozide	May significantly increase pimozide serum levels resulting in QTc prolongation.	Contraindicated. Consider alternative: olanzapine.
Prednisone	Prednisolone serum concentration may be increased with IDV/r coadministration.	Dose adjustment may be needed with long-term coadministration.
Propafenone	May significantly increase serum levels of propafenone.	Do not coadminister.
Proton Pump Inhibitors (PPI) (omeprazole)	No significant interaction.	Use standard dose of both drugs.
Quinidine	IDV AUC increased by 10% (NS) based on a single dose study. Quinidine serum levels not reported.	Manufacturer does not recommend dose adjustment; however, use with caution since this was a single dose study. Monitoring of EKG (QTc) and serum levels: Target: 2 to 5 mcg/mL.
Raltegravir (RAL)	IDV may increase RAL serum concentrations.	Usual dose likely.
Ranolazine	May significantly increase ranolazine serum concentrations.	Contraindicated. May increase risk of QTc prolongation.
Rifabutin (RFB)	RFB AUC increased by 204%; IDV AUC decreased by 32%.	Recommended dose: RFB 150 mg once daily (or 300 mg 3 ×/wk) + IDV 1000 mg q8h or RFB 150 mg every other day (or 150 mg 3 ×/wk) + IDV 800 mg + RTV 100 mg twice daily (recommended but no data).
Rifampin	IDV AUC decreased by 89%.	Do not coadminister IDV (even with the addition of RTV).
Rifapentine	IDV AUC decreased by 75%. Rifapentine AUC not affected.	Avoid coadministration. Consider using RFB.
Rosuvastatin	Other CYP3A4 inhibitor (i.e., erythromycin) did not affect rosuvastatin serum levels.	Applies to PIs and NNRTI: interaction unlikely, but close monitoring recommended due to limited clinical data.
Salmeterol	May increase salmeterol serum concentrations.	Avoid coadministration. Consider formoterol.
Saquinavir (SQV)	Increase SQV AUC by 4–7 fold; no effect on IDV.	No data. Possible *in vitro* antagonism.

Drug	Effect of Interaction	Recommendations/Comments
Sildenafil	May significantly increase sildenafil serum levels.	Use with caution. Do not exceed 25 mg of sildenafil in 48 hrs.
Simvastatin	May significantly increase simvastatin levels.	Contraindicated. Recommended alternatives include atorvastatin, pravastatin, fluvastatin, and rosuvastatin. Monitor for adverse effects due to limited clinical data with these agents.
Sirolimus	May significantly increase serum levels of sirolimus.	Applies to all PIs: Dose sirolimus based on serum level. A significant reduction in sirolimus dose when combined with any PI is likely to be necessary.
St. John's wort	IDV AUC decreased by 57%.	Contraindicated with all PIs and NNRTIs. Use an alternative antidepressant.
Tacrolimus	May significantly increase tacrolimus levels.	Dose tacrolimus based on serum levels. A significant reduction of tacrolimus dose with IDV coadministration is likely to be necessary.
Tadalafil	May increase serum levels of tadalafil.	Applies to all PIs: Start with 5 mg. Do not exceed 10 mg in 72 hrs. Consider sildenafil due to more clinical data and shorter half-life allowing for easier titration.
Tamoxifen	May increase serum levels of tamoxifen.	Applies to all PIs: No data. Close monitoring of tamoxifen-induced toxicity recommended.
Teniposide	May increase serum levels of teniposide.	Applies to all PIs: no data. Close monitoring of teniposide-induced toxicity recommended.
Terfenadine	May significantly increase terfenadine serum levels.	Removed from IDV contraindicated list since it is no longer available in the US However, the potential of an old terfenadine bottle still poses a risk for cardiac arrhythmias with coadministration. Recommended alternative antihistamine: loratadine, fexofenadine, desloratidine, or cetirizine.
Tetrahydrocannabinol (THC)	Based on data with NFV and IDV interactions are unlikely.	Applies to PIs and NNRTIs: interactions are unlikely but illicit drug use should be avoided for obvious reasons.
Tipranavir (TPV)	No data.	Avoid coadministration.
Trazodone	May increase serum levels of trazodone.	Applies to all PIs: use with caution. Consider alternative antidepressants (i.e., SSRI: escitalopram, citalopram, sertraline, or fluoxetine).

INDINAVIR *(cont.)*

Drug	Effect of Interaction	Recommendations/Comments
Triazolam	May significantly increase triazolam serum levels.	Concurrent administration contraindicated due to potential for prolonged sedation. Consider alternative benzodiazepines (lorazepam, oxazepamor, and temazepam).
Vardenafil	Vardenafil AUC increased by 16-fold. IDV AUC decreased by 30%.	Do not exceed vardenafil 2.5 mg in 24 hrs. Consider sildenafil due to more clinical data and less pronounced interaction.
Venlafaxine	IDV AUC decreased by 28%. Venlafaxine: no effect.	Clinical significance unknown. Small study PK that used unboosted IDV; the observed change may be within the PK variability of IDV. Consider alternative SSRI (i.e., escitalopram).
Verapamil	May increase serum levels of verapamil.	Applies to all PIs: data limited to an interaction study conducted with ATV and diltiazem, which resulted in doubling of diltiazem serum levels (this led to PR interval prolongation). All PIs have the potential of prolonging the PR interval with calcium channel blocker coadministration. Calcium channel blockers should be started with 50% of the dose and slowly titrated with close monitoring of BP and pulse.
Vinblastine	May increase serum levels of vinblastine.	Applies to all PIs: no data. Close monitoring of vinblastine-induced toxicity recommended.
Vincristine	May increase serum levels of vincristine.	Applies to all PIs: no data. Close monitoring of vincristine-induced toxicity recommended.
Vitamin C	IDV AUC decreased by 14% and Cmin by 32% when coadministered with vitamin C (1 mg/day).	Clinical significance unknown due to small sample size (n = 7). Boosting IDV with RTV (IDV/r 800/100 mg twice daily) will likely overcome this potential interaction. Unknown effect on the serum levels of other PIs and NNRTIs.
Voriconazole	No significant change voriconazole and IDV AUC. Voriconazole serum concentration may be decreased with IDV/r.	No significant interaction with unboosted IDV. Use standard dose of both drugs. WIth IDV/r, monitor voriconazole serum concentration.
Warfarin	Case report of increased INR.	Other PIs and NNRTIs may also affect warfarin requirements. Monitor INR closely with coadministration.

DRUG-DRUG INTERACTION – ITRACONAZOLE

Drug	Effect of Interaction	Recommendations/Comments
Alfuzosin	May significantly increase alfuzosin serum concentrations resulting in hypotension.	Avoid coadministration. Consider doxazosin and terazosin for BPH (with close monitoring).
Alprazolam	Alprazolam serum concentrations may be increased.	Avoid coadministration. Consider lorazepam, oxazepam, or temazepam.
Amlodipine	May increase amlodipine serum concentrations.	Use with close monitoring.
Antacid	Itraconazole serum concentrations decreased.	Avoid coadministration.
Astemizole	Risk of QTc prolongation may be increased.	Contraindicated.
Bismuth	Itraconazole absorption decreased.	Avoid coadministration.
Busulfan	Busulfan concentrations may be increased.	Monitor closely for potential ADR with coadministration.
Carbamazepine	Itraconazole serum concentrations may be decreased.	Monitor itraconazole concentrations closely with coadministration. Consider valproic acid or levetiracetam.
Cilostazol	Cilostazol concentrations may be increased.	Cilostazol dose may need to be decreased.
Cimetidine	Itraconazole absorption decreased.	Avoid coadministration.
Cisapride	Risk of QTc prolongation may be increased.	Contraindicated.
Clarithromycin	May increase concentrations of clarithromycin and itraconazole.	Use with close monitoring. May increase risk for QTc prolongation.
Clopidogrel	May decrease the efficacy of clopidogrel.	Avoid coadministration.
Cyclosporine	Cyclosporine serum concentrations may be increased.	Monitor cyclosporine concentrations closely with coadministration.
Darunavir/ ritonavir (DRV/r)	Itraconazole serum concentrations may be increased.	Itraconazole dose >200 mg is not recommended by some; consider monitoring itraconazole serum concentrations to guide dosing. PIs serum concentrations may be increased (clinical significance unknown).
Diazepam	Diazepam serum concentrations may be increased.	Avoid coadministration. Consider lorazepam, oxazepam, or temazepam.
Didanosine (ddI) (buffered)	Itraconazole absorption decreased.	Consider fluconazole or separate >2 hrs apart. No interaction with ddI EC.

ITRACONAZOLE *(cont.)*

Drug	Effect of Interaction	Recommendations/Comments
Digoxin	Digoxin serum concentrations may be increased.	Monitor digoxin serum concentrations with coadministration.
Diltiazem	Diltiazem serum concentrations may be increased.	Monitor.
Disopyramide	May increase risk of QTc prolongation.	Avoid coadministration.
Docetaxel	Docetaxel concentrations may be increased.	Monitor closely for potential ADR with coadministration.
Dofetilide	May significantly increase dofetilide serum concentrations.	Contraindicated.
Efavirenz (EFV)	Itraconazole serum concentrations may be decreased.	Monitor itraconazole concentrations closely with coadministration.
Eletriptan	Eletriptan may be increased.	Avoid coadministration. Consider sumatriptan.
Ergot Alkaloids	Ergot alkaloid serum concentrations may be increased.	Avoid coadministration.
Erythromycin	May increase concentrations of erythromycin and itraconazole.	Use with close monitoring. May increase risk for QTc prolongation.
Esomeprazole	Itraconazole absorption decreased.	Avoid coadministration.
Etravirine (ETR)	Itraconazole serum concentrations may be decreased.	Monitor itraconzole serum concentrations with coadministration.
Famotidine	Itraconazole absorption decreased.	Avoid coadministration.
Fentanyl	Fentanyl concentrations may be increased.	Use with close monitoring. Consider morphine.
Fosamprenavir/ ritanavir (FPV/r)	Itraconazole serum concentrations may be increased.	Itraconazole dose >200 mg is not recommended by some; consider monitoring itraconazole serum concentrations to guide dosing. PIs serum concentrations may be increased (clinical significance unknown).
Glimepiride	Risk of hypoglycemia may be increased.	Monitor.
Glipizide	Glipizide concentrations may be increased, resulting in hypoglycemia.	Monitor blood sugar closely with coadministration.

Drug	Effect of Interaction	Recommendations/Comments
Glucocorticosteroids (e.g., prednisone, budesonide, dexamethasone, and fluticasone)	Glucocorticosteroid concentrations may be increased.	Glucocorticoid dose may need to be decreased.
Glyburide	Glyburide concentrations may be increased, resulting in hypoglycemia.	Monitor blood sugar closely with coadministration.
Halofantrine	May increase risk of QTc prolongation.	Avoid coadministration.
Indinavir (IDV)	IDV serum concentrations may be increased.	Itraconazole dose >200 mg is not recommended by some; consider monitoring itraconazole serum concentrations to guide dosing. PIs serum concentrations may be increased and increase risk for IDV stones.
Isoniazid	May decrease itraconazole serum concentrations.	Monitor itraconazole serum concentrations with coadministration.
Lansoprazole	Itraconazole absorption decreased.	Avoid coadministration.
Levacetylmethadol (levomethadyl)	May significantly increase levacetylmethadol serum concentrations. May increase QTc prolongation.	Contraindicated.
Lopinavir/ritonavir (LPV/r)	Itraconazole serum concentrations may be increased.	Itraconazole dose >200 mg is not recommended by some; consider monitoring itraconazole serum concentrations to guide dosing. PIs serum concentrations may be increased (clinical significance unknown).
Lovastatin	May significantly increase lovastatin serum concentrations.	Contraindicated. Consider pravastatin, rosuvastatin, or atorvastatin with close monitoring.
Maraviroc (MVC)	MVC serum concentrations may be significantly increased.	Dose: MVC 150 mg twice daily.
Midazolam	Midazolam serum concentrations may be increased.	Contraindicated. Consider lorazepam, oxazepam, or temazepam.
Nevirapine (NVP)	Itraconazole serum concentrations may be decreased. NVP serum concentrations may be increased.	Monitor itraconazole concentrations closely with coadministration.
Nifedipine	May increase nifedipine serum concentrations.	Use with close monitoring.
Nisoldipine	May increase nisoldipine serum concentrations.	Contraindicated. May increase risk of CHF.

ITRACONAZOLE *(cont.)*

Drug	Effect of Interaction	Recommendations/Comments
Nizatidine	Itraconazole absorption decreased.	Avoid coadministration.
Omeprazole	Itraconazole absorption decreased.	Avoid coadministration.
Pantoprazole	Itraconazole absorption decreased.	Avoid coadministration.
Phenobarbital	Itraconazole serum concentrations may be decreased.	Monitor itraconazole concentrations closely with coadministration. Consider valproic acid or levetiracetam.
Phenytoin	Itraconazole serum concentrations may be decreased.	Monitor itraconazole concentrations closely with coadministration. Consider valproic acid or levetiracetam.
Pimozide	Risk of QTc prolongation may be increased.	Contraindicated.
Quinidine	Risk of QTc prolongation may be increased.	Contraindicated.
Rabeprazole	Itraconazole absorption decreased.	Avoid coadministration.
Raltegravir (RAL)	Interaction unlikely.	Usual dose.
Ranitidine	Itraconazole absorption decreased.	Avoid coadministration.
Ranolazine	May significantly increase ranolazine serum concentrations.	Avoid coadministration.
Rifabutin (RFB)	RFB serum concentrations s may be increased. Itraconazole AUC decreased by 70%.	Avoid coadministration.
Rifampin	Itraconazole serum concentrations may be significantly decreased.	Avoid coadministration.
Ritonavir (RTV)	Itraconazole serum concentrations may be increased.	Itraconazole dose >200 mg is not recommended by some; consider monitoring itraconazole serum concentrations to guide dosing PIs serum concentrations may be increased (clinical significance unknown).

Drug	Effect of Interaction	Recommendations/Comments
Saquinavir/ ritonavir (SQV/r)	Itraconazole serum concentrations may be increased.	Itraconazole dose > 200 mg is not recommended by some; consider monitoring itraconazole serum concentrations to guide dosing. PIs serum concentrations may be increased (clinical significance unknown).
Sildenafil	Sildenafil serum concentrations may be increased.	Use with close monitoring. Do not exceed 25 mg in 48 hrs recommended by some.
Simvastatin	May significantly increase simvastatin serum concentrations.	Contraindicated. Consider pravastatin, rosuvastatin, or atorvastatin with close monitoring.
Sirolimus	Sirolimus serum concentrations may be increased.	Monitor sirolimus concentrations closely with coadministration.
Tacrolimus	Tacrolimus serum concentrations may be increased.	Monitor tacrolimus concentrations closely with coadministration.
Tadalafil	Tadalafil serum concentrations may be increased.	Use with close monitoring Start with 5 mg. Do not exceed 10 mg in 72 hrs recommended by some.
Terfenadine	Risk of QTc prolongation may be increased.	Contraindicated. Alternative: fexofenadine.
Tipranavir/ ritonavir (TPV/r)	Itraconazole serum concentrations may be increased.	Itraconazole dose >200 mg is not recommended by some; consider monitoring itraconazole serum concentrations to guide dosing. PIs serum concentrations may be increased (clinical significance unknown).
Tolbutamide	Risk of hypoglycemia may be increased.	Monitor.
Triazolam	Triazolam serum concentrations may be increased.	Contraindicated. Consider lorazepam, oxazepam, or temazepam.
Vardenafil	Vardenafil serum concentrations may be increased.	Use with close monitoring. Do not exceed 2.5 mg in 24 hrs recommended by some.
Verapamil	Verapamil serum concentrations may be increased.	Monitor.
Vinca alkaloids	Vinca alkaloids concentrations may be increased.	Monitor closely for potential ADR with coadministration.
Warfarin	Anticoagulation may be increased.	Monitor INR closely with coadministration.

DRUG-DRUG INTERACTION – KETOCONAZOLE

Drug	Effect of Interaction	Recommendations/Comments
Alcohol	Disulfiram-type reaction may occur.	Avoid coadministration.
Alprazolam	Alprazolam serum levels may be increased.	May increase risk of sedation. Consider lorazepam, oxazepam, or temazepam.

KETOCONAZOLE *(cont.)*

Drug	Effect of Interaction	Recommendations/Comments
Antacid	May significantly decrease ketoconazole serum concentrations.	Separate administration time by >2 hrs.
Astemizole	Risk of QTc prolongation may be increased.	Contraindicated.
Atazanavir (ATV)	No significant interaction.	No dose adjustment necessary.
Bismuth	Ketoconazole serum concentrations may be decreased.	Avoid coadministration.
Carbamazepine	Ketoconazole serum concentrations may be decreased.	Monitor for therapeutic effect; ketoconazole dose may need to be increased.
Cimetidine	Ketoconazole serum concentrations may be decreased.	Avoid coadministration.
Cisapride	Risk of QTc prolongation may be increased.	Contraindicated.
Clarithromycin	Clarithromycin and ketoconazole serum concentrations may be increased.	Consider clarithromycin dose adjustment with CrCl <30 mL/min. Consider azithromycin with ketoconazole coadministration.
Cyclosporine	Cyclosporine serum concentrations may be significantly increased.	Monitor cyclosporine serum concentrations closely with dose adjustment.
Darunavir/ ritonavir (DRV/r)	DRV AUC increased by 42%. Ketoconazole AUC increased by 300%.	Ketoconazole dose >200 mg is not recommended.
Delavirdine (DLV)	DLV Cmin increased by 50%.	Clinical significance unknown. Use standard dose.
Diazepam	Diazepam serum levels may be increased.	May increase risk of sedation. Consider lorazepam, oxazepam, or temazepam.
Didanosine (ddI) (buffered suspension)	Ketoconazole serum concentrations may be decreased.	Use ddI EC. Consider fluconazole or separate >2 hrs apart.
Efavirenz (EFV)	EFV serum concentrations may be increased. Ketoconazole serum concentrations may be decreased.	Monitor for therapeutic efficacy and EFV CNS side effects.
Ergot Alkaloids	Ergot alkaloid serum concentrations may be increased.	Avoid coadministration.
Esomeprazole	Ketoconazole serum concentrations may be decreased.	Avoid coadministration.
Etravirine (ETR)	Ketoconazole serum concentrations may be decreased.	Monitor for therapeutic efficacy.

Drug	Effect of Interaction	Recommendations/Comments
Famotidine	Ketoconazole serum concentrations may be decreased.	Avoid coadministration.
Fosamprenavir (FPV)	Ketoconazole AUC increased by 44% (studied with APV).	Ketoconazole dose ≥ 400 mg/day is not recommended.
Indinavir (IDV)	IDV AUC increased by 68%.	IDV 600 mg q8h.
Isoniazid	Ketoconazole serum concentrations may be decreased.	Monitor for therapeutic effect; ketoconazole dose may need to be increased.
Lansoprazole	Ketoconazole serum concentrations may be decreased.	Avoid coadministration.
Lopinavir/ritonavir (LPV/r)	Ketoconazole AUC increased by 300%.	Ketoconazole dose >200 mg is not recommended.
Maraviroc (MVC)	MVC serum concentrations may be increased.	Dose: MVC 150 mg twice daily.
Methylprednisolone	Methylprednisolone metabolism decreased by 50%.	Methylprednisolone dose adjustment may be required when coadministration is expected to exceed 7 days.
Midazolam	Midazolam serum levels may be increased.	Contraindicated. Consider lorazepam, oxazepam, or temazepam.
Nelfinavir (NFV)	NFV AUC increased by 36%.	No dose adjustment necessary.
Nevirapine (NVP)	Ketoconazole AUC decreased by 63%.	Avoid coadministration.
Nizatidine	Ketoconazole serum concentrations may be decreased.	Avoid coadministration.
Omeprazole	Ketoconazole serum concentrations may be decreased.	Avoid coadministration.
Pantoprazole	Ketoconazole serum concentrations may be decreased.	Avoid coadministration.
Phenobarbital	Ketoconazole serum concentrations may be decreased.	Monitor.
Phenytoin	Ketoconazole serum concentrations may be decreased.	Monitor for therapeutic effect; ketoconazole dose may need to be increased.
Pimozide	Risk of QTc prolongation may be increased.	Contraindicated.
Quinidine	May significantly increase quinidine serum concentrations.	Contraindicated.
Rabeprazole	Ketoconazole serum concentrations may be decreased.	Avoid coadministration.
Raltegravir (RAL)	Interaction unlikely.	Use standard dose.

KETOCONAZOLE *(cont.)*

Drug	Effect of Interaction	Recommendations/Comments
Ranitidine	Ketoconazole serum concentrations may be decreased.	Avoid coadministration.
Rifabutin (RFB)	RFB serum concentrations may be increased. Ketoconazole serum concentrations may be decreased.	Monitor for therapeutic efficacy of ketoconazole and RFB toxicity (e.g., uveitis).
Rifampin	Ketoconazole serum concentrations decreased by 50%.	Avoid coadministration. Consider RFB.
Ritonavir (RTV)	Ketoconazole AUC increased by 300%.	Ketoconazole dose >200 mg is not recommended.
Saquinavir (SQV)	SQV AUC increased by 300%.	No dose adjustment necessary.
Sirolimus	Sirolimus serum concentrations may be significantly increased.	Monitor sirolimus serum concentrations closely with dose adjustment.
Tacrolimus	Tacrolimus serum concentrations may be significantly increased.	Monitor tacrolimus serum concentrations closely with dose adjustment.
Terfenadine	Risk of QTc prolongation may be increased.	Contraindicated.
Theophylline	Theophylline serum concentrations may be increased.	Monitor theophylline serum concentrations with dose adjustment.
TPV/r	Ketoconazole serum concentrations may be increased.	Ketoconazole dose >200 mg is not recommended.
Triazolam	Triazolam serum levels may be increased.	Contraindicated. Consider lorazepam, oxazepam, or temazepam.
Warfarin	Anticoagulation may be increased.	Monitor INR closely.

DRUG-DRUG INTERACTION – LAMIVUDINE (3TC)

Drug	Effect of Interaction	Recommendations/Comments
Abacavir (ABC)	3TC AUC decreased by 15%; Cmax decreased by 35%.	Not clinically significant. Use standard dose.
Methadone	3TC: no reported interaction. Methadone: no change.	Not clinically significant. Use standard dose.
Nelfinavir (NFV)	No effect on 3TC AUC.	Not clinically significant. Use standard doses of both.
TMP/SMX	3TC AUC increased by 44%.	Not clinically significant. Use standard dose.

Drug-Drug Interaction – Lopinavir/Ritonavir (LPV/r)

Drug	Effect of Interaction	Recommendations/Comments
Abacavir (ABC)	May increase serum levels of alprazolam.	Applies to all PIs: consider alternative benzodiazepine (i.e., lorazepam, temazepam, or oxazepam).
Alfuzosin	May significantly increase alfuzosin levels.	Contraindicated. Consider doxazosin and terazosin for BPH (with close monitoring).
Amiodarone	May significantly increase amiodarone serum level.	Applies to all PIs: data limited to case report of increased amiodarone levels with IDV coadministration. RTV, APV, and ATV manufacturers recommend against use of amiodarone, but all PIs have the same potential of significantly increasing amiodarone serum levels. If coadministration can not be avoided, monitor for amiodarone ADR (PFTs and TSH). Consider monitoring serum levels of amiodarone, but its long half-life may make titration difficult.
Amlodipine	May increase serum levels of amlodipine.	Applies to all PIs: data limited to an interaction study conducted with ATV and diltiazem, which resulted in doubling of diltiazem serum levels (this led to PR interval prolongation). All PIs have the potential of prolonging the PR interval with calcium channel blockers coadministration. Calcium channel blockers should be started with 50% of the dose and slowly titrated with close monitoring of BP and pulse.
Artemether (artemisinin)	May increase serum levels of artemether.	Data available only for EFV. Coadministration of EFV with artesunate + amodiaquine resulted in significant LFT elevations. Close monitoring for artemether toxicity (bone marrow suppression, bradycardia and seizure).
Astemizole	May significantly increase astemizole serum levels.	Contraindicated due to the potential for cardiac arrhythmias. Recommended alternative antihistamine: loratadine, fexofenadine, desloratadine, or cetirizine.
Atazanavir (ATV)	ATV geometric mean Cmin increased by 45% with LPV/r 400/100 mg twice daily coadministration (compared to ATV/r 300/100 mg once daily). LPV PK comparable to historical data.	Dose: ATV 300 mg once daily + LPV/r 400/100 mg twice daily. May increase risk of PR interval prolongation.

DRUG-DRUG INTERACTIONS

LOPINAVIR/RITONAVIR (cont.)

Drug	Effect of Interaction	Recommendations/Comments
Atorvastatin	Atorvastatin AUC increased by 488%.	Use with caution at lower end of dosing range (10–40 mg/day). Monitor for Sx of atorvastatin toxicity (rhabdomyolysis and myopathy). Consider alternative agents: pravastatin, fluvastatin, or rosuvastatin.
Azathioprine	Interaction unlikely.	Applies to all PIs and NNRTIs: use standard dose.
Bepridil	May significantly increase bepridil serum levels.	Applies to all PIs: no data. The manufacturer of ATV RTV, and APV does not recommend bepridil coadministration, this contraindication should extend to all PIs since a significant increase in bepridil serum level can result in pro-arrhythmic events such as VT, PVC, and VFib.
Bisoprolol	May increase risk of PR interval prolongation.	Coadminister with close clinical monitoring.
Bosentan	Bosentan AUC increased 48-fold (on day 4) and 5-fold (on day 10).	Coadminister bosentan only after RTV has reached steady-state. In patients on RTV >10 days: start bosentan at 62.5 mg once daily or every other day. In patients already on bosentan: d/c bosentan for >36 hrs prior to initiation of RTV-boosted PIs and restart bosentan at 62.5 mg once daily or every other day after RTV has reached steady-state (after 10 days).
Buprenorphine	No significant change in buprenorphine AUC.	Use standard dose.
Bupropion	Bupropion AUC decreased 46–57%.	Titrate bupropion based on clinical response.
Carbamazepine	LPV serum levels may be significantly decreased.	Consider alternative anticonvulsants (e.g., levetiracetam). With coadministration, monitor anticonvulsants level and consider TDM of LPV.
Chlordiazepoxide	May increase serum levels of chlordiazepoxide.	Applies to all PIs: consider an alternative benzodiazepine (lorazepam, temazepam, or oxazepam).
Cisapride	May significantly increase cisapride serum levels.	Contraindicated due to potential for cardiac arrhythmias. Recommended alternative: metoclopramide.

Drug	Effect of Interaction	Recommendations/Comments
Clarithromycin	Clarithromycin and LPV serum concentrations may increased.	Current recommendation is to use standard clarithromycin dose in patients with normal renal function, but patients at risk for QTc or PR interval prolongation should be closely monitored. For creatinine clearance 30–60 mL/min, administer clarithromycin 500 mg PO once daily. For creatine clearance <30 mL/min administer clarithromycin 250 mg PO once daily. Consider using azithromycin.
Clorazepate	May increase serum levels of clorazepate.	Applies to all PIs: Consider an alternative benzodiazepine (lorazepam, temazepam, or oxazepam).
Cyclophosphamide	May increase serum level of cyclophosphamide.	Applies to all PIs: Data limited to an interaction study conducted with IDV resulting in a 50% increase in cyclophosphamide serum levels. Since all PIs have the potential of increasing cyclophosphamide levels, close monitoring of cyclophosphamide-induced toxicity is recommended.
Cyclosporine	May significantly increase serum levels of cyclosporine.	Applies to all PIs: Monitor serum levels of cyclosporine closely with coadministration. Cyclosporine dose may need to be decreased.
Darunavir (DRV)	DRV AUC and Cmin decreased 53% and 65%, respectively. LPV AUC and Cmin increased 37% and 72%, respectively.	Avoid coadministration.
Dasatinib	Serum concentrations of dasatinib may be increased.	Lower doses of dasatinib may be needed.
Desipramine	Desipramine AUC may be increased. LPV not affected.	Clinical significance unknown. Monitor for desipramine adverse drug reaction and serum level (if available). Consider alternative antidepressant: escitalopram, citalopram, sertraline, or fluoxetine.
Digoxin	Digoxin AUC increased 81% with LPV/r coadministration.	Monitor digoxin plasma concentration closely with coadministration. May increase risk of PR interval prolongation.
Diltiazem	May increase serum levels of diltiazem.	Applies to all PIs: Data limited to an interaction study conducted with ATV, which resulted in doubling of diltiazem serum levels (this led to PR interval prolongation). All PIs have the potential of prolonging PR interval with diltiazem coadministration. Diltiazem should be started with 50% of the dose and slowly titrated with close monitoring of BP and pulse.

LOPINAVIR/RITONAVIR *(cont.)*

Drug	Effect of Interaction	Recommendations/Comments
Disopyramide	May increase disopyramide serum levels.	Applies to all PIs: no data. Monitor disopyramide serum levels (target: 2 to 7.5 mcg/mL).
Docetaxel	May increase serum levels of docetaxel.	Applies to all PIs: no data. Close monitoring of chemotherapy-induced toxicity recommended.
Dofetilide	May significantly increase serum levels of dofetilide.	Applies to all PIs: no data. Use with caution. Monitor QTc closely and adjust dofetilide dosing based on QTc prolongation and renal function. Consider an alternative class III antiarrhythmic such as bretylium or ibutilide.
Echinacea	LPV and RTV serum concentrations not affected with echinacea purpurea 500 mg 3 ×/day, but other CYP3A substrate (midazolam) reduced by echinacea co-administration.	Avoid if possible.
Efavirenz (EFV)	LPV/r AUC decreased by 19% and Cmin decreased by 39%; EFV levels unaffected.	Dose: LPV/r 500/125 mg twice daily + EFV 600 mg qhs, especially in patients with PI resistance. Standard doses may be acceptable in PI-naive patients.
Ergot Alkaloid	May significantly increase serum levels of ergotamine resulting in acute ergot toxicity.	Contraindicated. Consider alternative agent for migraine such as sumatriptan (but not eletriptan since it is a CYP3A4 substrate and significant drug-drug interaction occurred with CYP3A4 inhibitor).
Erythromycin	Erythromycin and LPV serum concentrations may increased.	May increase risk for QTc and PR interval prolongation. Avoid coadministration and consider using azithromycin.
Estazolam	May increase serum levels of estazolam.	Applies to all PIs: consider an alternative benzodiazepine (i.e., lorazepam, temazepam, or oxazepam).
Ethinyl Estradiol	Ethinyl estradiol AUC decreased by 42%.	Recommend an alternative or additional form of contraception.
Ethosuximide	May increase serum levels of ethosuximide.	Applies to all PIs: consider switching to valproic acid for the treatment of absence seizure.
Etoposide	May increase serum levels of etoposide.	Applies to all PIs: no data. Close monitoring of chemotherapy-induced toxicity recommended.

Drug	Effect of Interaction	Recommendations/Comments
Etravirine (ETR)	LPV AUC decreased 18%. ETR Cmin decreased by 45%.	Usual dose recommended. ETR Cmin reduction with LPV/r was comparable to observed reduction with DRV/r coadministration.
Ezetimibe	No significant change in LPV/r trough measurements after the addition of ezetimibe.	Separate administration time if possible. Observation pharmacokinetic substudy that needs confirmation.
Felodipine	May increase serum levels of felodipine.	Applies to all PIs: data limited to an interaction study conducted with ATV and diltiazem, which resulted in doubling of diltiazem serum level (this led to PR interval prolongation). All PIs have the potential of prolonging the PR interval with calcium channel blockers coadministration. Calcium channel blockers should be started with 50% of the dose and slowly titrated with close monitoring of BP and pulse.
Fentanyl	May significantly increase fentanyl serum levels.	Use with caution. Consider morphine.
Flecainide	May significantly increase serum levels of flecainide.	Contraindicated.
Fluconazole	Interaction unlikely.	Use standard doses for both drugs.
Flurazepam	May increase serum levels of flurazepam.	Applies to all PIs: consider an alternative benzodiazepine(i.e., lorazepam, temazepam, or oxazepam).
Fluticasone	With RTV coadministration fluticasone AUC and Cmax increased by 350-fold and 25-fold, respectively.	Data limited to RTV coadministration. With chronic RTV coadministration, plasma cortisol AUC decreased by 86%. Cushing's syndrome and adrenal suppression have been reported. Coadministration not recommended by manufacturer. Avoid long-term coadministration.
Food	Increases LPV AUC.	LPV/r tabs can be taken with or without food.
Fosamprenavir (FPV)	Decreased APV and LPV levels.	Not recommended by some. Consider FPV 1400 mg twice daily + LPV/r 600/150 mg (3 tabs) twice daily (and consider TDM).
Garlic Supplement	49% and 51% reduction of SQV Cmin and AUC, respectively when coadministered with garlic supplement (3.5 mg twice daily).	Studies only done with SQV but garlic may affect the serum levels of other PIs or NNRTIs. Coadministration of garlic supplements should be avoided with PIs and NNRTIs.

LOPINAVIR/RITONAVIR *(cont.)*

Drug	Effect of Interaction	Recommendations/Comments
Granisetron	May increase serum levels of granisetron.	Applies to all PIs: due to the large therapeutic index of granisetron, potential interaction is unlikely to be clinically significant.
Heroin (diamorphine)	Drug interactions unlikely.	Applies to PIs and NNRTIs: interaction unlikely but illicit drug use should be avoided for obvious reasons.
Ifosphamide	May increase serum levels of ifosphamide.	Applies to all PIs: no data. Close monitoring of chemotherapy-induced toxicity recommended.
Indinavir (IDV)	IDV AUC increased by 20% and Cmin increased by 46%; IDV Cmin increased by 247%.	Dose: IDV 600 mg or 666 mg twice daily + LPV/r 400/100 mg twice daily.
Irinotecan	May increase irinotecan serum levels.	Applies to all PIs: Coadministration of ATV is contraindicated by manufacturer. All PIs also have the potential for significant interaction with irinotecan, therefore coadministration should be done with extreme caution.
Itraconazole	CYP3A4 inhibitor and substrate-bidirectional inhibition with increase levels of PIs and itraconazole.	Use standard dose with itraconazole and LPV/r coadministration. Consider monitoring itraconazole levels.
Ketoconazole	LPV increased 13%. Ketoconazole increased by 3-fold.	Do not exceed ketoconazole 200 mg once daily with LPV/r coadministration.
Lamotrigine	Lamotrigine Cmin and AUC decreased 56% and 50%, respectively. LPV not affected.	Titrate lamotrigine dose to therapeutic effect.
Lidocaine	May increase antiarrhythmic serum levels.	Applies to all PIs: no data. Use with caution, monitor lidocaine serum levels (target: 1.5 to 6 mcg/mL) with coadministration.
Lovastatin	May significantly increase lovastatin levels.	Contraindicated. Recommended alternatives include pravastatin, rosuvastatin, and fluvastatin (and possibly atorvastatin —start at 10 mg once daily). Monitor for adverse effect due to limited clinical data.
Maraviroc (MVC)	MVC AUC increased 283%.	Dose: MVC 150 mg twice daily + LPV/r 400/100 mg twice daily.

Drug	Effect of Interaction	Recommendations/Comments
Mefloquine	May increase serum levels of mefloquine.	Applies to all PIs: monitor mefloquine serum levels. Monitor for mefloquine toxicity (i.e., dizziness, LFTs, and periodic ophthalmic examination).
Methadone	Methadone AUC decreased by 26%–36%.	No withdrawal Sx observed in 2 of 3 studies. Standard methadone dose recommended, but may need to increase methadone dose in a small subset of patients. Monitor QTc with high-dose methadone; coadministration may increase risk of QTc prolongation.
Metoprolol	May increase risk of PR interval prolongation.	Coadminister with close clinical monitoring.
Metronidazole	Disulfiram-like reaction.	Applies to LPV liquid formulation. Warn patients of LPV alcohol content (liquid). Use LPV/r caps.
Mexiletine	May increase antiarrhythmic serum levels.	Applies to all PIs: no data. Use with caution. Monitor EKG and serum levels. Serum levels exceeding 1.5 to 2 mcg/mL have been associated with an increased risk of toxicity.
Midazolam	May significantly increase midazolam levels.	Concurrent administration of oral midazolam is contraindicated. Consider alternative benzodiazepines (temazepam, oxazepam, or lorazepam). If LPV/r is coadministered with IV midazolam, close clinical monitoring for respiratory depression and/or prolonged sedation and dosage adjustment should be considered.
Milk Thistle	Data limited to an interaction study with milk thistle and IDV. IDV AUC: unchanged and IDV Cmin decreased by 47%.	Unknown effect on LPV serum levels. Avoid coadministration with PIs and NNRTIs until it can be further evaluated.
Mirtazapine	May increase serum levels of mirtazapine.	Applies to all PIs: use with caution. Consider an alternative antidepressant (i.e., SSRI: escitalopram, citalopram, sertraline, or fluoxetine).
Mycophenolate	Interaction unlikely. No significant interaction observed with NVP.	Applies to all PIs and NNRTI: no significant interaction observed with NVP. Use standard dose.
Nadolol	May increase risk of PR interval prolongation.	Coadminister with close clinical monitoring.
Nefazodone	May increase serum levels of nefazodone.	Applies to all PIs: use with caution. Consider an alternative antidepressant (i.e., SSRI: escitalopram, citalopram, sertraline, or fluoxetine).

LOPINAVIR/RITONAVIR *(cont.)*

Drug	Effect of Interaction	Recommendations/Comments
Nelfinavir (NFV)	LPV AUC decreased by 27% and Cmin decreased by 33% NFV Cmin increased by 113%.	Do not coadminister or consider LPV/r 600/150 mg (3 tabs) + NFV 1250 mg twice daily with TDM.
Nevirapine (NVP)	LPV AUC decreased by 22%. NVP levels unaffected.	Dose: LPV/r 500/125 mg twice daily + NVP standard dose, especially in patients with PI resistance. Standard doses may be acceptable for PI-naive patients.
Nifedipine	May increase serum levels of nifedipine.	Applies to all PIs: data limited to an interaction study conducted with ATV and diltiazem, which resulted in doubling of diltiazem serum levels (this led to PR interval prolongation). All PIs have the potential of prolonging the PR interval with calcium channel blockers coadministration. Calcium channel blockers should be started with 50% of the dose and slowly titrated with close monitoring of BP and pulse.
Nilotinib	Serum concentrations of Nilotinib may be increased.	Lower doses of nilotinib may be needed.
Nisoldipine	May increase serum levels of nisoldipine.	Applies to all PIs: data limited to an interaction study conducted with ATV and diltiazem, which resulted in doubling of diltiazem serum levels (this led to PR interval prolongation). All PIs have the potential of prolonging the PR interval with calcium channel blockers coadministration. Calcium channel blockers should be started with 50% of the dose and slowly titrated with close monitoring of BP and pulse.
Omeprazole	No change in LPV/r pharmacokinetics.	Use standard dose LPV/r tablet with omeprazole coadministration.
Paclitaxel	May increase serum levels of paclitaxel. Reports of toxicity associated with LPV/r and paclitaxel coadministration.	Monitor closely for paclitaxel-induced toxicity.
Phencyclidine (PCP)	May significantly increase serum levels of PCP.	Applies to all PIs: avoid all illicit drug use for obvious reasons.
Phenobarbital	LPV levels may be significantly decreased.	Consider alternative anticonvulsants (e.g., levetiracetam). Monitor anticonvulsants level when applicable and consider TDM of LPV.

Drug	Effect of Interaction	Recommendations/Comments
Phenytoin	LPV AUC decreased by 33%. Phenytoin AUC decreased by 31%.	Avoid coadministration. Monitor anticonvulsants levels. Consider alternative anticonvulsants (e.g., levetiracetam). Consider empirically increasing LPV/r to 600/150 mg (3 tabs) twice daily (with TDM).
Pimozide	May significantly increase pimozide serum levels resulting in QTc prolongation.	Contraindicated. Consider alternative: olanzapine.
Pravastatin	Pravastatin AUC increased 33%.	Use standard dose.
Prednisone	May increase prednisone serum concentration.	May require dose adjustment with long-term coadministration.
Propafenone	May significantly increase serum levels of propafenone.	Contraindicated.
Propranolol	May increase risk of PR interval prolongation.	Coadminister with close clinical monitoring.
Quinidine	May increase antiarrhythmic serum levels.	Applies to all PIs: no data. Contraindicated with RTV. With all PIs and NNRTI coadministration, monitor EKG (QTc) and serum levels: target: 2 to 5 mcg/mL.
Raltegravir (RAL)	Interaction unlikely.	No data with LPV/r. RTV (100 mg twice daily) did not affect RAL PK parameters. Consider usual dose with close monitoring of virologic efficacy.
Ranitidine	No interaction.	Use standard dose LPV/r tablet with ranitidine coadministration.
Ranolazine	May significantly increase ranolazine serum concentrations.	Avoid coadministration. May increase risk of QTc prolongation.
Rifabutin (RFB)	RFB AUC increased by 203%. LPV serum level increased 20% (NS).	Dose: LPV/r 2 tabs twice daily + RFB 150 mg every other day. In an observational study, RFB serum concentrations lower compared to historical controls. RFB TDM recommended with coadministration.
Rifampin	LPV/r AUC decreased by 75% and Cmin decreased by 99%.	Generally not recommended. With coadministration consider LPV/r 400/100 mg (3 caps) + RTV 300 mg twice daily (note: monitor LFTs, GI intolerance, and lipids). A more recent study of LPV/r 3 to 4 tabs twice daily + rifampin found high incidence of nausea, vomiting, and grade 4 LFTs elevation. RFB preferred w/ LPV/r coadministration.
Rifapentine	LPV serum levels may be significantly decreased.	Avoid coadministration. Consider using RFB.

LOPINAVIR/RITONAVIR *(cont.)*

Drug	Effect of Interaction	Recommendations/Comments
Rosiglitazone	LPV AUC increased by 20% and Cmin increased by 21%.	Use standard dose. Limited sample size (NS) (n = 4).
Rosuvastatin	Rosuvastatin AUC and Cmax increased 2.1 to 4.7-fold, respectively. LPV and RTV PK parameters not significantly affected.	Use with close monitoring due to limited clinical data. Use low-dose rosuvastatin and titrate slowly.
Salmeterol	May increase salmeterol serum concentrations.	Avoid coadministration. Consider formoterol.
Saquinavir (SQV)	SQV AUC increased by 836% and Cmin increased by 1700%.	Dose: SQV 1000 mg twice daily + LPV/r 400/100 mg twice daily.
Sildenafil	May increase sildenafil serum levels.	Applies to all PIs: Use with close monitoring. Do not exceed 25 mg in 48-hrs.
Simvastatin	May significantly increase simvastatin levels.	Contraindicated. Alternative HMG-CoA reductase inhibitor that may be used include pravastatin, cerivastatin, fluvastatin. Monitor for adverse effects due to limited clinical data.
Sirolimus	May significantly increase serum levels of sirolimus.	Applies to all PIs: dose sirolimus based on serum levels. A significantly reduction of sirolimus dose with all PIs coadministration is highly likely.
St. John's wort	May significantly decrease LPV serum levels.	Contraindicated. Studies only done with IDV but St. John's wort likely to increase metabolism of other PIs and NNRTIs. Use an alternative (more effective) antidepressant.
Tacrolimus	Tacrolimus increased 10-fold with coadministration. Several case reports of toxic serum levels of tacrolimus upon initiation of LPV/r.	Dose tacrolimus based on serum levels. A much lower dose (0.5–1 mg/wk or 1/20–1/10 of standard dose) may be sufficient with LPV/r coadministration.
Tadalafil	May increase serum level of tadalafil.	Applies to all PIs: start with 5 mg. Do not exceed 10 mg in 72 hrs. Consider sildenafil due to more clinical data and shorter half-life allowing for easier titration.
Tamoxifen	May increase serum level of tamoxifen.	Applies to all PIs: no data. Close monitoring of tamoxifen-induced toxicity recommended.
Teniposide	May increase serum level of teniposide.	Applies to all PIs: no data. Close monitoring of teniposide induced toxicity recommended.

Drug	Effect of Interaction	Recommendations/Comments
Terfenadine	May significantly increase terfenadine serum levels.	Contraindicated due to the potential for cardiac arrhythmias. Recommended alternative antihistamine: loratadine, fexofenadine, desloratidine, or cetirizine.
Tetrahydrocan-nabinol (THC)	Based on data with NFV and IDV interactions are unlikely.	Applies to PIs and NNRTIs: interactions are unlikely but illicit drug use should be avoided for obvious reasons.
Tipranavir (TPV)	LPV AUC decreased by 49% (studied dose TPV 500 mg + LPV/r 400/100 mg twice daily).	Not generally recommended. LPV/r 400/100 mg twice daily with TPV/r 500/200 mg twice daily (additional RTV 200 mg) resulted in "adequate" LPV Cmin, but significant interpatient variability and small sample size suggest confirmation of these findings before this dosing regimen can be recommended.
Trazodone	Trazodone AUC increased 2-4-fold with RTV co-administration. With boosted PIs, decrease trazodone dose by 50% with slow dose titration.	Use with caution with close monitoring for CNS and CV adverse effects.
Triazolam	May significantly increase triazolam serum levels.	Contraindicated. Consider alternative benzodiazepines (temazepam, oxazepam, or lorazepam).
Valproic Acid	May decrease valproic serum concentrations. LPV AUC increased by 75%.	Monitor for LPV associated ADR and valproic serum concentrations with coadministration.
Vardenafil	May significantly increase serum levels of vardenafil.	Applies to all PIs: do not exceed vardenafil 2.5 mg in 72 hrs (with RTV) or 2.5 mg in 24 hrs (with other PIs). Consider sildenafil due to more clinical data and less pronounced interaction. Avoid coadministration with IDV.
Verapamil	May increase serum levels of verapamil.	Applies to all PIs: data limited to an interaction study conducted with ATV and diltiazem, which resulted in doubling of diltiazem serum levels (this led to PR interval prolongation). All PIs have the potential of prolonging the PR interval with calcium channel blockers coadministration. Calcium channel blockers should be started with 50% of the dose and slowly titrated with close monitoring of BP and pulse.
Vinblastine	May increase serum levels of vinblastine.	Applies to all PIs: no data. Close monitoring of vinblastine-induced toxicity recommended.

LOPINAVIR/RITONAVIR *(cont.)*

Drug	Effect of Interaction	Recommendations/Comments
Vincristine	May increase serum levels of vincristine.	Applies to all PIs: no data. Close monitoring of vincristine-induced toxicity recommended.
Vitamin C	Data limited to interaction study with IDV and vitamin C (1 g/day): IDV AUC decreased by 14% and Cmin by 32%.	Clinical significance unknown. Other PI and NNRTI serum levels may be affected when coadministered with similar dose of vitamin C.
Voriconazole	May significantly decrease voriconazole AUC. Voriconazole may increase LPV.	Significant interaction with EFV and RTV (400 mg twice daily); contraindicated. Voriconazole AUC decreased 39% with RTV 200 mg/day coadministration; avoid coadministration with boosted PI. Consider another antifungal for aspergillosis (i.e., *AmBisome* or caspofungin) or use with TDM. Voriconazole dose may need to be increased.
Warfarin	A case report of increased warfarin requirement after RTV initiation.	Other PIs and NNRTIs may also affect warfarin requirements. Monitor INR closely with coadministration.

DRUG-DRUG INTERACTION – MARAVIROC (MVC)

Drug	Effect of Interaction	Recommendations/Comments
Atazanavir (ATV)	MVC AUC increased 257%.	Decrease MVC to 150 mg twice daily with ATV coadministration.
Atazanavir/ ritonavir (ATV/r)	MVC AUC increased 388%.	Decrease MVC to 150 mg twice daily with ATV/r coadministration.
Carbamezapine	MVC AUC may significantly decrease with carbamezapine coadministration.	Increase MVC to 600 mg twice daily with coadministration, or consider alternative anticonvulsant (i.e., valproic acid or levetiracetam). Monitor for postural hypotension during the 1st 2 wks.
Clarithromycin	May increase MVC serum concentrations.	Dose: MVC 150 mg twice daily.
Darunavir/ ritonavir (DRV/r)	MVC AUC increased 344% with coadministration.	Decrease MVC to 150 mg twice daily with DRV/r coadministration.
Delavirdine (DLV)	May increase MVC serum concentrations.	Dose: MVC 150 mg twice daily.
Efavirenz (EFV)	MVC AUC decreased by 45%.	Increase MVC to 600 mg twice daily with EFV coadministration. Monitor for postural hypotension during the 1st 2 wks.
Erythromycin	May increase MVC serum concentrations.	Dose: MVC 150 mg twice daily.

Drug	Effect of Interaction	Recommendations/Comments
Ethinyl Estradiol	No significant interaction.	Use standard doses. Consider an additional barrier form of contraception.
Itraconazole	May increase MVC serum concentrations.	Dose: MVC 150 mg twice daily.
Ketoconazole	MVC AUC increased 5-fold with coadministration.	Dose: MVC 150 mg twice daily.
Lopinavir/ritonavir (LPV/r)	MVC AUC increased 283%.	Decrease MVC to 150 mg twice daily with LPV/r coadministration.
Lopinavir/ritonavir + Efavirenz (LPV/r + EFV)	MVC AUC increased 153%.	Decrease MVC to 150 mg twice daily with LPV/r + EFV coadministration.
Levonorgestrel	No significant interaction.	Use standard doses. Consider an additional barrier form of contraception.
Midazolam	Midazolam AUC increased by 18%.	Unlikely to be clinically significant. Use standard doses.
Nefazodone	May increase MVC serum concentrations.	Dose: MVC 150 mg twice daily.
Nevirapine (NVP)	MVC serum concentration was not significantly affected compared to historical controls in a single dose study; however, MVC AUC may be decreased at steady state.	Limited data; consider MVC 300 mg twice daily + standard dose NVP.
Phenobarbital	MVC AUC may significantly decrease with phenobarbital coadministration.	Increase MVC to 600 mg twice daily with coadministration, or consider alternative anticonvulsant (i.e., valproic acid or levetiracetam). Monitor for postural hypotension during the 1st 2 wks.
Phenytoin	MVC AUC may significantly decrease with phenytoin coadministration.	Increase MVC dose to 600 mg twice daily with coadministration, or consider alternative anticonvulsant (i.e., valproic acid or levetiracetam). Monitor for postural hypotension during the 1st 2 wks.
Posaconazole	May increase MVC serum concentrations.	No data. Consider MVC 150 mg twice daily.
Rifabutin (RFB)	Modest impact of RFB on MVC exposure.	MVC to 300 mg twice daily with RFB coadministration.
Rifampin	MVC AUC decreased 66% with coadministration.	Limited clinical; avoid coadministration if possible. Increase MVC to 600 mg twice daily with coadministration. Monitor for postural hypotension during the 1st 2 wks.
Rifapentine	May significantly decrease MVC concentrations.	Avoid coadministration. Consider RFB with MVC coadministration.

DRUG-DRUG INTERACTIONS

MARAVIROC *(cont.)*

Drug	Effect of Interaction	Recommendations/Comments
Saquinavir/ ritonavir (SQV/r)	MVC AUC increased 732%.	Decrease MVC to 150 mg twice daily with SQV/r coadministration.
Saquinavir/ ritonavir + Efavirenz (SQV/r + EFV)	MVC AUC increased 400%.	Decrease MVC to 150 mg twice daily with SQV/r + EFV coadministration.
St. John's wort	May significantly decrease MVC concentrations.	Avoid coadministration.
Sulfamethoxazole- trimethoprim (TMP/SMX)	MVC AUC increased 10%.	Use standard dose. MVC 300 mg twice daily.
Tenofovir (TDF)	No significant interaction.	Use standard doses. MVC 300 mg twice daily.
Telithromycin	May increase MVC serum concentrations.	Dose: MVC 150 mg twice daily.
Tipranavir/ ritonavir (TPV/r)	No significant interaction.	Use standard doses. MVC 300 mg twice daily.
Voriconazole	May increase MVC serum concentrations.	No data. Consider MVC 150 mg twice daily.

DRUG-DRUG INTERACTION – METHADONE

Drug	Effect of Interaction	Recommendations/Comments
Abacavir (ABC)	Methadone clearance increased 23%. Abacavir decreased 34%.	Clinical significance unknown. Usual dose recommended.
Atazanavir (ATV)	No interaction.	No dose adjustment needed with unboosted ATV. Monitor for withdrawal with boosted ATV.
Carbamazapine	May significantly decrease methadone serum concentrations.	Monitor for withdrawal signs and Sx. May require methadone dose increase or switch to alternative anticonvulsant (e.g., valproic acid or levetiracetam).
Darunavir (DRV)	R-methadone (active isomer) area under the curve decreased 16%. S-methadone AUC decreased 36%. Evidence of opiate withdrawal was observed in 4/16 volunteers.	Monitor for withdrawal signs and Sx. May require methadone dose increase.
Didanosine (ddI) (buffered formulation)	ddI AUC decreased by 57%.	Avoid coadministration with buffered ddI. ddI EC preferred formulation due to a lack of interaction with methadone.

Drug	Effect of Interaction	Recommendations/Comments
Efavirenz (EFV)	Methadone AUC decreased by 52%.	Increase in methadone dose often needed. Titrate methadone to effect.
Etravirine (ETR)	No significant change in S-methadone and R-methadone AUC. ETR pharmacokinetic parameters were comparable to historical control.	Use standard dose. Monitor for withdrawal.
Fluconazole	Fluconazole increases methadone AUC by 35%, but no sign of toxicity observed.	Monitor patients for effects of increased methadone effects when adding or discontinuing fluconazole.
Fosamprenavir (FPV)	Not studied but may decrease serum levels of APV and methadone. No withdrawal symptoms observed with APV coadministration.	Dose adjustments unlikely to be needed.
Indinavir (IDV)	No interaction.	No dose adjustment needed.
Lopinavir/ritonavir (LPV/r)	May decrease methadone concentrations 26%–36%.	Conflicting data: monitor for need to increase methadone dose. Some patients may require an increase in methadone dose.
Maraviroc (MVC)	Interaction unlikely.	Use standard dose.
Nelfinavir (NFV)	Decreased in methadone levels, but active isomer not significantly affected.	Dose adjustments unlikely to be needed.
Nevirapine (NVP)	Methadone AUC decreased by 46%.	Increase in methadone dose often needed. Titrate methadone to effect.
Phenobarbital	May significantly decrease methadone serum concentrations.	Monitor for withdrawal signs and Sx. May require methadone dose increase or switch to an alternative anticonvulsant (e.g., valproic acid or levetiracetam).
Phenytoin	May significantly decrease methadone serum concentrations.	Monitor for withdrawal signs and Sx. May require methadone dose increase or switch to alternative anticonvulsant (e.g., valproic acid or levetiracetam).
Raltegravir (RAL)	Interaction unlikely.	Use standard dose.
Rifabutin (RFB)	No change in methadone levels.	Preferred rifamycin with methadone coadministration.
Rifampin	Decreases methadone AUC by up to 65%.	Avoid coadministration. Monitor patients for withdrawal symptoms. Dose adjustments may be needed. Consider RFB with methadone coadministration.

METHADONE *(cont.)*

Drug	Effect of Interaction	Recommendations/Comments
Ritonavir (RTV)	Methadone AUC decreased 36% (studied with RTV 500 mg q12h).	With lower RTV dose, interaction dependent on coadministered PIs.
Saquinavir (SQV)	S-methadone AUC decreased 25%. R-methadone AUC decreased 20% (studied with SQV/RTV 400/400 mg twice daily).	Use standard SQV/r dose. Monitor for withdrawal with coadministration.
Stavudine (d4T)	d4T AUC decreased by 27%.	Interaction may not be clinically significant; dose adjustment not needed.
Tenofovir (TDF)	No effect.	Use standard dose.
Tipranavir/ ritonavir (TPV/r)	Methadone (active) AUC decreased by 50%.	Monitor for withdrawal signs and Sx. Methadone stereoisomer not specified, but may require methadone dose increase.
Voriconazole	Methadone AUC by up to 57%.	Monitor pats for effects of increased methadone effects when adding or discontinuing voriconazole.
Zidovudine (AZT)	AZT AUC increased by 43%.	Clinical implications unknown; monitor for symptoms of AZT toxicity.

DRUG-DRUG INTERACTION – METRONIDAZOLE

Drug	Effect of Interaction	Recommendations/Comments
Barbiturates	May decrease metronidazole serum concentrations.	Monitor for clinical response to metronidazole with coadministration.
Lithium	Lithium serum concentrations may be increased.	Monitor lithium serum concentrations closely with coadministration.
Lopinavir/ Lopinavir (LPV/r)	Alcohol content in the LPV/r liquid formulation may cause a disulfiram-like reaction.	Avoid coadministration (liquid formulation of LPV/r).
Phenytoin	Phenytoin serum concentrations may be increased.	Monitor phenytoin serum concentrations with coadministration.
Ritonavir (RTV)	Alcohol content in the RTV liquid formulation may cause a disulfiram-like reaction.	Avoid coadministration.
Tipranavir (TPV)	Alcohol content in the TPV caps formulation may cause a disulfiram-like reaction.	Avoid coadministration.
Warfarin	INR may be increased.	Monitor INR closely with coadministration.

DRUG-DRUG INTERACTION – NELFINAVIR (NFV)

Drug	Effect of Interaction	Recommendations/Comments
Alfuzosin	May increase alfuzosin serum concentrations.	Contraindicated. Consider doxazosin and terazosin for BPH (with close monitoring).
Alprazolam	May increase serum levels of alprazolam.	Applies to all PIs: consider alternative benzodiazepine (i.e., lorazepam, oxazepam, or temazepam).
Amiodarone	May significantly increase amiodarone serum levels.	Applies to all PIs: data limited to case report of increased amiodarone levels with IDV coadministration. RTV, APV, and ATV manufacturers recommend against use of amiodarone, but all PIs have the same potential of significantly increasing amiodarone serum levels. If coadministration cannot be avoided, monitor for amiodarone ADR (PFTs and TSH). Consider monitoring serum levels of amiodarone, but its long half-life may make titration difficult.
Amlodipine	May increase serum levels of amlodipine.	Applies to all PIs: data limited to an interaction study conducted with ATV and diltiazem, which resulted in doubling of diltiazem serum levels (this led to PR interval prolongation). All PIs have the potential of prolonging PR interval with calcium channel blocker coadministration. Calcium channel blockers should be started with 50% of the dose and slowly titrated with close monitoring of BP and pulse.
Artemether (artemisinin)	May increase serum levels of artemether.	Applies to all PIs: close monitoring for artemether toxicity (bone marrow suppression, bradycardia, and seizure).
Astemizole	May significantly increase astemizole serum levels.	Contraindicated due to the potential for cardiac arrhythmias. Recommended alternative antihistamine: loratadine, fexofenadine, desloratidine, or cetirizine.
Atorvastatin	Atorvastatin AUC increased by 74%.	Use with caution. Monitor for adverse effects (LFTs and CPK). Consider alternative agents: pravastatin, fluvastatin, or rosuvastatin.
Azathioprine	Interaction unlikely.	Applies to all PIs and NNRTI: use standard dose.
Azithromycin	NFV not significantly affected. Azithromycin AUC increased by 100%.	Monitor for azithromycin adverse drug reaction (reversible ototoxicity and elevated LFTs).

NELFINAVIR *(cont.)*

Drug	Effect of Interaction	Recommendations/Comments
Bepridil	May significantly increase bepridil serum levels.	Applies to all PIs: no data. The manufacturer of ATV, RTV, and FPV does not recommend bepridil coadministration. This contraindication should extend to all PIs since a significant increase in bepridil serum level can result in pro-arrhythmic events such as VT, PVC, and VFib.
Bosentan	May significantly increase bosentan serum concentrations.	Significant bosentan dose reduction needed.
Bupropion	May increase bupropion serum levels slightly.	Not likely to be clinically significant. Start with the lowest possible dose of bupropion. In a small case series, no seizures reported with coadministration.
Carbamazepine	May significantly decrease serum levels of NFV.	Consider alternative anticonvulsants (i.e., valproic acid, lamotrigine, levetiracetam, or topiramate). Monitor carbamazepine levels and consider TDM of NFV.
Caspofungin	Caspofungin serum levels were not affected. NFV not measured.	Use standard dose.
Chlordiazepoxide	May increase serum levels of chlordiazepoxide.	Applies to all PIs: consider alternative benzodiazepine (lorazepam, oxazepam, or temazepam).
Cisapride	May significantly increase cisapride serum levels.	Contraindicated due to potential for cardiac arrhythmias. Recommended alternative: metoclopramide.
Clorazepate	May increase serum levels of clorazepate.	Applies to all PIs: consider an alternative benzodiazepine (lorazepam, oxazepam, or temazepam).
Cyclophosphamide	May increase serum levels of cyclophosphamide.	Applies to all PIs: data limited to an interaction study conducted with IDV resulting in a 50% increase in cyclophosphamide serum levels. Since all PIs have the potential of increasing cyclophosphamide levels, close monitoring of cyclophosphamide-induced toxicity is recommended.
Cyclosporine	May significantly increase serum levels of cyclosporine.	Applies to all PIs: monitor serum levels of cyclosporine closely with coadministration. Cyclosporine dose may need to be decreased.
Depo-medroxy-progesterone Acetate (DMPA)	NFV and M8 metabolite were not affected. DMPA levels were not reported.	No evidence of ovulation occurring based on progesterone levels through wk 12. Use standard dose with coadministration.

Drug	Effect of Interaction	Recommendations/Comments
Diazepam	May increase diazepam serum concentrations.	Diazepam dose reduction may be needed. Consider lorazepam, temazepam, or oxazepam.
Diltiazem	May increase serum levels of diltiazem.	Applies to all PIs: data limited to an interaction study conducted with ATV, which resulted in doubling of diltiazem serum levels (this led to PR interval prolongation). All PIs have the potential of prolonging the PR interval with diltiazem coadministration. Diltiazem should be started with 50% of the dose and slowly titrated with close monitoring of BP and pulse.
Disopyramide	May increase disopyramide serum levels.	Applies to all PIs: no data. Monitor disopyramide serum levels (target: 2 to 7.5 mcg/mL).
Docetaxel	May increase serum levels of docetaxel.	Applies to all PIs: no data. Close monitoring of chemotherapy-induced toxicity recommended.
Dofetilide	May significantly increase serum levels of dofetilide.	No data. Applies to all PIs: No data. Use with caution. Monitor QTc closely and adjust dofetilide dosing based on QTc prolongation and renal function. Consider an alternative class III antiarrhythmic such as bretylium or ibutilide.
Dronabinol	No significant interaction.	Use standard dose.
Echinacea	May decrease NFV serum levels. Echinacea decreased CYP3A4 substrate (midazolam) by 23%.	Clinical significance unknown but should be avoided with all PIs and NNRTIs until its safety is further evaluated.
Efavirenz (EFV)	NFV AUC increased by 20%. EFV levels unchanged.	No significant drug interaction. Use standard doses of both drugs.
Ergot Alkaloid	May significantly increase serum levels of ergotamine resulting in acute ergot toxicity.	Contraindicated. Consider alternative agent for migraine such as sumatriptan (but not eletriptan since it is a CYP3A4 substrate and significant drug-drug interaction occurred with CYP3A4 inhibitor).
Estazolam	May increase serum levels of estazolam.	Applies to all PIs: consider alternative benzodiazepines (lorazepam, oxazepam, or temazepam).
Ethinyl Estradiol and Northindrone	Ethinyl estradiol AUC decreased by 47%, northindrone decreased by 18%.	Advise patients to use additional or alternative method of contraception.
Ethosuximide	May increase serum levels of ethosuximide.	Applies to all PIs: consider switching to valproic acid for the treatment of absence seizure.

NELFINAVIR *(cont.)*

Drug	Effect of Interaction	Recommendations/Comments
Etoposide	May increase serum levels of etoposide.	Applies to all PIs: no data. Close monitoring of chemotherapy-induced toxicity recommended.
Etravirine (ETR)	NFV serum concentrations may be increased.	Consider usual dose, but no PK data.
Felodipine	May increase serum levels of felodipine.	Applies to all PIs: data limited to study conducted with ATV and diltiazem, which resulted in doubling of diltiazem serum levels (this led to PR interval prolongation). All PIs have the potential of prolonging the PR interval with calcium channel blocker coadministration. Calcium channel blockers should be started with 50% of the dose and slowly titrated with close monitoring of BP and pulse.
Fentanyl	May increase fentanyl serum levels.	Use with caution. Consider morphine.
Flecainide	May increase antiarrhythmic serum levels.	Applies to all PIs: avoid coadministration; if necessary, monitor flecainide trough levels with coadministration. Target: 200–1000 ng/mL. Toxicity is frequent with trough serum levels above 1000 ng/mL.
Fluconazole	NFV AUC increased by 30%.	Use standard dose.
Flurazepam	May increase serum levels of flurazepam.	Applies to all PIs: consider alternative benzodiazepines (lorazepam, oxazepam, or temazepam).
Fluticasone	Fluticasone may be significantly increased.	Avoid long term coadministration. Consider beclomethasone.
Food	NFV AUC increased by 2-fold with 125 kcal with 20% fat meal. NFV AUC increased 5-fold 1000 kcal with 50% fatty meal.	NFV must be taken with a fatty meal (a minimum of 500 kcal with 20% fat).
Fosamprenavir (FPV)	APV increased 1.5-fold.	Insufficient data for dose recommendation.
Garlic Supplement	49% and 51% reduction of SQV Cmin and AUC, respectively.	Studies only done with SQV. Effect of garlic on the PK parameters of NFV is not known. Avoid coadministration with PIs and NNRTIs until it can be further studied.
Granisetron	May increase serum levels of granisetron.	Applies to all PIs: due to the large therapeutic index of granisetron, potential interaction is unlikely to be clinically significant.

Drug	Effect of Interaction	Recommendations/Comments
Heroin (diamorphine)	Drug interactions unlikely.	Applies to PIs and NNRTIs: interaction unlikely but illicit drug use should be avoided for obvious reasons.
Indinavir (IDV)	IDV AUC increased by 51%; NFV AUC increased by 83%.	Limited data for dosing IDV 1200 mg twice daily + NFV 1250 mg twice daily.
Ifosphamide	May increase serum levels of ifosphamide.	Applies to all PIs: no data. Close monitoring of chemotherapy-induced toxicity recommended.
Irinotecan	May increase irinotecan serum levels.	Applies to all PIs: coadministration of ATV is contraindicated by manufacturer. All PIs also have the potential for significant interaction with irinotecan, therefore the coadministration should be done with extreme caution.
Itraconazole	CYP3A4 inhibitor and substrate-bidirectional inhibition with the potential to increase levels of itraconazole and coadministered PI.	No data with NFV. Standard dose NFV likely. Consider monitoring itraconazole with coadministration.
Ketoconazole	NFV AUC increased by 35%.	Use standard dose.
Lidocaine	May increase antiarrhythmic serum levels.	Applies to all PIs: no data. Use with caution, monitor lidocaine serum levels (target: 1.5 to 6 mcg/mL) with coadministration.
Lopinavir/ritonavir (LPV/r)	LPV AUC decreased by 27%; NFV Cmin increased by 113%.	Avoid coadministration or consider increasing LPV/r dose to 3 tabs twice daily with NFV coadministration (no data).
Lovastatin	May significantly increase lovastatin levels.	Contraindicated. Recommended alternatives include pravastatin, rosuvastatin, and fluvastatin (and possibly atorvastatin—start with 10 mg/day and monitor for myopathy).
Maraviroc (MVC)	May increase serum concentrations of MVC.	No data, but dose reduction of MVC to 150 mg twice daily should be considered.
Mefloquine	May increase serum levels of mefloquine.	Applies to all PIs: consider monitoring mefloquine levels and mefloquine-induced toxicity (i.e., dizziness, LFTs, and periodic ophthalmic examination).
Methadone	Decreased serum levels of inactive methadone (S)-isomer. No change in active methadone R-isomer.	Use standard dose. No withdrawal symptoms observed.

NELFINAVIR (cont.)

Drug	Effect of Interaction	Recommendations/Comments
Mexiletine	May increase antiarrhythmic serum levels.	Applies to all PIs: no data. Use with caution. Monitor EKG and serum levels. Serum levels exceeding 1.5 to 2 mcg/mL have been associated with an increased risk of toxicity.
Midazolam	May significantly increase midazolam levels.	Do not coadminister. Consider alternative benzodiazepines (temazepam, oxazepam, or lorazepam).
Milk Thistle	Data limited to interaction study with milk thistle and IDV. IDV AUC: unchanged; IDV Cmin: decreased by 25%.	Clinical significance unknown. Unknown effect on the metabolism of other PIs or NNRTIs. Avoid coadministration with PIs and NNRTIs until it can be further evaluated.
Mirtazapine	May increase serum levels of mirtazapine.	Applies to all PIs: use with caution. Consider an alternative antidepressant (i.e., SSRI: escitalopram, citalopram, sertraline, or fluoxetine).
Mycophenolate	NFV AUC decreased by 32%; NFV-M8 metabolite decreased by 32%.	Clinical significance unknown. Proper dosing has not been established. Consider an alternative boosted PI.
Nefazodone	May increase serum levels of nefazodone.	Applies to all PIs: use with caution. Consider an alternative antidepressant (i.e., SSRI: escitalopram, citalopram, sertraline, or fluoxetine).
Nevirapine (NVP)	No significant drug interaction.	Use standard dose of both drugs.
Nifedipine	May increase serum levels of nifedipine.	Applies to all PIs: data limited to an interaction study conducted with ATV and diltiazem, which resulted in doubling of diltiazem serum levels (this led to PR interval prolongation). All PIs have the potential of prolonging PR interval with calcium channel blocker coadministration. Calcium channel blockers should be started with 50% of the dose and slowly titrated with close monitoring of BP and pulse.
Nisoldipine	May increase serum levels of nisoldipine.	Applies to all PIs: data limited to an interaction study conducted with ATV and diltiazem, which resulted in doubling of diltiazem serum levels (this led to PR interval prolongation). All PIs have the potential of prolonging PR interval with calcium channel blocker coadministration. Calcium channel blockers should be started with 50% of the dose and slowly titrated with close monitoring of BP and pulse.

Drug	Effect of Interaction	Recommendations/Comments
Paclitaxel	May increase paclitaxel serum levels.	Applies to all PIs: since all PIs have the potential of significantly increasing paclitaxel serum levels, close monitoring of paclitaxel-induced toxicity is recommended.
Phencyclidine (PCP)	May significantly increase serum levels of PCP.	Applies to all PIs. Illicit drug use should be avoided for obvious reasons.
Phenobarbital	May significantly decrease serum levels of NFV.	Consider alternative anticonvulsants (i.e., valproic acid, lamotrigine, levetiracetam, or topiramate). Monitor phenobarbital levels and consider TDM of NFV.
Phenytoin	Phenytoin AUC decreased by 20%–40%; no change in NFV AUC.	Monitor phenytoin levels, may need to increase phenytoin dose. Consider valproic acid or levetiracetem.
Pimozide	May significantly increase pimozide serum levels resulting in QTc prolongation.	Contraindicated. Consider alternative: olanzapine.
Pravastatin	Pravastatin AUC decreased with coadministration.	Clinical significance unknown. May need to increase dose of pravastatin.
Propafenone	May increase antiarrhythmic serum levels.	Applies to all PIs: no data. Coadministration should be avoided. Serum levels are not routinely recommended due to the poor correlation with efficacy and toxicity.
Proton Pump Inhibitors (PPI)	NFV and M8 metabolite AUC decreased by 36% and 92%, respectively.	Contraindicated.
Quinidine	May increase antiarrhythmic serum levels.	Applies to all PIs: no data. Contraindicated with RTV. With all Ps and NNRTI coadministration, monitor EKG (QTc) and serum levels: target: 2 to 5 mcg/mL.
Raltegravir (RAL)	NFV may induce RAL's metabolism.	RAL 400 mg twice daily currently recommended, but no PK data.
Ranolazine	May significantly increase ranolazine serum concentrations.	Contraindicated. May increase risk of QTc prolongation.
Rifabutin (RFB)	NFV AUC decreased by 32%; RFB levels increased by 207%.	If coadministration required, dose NFV to 1000 mg PO 3 ×/day with RFB to 150 mg PO once daily or 300 mg 3 ×/wk.
Rifampin	NFV AUC decreased by 82%.	Coadministration not recommended.
Rifapentine	NFV serum levels may be significantly decreased.	Avoid coadministration. Consider using RFB.

NELFINAVIR (cont.)

Drug	Effect of Interaction	Recommendations/Comments
Ritonavir (RTV)	NFV AUC increased by 150%, Cmax by 95%.	Limited data: RTV 400 mg twice daily and NFV 500 mg or 750 mg twice daily. Generally not combined since boosting with RTV will yield only minimal PK enhancement of NFV serum concentrations at the expense of GI intolerance.
Rosiglitazone	NFV AUC increased by 14% and Cmin increased by 18% (NS) (n = 3).	No significant interaction. Use standard dose.
Rosuvastatin	Other CYP3A4 inhibitor (i.e., erythromycin) did not affect rosuvastatin serum level.	Applies to PIs and NNRTI. In one study, rosuvastatin AUC and Cmax increased when coadministered with LPV. Clinical significance unknown and no data available with other PIs and NNRTIs. Close monitoring recommended due to limited clinical data.
Saquinavir (SQV)	SQV sgc AUC increased by 3–5 fold; NFV AUC increased by 18% and Cmax not altered.	Dose NFV 1250 mg twice daily + SQV 1200 mg twice daily or NFV 750 mg 3 ×/day + SQV 800 mg 3 ×/day.
Sildenafil	May increase sildenafil levels. No change in NFV serum levels.	Use with caution. Do not exceed 25 mg of sildenafil in 48 hrs.
Simvastatin	Simvastatin AUC increased by 506%.	Contraindicated. Alternatives include pravastatin, fluvastatin, and atorvastatin (start with 10 mg/day). Monitor for ADRs due to limited clinical data.
Sirolimus	Case report of sirolimus Cmin increased by 5-fold with NFV coadministration.	Dose sirolimus based on serum levels. A significantly reduction of sirolimus dose with NFV coadministration is recommended.
St. John's wort	May significantly decrease NFV serum levels.	Contraindicated. Studies done with IDV and NVP but St. John's wort may affect the metabolism of other PIs and NNRTIs. Use an alternative (more effective) antidepressant.
Tacrolimus	Case report of increased tacrolimus serum levels with NFV coadministration.	Dose tacrolimus based on serum levels. A significantly reduction of tacrolimus dose with NFV coadministration is recommended.
Tadalafil	May increase serum levels of tadalafil.	Applies to all PIs: start with 5 mg. Do not exceed 10 mg in 72 hrs. Consider sildenafil due to more clinical data and shorter half-life allowing for easier titration.

Drug	Effect of Interaction	Recommendations/Comments
Tamoxifen	May increase serum levels of tamoxifen.	Applies to all PIs: no data. Close monitoring of tamoxifen-induced toxicity recommended.
Teniposide	May increase serum levels of teniposide.	Applies to all PIs: no data. Close monitoring of teniposide-induced toxicity recommended.
Terfenadine	May significantly increase terfenadine serum levels.	Contraindicated due to the potential for cardiac arrhythmias. Recommended alternative antihistamine: loratadine, fexofenadine, desloratidine, or cetirizine.
Tetrahydrocannabinol (THC)	No interactions.	No drug interactions but illicit drug use should be avoided for obvious reasons.
Trazodone	May increase serum levels of trazodone.	Applies to all PIs: use with caution. Consider an alternative antidepressant (i.e., SSRI: escitalopram, citalopram, sertraline, or fluoxetine).
Triazolam	May significantly increase triazolam serum levels.	Contraindicated. Consider alternative benzodiazepines (temazepam, oxazepam, or lorazepam).
Vardenafil	May significantly increase serum levels of vardenafil.	Applies to all PIs: do not exceed vardenafil 2.5 mg in 72 hrs (with RTV) or 2.5 mg in 24 hrs (with other PIs). Consider sildenafil due to more clinical data and less pronounced interaction. Avoid coadministration with IDV.
Verapamil	May increase serum levels of verapamil.	Applies to all PIs: data limited to an interaction study conducted with ATV and diltiazem, which resulted in doubling of diltiazem serum levels (this led to PR interval prolongation). All PIs have the potential of prolonging the PR interval with calcium channel blockers coadministration. Calcium channel blockers should be started with 50% of the dose and slowly titrated with close monitoring of BP and pulse.
Vinblastine	May increase serum levels of vinblastine.	Applies to all PIs: no data. Close monitoring of vinblastine-induced toxicity recommended.
Vincristine	May increase serum levels of vincristine.	Applies to all PIs: no data. Close monitoring of vincristine-induced toxicity recommended.
Vitamin C	Data limited to interaction study with IDV and vitamin C (1 g/day): IDV AUC decreased by 14% and Cmin by 32%.	Clinical significance unknown. Data not available for other PIs or NNRTIs.

NELFINAVIR *(cont.)*

Drug	Effect of Interaction	Recommendations/Comments
Voriconazole	May decrease voriconazole AUC. Voriconazole may increase NFV levels.	Significant interaction with EFV and RTV (400 mg twice daily) but not IDV, data with other PIs and NNRTIs are not available and should be used with caution. In severe cases of invasive aspergillosis where voriconazole is clearly the first-line agent, the authors recommend voriconazole TDM ($\pm$ addition of another antifungal for aspergillosis i.e., *AmBisome* or caspofungin). Target voriconazole Cmin >2 mcg/mL.
Warfarin	Case report of increased INR when coadministered with IDV.	Other PIs and NNRTIs may affect warfarin requirements. Monitor INR closely.

DRUG-DRUG INTERACTION – NEVIRAPINE (NVP)

Drug	Effect of Interaction	Recommendations/Comments
Amiodarone	Serum levels of amiodarone may be decreased.	Clinical significance unknown. Dose adjustment of coadministered drug may be needed with titration to effect.
Artemether (artemisinin)	May decrease serum levels of artemether.	Applies to EFV and NVP. Coadministration of artesunate and amodiaquine may result in significant LFT elevations. Close monitoring of artemether therapeutic efficacy recommended (i.e., parasite count on blood smear and clinical signs and symptoms of clinical improvement).
Atazanavir (ATV)	ATV decreased 42%. NVP increased by 46% (compared with historical control).	Coadministration not recommended.
Azathioprine	Interaction unlikely.	Applies to all PIs and NNRTIs: use standard dose.
Carbamazepine	May decrease serum levels of NVP and carbamazepine.	Consider alternative anticonvulsants (i.e., valproic acid, lamotrigine, levetiracetam, or topiramate). With coadministration, monitor anticonvulsants level and consider TDM of NNRTIs.
Caspofungin	May decrease caspofungin serum levels.	Monitor for caspofungin for therapeutic failure, may need to increase dose to 70 mg/day.
Cimetidine	NVP Cmin increased by 21%.	No significant interaction. Use standard dose.

Drug	Effect of Interaction	Recommendations/Comments
Clarithromycin	Clarithromycin AUC decreased by 29% but 14-hydroxy clarithromycin AUC increased by 27%. NVP AUC increased by 26%.	No dose modification needed. Consider azithromycin for treatment or prophylaxis of MAC.
Clonazepam	May decrease serum levels of clonazepam.	Consider alternative anticonvulsants (i.e., valproic acid, levetiracetam, or topiramate).
Cocaine	May theoretically increase serum levels of hepatotoxic metabolite.	Avoid illicit drug use for obvious reasons.
Cyclophosphamide	Serum concentrations of coadministered drug may be decreased.	Clinical significance unknown. Monitor serum concentrations of immunosuppressant with dose adjustment if needed.
Cyclosporine	Serum concentrations of cyclosporine drug may be significantly decreased.	Clinical significance unknown. Monitor serum concentrations of immunosuppressant with dose adjustment if needed.
Darunavir/ ritonavir (DRV/r)	Based on observational data, NVP AUC decreased by 27%. No change in DRV AUC.	Dose: DRV/r 600/100 mg twice daily plus standard dose NVP.
Depo-medroxy- progesterone Acetate (DMPA)	NVP AUC slightly increased with DMPA coadministration. DMPA levels were not reported.	No evidence of ovulation based on progesterone levels through wk 12. Small increase in NVP AUC not likely to be significant.
Diltiazem	NVP may decrease diltiazem serum concentrations.	Titrate diltiazem to therapeutic effect with NVP coadministration.
Disopyramide	Serum concentrations of disopyramide may be decreased.	No data. Clinical significance unknown. Monitor disopyramide serum concentrations (target: 2 to 7.5 mcg/mL).
Docetaxel	May decrease serum concentrations of docetaxel.	Applies to EFV and NVP: no data. Docetaxel dose may need to be increased.
Echinacea	May decrease NVP serum level. Echinacea (400 mg 4 ×/day) decreased CYP3A4 substrate (midazolam) by 23%.	Clinical significance unknown but should be avoided until the safety of this combination is further evaluated.
Efavirenz (EFV)	EFV AUC: decreased by 22%; Cmin: decreased by 36%.	Coadministration not recommended due to overlapping resistance profile and potential for increased toxicity.
Ergot Alkaloid	Serum levels of coadministered drug may be decreased.	Clinical significance unknown. Consider sumatriptan.
Ethinyl Estradiol/ Norethindrone	Ethinyl estradiol: AUC decreased by 23%; norethindrone: AUC decreased by 18%.	Patients should use alternative form of birth control methods (i.e., barrier contraceptive method).

NEVIRAPINE *(cont.)*

Drug	Effect of Interaction	Recommendations/Comments
Ethosuximide	May decrease serum levels of ethosuximide.	Consider switching to valproic acid for treatment of absence seizure.
Etoposide	May decrease serum concentrations of etoposide.	Applies to EFV and NVP: no data. Etoposide dose may need to be increased.
Fentanyl	Serum concentrations of coadministered drug may be decreased.	Clinical significance unknown. Dose adjustment of coadministered drug may be needed. Consider other opiates (i.e., morphine or oxycodone).
Fluconazole	NVP clearance decreased by 2-fold; no significant effect on fluconazole levels.	Data limited to an interaction study with 24 HIV+ patients; 25% developed elevated transaminates (5 × UNL). Recommend monitoring for liver toxicity and NVP levels.
Food	NVP AUC not affected.	Administer NVP with or without food.
Fosamprenavir (FPV)	May decrease APV levels.	Clinical significance unknown. Dose: FPV/r 700/100 mg twice daily with coadministration (limited data).
Garlic Supplement	No data.	Studies only done with SQV resulting in reduction of SQV levels. Avoid coadministration.
Heroin (diamorphine)	Drug interaction unlikely.	Applies to PIs and NNRTIs: interaction unlikely but illicit drug use should be avoided for obvious reasons.
Indinavir (IDV)	IDV AUC: decreased by 28%.	Clinical trials demonstrated good efficacy with standard dose. Consider increasing the dose of IDV to 1000 mg q8h (or IDV/r 800/100 mg twice daily) with NVP coadministration.
Ifosphamide	May decrease serum concentrations of ifosphamide.	Applies to EFV and NVP: no data. Ifosphamide dose may need to be increased.
Itraconazole	Serum concentrations of itraconazole may be decreased.	Clinical significance unknown. Dose adjustment of coadministered drug may be needed.
Ketoconazole	Ketoconazole AUC decreased by 72%; NVP levels increased by 15%–30%.	Coadministration not recommended. Consider alternative antifungal (i.e., fluconazole).
Lidocaine (systemic)	Serum concentrations of lidocaine may be decreased.	No data. Clinical significance unknown. Dose adjustment of coadministered drug may be needed. Monitor serum levels (target: 1.5 to 6 mcg/mL) with coadministration.

Drug	Effect of Interaction	Recommendations/Comments
Lopinavir/ritonavir (LPV/r)	LPV AUC: decreased by 22%; Cmin: decreased by 55%.	Consider increasing dose of LPV to 600/150 mg (3 tabs) twice daily or 6.5 mL twice daily, especially in patients with PI resistance. Standard doses may be adequate in PI-naive patients.
Maraviroc (MVC)	MVC serum concentration was not significantly affected compared to historical controls in a single dose study; however, MVC AUC may be decreased at steady state.	Consider MVC 300 mg twice daily plus NVP 200 mg twice daily.
Mefloquine	May decrease serum concentrations of mefloquine.	Monitor mefloquine serum concentrations. Close monitoring of mefloquine therapeutic efficacy (i.e., parasite count on blood smear and clinical signs and Sx of clinical improvement).
Methadone	Methadone AUC: decreased by 46%–51%.	Monitor for signs and Sx of methadone withdrawal (methadone withdrawal observed one wk into therapy); some patients may need an increase in the methadone dose.
Milk Thistle	No data.	Data limited to an interaction study with milk thistle and IDV. IDV AUC unchanged; IDV Cmin decreased by 47%. Clinical significance unknown. Avoid coadministration.
Mycophenolate	NVP clearance increased by 27%.	Clinical significance unknown. Unlikely to be significant.
Nelfinavir (NFV)	No significant drug interaction.	Dose: NVP 200 mg twice daily + NFV 1250 mg twice daily.
Nifedipine	NVP may decrease nifedipine serum concentrations.	Titrate nifedipine to therapeutic effect with NVP coadministration.
Paclitaxel	Case report states no dose adjustments necessary if KS treated with paclitaxel dose of 100 mg/m^2.	Monitor for chemotherapeutic response.
Phenobarbital	May decrease serum concentrations of NVP and phenobarbital.	Consider alternative anticonvulsants (i.e., valproic acid, lamotrigine, levetiracetam, or topiramate). With coadministration, monitor anticonvulsants levels.
Phenytoin	May decrease serum levels of NVP and phenytoin.	Consider alternative anticonvulsants (i.e., valproic acid, lamotrigine, levetiracetam, or topiramate). With coadministration, monitor anticonvulsants level and consider TDM of NVP.

DRUG-DRUG INTERACTIONS

NEVIRAPINE (cont.)

Drug	Effect of Interaction	Recommendations/Comments
Rifabutin (RFB)	RFB AUC increased by 16% (NS) NVP AUC unchanged.	Unlikely to be clinically significant. Monitor for RFB-associated ADRs. Standard dose: RFB 300 mg/day or 300 mg 3 ×/wk.
Rifampin	NVP Cmin: decreased by 37%–68%; NVP AUC: decreased by 37%–58%. Rifampin AUC increased 11% (NS).	Coadministration not recommended. RFB with NVP OR rifampin with EFV can be considered. NVP dose escalation not needed if rifampin at steady-state. Case series of favorable outcome with NVP 200 mg twice daily with rifampin 600 mg once daily has been published (Oliva et al. *AIDS* 2003;17:637), but higher rates of virologic failure reported in large cohorts (Boulle A. *JAMA* 2008;300:530). Although NVP 300 mg twice daily may result in better PK, a randomized trial comparing standard-dose NVP (200 mg twice daily) to a higher dose (300 mg twice daily) among patients on rifampin demonstrated increased risk of NVP hypersensitivity among patients receiving high-dose NVP.
Rifapentine	NVP serum levels may be significantly decreased.	Avoid coadministration. Consider using RFB.
Ritonavir (RTV)	RTV AUC decreased by 11%.	Not clinically significant. Use standard dose.
Rosiglitazone	NVP AUC decreased by 31%, Cmin decreased by 36% (p = 0.032) (n = 4).	Clinical significance unknown. Consider alternative agent EFV (no interaction).
Rosuvastatin	Interaction unlikely.	Data limited to one drug interaction study with LPV and TPV showing that rosuvastatin were increased. LPV and RTV PK parameters were not significantly affected. Effect on NVP PK unknown. Close monitoring recommended due to limited clinical data.
Saquinavir (SQV)	SQV AUC: decreased by 38%.	Boost SQV with RTV (SQV 1000 mg + RTV 1000 mg twice daily).
Sirolimus	May significantly decrease serum concentrations of sirolimus.	Applies to EFV and NVP: dose sirolimus based on serum concentrations. May need to increase sirolimus dose.
St. John's wort	NVP clearance: increased by 35%.	Do not coadminister.
Tacrolimus	May significantly decrease serum concentrations of tacrolimus.	Applies to EFV and NVP: dose tacrolimus based on serum concentrations. May need to increase tacrolimus dose.

Drug	Effect of Interaction	Recommendations/Comments
Teniposide	May decrease serum concentrations of teniposide.	Applies to EFV and NVP: no data. Monitor for chemotherapeutic response. Teniposide dose may need to be increased.
Tetrahydrocannabinol (THC)	Based on data with NFV and IDV interactions are unlikely.	Applies to PIs and NNRTIs: interactions are unlikely but illicit drug use should be avoided for obvious reasons.
Tipranavir (TPV)	May decrease TPV serum concentrations. No change in NVP concentrations (observational data).	Dose: TPV/r 500/200 mg twice daily plus standard dose NVP.
Verapamil	NVP may decrease verapamil serum concentrations.	Titrate verapamil to therapeutic effect with NVP coadministration.
Vinblastine	May decrease serum concentrations of vinblastine.	Applies to EFV and NVP: no data. Monitor for chemotherapeutic response. Vinblastine dose may need to be increased.
Vincristine	May decrease serum concentrations of vincristine.	Applies to EFV and NVP: no data. Monitor for chemotherapeutic response. Vincristine dose may need to be increased.
Voriconazole	Serum concentrations of voriconazole may be significantly decreased. Voriconazole may increase NVP serum concentrations.	Avoid or use with voriconazole TDM. D (target Cmin >2 mcg/mL). Dose adjustment of voriconazole may be needed.
Warfarin	Warfarin plasma concentrations may be increased (per manufacturer), but case reports of need for increased dose of warfarin in patients taking NVP have been published.	Clinical significance unknown. Monitor INR closely with NVP coadministration.

Drug-Drug Interaction – Posaconazole

Drug	Effect of Interaction	Recommendations/Comments
Alprazolam	Alprazolam serum concentrations may be increased.	Consider lorazepam, oxazepam, or temazepam.
Amiodarone	Amiodarone serum concentrations may be increased.	Avoid or use with close monitoring.
Amlodipine	Amlodipine serum concentrations may be increased.	Avoid or use with close monitoring.
Astemizole	Risk of QTc prolongation may be increased.	Contraindicated.

POSACONAZOLE *(cont.)*

Drug	Effect of Interaction	Recommendations/Comments
Atazanavir (ATV)	May increase posaconazole and ATV serum concentrations. Posaconazole increased ATV AUC by ~3-fold.	Clinical significance unclear; use standard doses with close monitoring. Use with caution in patients with QTc prolongation.
Bismuth	No significant interaction.	No dose adjustment necessary.
Carbamazepine	Carbamazepine serum concentrations may be increased.	Monitor carbamazepine serum concentrations closely with coadministration.
Cimetidine	Posaconazole AUC decreased by 39%.	Avoid coadministration. Use an alternative H2 blocker.
Cisapride	Risk of QTc prolongation may be increased.	Contraindicated.
Cyclosporine	Cyclosporine serum concentrations may be increased.	Reduce cyclosporine dose by 25% with TDM.
Diazepam	Diazepam serum concentrations may be increased.	Consider lorazepam, oxazepam, or temazepam.
Digoxin	May increase digoxin serum concentrations.	Monitor digoxin serum concentrations with coadministration.
Diltiazem	Diltiazem serum concentrations may be increased.	Avoid or use with close monitoring.
Dofetilide	Dofetilide serum concentrations may be increased.	Avoid or use with close monitoring.
Efavirenz (EFV)	May increase EFV serum concentrations.	Clinical significance unclear. Avoid concomitant use unless the benefit outweighs the risks.
Ergot Alkaloids	Ergot alkaloid serum levels may be increased.	Contraindicated.
Esomeprazole	May decrease posaconazole.	Use with caution. Posaconazole TDM recommended.
Etravirine (ETR)	May decrease posaconazole serum concentrations.	Use with close monitoring for therapeutic efficacy.
Famotidine	No significant interaction.	No dose adjustment necessary.
Felodipine	Felodipine serum concentrations may be increased.	Avoid or use with close monitoring.
Glimepiride	No significant interaction.	No dose adjustment necessary.
Glipizide	No significant interaction.	No dose adjustment necessary.
Glyburide	No significant interaction.	No dose adjustment necessary.
Halofantrine	Risk of QTc prolongation may be increased.	Contraindicated.
Indinavir (IDV)	May increase posaconazole serum concentrations.	Clinical significance unclear; use standard doses.

Drug	Effect of Interaction	Recommendations/Comments
Irinotecan	Irinotecan serum concentrations may be increased.	Avoid or use with close monitoring.
Lansoprazole	May decrease posaconazole.	Use with caution. Posaconazole TDM recommended.
Lopinavir/ritonavir (LPV/r)	Posaconazole serum concentrations may be decreased.	Use with close monitoring for therapeutic efficacy.
Lovastatin	Lovastatin serum concentrations may be increased.	Consider pravastatin, atorvastatin, and rosuvastatin.
Maraviroc (MVC)	May increase MVC serum concentrations.	Consider MVC 150–300 mg twice daily.
Midazolam	Midazolam AUC increased by 83%.	Consider lorazepam, oxazepam, or temazepam.
Nelfinavir (NFV)	Posaconazole serum concentrations may be decreased.	Use with close monitoring for therapeutic efficacy.
Nifedipine	Nifedipine serum concentrations may be increased.	Avoid or use with close monitoring.
Nisoldipine	Nisoldipine serum concentrations may be increased.	Avoid or use with close monitoring.
Nizatidine	No significant interaction.	No dose adjustment necessary.
Omeprazole	May decrease posaconazole.	Use with caution. Posaconazole TDM recommended.
Pantoprazole	May decrease posaconazole.	Use with caution. Posaconazole TDM recommended.
Phenytoin	Posaconazole AUC decreased by 50%.	Avoid coadministration unless the benefit outweighs the risks.
Pimozide	Risk of QTc prolongation may be increased.	Contraindicated.
Quinidine	Risk of QTc prolongation may be increased.	Contraindicated.
Rabeprazole	May decrease posaconazole.	Use with caution. Posaconazole TDM recommended.
Raltegravir (RAL)	Interaction unlikely.	Use standard doses.
Ranitidine	No significant interaction.	No dose adjustment necessary.
Rifabutin (RFB)	RFB AUC increased by 72%. Posaconazole AUC decreased by 49%.	Avoid coadministration unless the benefit outweighs the risks. Monitor for sign and symptoms of uveitis.
Rifampin	May significantly decrease posaconazole serum concentrations.	Avoid coadministration.
Ritonavir (RTV)	May increase RTV serum concentrations.	No dose adjustment necessary when RTV dose is 100–200 mg/day.

POSACONAZOLE *(cont.)*

Drug	Effect of Interaction	Recommendations/Comments
Sildenafil	Sildenafil serum concentrations may be increased.	Avoid or use with close monitoring.
Simvastatin	Simvastatin serum concentrations may be increased.	Consider pravastatin, atorvastatin, and rosuvastatin.
Sirolimus	Sirolimus serum concentrations may be increased.	Contraindicated per manufacturer, but with a 50% empiric dose reduction of sirolimus, therapeutic sirolimus serum concentrations achieved (Koo S, et al. ICAAC 2009, A1–592).
Tacrolimus	Tacrolimus serum concentrations may be increased.	Reduce tacrolimus dose to 1/3 of original dose with TDM.
Tadalafil	Tadalafil serum concentrations may be increased.	Avoid or use with close monitoring.
Terfenadine	Risk of QTc prolongation may be increased.	Contraindicated.
Tipranavir/ ritonavir (TPV/r)	Posaconazole serum concentrations may be decreased.	Use with close monitoring for therapeutic efficacy.
Triazolam	Triazolam serum concentrations may be increased.	Consider lorazepam, oxazepam, or temazepam.
Vardenafil	Vardenafil serum concentrations may be increased.	Avoid or use with close monitoring.
Verapamil	Verapamil serum concentrations may be increased.	Avoid or use with close monitoring.
Vinblastine	Vinblastine serum concentrations may be increased.	Avoid or use with close monitoring for neuropathy. Consider dose adjustment.
Vincristine	Vincristine serum concentrations may be increased.	Avoid or use with close monitoring for neuropathy. Consider dose adjustment.

DRUG-DRUG INTERACTION – RALTEGRAVIR (RAL)

Drug	Effect of Interaction	Recommendations/Comments
Antacid (e.g., *Maalox*)	RAL AUC and Cmin decreased by 24% and 67%, respectively.	Avoid coadministration. Administer RAL 2–4 hrs before antacid administration.

Drug	Effect of Interaction	Recommendations/Comments
Atazanavir (ATV)	With ATV/r, RAL AUC and Cmin increased 41% and 77%, respectively. Unboosted ATV 300 mg twice daily + RAL 400 mg twice daily resulted in ATV AUC and Cmin reduction of 17% and 29%, respectively. Mean QTc was not increased, but QRS interval increased 11 ms (range 2–25 ms).	Recommended dose ATV/r 300/100 mg once daily plus RAL 400 mg twice daily. The clinical significance of QRS interval increase and lower ATV concentrations observed with ATV 300 mg twice daily + RAL 400 mg twice daily remains to be determined. With RAL coadministration, use boosted ATV/r 300/100 mg once daily.
Efavirenz (EFV)	RAL AUC decreased by 36%, but Cmin not significantly affected.	Use standard dose RAL.
Etravirine (ETR)	RAL PK unchanged. ETR AUC increased 10%.	Use standard dose.
Fosamprenavir (FPV)	RAL and APV AUC decreased 37% and 36%, respectively (with unboosted FPV). RAL AUC decreased 55% (with FPV/r 700/100 mg twice daily).	Clinical significance unknown. Avoid unboosted FPV with RAL coadministration. Use FPV/r with close monitoring or consider alternative boosted PI with RAL coadministration.
Lopinavir/ritonavir (LPV/r)	RAL Cmin decreased 30%.	Use standard dose.
Maraviroc (MVC)	RAL PK unchanged.	Use standard dose.
Methadone	No change in RAL and methadone PK.	Use standard dose.
Nevirapine (NVP)	May decrease RAL serum concentrations.	Use standard dose RAL with close monitoring of virologic efficacy.
Omeprazole	RAL AUC and Cmin increased by 3-fold and 1.5-fold, respectively.	Unclear clinical significance. Use standard dose.
Phenobarbital	Phenobarbital may significantly decrease RAL serum concentrations.	Avoid coadministration. Consider valproic acid or levetiracetam.
Phenytoin	Phenytoin may significantly decrease RAL serum concentrations.	Avoid coadministration. Consider valproic acid or levetiracetam.
Rifabutin (RFB)	RFB reduces RAL trough by 20%, but RAL AUC not affected.	Use RAL 400 mg twice daily plus RFB 300 mg once daily.
Rifampin	Rifampin decreases RAL AUC and Cmin by 40% and 61%, respectively.	Increasing RAL to 800 mg twice daily resulted in adequate AUC, but Cmin was decreased by 53%. Limited clinical data. Avoid coadministration if possible. Consider RFB with RAL coadministration.
Ritonavir (RTV)	RAL PK unchanged.	Use standard dose.

RALTEGRAVIR *(cont.)*

Drug	Effect of Interaction	Recommendations/Comments
Sirolimus	Drug interaction unlikely.	Case report of safe coadministration of RAL and sirolimus. Use standard dose.
St. John's wort	May decrease RAL serum concentrations.	Avoid coadministration until PK data becomes available.
Tacrolimus	No significant interaction.	Case series of favorable outcome in patients treated with RAL-based regimen s/p solid organ transplant on tacrolimus. Use standard dose.
Tenofovir (TDF)	RAL AUC increased 49%.	Standard dose.
Tipranavir/ ritonavir (TPV/r)	RAL Cmin decreased by 55%, but AUC decreased by 24% (NS).	Use with close monitoring of virologic efficacy. Clinical significance unclear; comparable efficacy observed in subgroup of patients who received TPV/r plus RAL relative to patients not receiving TPV/r. Hepatic necrolysis reported in 3 patients on TPV/r + RAL: monitor transaminases.

DRUG-DRUG INTERACTION – RIFABUTIN (RFB)*

Drug	Effect of Interaction	Recommendations/Comments
Amprenavir (APV)	RFB AUC increased by 193% and Cmin increased by 271% with RFB 150 mg coadministration. APV AUC decreased by 15% and Cmin decreased by 15%.	Switch to FPV. Recommended dosing: RFB 150 mg every other day (or 150 mg 3 × wk) with FPV/r 700/100 mg twice daily.
Atazanavir (ATV)	RFB AUC increased by 110% and Cmin increased by 243% with RFB 150 mg q day coadministration. ATV AUC increased by 191%.	Recommended dosing: ATV 400 mg once daily OR ATV/r 300/100 mg once daily with RFB 150 mg 3 ×/wk.
Bisoprolol	RFB may decrease serum concentrations of coadministered drug.	Titrate to effect.
Clarithromycin	RFB AUC increased by 56% and clarithromycin AUC decreased by 50%.	Clinical significance unknown since clarithromycin intracellular level is likely to be higher. Monitor for uveitis. Consider switching to azithromycin.
Corticosteroids	RFB may decrease serum concentrations of coadministered drug.	Corticosteroid dose may need to be increased.
Cyclosporine	RFB may decrease serum concentrations of coadministered drug.	Monitor cyclosporine serum concentrations closely with coadministration. Cyclosporine dose will likely need to be increased.

*For the treatment of TB, most experts recommend rifabutin 150 mg every day with PI/r. Consider TDM.

Drug	Effect of Interaction	Recommendations/Comments
Darunavir (DRV)	RFB serum concentrations may be increased. The RFB PK parameters are comparable between RFB 150 mg every other day plus DRV/r 600/100 mg twice daily and RFB 300 mg once daily.	Dose: RFB dose reduction (RFB 150 mg every other day with DRV/r coadministration).
Delavirdine (DLV)	RFB AUC increased by 100% and DLV AUC decreased by 80%.	Contraindicated.
Diazepam	RFB may decrease serum concentrations of coadministered drug.	Titrate to effect.
Digoxin	RFB may decrease coadministered drug.	Monitor digoxin serum concentrations with coadministration.
Disopyramide	RFB may decrease coadministered drug.	Monitor for therapeutic efficacy.
Doxycycline	RFB may decrease serum concentrations of coadministered drug.	Consider an alternative antibiotic.
Efavirenz (EFV)	RFB AUC decreased by 38%. No change in EFV AUC.	Recommended dosing: increase RFB to 450 mg/day OR 600 mg 3 ×/wk with standard dose EFV 600 mg qhs.
Etravirine (ETR)	ETR AUC and Cmin decreased 37% and 35%, respectively. RFB AUC decreased 17%.	Clinical significance unclear. Dose: ETR 200 mg twice daily plus RFB 300 mg once daily. Avoid coadministration of DRV/r or SQV/r with RFB and ETR due to potential additive decrease in ETR exposure.
Fluconazole	Fluconazole increases RFB AUC by 80%. Fluconazole AUC not affected.	Monitor for uveitis.
Fosamprenavir (FPV)	RFB AUC increased by 193% and Cmin increased by 271% with RFB 150 mg coadministration. APV AUC decreased by 15% and Cmin decreased by 15%.	Switch to FPV. Recommended dosing: RFB 150 mg every other day (or 150 mg 3 × wk) with FPV/r 700/100 mg twice daily.
Indinavir (IDV)	RFB AUC increased by 204% and IDV AUC decreased by 32%.	Recommended dosing: RFB 150 mg every other day (OR 150 mg 3 ×/wk) with IDV/r 800/100 mg twice daily (recommended but no data) OR RFB 150 mg once daily (OR 300 mg 3 ×/wk) with IDV 1000 mg q8h (twice daily dosing with RTV boosting preferred).
Itraconazole	RFB may decrease coadministered drug.	Monitor itraconazole serum concentrations and signs and symptoms of uveitis with coadministration.

RIFABUTIN (cont.)

Drug	Effect of Interaction	Recommendations/Comments
Ketoconazole	RFB may decrease ketoconazole. Ketoconazole may increase RFB.	Monitor for uveitis with coadministration.
Levothyroxine	RFB may decrease serum concentrations of coadministered drug.	Monitor T3/T4 with coadministration.
Lopinavir/ritonavir (LPV/r)	RFB AUC increased by 203%. LPV serum level increased by 20% (NS).	Recommended dosing: LPV/r 2 tabs (400/100 mg) twice daily with RFB 150 mg every other day (OR 150 mg 3 ×/wk). In an observational study, RFB serum concentrations lower compared to historical controls. RFB TDM recommended with coadministration.
Maraviroc (MVC)	MVC serum concentrations may be decreased.	No data. Dose: MVC 600 mg twice daily.
Methadone	No significant interactions.	Use standard dose.
Metoprolol	RFB may decrease serum concentrations of coadministered drug.	Titrate to effect.
Mexiletine	RFB may decrease coadministered drug.	Monitor for therapeutic efficacy.
Midazolam	RFB may decrease serum concentrations of coadministered drug.	Titrate to effect.
Nelfinavir (NFV)	NFV AUC decreased by 32%. RFB concentrations increased by 207%.	Recommended dosing NFV 1000 mg 3 ×/day with RFB 150 mg once daily (OR 300 mg 3 ×/wk).
Nevirapine (NVP)	RFB AUC increased by 16% (NS). NVP AUC unchanged.	Unlikely to be clinically significant. Recommended dosing: RFB 300 mg/day (OR 300 mg 3 ×/wk).
Oral Contraceptives and Estrogens	RFB may decrease serum concentrations of coadministered drug.	Consider an alternative barrier form of contraception with coadministration.
Posaconazole	May significantly decrease voriconazole serum concentrations.	Avoid coadministration.
Propranolol	RFB may decrease serum concentrations of coadministered drug.	Titrate to effect.
Quinidine	RFB may decrease serum concentrations of coadministered drug.	Monitor for therapeutic efficacy.
Quinine	RFB may decrease serum concentrations of coadministered drug.	Monitor for therapeutic efficacy.

Drug	Effect of Interaction	Recommendations/Comments
Raltegravir (RAL)	Significant interaction unlikely.	No data. Use standard dose.
Ritonavir (RTV)	RFB AUC increased by 400%.	Recommended dose: RFB 150 mg every other day (OR 150 mg 3 ×/wk) with standard dose of RTV (rarely used).
Saquinavir (SQV)	SQV AUC decreased by 43%.	Do not coadminister SQV with RFB as sole PI. Recommended dosing: consider SQV/r 1000/100 mg twice daily with RFB 150 mg every other day (no data, but likely to attain adequate serum concentrations).
Sirolimus	RFB may significantly decrease sirolimus serum concentrations.	Monitor sirolimus serum concentrations closely with coadministration. Sirolimus dose will need to be increased.
Tacrolimus	RFB may significantly decrease tacrolimus serum concentrations.	Monitor tacrolimus serum concentrations closely with coadministration. Tacrolimus dose will likely need to be increased.
Theophylline	RFB may decrease serum concentrations of coadministered drug.	Monitor theophylline serum concentrations with coadministration.
Tipranavir (TPV)	RFB AUC increased 190%. No significant change in TPV.	Dose reduce RFB to 150 mg every other day.
Tocainide	RFB may decrease serum concentrations of coadministered drug.	Monitor for therapeutic efficacy.
Triazolam	RFB may decrease serum concentrations of coadministered drug.	Titrate to effect.
Verapamil	RFB may decrease coadministered drug.	Titrate to effect.
Voriconazole	May significantly decrease voriconazole serum concentrations.	Contraindicated.
Warfarin	RFB may decrease serum concentrations of coadministered drug.	Monitor INR closely with coadministration. Warfarin dose may need to be increased.

DRUG-DRUG INTERACTION – RIFAMPIN

Drug	Effect of Interaction	Recommendations/Comments
Aluminum-Containing Antacids	Controversial but may decrease oral absorption of rifampin; some studies found no effect.	Consider separate oral administration by 4 hrs.

RIFAMPIN (cont.)

Drug	Effect of Interaction	Recommendations/Comments
Aminosalicylic Acid Granules	Absorption of rifampin may be impaired by the bentonite excipient.	Separate administration by 8–12 hrs intervals.
Amiodarone	Amiodarone serum concentrations may be significantly decreased.	Monitor EKG with coadministration. Amiodarone dose may need to be increased.
Amlodipine	Amlodipine serum concentrations may be significantly decreased.	Titrate to effect.
Aprepitant	Aprepitant serum concentrations may be decreased.	Apretitant dose may need to be increased.
Atazanavir (ATV)	ATV/r Cmin decreased 60%–93%.	Contraindicated. Use RFB with coadministration.
Atorvastatin	Atorvastatin decreased by 80%.	Titrate to effect. Pravastatin or rosuvastatin less likely to interact with rifampin.
Atovaquone	Atovaquone AUC decreased by approximately 50%.	Avoid coadministration. Consider aerosolized pentamidine (AP) for PCP prophylaxis.
Bisoprolol	Bisoprolol serum concentrations may be significantly decreased.	Bisoprolol dose may need to be increased.
Bosentan	Bosentan AUC decreased 60%.	May need to increase bosentan dose.
Buprenorphine	Buprenorphine serum concentrations may be decreased.	Titrate buprenorphine to effect.
Caspofungin	Caspofungin trough concentrations decreased 30%.	Use caspofungin 70 mg with rifampin coadministration.
Chlorpropamide	Chlorpropamide serum concentrations decreased by up to 50%.	Monitor blood glucose control with coadministration. Consider a shorter acting hypoglycemic agent.
Clarithromycin	Clarithromycin serum concentrations may be significantly decreased.	Consider azithromycin.
Cyclosporine	Cyclosporine serum concentrations may be significantly decreased.	Monitor cyclosporine serum concentrations closely with coadministration. Cyclosporine dose may need to be increased.
Dapsone	Dapsone serum concentrations may be decreased.	For PCP prophylaxis, if unable to tolerate TMP/SMX, consider using AP.
Darunavir/ ritonavir (DRV/r)	DRV serum concentrations may be significantly decreased.	Contraindicated. Use RFB with coadministration.

Drug	Effect of Interaction	Recommendations/Comments
Dasatinib	Dasatinib AUC decreased 82%.	Higher dasatinib dose is recommended at steady-state (2 wks).
Dexamethasone	Dexamethasone serum concentrations may be significantly decreased.	Dexamethasone dose may need to be increased.
Diazepam	Diazepam serum concentrations may be significantly decreased.	Titrate to effect.
Digoxin	Digoxin serum concentrations may be decreased by 30% to 60%.	Monitor digoxin serum concentrations with coadministration.
Diltiazem	Diltiazem serum concentrations may be significantly decreased.	Titrate to effect.
Disopyramide	Disopyramide half-life decreased by 40%.	Monitor EKG with coadministration. Disopyramide dose may need to be increased.
Doxycycline	Doxycycline serum concentrations may be decreased.	Clinical significance unclear.
Efavirenz (EFV)	EFV AUC decreased 26%. No change in rifampin area under the curve.	Recommended dosing: EFV 600–800 mg/day in patients >50kg with rifampin 600 mg once daily (monitor for EFV central nervous system side effects). May decrease to EFV 600 mg/day if 800 mg dose not easily tolerated.
Erlotinib	Erlotinib AUC decreased by approximately 67% to 80%.	Higher dose of erlotinib may be needed.
Etravirine (ETR)	ETR serum concentrations may be significantly decreased.	Avoid coadministration until more data becomes available.
Everolimus	Everolimus AUC decreased by 58%.	Monitor everolimus serum concentrations closely with coadministration. Dose may need to be increased.
Fluconazole	Fluconazole serum concentrations decreased by 23%–56%.	Consider switching to RFB with coadministration.
Fosamprenavir (FPV)	No data, but significant decrease in APV serum concentrations expected. When studied with APV, AUC decreased 82%; Cmin decreased 92%.	Contraindicated. Use RFB with coadministration.
Glimepiride	Glimepiride serum concentrations may be significantly decreased.	Monitor glucose control with coadministration.

RIFAMPIN *(cont.)*

Drug	Effect of Interaction	Recommendations/Comments
Glyburide	Glyburide serum concentrations may be significantly decreased.	Monitor glucose control with coadministration.
Indinavir (IDV)	IDV AUC decreased 90%.	Contraindicated. Use RFB with coadministration.
Itraconazole	Itraconazole serum concentrations may be significantly decreased.	Avoid coadministration. Consider RFB with monitoring of itraconazole serum concentrations and monitor for uveitis.
Ketoconazole	Ketoconazole serum concentrations decreased by 50%.	Avoid coadministration. Consider RFB.
Lamotrigine	Lamotrigine AUC decreased by approximately 40%.	Titrate to effect.
Levothyroxine	Levothyroxine serum concentrations may be significantly decreased.	Monitor TSH. May need higher levothyroxine dose with coadministration.
Linezolid	Linezolid AUC decreased 32% with coadministration.	Clinical significance unknown. Consider linezolid 600 mg q8h for severe infections.
Lopinavir/ritonavir (LPV/r)	LPV AUC decreased 75%, and Cmin decreased 99%.	Coadministration not recommended. Although studies used LPV/r 400/100 mg twice daily (2 tabs) plus RTV 300 mg twice daily or LPV/r 3 to 4 tabs twice daily to overcome this interaction, high incidence of nausea, vomiting, and grade 4 LFTs elevation were common. Consider RFB with LPV/r coadministration.
Lovastatin	Lovastatin serum concentrations may be significantly decreased.	Titrate to effect. Pravastatin or rosuvastatin less likely to interact with rifampin.
Maraviroc (MVC)	MVC AUC decreased by 63%.	Increase MVC dose to 600 mg twice daily with rifampin coadministration.
Mefloquine	Mefloquine AUC decreased 68%.	Consider an alternative antimalarial drug.
Methadone and Other Opiate Agonists	Opiate serum concentrations may be significantly decreased. Methadone AUC decreased 30%–65%.	Monitor for signs and symptoms of withdrawal and titrate opiate to effect.
Metoprolol	Metoprolol serum concentrations decreased by 33%.	Titrate to effect.
Mexiletine	Mexiletine half-life decreased by 5–9 hrs.	Monitor EKG with coadministration. Mexiletine dose may need to be increased.
Midazolam	Midazolam serum concentrations may be significantly decreased.	Titrate to effect.

Drug	Effect of Interaction	Recommendations/Comments
Montelukast	Montelukast AUC decreased by 40%.	Dose of montelukast may need to be increased.
Morphine	Morphine AUC decreased by 45%.	Titrate to effect.
Moxifloxacin	Moxifloxacin serum concentrations decreased by approximately 30%.	Monitor for therapeutic efficacy. Consider levofloxacin.
Mycophenolate Mofetil	Mycophenolate AUC decreased 67%.	Mycophenolate dose may need to be increased.
Nelfinavir (NFV)	NFV AUC decreased 82%.	Contraindicated. Use RFB with coadministration.
Nevirapine (NVP)	NVP Cmin decreased 37%–68%. NVP AUC decreased 37%–58%. Rifampin area under the curve increased 11% (not significant).	Avoid coadministration.
Nifedipine	Nifedipine serum concentrations may be decreased up to 70%.	Titrate to effect.
Nilotinib	Nilotinib AUC decreased by 80%.	Avoid coadministration.
Oral Contraceptives	Ethinyl estradiol Cmin decreased by 79%. Norethindrone Cmin decreased by 89%.	Use an alternative or additional barrier form of contraception. Despite these PK interactions, all subjects remained anovulatory as indicated by undetectable progesterone levels.
Phenytoin	Phenytoin serum concentrations may be decreased.	Monitor phenytoin serum concentrations closely with coadministration.
Pioglitazone	Pioglitazone AUC decreased 54%.	Monitor glucose control with coadministration. Pioglitazone dose may need to be increased.
Posaconazole	Posaconazole serum concentrations may be significantly decreased.	Contraindicated. RFB may be considered if benefit outweighs the risks. Use with close monitoring of posaconazole serum concentrations and monitor for sign and symptoms of uveitis.
Praziquantel	Praziquantel serum concentrations may be significantly decreased.	Avoid coadministration.
Prednisone	Prednisone serum concentrations decreased by up to 60%.	Prednisone dose may need to be increased.
Propafenone	Propafenone serum concentrations may be significantly decreased.	Monitor EKG with coadministration. Propafenone dose may need to be increased.

RIFAMPIN (cont.)

Drug	Effect of Interaction	Recommendations/Comments
Propranolol	Propranolol serum concentrations may be significantly decreased.	Titrate to effect.
Quinidine	Quinidine serum concentrations may be significantly decreased.	Monitor quinidine serum concentrations. May need to increase quinidine dose.
Quinine	Quinine serum concentrations may be significantly decreased.	Quinine dose may need to increased.
Raltegravir (RAL)	RAL AUC and Cmin decreased by 40% and 61%, respectively. Increasing RAL to 800 mg twice daily resulted in adequate AUC but Cmin was decreased by 53%.	Increase RAL dose to 800 mg twice daily with close monitoring of virologic efficacy. Consider using RFB with coadministration.
Ranolazine	Ranolazine AUC decreased 95%.	Contraindicated.
Repaglinide	Repaglinide AUC decreased 57%.	Titrate to effect.
Ritonavir (RTV)	RTV AUC decreased 35%.	RTV standard dosage recommended by manufacturer, but coadministration with rifampin should be avoided.
Rosiglitazone	Rosiglitazone AUC decreased by 54%.	Monitor glucose control with coadministration.
Saquinavir (SQV)	SQV AUC decreased 70% (SQV soft gel capsules without RTV boosting).	Contraindicated due to the high incidence of hepatitis with SQV 1000 mg + RTV 100 mg twice daily.
Simvastatin	Simvastatin serum concentrations decreased by 56% to 94%.	Titrate to effect. Pravastatin or rosuvastatin less likely to interact with rifampin.
Sirolimus	Sirolimus serum concentrations decreased 82%.	Monitor sirolimus serum concentrations closely with coadministration. Sirolimus dose may need to be increased.
Tacrolimus	Tacrolimus serum concentrations may be significantly decreased.	Monitor tacrolimus serum concentrations closely with coadministration. Tacrolimus dose may need to be increased.
Tamoxifen	Tamoxifen AUC decreased 86%.	Higher dose may be needed.
Telithromycin	Telithromycin AUC decreased 79%.	Avoid coadministration.
Temsirolimus	Temsirolimus AUC decreased up to 56%.	Monitor temsirolimus serum concentration with dose titration.

Drug	Effect of Interaction	Recommendations/Comments
Theophylline	Theophylline serum concentrations decreased 18%.	Monitor theophylline serum concentrations. Theophylline dose may need to be increased.
Tipranavir/ ritonavir (TPV/r)	May significantly decrease TPV serum concentrations.	Contraindicated. Use RFB with coadministration.
Tocainide	Tocainide AUC decreased 28%.	Tocainide dose may need to be increased.
Tolbutamide	Tolbutamide serum concentrations may be significantly decreased.	Monitor blood glucose control with coadministration.
Triazolam	Triazolam serum concentrations may be significantly decreased.	Titrate to effect.
Verapamil	Verapamil serum concentrations may be significantly decreased.	Titrate to effect.
Voriconazole	Voriconazole serum concentrations decreased.	Both rifampin and RFB are contraindicated with voriconazole.
Warfarin	Warfarin serum concentrations may be significantly decreased.	Monitor INR closely. May need higher warfarin dose.
Zidovudine (AZT)	AZT AUC decreased 47%. Intracellular concentrations not measured.	Consider switching to RFB.

DRUG-DRUG INTERACTION – RILPIVIRINE

Drug	Effect of Interaction	Recommendations/Comments
Amiodarone	May prolong QTc	Avoid co-administration
Antacids	RPV concentrations may be significantly decreased.	Antacid should be administered >2 hrs before or 4 hours after RPV.
Astemizole	May prolong QTc	Avoid co-administration
Atorvastatin	Hydroxy metabolites increased by 23-39%. Clinical significance unknown.	Use standard dose atorvastatin.
ddI	No drug interaction	ddI is dosed on an empty stomach and RPV must be taken with a meal. No significant interaction if ddI taken 2 hours before RPV; RPV concentrations not affected.
Disopyramide	May prolong QTc	Avoid co-administration
DRV/r	RPV AUC increased 130%	Use standard dose. Monitor QTc in patients at risk for QTc prolongation.

RILPIVIRINE (cont.)

Drug	Effect of Interaction	Recommendations/Comments
Erythromycin	May increase RPV concentrations and prolong QTc	Avoid co-administration
Ethinyl estradiol/norethindrone	AUC increased 14% and norethindrone decreased 11%. Clinical significance unknown.	Use an additional barrier form of contraception.
Fluconazole	May increase RPV concentrations.	Monitor for QTc prolongation and antifungal efficacy.
H2 blockers	RPV concentrations may be significantly decreased.	H2 blockers must be given 12hrs before or 4 hrs after RPV.
Haloperidol	May prolong QTc	Avoid co-administration
Itraconazole	May increase RPV concentrations.	Monitor for QTc prolongation and antifungal efficacy.
Ketoconazole	Increases RPV AUC 49% and ketoconazole AUC decreased by 24%.	Monitor for QTc prolongation and antifungal efficacy.
LPV/r	RPV AUC increased 52%	Use standard dose. Monitor QTc in patients at risk for QTc prolongation.
Macrolide antibiotics (e.g. clarithromycin, troleandomycin, erythromycin)	May increase RPV concentrations and prolong QTc	Monitor for QTc prolongation. Consider azithromycin with co-administration.
Methadone (active R-isomer)	Methadone AUC decreased by 26%	Monitor for withdrawal symptoms. Monitor for QTc prolongation with high dose methadone.
Omeprazole	RPV AUC decreased 40%	Contraindicated. All PPIs may also significantly decrease RPV absorption and are contraindicated. If acid suppression is needed, H2 blockers can be considered.
Pimozide	May prolong QTc	Avoid co-administration
Posaconazole	May increase RPV concentrations.	Monitor for QTc prolongation and antifungal efficacy.
Procaindamide	May prolong QTc	Avoid co-administration
Rifabutin	RPV AUC decreased by 46%	Contraindicated. Avoid co-administration
Rifampin	RPV AUC decreased by 80%	Contraindicated. Avoid co-administration
Sildenafil	No significant interaction	Use standard dose
Sotalol	May prolong QTc	Avoid co-administration
TDF	AUC increased 23%	RPV concentrations not affected.
Terfenadine	May prolong QTc	Avoid co-administration

Drug	Effect of Interaction	Recommendations/Comments
Tricyclic antidepressant	May prolong QTc	Avoid co-administration
Voriconazole	May increase RPV concentrations.	Monitor for QTc prolongation and antifungal efficacy.

DRUG-DRUG INTERACTION – RITONAVIR (RTV)

Drug	Effect of Interaction	Recommendations/Comments
Alfuzosin	May significantly increase alfuzosin levels.	Contraindicated. Consider doxazosin and terazosin for BPH (with close monitoring).
Alprazolam	Alprazolam clearance decreased by 59% (single-dose study); alprazolam AUC decreased by 12% (steady-state).	Use with caution. With coadministration, alprazolam should be administered at the lowest possible dose with slow titration. Alternative benzodiazepines that can be used: temazepam, oxazepam, or lorazepam.
Amiodarone	May significantly increase amiodarone serum levels.	Contraindicated.
Amitriptyline	May increase serum levels of amitriptyline.	Use with caution. Consider an alternative antidepressant (i.e., SSRI: escitalopram, citalopram, sertraline, or fluoxetine).
Amlodipine	May increase serum levels of amlodipine.	Applies to all PIs: data limited to an interaction study conducted with ATV and diltiazem, which resulted in doubling of diltiazem serum levels (this led to PR interval prolongation). All PIs have the potential of prolonging the PR interval with calcium channel blockers coadministration. Calcium channel blockers should be started with 50% of the dose and slowly titrated with close monitoring of BP and pulse.
Amphetamine (including methamphetamine)	May increase serum levels of amphetamine.	Avoid all illicit drug use with RTV.
Artemether (artemisinin)	May increase serum levels of artemether.	Coadministration of EFV with artesunate plus amodaquine may result in significant LFT elevations. Unknown effect of artemeter on other Ps and NNRTIs. Close monitoring for artemether toxicity (bone marrow suppression, bradycardia, and seizure).
Astemizole	May significantly increase astemizole serum levels.	Contraindicated due to the potential for cardiac arrhythmias. Recommended alternative antihistamine: loratadine, fexofenadine, desloratidine, or cetirizine.

RITONAVIR (cont.)

Drug	Effect of Interaction	Recommendations/Comments
Atazanavir (ATV)	ATV AUC and Cmin increased 238% and 1089%, respectively.	Dose: ATV/r 300/100 mg once daily. With EFV, use ATV/r 400/100 mg once daily (only in patients without PI resistance).
Atorvastatin	Atorvastatin AUC increased by 450% (studied with RTV/SQV).	Use with caution. Begin with lowest possible dose of atorvastatin (10 mg/day), and avoid doses >40 mg/day. Consider pravastatin, fluvastatin, or rosuvastatin.
Azathioprine	Interaction unlikely.	Applies to all PIs and NNRTIs: use standard dose.
Bepridil	May significantly increase bepridil serum levels.	Contraindicated.
Bosentan	With LPV/r coadministration, bosentan AUC increased 48-fold (on day 4) and 5-fold (on day 10).	Coadminister bosentan only after RTV has reached steady-state. In patients on RTV >10 days: start bosentan at 62.5 mg once daily or every other day. In patients already on bosentan: d/c bosentan for >36 hrs prior to initiation of RTV-boosted PIs and restart bosentan at 62.5 mg once daily or every other day after RTV has reached steady-state (after 10 days).
Bupropion	May increase bupropion concentration (initially), but decrease concentrations (at steady-state).	Titrate bupropion dose to therapeutic effect. In a small case series no seizures reported with coadministration.
Carbamazepine	May decrease serum levels of RTV. RTV may increase serum levels of carbamazepine.	Consider alternative anticonvulsants (i.e., valproic acid, lamotrigine, levetiracetam, or topiramate). Carbamazepine toxicity has been reported with coadministration. With coadministration, monitor anticonvulsants levels closely.
Carvedilol	May increase carvedilol serum levels.	Carvedilol levels may be increased with RTV. Monitor closely with coadministration. Consider alternative beta-blocker such as atenolol since it is primarily excreted unchanged in the urine with limited interaction with RTV.
Chlordiazepoxide	May increase serum levels of chlordiazepoxide.	Applies to all PIs: consider an alternative benzodiazepine (i.e., lorazepam, oxazepam, or temazepam).
Cisapride	May significantly increase cisapride serum levels.	Contraindicated due to potential for cardiac arrhythmias. Recommended alternative: metoclopramide.

Drug	Effect of Interaction	Recommendations/Comments
Clarithromycin	Clarithromycin AUC increased by 77%, Cmin increased by 182%.	Reduce clarithromycin dose by 50% in end stage renal disease. May increase risk of QTc prolongation with RTV 400 mg twice daily. Consider using azithromycin.
Clomipramine	May increase serum levels of clomipramine.	Clinical significance unknown. Consider an alternative antidepressant (i.e., SSRI: escitalopram, citalopram, sertraline, or fluoxetine).
Clorazepate	May increase serum levels of clorazepate.	Applies to all PIs: consider an alternative benzodiazepine (i.e., lorazepam, oxazepam, or temazepam).
Cocaine	May theoretically increase serum levels of hepatotoxic metabolite.	Applies to all PIs and NNRTIs. illicit drug use should be avoided for the obvious reasons.
Cyclophosphamide	May increase serum levels of cyclophosphamide.	Applies to all PIs: data limited to an interaction study conducted with IDV resulting in a 50% increase in cyclophosphamide serum level. Since all PIs have the potential of increasing cyclophosphamide levels, close monitoring of cyclophosphamide-induced toxicity is recommended.
Cyclosporine	May significantly increase serum levels of cyclosporine.	Applies to all PIs: monitor serum level of cyclosporine closely with coadministration. Cyclosporine dose may need to be decreased.
Darunavir (DRV)	DRV AUC increased 14-fold.	Dose: DRV/r 600/100 mg twice daily.
Didanosine ddI (buffered)	Decreased RTV absorption.	Use ddI EC or separate administration by >2 hrs.
Desipramine	Desipramine AUC increased by 145%.	If available, monitor desipramine levels. Consider escitalopram, citalopram, sertraline, or fluoxetine.
Digoxin	Digoxin AUC increased 49%.	Reduction in the digoxin dose may bee need with all boosted PI coadministration. Monitor for PR interval prolongation.
Diltiazem	May increase serum level of diltiazem.	Data limited to an interaction study conducted with ATV, which resulted in doubling of diltiazem serum levels (this led to PR interval prolongation). All PIs have the potential of prolonging the PR interval with diltiazem coadministration. Diltiazem should be started with 50% of the dose and slowly titrated with close monitoring of BP and pulse.
Disopyramide	May increase disopyramide serum levels.	Applies to all PIs: no data. Monitor disopyramide serum levels (target: 2 to 7.5 mcg/mL).

RITONAVIR *(cont.)*

Drug	Effect of Interaction	Recommendations/Comments
Docetaxel	May increase serum levels of docetaxel.	Applies to all PIs: no data. Close monitoring of chemotherapy-induced toxicity recommended.
Dofetilide	May significantly increase serum level of dofetilide.	Applies to all PIs: no data. Use with caution. Monitor QTc closely and adjust dofetilide dosing based on QTc prolongation and renal function. Consider an alternative class III antiarrhythmic such as bretylium or ibutilide.
Dolasetron	May increase serum levels of dolesetron.	Due to the large therapeutic index of dolasetron, potential interaction is unlikely to be clinically significant.
Doxepine	May increase serum levels of doxepine.	Use with caution. Consider an alternative antidepressant (i.e., SSRI: escitalopram, citalopram, sertraline, or fluoxetine).
Echinacea	May decrease RTV serum level. Echinacea (400 mg 4 × days) decreased CYP3A4 substrate (midazolam) by 23%.	Applies to all PIs and NNRTIs. Clinical significance unknown but should be avoided until the safety of this combination is further evaluated.
Efavirenz (EFV)	RTV AUC increased 18%. EFV AUC increased 21%.	Dose: standard dose for both drugs.
Ergot Alkaloid	May significantly increase ergotamine serum level. Acute ergotism has been reported with coadministration.	Contraindicated. Consider alternative agent for migraine such as sumatriptan (but not eletriptan since it is a CYP3A4 substrate and significant drug-drug interaction occurred with CYP3A4 inhibitor).
Escitalopram	No significant change in serum levels.	No significant interaction. Use standard dose.
Estazolam	May increase serum levels of estazolam.	Applies to all PIs: consider an alternative benzodiazepine (i.e., lorazepam, temazepam, or flurazepam).
Ethinyl estradiol	Ethinyl estradiol decreased by 40%.	Use alternative method of contraception.
Ethosuximide	May increase serum levels of ethosuximide.	Applies to all PIs: consider switching to valproic acid for the treatment of absence seizure.
Etoposide	May increase serum levels of etoposide.	Applies to all PIs: no data. Close monitoring of chemotherapy-induced toxicity recommended.
Etravirine (ETR)	ETR area under curve decreased 46% with high-dose RTV, not significant interaction with low-dose RTV.	High-dose RTV not recommended, but DRV/r, FPV/r, SQV/r, LPV/r, and ATV/r may be coadministered at standard dose.

Drug	Effect of Interaction	Recommendations/Comments
Felodipine	May increase serum levels of felodipine.	Applies to all PIs: data limited to an interaction study conducted with ATV and diltiazem, which resulted in doubling of diltiazem serum levels (this led to PR interval prolongation). All PIs have the potential of prolonging the PR interval with calcium channel blocker coadministration. Calcium channel blockers should be started with 50% of the dose and slowly titrated with close monitoring of BP and pulse.
Fentanyl	Fentanyl clearance decreased by 67%.	Avoid concurrent administration of fentanyl. Morphine may be a safer alternative.
Flecainide	May significantly increase flecainide serum level.	Contraindicated.
Fluconazole	RTV AUC increased by 12%.	Interaction not significant. Use standard doses for both drugs.
Fluoxetine	RTV AUC increased by 19%.	Use standard dose. Serotonin syndrome has been reported but clear association is unclear [*AIDS 2001;15:1281*].
Flurazepam	May increase serum levels of flurazepam.	Applies to all PIs: consider an alternative benzodiazepine (i.e., lorazepam, temazepam, or flurazepam).
Fluticasone	Fluticasone AUC and Cmax increased by 350-fold and 25-fold, respectively.	With chronic administration plasma cortisol AUC decreased by 86%. Cushing's syndrome and adrenal insufficiency have been reported. Coadministration not recommended by manufacturer. Avoid long-term coadministration.
Fluvoxamine	May increase serum levels of fluvoxamine.	Clinical significance unknown. Consider an alternative antidepressant (i.e., SSRI: escitalopram, citalopram, sertraline, or fluoxetine).
Food (with 15g fat)	RTV AUC increased by 15%.	Minimal PK benefit with food; improves GI tolerance.
Fosamprenavir (FPV)	FPV AUC increased by 2-fold; Cmin increased by 4-fold with once daily; and Cmin increased by 6-fold with twice daily.	FPV/r 700/100 mg twice daily or FPV/r 1400/200 mg once daily (once daily dosing for PI-naive only). FPV/r 1400/300 mg once daily with EFV coadministration. FPV/r 1400/100 mg once daily under study in PI-naive patients.
Garlic Supplement	49% and 51% reduction of SQV AUC Cmin and AUC, respectively.	Studies only done with SQV but garlic supplements may effect serum levels of other PIs or NNRTIs. Avoid coadministration of garlic supplements with PIs and NNRTIs.

RITONAVIR *(cont.)*

Drug	Effect of Interaction	Recommendations/Comments
GHB (gamma-hydroxybutyrate)	Case report of prolonged and severe agitation attributed to interaction between GHB and RTV.	All illicit drug use should be avoided for obvious reasons. Warn patients of severe drug interaction with RTV.
Granisetron	May increase serum level of granisetron.	Applies to all PIs: due to the large therapeutic index of granisetron, potential interaction is unlikely to be clinically significant.
Haloperidol	May increase serum level of haloperidol.	Consider an alternative neuroleptic: olanzapin.
Heroin (diamorphine)	Drug interactions unlikely.	Applies to PIs and NNRTIs: interaction unlikely but illicit drug use should be avoided for obvious reasons.
Ifosphamide	May increase serum levels of ifosphamide.	Applies to all PIs: no data. Close monitoring of chemotherapy-induced toxicity recommended.
Imipramine	May increase serum levels of imipramine.	Use with caution. Consider an alternative antidepressant (i.e., SSRI: escitalopram, citalopram, sertraline, or fluoxetine).
Indinavir (IDV)	IDV AUC increased by 2 to 5-fold. Cmin increased by 400%.	Dosing recommendation: IDV/RTV 400/400 mg twice daily (more GI intolerance but less nephrolithiasis). IDV/r 800/100 mg twice daily (less GI intolerance but more nephrolithiasis). IDV/r 800/200 mg twice daily (highest incidence of nephrolithiasis, use only if EFV is coadministered).
Irinotecan	May increase irinotecan serum levels.	Applies to all PIs: coadministration of ATV is contraindicated by manufacturer. All PIs also have the potential for significant interaction with irinotecan, therefore coadministration should be done with extreme caution.
Itraconazole	CYP3A4 inhibitor and substrate-bidirectional inhibition with increase levels of PIs and itraconazole.	Monitor itraconazole serum level with RTV coadministration. May need itraconazole dose reduction.
Ketamine	May cause chemical hepatitis.	Avoid. All illicit drug use should be avoided for obvious reasons.
Ketoconazole	Ketoconazole AUC increased by greater than 3-fold.	May need to decrease ketoconazole dose (do not exceed 200 mg/day).
Lidocaine	May increase antiarrhythmic serum levels.	Applies to all PIs: no data. Use with caution, monitor lidocaine serum level (target: 1.5 to 6 mcg/mL) with coadministration.

Drug	Effect of Interaction	Recommendations/Comments
Lovastatin	May significantly increase lovastatin levels.	Contraindicated. Recommended alternatives include pravastatin, rosuvastatin, and fluvastatin (and possibly atorvastatin— start with 10 mg/day). Monitor for adverse effect due to limited clinical data.
Maraviroc (MVC)	MVC AUC increased 161%.	Dose: decrease MVC to 150 mg twice daily.
MDMA	Fatal case report attributed to drug interactions with RTV resulting in 10-fold increase in MDMA serum levels.	Case report limited to RTV. Unknown effect of other PIs and NNRTIs on MDMA serum levels. Avoid all illicit drug use for obvious reasons.
Mefloquine	RTV AUC decreased by 31% and Cmin by 43% (with RTV 200 mg at steady-state).	Clinical significance unknown but may consider increasing RTV dose.
Meperidine	Meperidine AUC decreased by 67%, nor-meperidine AUC increased by 47%.	Avoid concurrent administration of meperidine. Morphine may be a safer alternative.
Methadone	Methadone levels decreased by 37%, S-Methadone AUC decreased by 25%, R-Methadone AUC decreased by 20%.	Decrease in methadone AUC is unlikely to be significant since S-methadone(inactive) is more affected. No withdrawal symptoms observed. Use standard methadone dose.
Metoclopramide	May increase serum level of metoclopramide.	No data. Start with a low dose and titrate to effect.
Metoprolol	May increase metoprolol serum level.	Monitor closely with coadministration. It is unknown whether other PIs and NNRTIs can affect metoprolol serum concentrations. Consider alternative beta-blocker such as atenolol since it is primarily excreted unchanged in the urine with limited interaction with RTV.
Metronidazole	Disulfiram-like reaction.	Applies to RTV (liquid). Warn patients of the alcohol content in RTV liquid. Use RTV capsule.
Mexiletine	May increase antiarrhythmic serum levels.	Applies to all PIs: no data. Use with caution. Monitor EKG and serum levels. Serum levels exceeding 1.5 to 2 mcg/mL have been associated with an increased risk of toxicity.
Midazolam	May significantly increase midazolam levels.	Concurrent administration of midazolam is contraindicated. Alternative benzodiazepine can be used (temazepam, oxazepam, and lorazepam).

RITONAVIR *(cont.)*

Drug	Effect of Interaction	Recommendations/Comments
Milk Thistle	Data limited to an interaction study with milk thistle and IDV. IDV AUC: unchanged; IDV Cmin: decreased by 47%.	Clinical significance unknown. Unknown effect of the metabolism of other PIs or NNRTIs. Avoid coadministration with PIs and NNRTIs until it can be further evaluated.
Mirtazapine	May increase serum levels of mirtazapine.	Use with caution. Consider an alternative antidepressant (i.e., SSRI: escitalopram, citalopram, sertraline, or fluoxetine).
Mycophenolate	Interaction unlikely. No significant interaction observed with NVP.	Applies to all PIs and NNRT: no significant interaction observed with NVP. Use standard dose.
Nefazodone	May increase serum levels of nefazodone.	Applies to all PIs: use with caution. Consider an alternative antidepressant (i.e., SSRI: escitalopram, citalopram, sertraline, or fluoxetine).
Nelfinavir (NFV)	NFV AUC increased by 1.5 fold (152%).	NFV not generally coadministered since there is only a modest increase in NFV exposure.
Nevirapine (NVP)	RTV AUC decreased 11%.	Dose: standard dose for both drugs.
Nifedipine	May increase serum level of nifedipine.	Applies to all PIs: data limited to an interaction study conducted with ATV and diltiazem, which resulted in doubling of diltiazem serum levels (this led to PR interval prolongation). All PIs have the potential of prolonging the PR interval with calcium channel blocker coadministration. Calcium channel blockers should be started with 50% of the dose and slowly titrated with close monitoring of BP and pulse.
Nisoldipine	May increase serum levels of nisoldipine.	Applies to all PIs: data limited to an interaction study conducted with ATV and diltiazem, which resulted in doubling of diltiazem serum levels (this led to PR interval prolongation). All PIs have the potential of prolonging PR interval with calcium channel blockers coadministration. Calcium channel blockers should be started with 50% of the dose and slowly titrated with close monitoring of BP and pulse.
Nortriptyline	May increase serum levels of nortriptyline.	Use with caution. Consider an alternative antidepressant (i.e., SSRI: escitalopram, citalopram, sertraline, or fluoxetine).
Olanzapine	Olanzapine AUC decreased by 53%.	Olanzapine dose may need to be increased. Monitor and adjust as necessary.

Drug	Effect of Interaction	Recommendations/Comments
Ondansetron	May increase serum levels of ondansetron.	Due to the large therapeutic index of ondansetron, potential interaction is unlikely to be clinically significant.
Paclitaxel	May increase paclitaxel serum levels.	Applies to all PIs: since all PIs have the potential of significantly increasing paclitaxel serum level, close monitoring of paclitaxel-induced toxicity is recommended.
Paroxetine	May increase serum levels of paroxetine.	Clinical significance unknown. consider an alternative antidepressant (i.e., SSRI: escitalopram, citalopram, sertraline, or fluoxetine).
Perphenazine	May increase serum levels of perphenazine.	Consider an alternative neuroleptic: olanzapine.
Phencyclidine (PCP)	May significantly increase serum levels of PCP.	Applies to all PIs. Illicit drug use should be avoided for the obvious reason.
Phenobarbital	May decrease serum levels of RTV. RTV may increase serum levels of phenobarbital.	Consider alternative anticonvulsants (i.e., valproic acid, levetiracetam, lamotrigine, topiramate). Monitor anticonvulsants levels and consider TDM of RTV.
Phenytoin	May decrease serum levels of RTV. RTV may increase serum levels of phenytoin.	Consider alternative anticonvulsants (i.e., valproic acid, lamotrigine, levetiracetam, or topiramate). Monitor anticonvulsant levels and consider TDM of RTV.
Pimozide	May significantly increase pimozide serum levels resulting in QTc prolongation.	Contraindicated. Consider alternative: olanzapine.
Pravastatin	No change in RTV AUC, but pravastatin levels decreased by 50% with SQV/RTV.	Clinical significance unknown. Start with standard dose of pravastatin; titrate to effect.
Prednisone	Prednisolone AUC increase 30%–40% with with RTV (200 mg twice daily) coadministration.	Dose adjustment may be needed with long-term coadministration.
Propafenone	May significantly increase propafenone serum levels.	Contraindicated.
Propranolol	May increase propranolol serum levels.	Monitor closely with coadministration. It is unknown whether other PIs and NNRTIs affect propranolol serum levels. Consider alternative beta-blocker such as atenolol since it is primarily excreted unchanged in the urine with limited interaction with RTV.
Propoxyphene	May significantly increase propoxyphene serum levels.	Avoid concurrent administration.

RITONAVIR *(cont.)*

Drug	Effect of Interaction	Recommendations/Comments
Quinidine	May significantly increase quinidine levels.	Contraindicated.
Raltegravir (RAL)	No interactions.	Dose: standard dose for both drugs.
Ranolazine	May significantly increase ranolazine serum concentrations.	Contraindicated. May increase risk of QTc prolongation.
Rifabutin (RFB)	RFB AUC increased by 400%.	Recommended dose: RFB 150 mg every other day or 150 mg 3 ×/wk with standard dose RTV.
Rifampin	RTV AUC decreased by 35%.	Recommended dose: rifampin 600 mg once daily with standard dose RTV.
Rifapentine	RTV serum levels may be significantly decreased.	Avoid coadministration. Consider using RFB or rifampin with SQV 400 mg + RTV 400 mg twice daily.
Risperidone	Risperidone serum levels may be increased.	A case report of reversible coma associated with RTV-risperidone coadministration. Consider risperidone dose reduction with coadministration or use alternative neuroleptic (i.e., olanzapine).
Rosuvastatin	Other CYP3A4 inhibitor (i.e., erythromycin) did not affect rosuvastatin serum levels. Rosuvastatin AUC and Cmax were increased 2.1 to 4.7-fold, respectively. LPV and RTV PK parameters were not significantly affected.	Clinical significance of rosuvastatin effects on RTV PK unknown. This drug interaction study had important design limitations that could had affected the results. Unknown effect of rosuvastatin on other PIs and NNRTIs. Close monitoring recommended due to limited clinical data.
Salmeterol	May increase salmeterol serum concentrations.	Avoid coadministration. Consider formoterol.
Saquinavir (SQV)	SQV AUC increased by 20-fold.	Recommended doses: SQV/r 1000/100 mg twice daily. SQV/RTV 400/400 mg twice daily rarely used due to GI intolerance. SQV/r 2000/100 mg once daily (limited clinical data).
Sildenafil	Sildenafil AUC increased by 11-fold, Cmax increased by 300%.	Caution with concurrent use. Do not exceed 25 mg of sildenafil in a 48-hr period.
Simvastatin	May significantly increase simvastatin levels.	Contraindicated. Alternatives that may be used include atorvastatin (start with 10 mg/day), pravastatin, rosuvastatin, or fluvastatin. Monitor for adverse effect due to limited clinical data.

Drug	Effect of Interaction	Recommendations/Comments
Sirolimus	May significantly increase serum levels of sirolimus.	Applies to all PIs: dose sirolimus based on serum levels. A significant reduction of sirolimus dose with all PIs coadministration is highly likely.
St. John's wort	May decrease RTV serum levels.	Contraindicated. Studies done with IDV and NVP but St. John's wort likely to increase the metabolism of other PIs and NNRTIs. Use an alternative (more effective) antidepressant.
Tacrolimus	May significantly increase serum levels of tacrolimus.	Applies to all PIs: dose tacrolimus based on serum levels. A significantly reduction of tacrolimus dose with all PIs coadministration is recommended.
Tadalafil	Tadalafil AUC increased by 124% (with RTV 200 mg twice daily).	Start with 5 mg. Do not exceed 10 mg in 72 hrs. Consider sildenafil due to more clinical data and shorter half-life allowing for easier titration.
Tamoxifen	May increase serum levels of tamoxifen.	Applies to all PIs: no data. Close monitoring of tamoxifen-induced toxicity recommended.
Teniposide	May increase serum levels of teniposide.	Applies to all PIs: no data. Close monitoring of teniposide-induced toxicity recommended.
Terfenadine	May significantly increase terfenadine serum levels.	Contraindicated due to the potential for cardiac arrhythmias. Recommended alternative antihistamine: loratadine, fexofenadine, desloratidine, or cetirizine.
Tetrahydrocannabinol (THC)	Based on data with NFV and IDV, interactions are unlikely.	Applies to PIs and NNRTIs: interactions are unlikely but illicit drug use should be avoided for obvious reasons.
Theophylline	Theophylline AUC: decreased by 43%; Cmin: decreased by 57%.	Monitor theophylline levels; dose may need to be increased if sub therapeutic.
Thioridazine	May increase serum levels of thioridazine.	Consider an alternative neuroleptic: olanzapine.
Tipranavir (TPV)	TPV AUC increased 11-fold.	Dose: TPV/r 500/200 mg twice daily.
Trazodone	Trazodone AUC increased by 2.4-fold and Cmax by 34%.	Monitor for CNS and CV adverse effects. Consider decreasing trazodone dose by 50% with slow-dose titration.
Triazolam	May significantly increase serum levels of triazolam.	Applies to all PIs: avoid coadministration. Consider alternative benzodiazepine (lorazepam, oxazepam, or temazepam).
Vardenafil	Vardenafil AUC increased by 49-fold. RTV AUC decreased by 20%.	Do not exceed vardenafil 2.5 mg in 72 hrs. Consider sildenafil due to more clinical data and less pronounced interaction.

RITONAVIR *(cont.)*

Drug	Effect of Interaction	Recommendations/Comments
Venlafaxine	May increase serum levels of venlafaxine.	Consider an alternative antidepressant (i.e., SSRI: escitalopram, citalopram, sertraline, or fluoxetine).
Verapamil	May increase serum levels of verapamil.	Applies to all PIs: data limited to an interaction study conducted with ATV and diltiazem, which resulted in doubling of diltiazem serum levels (this led to PR interval prolongation). All PIs have the potential of prolonging the PR interval with calcium channel blocker coadministration. Calcium channel blockers should be started with 50% of the dose and slowly titrated with close monitoring of BP and pulse.
Vinblastine	May increase serum levels of vinblastine.	Applies to all PIs: no data. Close monitoring of vinblastine-induced toxicity recommended.
Vincristine	May increase serum levels of vincristine.	Applies to all PIs: no data. Close monitoring of vincristine-induced toxicity recommended.
Vitamin C	Data limited to interaction study with IDV and vitamin C (1 g/day): IDV AUC decreased by 14% and Cmin by 32%.	Clinical significance unknown. Other PIs and NNRTIs serum concentrations may be affected when coadministered with similar dose of vitamin C.
Voriconazole	RTV (400 mg twice daily) decreased steady-state voriconazole AUC by 82%. RTV levels was not affected by voriconazole. RTV (100 mg twice daily) decreased steady-state voriconazole AUC by 39%.	RTV (400 mg twice daily) contraindicated with voriconazole. Avoid coadministration with boosted PI. Consider another anti-fungal for aspergillosis (i.e., *AmBisome* or caspofungin) or use with TDM.
Warfarin	Case report of increased warfarin requirement after RTV initiation.	Other PIs and NNRTIs may also affect warfarin requirements. Monitor INR closely with coadministration.

DRUG-DRUG INTERACTION – SAQUINAVIR (SQV)

Drug	Effect of Interaction	Recommendations/Comments
Alfuzosin	May increase alfuzosin serum concentrations.	Avoid coadministration. Consider doxazosin and terazosin for BPH (with close monitoring).
Alprazolam	May increase serum level of alprazolam.	Avoid coadministration. Consider an alternative benzodiazepine (i.e., lorazepam, oxazepam, or temazepam).

Drug	Effect of Interaction	Recommendations/Comments
Amiodarone	May significantly increase amiodarone serum level.	Avoid coadministration. Data limited to case report of increased amiodarone concentrations with IDV coadministration. RTV, FPV, SQV, and ATV manufacturer recommends against use of amiodarone, but all PIs have the same potential of significantly increasing amiodarone serum concentrations and increasing QTc interval. If coadministration cannot be avoided, monitor for amiodarone ADRs (PFTs, TSH). Consider monitoring serum concentrations of amiodarone, but its long half-life may make titration difficult.
Amlodipine	May increase serum level of amlodipine.	Applies to all PIs: data limited to an interaction study conducted with ATV and diltiazem, which resulted in doubling of diltiazem serum level (this led to PR interval prolongation). All PIs and have the potential of prolonging PR interval with calcium channel blocker coadministration. Calcium channel blockers should be started with 50% of the recommended dose and slowly titrated with close monitoring of BP and pulse.
Artemether (artemisinin)	May increase serum level of artemether.	Applies to all PIs: close monitoring for artemether toxicity (bone marrow suppression, bradycardia, and seizure).
Astemizole	May significantly increase astemizole serum level.	Contraindicated due to the potential for cardiac arrhythmias. Recommended alternative antihistamine: loratadine, fexofenadine, desloratidine, or cetirizine.
Atorvastatin	Atorvastatin increased by 450% (studied with RTV/SQV).	Use with caution. Use lowest possible dose of atrovastatin (10 mg). Consider pravastatin or rosuvastatin.
Azathioprine	Interaction unlikely.	Applies to all PIs and NNRTIs: use standard dose.
Bepridil	May significantly increase bepridil serum level.	Applies to all PIs: no data. The manufacturer of ATV, RTV, and APV does not recommend bepridil coadministration. This contraindication should be extended to all PIs since a significant increase in bepridil serum level can result in pro-arrhythmic events such as VT, PVC, and VFib.
Beta-blockers	May increase risk of PR interval prolongation.	Use with close monitoring.

SAQUINAVIR *(cont.)*

Drug	Effect of Interaction	Recommendations/Comments
Carbamazepine	May decrease serum levels of SQV.	Consider alternative anticonvulsants (i.e., valproic acid, lamotrigine, levetiracetam, or topiramate). Monitor anticonvulsant levels and SQV Cmin with coadministration.
Chlordiazepoxide	May increase serum level of chlordiazepoxide.	Applies to all PIs: consider an alternative benzodiazepine (i.e., lorazepam, temazepam, or oxazepam).
Cisapride	May significantly increase cisapride serum level.	Contraindicated due to potential for cardiac arrhythmias. Recommended alternative: metoclopramide.
Clarithromycin	Clarithromycin increases SQV AUC 177% and SQV increases clarithromycin AUC 45%.	Use standard doses.
Clorazepate	May increase serum level of clorazepate.	Applies to all PIs: consider an alternative benzodiazepine (i.e., lorazepam, temazepam, or oxazepam).
Cyclophosphamide	May increase serum level of cyclophosphamide.	Applies to all PIs: data limited to an interaction study conducted with IDV resulting in a 50% increase in cyclophosphamide serum level. Since all PIs have the potential of increasing cyclophosphamide levels, close monitoring of cyclophosphamide-induced toxicity is recommended.
Cyclosporine	Cyclosporine Cmin: increased 300%.	Case report of significant increase of cyclosporine levels. Monitor serum level of cyclosporine closely with coadministration. Cyclosporine dose may need to be decreased.
Darunavir (DRV)	DRV AUC decreased 26%.	Avoid coadministration.
Dexamethasone	May decrease SQV serum levels.	Clinical significance unknown.
Digoxin	Digoxin AUC and Cmax increased by 49% and 27%, respectively.	Reduce digoxin dose with SQV/r coadministration. Magnitude of interaction higher in females (AUC increased 74% in females vs 33% in males). Use with close monitoring. Significant increased in PR prolongation observed.

Drug	Effect of Interaction	Recommendations/Comments
Diltiazem	May increase serum level of diltiazem.	Applies to all PIs: data limited to an interaction study conducted with ATV, which resulted in doubling of diltiazem serum level (this led to PR interval prolongation). All PIs have the potential of prolonging PR interval with diltiazem coadministration. Diltiazem should be started with 50% of the recommended dose and slowly titrated with close monitoring of BP and pulse.
Disopyramide	May increase disopyramide serum levels.	Applies to all PIs: no data. Monitor disopyramide serum level (target: 2–7.5 mcg/mL).
Docetaxel	May increase serum level of docetaxel.	Applies to all PIs: no data. Close monitoring of chemotherapy-induced toxicity recommended.
Dofetilide	May significantly increase serum level of dofetilide and increase QTc.	Applies to all PIs: no data, but coadministration should be avoided. Monitor QTc closely and adjust dofetilide dosing based on QTc prolongation and renal function. Consider an alternative class III antiarrhythmic such as bretylium or ibutilide.
Echinacea	May decrease SQV serum level. Echinacea decreased (400 mg 4 ×/day) CYP3A4 substrate (midazolam) by 23%.	Clinical significance unknown but should avoided with PIs and NNRTIs until the safety of this combination is further evaluated.
Ergot Alkaloid	May significantly increase serum level of ergotamine resulting in acute ergot toxicity.	Contraindicated. Consider alternative agent for migraine such as sumatriptan (but not eletriptan since it is a CYP3A4 substrate and significant drug-drug interaction occurred with CYP3A4 inhibitor).
Estazolam	May increase serum level of estazolam.	Applies to all PIs: consider an alternative benzodiazepine (i.e., lorazepam, oxazepam, or temazepam).
Ethosuximide	May increase serum levels of ethosuximide.	Applies to all PIs: consider switching to valproic acid for the treatment of absence seizure.
Etoposide	May increase serum level of etoposide.	Applies to all PIs: no data. Close monitoring of chemotherapy induced toxicity recommended.
Etravirine (ETR)	ETR AUC decreased 33%.	Clinical significance unknown. SQV/r 1000/100 mg twice daily plus standard dose ETR likely.

SAQUINAVIR *(cont.)*

Drug	Effect of Interaction	Recommendations/Comments
Fatty Food	SQV AUC increased 18-fold.	SQV should be taken with food.
Felodipine	May increase serum level of felodipine.	Applies to all PIs: data limited to an interaction study conducted with ATV and diltiazem, which resulted in doubling of diltiazem serum level (this led PR interval prolongation). All PIs has the potential of prolonging PR interval with calcium channel blockers coadministration. Calcium channel blockers should be started with 50% of the dose and slowly titrated with close monitoring of BP and pulse.
Fentanyl	May increase fentanyl serum level.	Use with caution. Consider morphine.
Flecainide	May increase antiarrhythmic serum levels.	Applies to all PIs: avoid coadministration; if necessary, monitor flecainide trough level with coadministration. Target: 200–1000 ng/mL. Toxicity is frequent with trough serum levels above 1000 ng/mL.
Fluconazole	No significant interaction.	Usual dose recommended.
Flurazepam	May increase serum level of flurazepam.	Applies to all PIs: consider an alternative benzodiazepine (i.e., lorazepam, oxazepam, or temazepam).
Fluticasone	Fluticasone AUC increased 350-fold (studied with RTV 100 mg q12h).	Avoid long-term coadministration. Consider beclomethasone.
Fosamprenavir (FPV)	SQV AUC decreased 14% (NS).	Consider SQV/r 1000/100–200 mg twice daily + FPV 700 mg twice daily.
Garlic Supplement	SQV Cmin decreased by 49%; AUC: decreased 51%; after 10-days washout period, pharmacokinetic values returned to only 60%–70% of baseline.	Coadministration not recommended.
Granisetron	May increase serum level of granisetron.	Applies to all PIs: due to the large therapeutic index of granisetron, potential interaction is unlikely to be clinically significant.
Grapefruit Juice	SQV AUC: increased 50% (grapefruit juice 200 mL from concentrate).	May be a beneficial interaction.
Heroin (diamorphine)	Drug interactions unlikely.	Applies to PIs and NNRTIs: interaction unlikely but illicit drug use should be avoided for obvious reasons.

Drug	Effect of Interaction	Recommendations/Comments
Ifosfamide	May increase serum level of ifosphamide.	Applies to all PIs: no data. Close monitoring of chemotherapy-induced toxicity recommended.
Indinavir (IDV)	SQV AUC increased 4–7-fold; no effect on IDV.	*In vitro* antagonism. Clinical significance unknown. Avoid coadministration.
Irinotecan	May increase irinotecan serum level.	Not recommended. All PIs also have the potential for significant interaction with irinotecan, therefore the coadministration should be done with extreme caution.
Itraconazole	SQV: no significant change. Itraconazole level: no significant change.	No significant change. Use standard dose of both drugs.
Ketoconazole	SQV AUC increased 30%.	Use standard dose. If SQV coadministered with RTV, do not exceed ketoconazole 200 mg/day.
Lidocaine	May increase antiarrhythmic serum levels.	Applies to all PIs: no data, but coadministration should be avoided.
Lopinavir/ ritonavir (LPV/r)	SQV AUC: increased 836%; Cmin: increased 1700%.	Dose: SQV 800–1000 mg twice daily + LPV/r 400/100 mg twice daily.
Lovastatin	May increase lovastatin serum level.	Contraindicated. Recommended alternatives include pravastatin (but pravastatin AUC decreased by 50% with SQV/r), fluvastatin, and rosuvastatin (and possibly atorvastatin). Monitor for adverse effects due to limited clinical data with these agents.
Maraviroc (MVC)	MVC AUC increased 732%.	Recommended dose: SQV/r 1000/100 mg twice daily + MVC 150 mg twice daily.
Mefloquine	May increase serum levels of mefloquine.	Applies to all PIs: if available consider mefloquine serum level monitoring. Monitor for mefloquine toxicity (i.e., dizziness, LFTs, and periodic ophthalmic examination).
Methadone	S-methadone AUC: decreased 25%; R-methadone (active) AUC: decreased 20% (studied with SQV/RTV).	Monitor for withdrawal symptoms but unlikely to be significant. Methadone dose may need to be increased if patient experiences withdrawal Sx.
Mexiletine	May increase antiarrhythmic serum levels.	Applies to all PIs: no data. Use with caution. Monitor EKG and serum level. Serum levels exceeding 1.5–2 mcg/mL have been associated with an increased risk of toxicity.

SAQUINAVIR (cont.)

Drug	Effect of Interaction	Recommendations/Comments
Midazolam	May increase midazolam serum level.	Concurrent administration contraindicated due to potential for prolonged sedation. Use alternative: lorazepam, oxazepam, or temazepam. Single dose midazolam may be used (chronic use not recommended).
Milk Thistle	Unknown.	Data limited to an interaction study with milk thistle and IDV. IDV AUC unchanged and IDV Cmin decreased by 47%. Avoid coadministration. No data available for other PIs and NNRTIs.
Mirtazapine	May increase serum level of mirtazapine.	Applies to all PIs: use with caution. Consider an alternative antidepressant (i.e., SSRI: escitalopram, citalopram, sertraline, or fluoxetine).
Mycophenolate	Interaction unlikely. No significant interaction observed with NVP.	Applies to all PIs and NNRTIs: no significant interaction observed with NVP. Use standard dose.
Nefazodone	May increase serum level of nefazodone.	Applies to all PIs: use with caution. Consider an alternative antidepressant (i.e., SSRI: escitalopram, citalopram, sertraline, or fluoxetine).
Nelfinavir (NFV)	SQV AUC increased by 3 to 5-fold. NFV AUC increased by 20%.	Consider: SQV 1200 mg twice daily + NFV 1250 mg twice daily (limited clinical experience and rarely used).
Nifedipine	May increase serum level of nifedipine.	Applies to all PIs: data limited to an interaction study conducted with ATV and diltiazem, which resulted in doubling of diltiazem serum level (this led PR interval prolongation). All PIs have the potential of prolonging PR interval with calcium channel blocker coadministration. Calcium channel blockers should be started with 50% of the dose and slowly titrated with close monitoring of BP and pulse.
Nisoldipine	May increase serum level of nisoldipine.	Applies to all PIs: data limited to an interaction study conducted with ATV and diltiazem, which resulted in doubling of diltiazem serum level (this led PR interval prolongation). All PIs have the potential of prolonging PR interval with calcium channel blocker coadministration. Calcium channel blockers should be started with 50% of the recommended dose and slowly titrated with close monitoring of BP and pulse.

Drug	Effect of Interaction	Recommendations/Comments
Oral Contraceptives	No data for NFV. Ethinyl estradiol AUC decreased by 47%, Norethindrone decreased by 18%.	Recommend an alternative form of contraception.
Paclitaxel	May increase paclitaxel serum level.	Applies to all PIs: since all PIs have the potential of significantly increasing paclitaxel serum level, close monitoring of paclitaxel-induced toxicity is recommended.
Phencyclidine (PCP)	May significantly increase serum level of PCP.	Applies to all PIs: avoid all illicit drug use with PIs.
Phenobarbital	May decrease serum levels of SQV.	Consider alternative anticonvulsants (i.e., valproic acid, lamotrigine, levetiracetam, or topiramate). Monitor anticonvulsant levels and SQV Cmin with coadministration.
Phenytoin	May decrease serum levels of SQV.	Consider alternative anticonvulsants (i.e., valproic acid, lamotrigine, levetiracetam, or topiramate). Monitor anticonvulsant levels and SQV Cmin with coadministration.
Pimozide	May significantly increase pimozide serum level resulting in QTc prolongation.	Contraindicated. Consider alternative: olanzapine.
Pravastatin	Pravastatin AUC decreased by 50% (studied with SQV/RTV).	Clinical significance unknown. May need to increase dose of pravastatin.
Prednisone	Prednisolone serum concentration may be increased with SQV/r coadministration.	Dose adjustment may be needed with long-term coadministration.
Propafenone	May increase antiarrhythmic serum levels.	Applies to all PIs: no data. Coadministration should be avoided. Serum levels are not routinely recommended due to the poor correlation with efficacy and toxicity.
Proton Pump Inhibitors (PPI) (e.g., omeprazole)	SQV AUC increased 82%.	Usual dose recommended.
Quinidine	May increase antiarrhythmic serum concentrations and increase QTc prolongation.	Avoid coadministration. May increase risk of QTc prolongation. Contraindicated with RTV. With all PIs and NNRTIs coadministration, monitor EKG (QTc) and serum concentrations: target: 2–5 mcg/mL.
Raltegravir (RAL)	Interaction unlikely.	Data with RTV (100 mg twice daily) did not affect RAL PK parameters. SQV/r 1000/100 mg twice daily plus standard dose RAL likely.

SAQUINAVIR *(cont.)*

Drug	Effect of Interaction	Recommendations/Comments
Ranitidine	No significant interaction.	Use standard dose.
Ranolazine	May significantly increase ranolazine serum concentrations.	Contraindicated. May increase risk of QTc prolongation.
Rifabutin (RFB)	SQV AUC decreased by 43%.	Do not coadminister SQV with RFB as a sole PI. Consider RTV 400 mg twice daily + SQV 400 mg twice daily with RFB 150 mg 3 ×/wk OR SQV 1000 mg + RTV 100 mg twice daily with RFB 150 mg every other day (no data, but likely to attain good PK).
Rifampin	Rifampin: SQV AUC: decreased by 84%.	Coadministration of rifampin with SQV (as sole PI) is not recommended due to significant decrease in SQV PK parameters. Boosting SQV with RTV is not recommended due to high incidence (39.3%) of hepatotoxicity.
Rifapentine	SQV serum levels may be significantly decreased.	Avoid coadministration. Consider using RFB.
Ritonavir (RTV)	SQV AUC increased by 20-fold.	Recommended doses: SQV/r 1000/100 mg twice daily. SQV/RTV 400/400 mg twice daily (higher rate of GI intolerance and hepatotoxicity). SQV/r 2000/100 mg once daily (limited clinical data).
Rosuvastatin	Other CYP3A4 inhibitor (i.e., erythromycin) did not affect rosuvastatin serum level.	Applies to PIs and NNRTIs: interaction unlikely, but close monitoring recommended due to limited clinical data.
Salmeterol	May increase salmeterol concentrations.	Avoid coadministration. Consider formoterol.
Sildenafil	Sildenafil AUC increased by 210% (with SQV 1200 mg three times daily).	Use with caution. Do not exceed 25 mg of sildenafil in 48-hr period.
Simvastatin	Simvastatin AUC: increased 3059% (studied with SQV/RTV).	Contraindicated. Recommended alternatives include atorvastatin, pravastatin (but pravastatin AUC decreased by 50% with SQV/r), fluvastatin, and rosuvastatin. Monitor for adverse effects due to limited clinical data with these agents.
Sirolimus	May significantly increase serum level of sirolimus.	Applies to All PIs: dose sirolimus based on serum level. A significantly reduction of sirolimus dose with all PIs coadministration is highly likely.
St. John's wort	May decrease SQV serum level.	Contraindicated. Use an alternative (more effective) antidepressant.

Drug	Effect of Interaction	Recommendations/Comments
Tacrolimus	May significantly increase serum level of tacrolimus.	Applies to all PIs: dose tacrolimus based on serum level. A significant reduction of tacrolimus dose with all PIs coadministration is recommended.
Tadalafil	May increase serum level of tadalafil.	Applies to All PIs: start with 5 mg. Do not exceed 10 mg in 72 hrs. Consider sildenafil due to more clinical data and shorter half-life allowing for easier titration.
Tamoxifen	May increase serum level of tamoxifen.	Applies to all PIs: no data. Close monitoring of tamoxifen-induced toxicity recommended.
Teniposide	May increase serum level of teniposide.	Applies to all PIs: no data. Close monitoring of teniposide-induced toxicity recommended.
Terfenadine	Terfenadine AUC: increased by 368%; Cmax: increased by 253%.	Contraindicated due to the potential for cardiac arrhythmias. Recommended alternative antihistamine: loratadine, fexofenadine, desloratidine, or cetirizine.
Tetrahydrocan-nabinol (THC)	Based on data with NFV and IDV interactions are unlikely.	Applies to PIs and NNRTIs: interactions are unlikely but illicit drug use should be avoided for obvious reasons.
Trazodone	May increase serum level of Trazodone and increase risk for QTc prolongation.	Applies to All PIs: use with caution. Consider an alternative antidepressant (i.e., SSRI: escitalopram, citalopram, sertraline, or fluoxetine).
Triazolam	May significantly increase triazolam serum level.	Contraindicated. Alternative benzodiazepine may be used (temazepam, oxazepam, or lorazepam).
Vardenafil	May significantly increase serum level of vardenafil.	Applies to all PIs: do not exceed vardenafil 2.5 mg in 72 hrs (with RTV) or 2.5 mg in 24 hrs (with other PIs). Consider sildenafil due to more clinical data and less pronounced interaction. Avoid coadministration with IDV.
Verapamil	May increase serum level of verapamil.	Applies to all PIs: data limited to an interaction study conducted with ATV and diltiazem, which resulted in doubling of diltiazem serum level (this led PR interval prolongation). All PIs have the potential of prolonging PR interval with calcium channel blocker coadministration. Calcium channel blockers should be started with 50% of the dose and slowly titrated with close monitoring of BP and pulse.
Vinblastine	May increase serum level of vinblastine.	Applies to all PIs: no data. Close monitoring of vinblastine-induced toxicity recommended.

SAQUINAVIR *(cont.)*

Drug	Effect of Interaction	Recommendations/Comments
Vincristine	May increase serum level of vincristine.	Applies to all PIs: no data. Close monitoring of vincristine-induced toxicity recommended.
Voriconazole	May decrease voriconazole AUC with SQV/r. Voriconazole may increase coadministered SQV.	Significant interaction with EFV and RTV (400 mg twice daily); contraindicated. Voriconazole AUC decreased 39% with RTV 100 mg twice daily coadministration; avoid coadministration with boosted PI. Consider another antifungal for aspergillosis (i.e., *AmBisome* or caspofungin) or use with TDM. Higher dose of voriconazole may be needed.

DRUG-DRUG INTERACTION – STAVUDINE (d4T)

Drug	Effect of Interaction	Recommendations/Comments
Cisplatin	May increase risk of peripheral neuropathy.	Monitor for peripheral neuropathy. Irreversible neuropathy with continued use. Avoid long-term coadministration.
Didanosine (ddI) (EC and buffered)	Additive toxicity (peripheral neuropathy, lactic acidosis, and pancreatitis).	Do not coadminister, especially in pregnancy.
Disulfiram	May increase risk of peripheral neuropathy.	Monitor for peripheral neuropathy. Irreversible neuropathy with continued use. Avoid long-term coadministration.
Fluconazole	d4T AUC: no significant change.	No significant interaction.
Gold Compounds	May increase risk of peripheral neuropathy.	Monitor for peripheral neuropathy. Irreversible neuropathy with continued use. Avoid long-term coadministration.
Hydralazine	May increase risk of peripheral neuropathy.	Monitor for peripheral neuropathy. Irreversible neuropathy with continued use. Avoid long-term coadministration.
Indinavir (IDV)	d4T AUC: increased by 25%.	Unlikely to be significant. Use standard dose.
Isoniazid	May increase risk of peripheral neuropathy.	Give isoniazid with pyridoxine to decrease the risk of neuropathy. Monitor for peripheral neuropathy. Irreversible neuropathy with continued use. Avoid long-term coadministration.
Methadone	d4T AUC: decreased by 23%; Methadone: no change.	Unlikely to be significant. Use standard dose.

Drug	Effect of Interaction	Recommendations/Comments
Metronidazole (long term)	May increase risk of peripheral neuropathy (rare).	Monitor for peripheral neuropathy. Irreversible neuropathy with continued use. Avoid long-term coadministration.
Pyridoxine (vitamin B6), high dose	May increase risk of peripheral neuropathy.	Monitor for peripheral neuropathy. Irreversible neuropathy with continued use. Avoid long-term coadministration.
Ribavirin	*In vitro* antagonism but not *in vivo*.	Not clinically significant. No *in vivo* antagonism observed.
Rifabutin (RFB)	d4T AUC: no significant change.	No significant interaction. Use standard dose.
Thalidomide	May increase risk of peripheral neuropathy.	Monitor for peripheral neuropathy. Irreversible neuropathy with continued use. Avoid long-term coadministration.
Vincristine	May increase risk of peripheral neuropathy.	Monitor for peripheral neuropathy. Irreversible neuropathy with continued use. Avoid long-term coadministration.
Zidovudine (AZT)	In *vitro* and in *avivo* antagonism.	Do not coadminister.

DRUG-DRUG INTERACTION – TENOFOVIR (TDF)

Drug	Effect of Interaction	Recommendations/Comments
Abacavir (ABC)	No evidence of drug-drug interactions.	ABC + TDF + 3TC once daily associated with suboptimal viral suppression. Effect probably due to increased selection for resistance (K65R) rather than drug interaction. Preliminary analysis of AZT/ABC/3TC + TDF as a twice daily regimen showed more favorable results, though unclear whether better than AZT/3TC/ABC alone. Do not coadminister ABC+TDF +3TC without a PI or thymidine analog.
Atazanavir (ATV)	ATV: AUC decreased by 25%; Cmin decreased by 26% (with RTV); TDF not measured. ATV AUC decreased by 25% and Cmin decreased by 40% (without RTV); TDF AUC: increased by 24%.	With coadministration, use ATV/r 300/100 mg once daily. Avoid unboosted ATV and use boosted ATV with caution.
Darunavir (DRV)	TDF AUC increased 22%.	Unlikely to be clinically significant, but monitor for TDF-associated nephrotoxicity. Use standard dose of both TDF and DRV/r.

TENOFOVIR *(cont.)*

Drug	Effect of Interaction	Recommendations/Comments
Didanosine (ddI)	ddI EC AUC: increased by 48% (fasted); ddI EC AUC: increased by 60% (fed state). TDF: No change.	Dose adjust ddI EC to 250 mg once daily (for >60 kg) or 200 mg once daily (for <60 kg) with TDF coadministration. Suboptimal virologic response in 91% of patients treated with ddI + TDF + 3TC once daily. Do not use ddI + TDF + 3TC as a triple-NRTI regimen.
Emtricitabine (FTC)	No significant drug interaction.	Use standard dose, usually in coformulated version (TDF/FTC or TDF/FTC/EFV).
Etravirine (ETR)	ETR AUC decreased by 19%, TDF AUC increased by 15%.	Use standard dose.
Food	Increased bioavailability with food (AUC increased 60%), especially high-fat meals, but levels adequate in fasting state.	Take with or without food.
Ganciclovir	May theoretically increase serum concentrations of TDF and/or ganciclovir.	No data. Monitor for dose-related toxicities.
Lopinavir/ ritonavir (LPV/r)	TDF AUC increased by 34%.	Unlikely to be clinically significant, but monitor for TDF-associated nephrotoxicity. Use standard dose of both TDF and LPV/r.
Norgestimate/ Ethinyl Estradiol	No significant drug interaction.	Use standard dose.
Probenecid	TDF levels may be increased due to probenecid-induced inhibition of the renal tubular secretion.	Clinical significance unknown.
Valganciclovir	May theoretically increase serum concentrations of TDF and/or ganciclovir.	No data. Monitor for dose-related toxicities.

DRUG-DRUG INTERACTION – TIPRANAVIR (TPV)

Drug	Effect of Interaction	Recommendations/Comments
Abacavir (ABC)	ABC AUC decreased by approximately 40%.	Clinical significance unknown. ABC intracellular triphosphate levels not measured.
Alfuzosin	May significantly increase alfuzosin serum concentrations.	Avoid coadministration. Consider tamsulosin or doxazosin.
Alprazolam	May increase serum level of alprazolam.	Consider an alternative benzodiazepine (lorazepam, temazepam, or oxazepam).

Drug	Effect of Interaction	Recommendations/Comments
Amiodarone	May significantly increase amiodarone serum level.	Contraindicated.
Amlodipine	May increase serum level of amlodipine.	Applies to all PIs: data limited to an interaction study conducted with ATV and diltiazem, which resulted in doubling of diltiazem level, which led to PR interval prolongation. All PIs have potential of prolonging PR interval with calcium channel blocker coadministration.
Antacids	TPV AUC decreased by approximately 30%.	Avoid coadministration or separate administration time by 2 hrs.
Artemether (artemisinin)	May increase serum level of artemether.	Data only available for EFV. Coadministration of EFV with artesunate + amodiaquine resulted in significant LFT elevations. Close monitoring for artemether toxicity (bone marrow suppression, bradycardia, and seizure).
Aspirin	May increase risk of bleeding.	Avoid coadministration or use with caution.
Astemizole	May significantly increase astemizole serum level.	Contraindicated.
Atazanavir (ATV)	ATV AUC decreased by 39% and Cmin decreased by 70%. TPV AUC increased by 11% and Cmin increased by 59%.	Avoid coadministration.
Atorvastatin	TPV/r increased atorvastatin AUC by 9-fold.	Caution with coadministration start with atorvastatin 10 mg/day or consider alternative HMG CoA reductase inhibitor such as rosuvastatin or pravastatin.
Azathioprine	Interaction unlikely.	Applies to all PIs and NNRTI: use standard dose.
Bepridil	May significantly increase bepridil serum level.	Contraindicated.
Bosentan	May significantly increase bosentan serum concentrations.	Coadminister bosentan only after RTV dosing has reached steady-state. In patients on RTV >10 days: start bosentan at 62.5 mg once daily or every other day. In patients already on bosentan: d/c bosentan for >36 hrs prior to initiation of RTV-boosted PIs and restart bosentan at 62.5 mg once daily or every other day after RTV has reached steady-state (after 10 days).
Buprenorphine	Compared to historical control, TPV Cmin decreased by 40%.	Clinical significance unknown. Use standard dose.

TIPRANAVIR *(cont.)*

Drug	Effect of Interaction	Recommendations/Comments
Bupropion	Bupropion AUC decreased 46%.	Titrate bupropion to therapeutic effect.
Carbamazepine	May decrease serum concentrations of PIs and NNRTIs. Carbamazepine AUC increased 26%.	Applies to all PIs and NNRTIs: consider alternative anticonvulsants (i.e., valproic acid, lamotrigine, levetiracetam, or topiramate). Monitor carbamazepine concentrations or consider TDM of PIs and NNRTIs.
Chlordiazepoxide	May increase serum level of chlordiazepoxide.	Applies to all PIs: consider an alternative benzodiazepine (i.e., lorazepam, oxazepam, or temazepam).
Cisapride	May significantly increase ergotamine serum level.	Contraindicated.
Clarithromycin	TPV AUC increased 66%. Clarithromycin AUC increased 19%.	Use standard dose TPV/r. Consider clarithromycindose adjustment in renal failure. Cr CL 30–60 mL/min = 50% of dose. Cr CL <30 mL/min = 25% of dose.
Clopidogrel	May increase risk of bleeding.	Avoid coadministration or use with caution.
Clorazepate	May increase serum level of clorazepate.	Applies to all PIs: consider an alternative benzodiazepine (lorazepam, oxazepam, temazepam).
Cyclophosphamide	May increase serum level of cyclophosphamide.	Applies to all PIs: data limited to an interaction study conducted with IDV resulting in 50% increase in cyclophosphamide levels. Since all PIs have the potential of increasing cyclophosphamide levels, close monitoring of cyclophosphamide-induced toxicity is recommended.
Cyclosporine	May significantly increase or decrease serum level of cyclosporine.	Applies to All PIs: monitor serum level of cyclosporine closely with coadministration.
Darunavir (DRV)	May decrease DRV serum concentrations.	No data; avoid coadministration.
Desipramine	Desipramine levels may be increased.	Use with caution. Consider dose reduction with close monitoring.
Didanosine (ddI)	ddI AUC decreased by 33% with TPV/r 250/200 mg twice daily coadministration.	Clinical significance unknown. Consider separating administration time by at least 2 hrs. ddI buffer may also decrease TPV serum level; separate administration time by at least 2 hrs.
Digoxin	May decrease digoxin concentrations secondary to Pgp induction.	No data. Monitor digoxin serum concentration with coadministration.

Drug	Effect of Interaction	Recommendations/Comments
Diltiazem	May increase serum level of diltiazem.	Applies to all PIs: data limited to an interaction study conducted with ATV that resulted in doubling of diltiazem levels, which led to PR interval prolongation. All PIs have potential of prolonging PR interval with diltiazem coadministration.
Disopyramide	May increase disopyramide serum levels.	Applies to all PIs: no data. Monitor disopyramide serum level (target: 2–7.5 mcg/mL).
Disulfiram	May result in disulfiram-like reaction.	Avoid coadministration due to the alcohol content in the TPV/r capsules.
Docetaxel	May increase serum level of docetaxel.	Applies to all PIs: no data. Close monitoring of chemotherapy-induced toxicity recommended.
Dofetilide	May significantly increase serum level of dofetilide.	Applies to all PIs: no data. Use with caution. Monitor QTc closely and adjust dofetilide dosing based on QTc prolongation and renal function. Consider an alternative class III antiarrhythmic such as bretylium or ibutilide.
Efavirenz (EFV)	PK profile of TPV/r unchanged by EFV following single dose; EFV levels also unchanged. Increases in TPV AUC, Cmax, and C12h seen at steady-state with EFV.	Unclear from abstract if EFV levels were measured at steady-state (Roszko PJ, et al. 2nd IAS, Paris, abstract 865, 2003). Phase III trials currently using TPV/r 500/200 mg with coadministration of EFV 600 mg qhs.
Enfuvirtide (ENF)	TPV Cmin increased 45%.	Clinical significance unknown. Use standard dose.
Ergotamine	May significantly increase ergotamine serum level.	Contraindicated.
Estazolam	May increase serum level of estazolam.	Applies to all PIs: consider an alternative benzodiazepine (lorazepam, oxazepam, or temazepam).
Ethinyl Estradiol	EE AUC decreased by 50%.	Alternative form of contraception should be used. 33% incidence of rash in healthy volunteer study.
Ethosuximide	May increase serum levels of ethosuximide.	Applies to all PIs: consider switching to valproic acid for the treatment of absence seizure.
Etoposide	May increase serum level of etoposide.	Applies to all PIs: no data. Close monitoring of chemotherapy-induced toxicity recommended.
Etravirine (ETR)	ETR AUC decreased by 76%. TPV and RTV AUC increased by 18% and 23%, respectively.	Avoid coadministration.

TIPRANAVIR *(cont.)*

Drug	Effect of Interaction	Recommendations/Comments
Felodipine	May increase serum level of felodipine.	Applies to all PIs: data limited to an interaction study conducted with ATV and diltiazem that resulted in doubling of diltiazem serum level, which led to PR interval prolongation. All PIs have potential of prolonging PR interval with calcium channel blocker coadministration.
Flecainide	May increase antiarrhythmic serum levels.	Contraindicated.
Fluconazole	TPV AUC increased by 50%. No change in fluconazole levels.	Use standard dose TPV/r. Avoid fluconazole >200 mg once daily. Monitor liver function closely.
Flurazepam	May increase serum level of flurazepam.	Applies to all PIs: consider an alternative benzodiazepine (lorazepam, oxazepam, or temazepam).
Fluticasone	May significantly increase fluticasone serum concentrations.	Avoid coadministration. Consider beclomethasone.
Fosamprenavir (FPV)	May significantly decrease APV serum concentrations.	Avoid coadministration.
Granisetron	May increase serum level of granisetron.	Applies to all PIs: due to large therapeutic index of granisetron, potential interaction unlikely to be clinically significant.
Heroin (diamorphine)	Drug interactions unlikely.	Applies to PIs and NNRTIs: interaction unlikely but illicit drug use should be avoided for obvious reasons.
Hypoglycemics	TPV/r may increase or decrease hypoglycemic agents (glimepiride, glipizide, glyburide, pioglitazone, repaglinide, and tolbutamide).	Careful glucose monitoring is recommended with coadministration.
Ifosphamide	May increase serum level of ifosphamide.	Applies to all PIs: no data. Close monitoring of chemotherapy-induced toxicity recommended.
Indinavir (IDV)	May decrease IDV serum concentrations.	No data; avoid coadministration.
Irinotecan	May increase irinotecan serum level.	Applies to all PIs: coadministration of ATV contraindicated by manufacturer. All PIs also have potential for significant interaction with irinotecan; therefore, coadminister with extreme caution.
Itraconazole	Itraconazole levels may be increased.	Doses higher than 200 mg not recommended.

Drug	Effect of Interaction	Recommendations/Comments
Ketoconazole	Ketoconazole levels may be increased.	Doses higher than 200 mg not recommended.
Lidocaine	May increase antiarrhythmic serum levels.	Applies to all PIs: no data. Use with caution, monitor lidocaine serum level (target: 1.5–6 mcg/mL) with coadministration.
Lopinavir/ ritonavir (LPV/r)	LPV AUC decreased by 55%.	Not recommended.
Lovastatin	May significantly increase lovastatin serum concentrations.	Contraindicated. Consider pravastatin, atorvastatin (start with 10 mg), or rosuvastatin (start with 5 mg).
Maraviroc (MCV)	No significant interaction.	Use standard dose.
Mefloquine	May increase serum levels of mefloquine.	Applies to all PIs: if available, consider mefloquine serum level monitoring. Monitor for mefloquine toxicity (i.e., dizziness, LFTs, and periodic ophthalmic examination).
Meperidine	Increased normeperidine levels.	Avoid coadministration.
Methadone	Methadone decreased by 50%.	Monitor for withdrawal signs and symptoms. Methadone stereoisomer not specified but may require methadone dose increase.
Metronidazole	May result in disulfiram-like reaction.	Avoid coadministration due to the alcohol content in the TPV/r capsules.
Mexiletine	May increase serum levels of mexiletine.	Applies to all PIs: no data. Use with caution. Monitor EKG and serum level. Serum levels exceeding 1.5–2 mcg/mL have been associated with an increased risk of toxicity.
Midazolam	May significantly increase midazolam serum level.	Contraindicated with oral midazolam. Consider alternative benzodiazepine (e.g., lorazepam, oxazepam, or temazepam). If TPV/r is coadministered with IV midazolam, close clinical monitoring for respiratory depression and/or prolonged sedation and dosage adjustment should be considered.
Mirtazapine	May increase serum level of mirtazapine.	Applies to all PIs: use with caution. Consider an alternative antidepressant (i.e., SSRI: escitalopram, citalopram, sertraline, or fluoxetine).
Mycophenolate	Interaction unlikely.	Applies to all PIs and NNRTIs.

TIPRANAVIR *(cont.)*

Drug	Effect of Interaction	Recommendations/Comments
Nefazodone	May increase serum level of nefazodone.	Applies to all PIs: use with caution. Consider alternative antidepressant (i.e., SSRI: escitalopram, citalopram, sertraline, or fluoxetine).
Nelfinavir (NFV)	NFV active metabolites may be decreased.	No data; avoid coadministration.
Nevirapine (NVP)	NVP AUC not significantly decreased. TPV PK not reported.	Consider standard dose.
Nifedipine	May increase serum level of nifedipine.	Applies to all PIs: data limited to an interaction study conducted with ATV and diltiazem that resulted in doubling of diltiazem serum level, which led to PR interval prolongation. All PIs have potential of prolonging PR interval with calcium channel blocker coadministration.
Nisoldipine	May increase serum level of nisoldipine.	Applies to all PIs: Data limited to an interaction study conducted with ATV and diltiazem that resulted in doubling of diltiazem serum levels, which led to PR interval prolongation. All PIs and have potential of prolonging PR interval with calcium channel blocker coadministration.
NSAIDs	May increase risk of bleeding.	Avoid coadministration or use with caution.
Omeprazole	Omeprazole concentrations may be decreased at steady state. No change in TPV concentrations.	Clinical significance unknown. Titrate omeprazole dose to therapeutic effect.
Paclitaxel	May increase paclitaxel serum level.	Applies to all PIs: since all PIs have potential of significantly increasing paclitaxel serum level; close monitoring of paclitaxel-induced toxicity recommended.
Phencyclidine (PCP)	May significantly increase serum level of PCP.	Applies to all PIs: avoid all illicit drug use with PIs.
Phenobarbital	May decrease serum level of PIs and NNRTIs. PIs and NNRTIs may increase or decrease phenobarbital serum levels.	Applies to all PIs and NNRTIs: consider alternative anticonvulsants (i.e., valproic acid, lamotrigine, levetiracetam, or topiramate). With coadministration, monitor anticonvulsant levels and consider TDM of PIs and NNRTIs.

Drug	Effect of Interaction	Recommendations/Comments
Phenytoin	May decrease serum level of PIs and NNRTIs. PIs and NNRTIs may increase or decrease phenytoin serum level.	Applies to all PIs and NNRTIs: consider alternative anticonvulsants (i.e., valproic acid, lamotrigine, levetiracetam, or topiramate). With coadministration, monitor anticonvulsant levels and consider TDM of PIs and NNRTIs.
Pimozide	May significantly increase pimozide serum level.	Contraindicated.
Propafenone	May increase antiarrhythmic serum levels.	Contraindicated.
Quinidine	May increase antiarrhythmic serum levels.	Contraindicated.
Raltegravir (RAL)	TPV/r decreased RAL Cmin by 55%, but did not affect AUC.	Not clinically significant in a small subset of patients receiving TPV/r plus RAL. Use standard dose. 3 cases of hepatic cytolysis reported in patients switched from RAL + ENF to RAL + TPV/r: monitor transaminases.
Ranolazine	May increase ranolazine serum concentrations and risk of QTc prolongation.	Contraindicated.
Rifabutin (RFB)	RFB AUC increased 190%. No change in TPV levels.	Dose RFB 150 mg every other day with TPV/r coadministration.
Rifampin	May significantly decrease serum level of TPV.	Contraindicated. Consider use with RFB.
Rifapentine	TPV serum levels may be significantly decreased.	Avoid coadministration. Consider using RFB.
Rosuvastatin	Rosuvastatin AUC increased 37%.	With coadministration, start with rosuvastatin 5 mg and titrate slowly.
Salmeterol	May increase salmeterol serum concentrations.	Avoid coadministration. Consider formoterol.
Saquinavir (SQV)	SQV AUC decreased 76%.	Do not coadminister.
Sildenafil	May increase sildenafil serum level.	Applies to all PIs: use with close monitoring. Do not exceed 25 mg in a 48-hr period.
Simvastatin	May significantly increase simvastatin serum concentrations.	Contraindicated. Consider pravastatin, atorvastatin (start with 10 mg), or rosuvastatin (start with 5 mg).
Sirolimus	May significantly increase or decrease serum level of sirolimus.	Applies to all PIs: dose sirolimus based on serum level.
St. John's wort	May decrease TPV serum concentrations.	Contraindicated.

TIPRANAVIR *(cont.)*

Drug	Effect of Interaction	Recommendations/Comments
Tacrolimus	May significantly increase or decrease serum level of tacrolimus.	Applies to All PIs: dose tacrolimus based on serum level.
Tadalafil	May increase serum level of tadalafil.	Applies to all PIs: start with 5 mg. Do not exceed 10 mg in 72 hrs. Consider sildenafil due to more clinical data and shorter half-life allowing for easier titration.
Tamoxifen	May increase serum level of tamoxifen.	Applies to all PIs: no data. Close monitoring for tamoxifen-induced toxicity recommended.
Teniposide	May increase serum level of teniposide.	Applies to all PIs: no data. Close monitoring of teniposide-induced toxicity recommended.
Tenofovir (TDF)	17% decrease in TPV AUC at the 500/100 mg dose and an 11% decrease in TPV AUC with 750/200 mg.	Unlikely to be significant. Use standard dose.
Terfenadine	May significantly increase terfenadine serum level.	Contraindicated.
Tetrahydrocan-nabinol (THC)	Based on data with NFV and IDV, interactions unlikely.	Applies to PIs and NNRTIs: interactions are unlikely.
Ticlopidine	May increase risk of bleeding?	Avoid coadministration or use with caution.
Trazodone	May increase serum level of trazodone.	Applies to all PIs: use with caution. Consider an alternative antidepressant (i.e., SSRI: escitalopram, citalopram, sertraline, or fluoxetine).
Triazolam	May significantly increase serum level of triazolam.	Contraindicated. Consider alternative benzodizepine (e.g., lorazepam, oxazepam, and temazepam).
Vardenafil	May significantly increase serum level of vardenafil.	Applies to all PIs: do not exceed vardenafil 2.5 mg in 72 hrs (with RTV) or 2.5 mg in 24 hrs (with other PIs). Consider sildenafil due to more clinical data and less pronounced interaction. Avoid coadministration with IDV.
Verapamil	May increase serum level of verapamil.	Applies to all PIs: data limited to an interaction study conducted with ATV and diltiazem that resulted in doubling of diltiazem serum level, which led to PR interval prolongation. All PIs have potential for prolonging PR interval with calcium channel blocker coadministration.

Drug	Effect of Interaction	Recommendations/Comments
Vinblastine	May increase serum level of vinblastine.	Applies to all PIs: no data. Close monitoring of vinblastine-induced toxicity recommended.
Vincristine	May increase serum level of vincristine.	Applies to all PIs: no data. Close monitoring of vincristine-induced toxicity recommended.
Voriconazole	May decrease Voriconazole AUC. Voriconazole may increase TPV AUC.	Significant interaction with EFV and RTV (400 mg twice daily) but not IDV; data with other PIs and NNRTIs not available and should be used with caution with close monitoring for therapeutic efficacy. Consider adding another antifungal for aspergillosis (i.e., *AmBisome* or caspofungin).
Warfarin	May increase risk of bleeding.	Use with caution, with close monitoring of INR.
Zidovudine (AZT)	AZT AUC decreased by approx. 42% with TPV/r 250/200 mg twice daily coadministration.	Clinical significance unknown. Intracellular AZT levels not measured.

DRUG-DRUG INTERACTION – VORICONAZOLE

Drug	Effect of Interaction	Recommendations/Comments
Alprazolam	Alprazolam serum concentrations may be increased.	Consider lorazepam, oxazepam, or temazepam.
Amlodipine	Amlodipine serum concentrations may be increased.	Monitor.
Astemizole	Risk of QTc prolongation may be increased.	Contraindicated.
Atazanavir (ATV)	Interaction unlikely with unboosted ATV. Voriconazole AUC may be decreased with ATV/r.	Consider voriconazole TDM (target Cmin >2.05 mcg/mL) with ATV /r coadministration.
Azithromycin	No significant interaction.	No dose adjustment necessary.
Carbamazepine	Voriconazole serum concentrations may be decreased.	Contraindicated.
Cimetidine	No significant interaction.	No dose adjustment necessary.
Cisapride	Risk of QTc prolongation may be increased.	Contraindicated.
Clopidogrel	May decrease the efficacy of clopidogrel.	Avoid coadministration.
Cyclosporine	Cyclosporine AUC increased by 70%.	Reduce cyclosporine dose by 50% with close TDM.

Voriconazole *(cont.)*

Drug	Effect of Interaction	Recommendations/Comments
Darunavir (DRV)	Voriconazole serum concentrations may be decreased.	Avoid coadministration. Consider voriconazole TDM (target Cmin >2.05 mcg/mL) with DRV/r coadministration.
Diazepam	Diazepam serum concentrations may be increased.	Consider lorazepam, oxazepam, or temazepam.
Digoxin	No significant interaction.	No dose adjustment necessary.
Diltiazem	Diltiazem serum concentrations may be increased.	Monitor.
Efavirenz (EFV)	EFV AUC increased by 44%. Voriconazole steady state serum levels decreased by 77%.	Avoid coadministration at standard doses. Voriconazole 400 mg twice daily plus EFV 300 mg qhs recommended with coadministration.
Ergot Alkaloids	Ergot alkaloid serum concentrations may be increased.	Contraindicated.
Erythromycin	No significant interaction.	No dose adjustment necessary.
Etravirine (ETR)	May increase voriconazole serum concentrations.	Consider voriconazole TDM (target Cmin >2.05 mcg/mL and Cmax <6 mcg/mL) with ETR coadministration.
Felodipine	Felodipine serum concentrations may be increased.	Monitor.
Fosamprenavir (FPV)	May decrease voriconazole serum concentrations.	Avoid coadministration. Consider voriconazole TDM (target Cmin >2.05 mcg/mL) with FPV /r coadministration.
Glimepiride	Glimepiride serum concentrations may be increased.	Monitor glucose closely with coadministration.
Glipizide	Glipizide serum concentrations may be increased.	Monitor glucose closely with coadministration.
Glyburide	Glyburide serum concentrations may be increased.	Monitor glucose closely with coadministration.
Indinavir (IDV)	No significant interaction with unboosted IDV.	No dose adjustment necessary with unboosted IDV. Consider voriconazole TDM with IDV/r coadministration.
Lopinavir/ritonavir (LPV/r)	Voriconazole serum concentrations may be decreased.	Avoid coadministration. Consider voriconazole TDM (target Cmin >2.05 mcg/mL) with LPV/r coadministration.
Lovastatin	Lovastatin serum concentrations may be increased.	Consider pravastatin, atorvastatin, or rosuvastatin.
Maraviroc (MVC)	May increase MVC serum concentrations.	No data; consider MVC 150 or 300 mg twice daily with coadministration.

Drug	Effect of Interaction	Recommendations/Comments
Methadone	R- methadone AUC increased by 47%.	Monitor for increased sedation. May need to dose adjust methadone with coadministration.
Methylprednisolone	No significant interaction.	No dose adjustment necessary.
Midazolam	Midazolam serum concentrations may be increased.	Consider lorazepam, oxazepam, or temazepam.
Mycophenolic Acid	No significant interaction.	No dose adjustment necessary.
Nevirapine (NVP)	Voriconazole serum concentrations may be decreased.	Consider voriconazole TDM (target Cmin >2.05 mcg/mL) with NVP coadministration.
Nifedipine	Nifedipine serum concentrations may be increased.	Monitor.
Nisoldipine	Nisoldipine serum concentrations may be increased.	Monitor.
Omeprazole	Omeprazole AUC increased by 400%.	Reduce omeprazole dose by 50%.
Pentobarbital	Voriconazole serum concentrations may be decreased.	Contraindicated.
Phenobarbital	Voriconazole serum concentrations may be decreased.	Contraindicated.
Phenytoin	Phenytoin AUC increased by 80%. Voriconazole AUC decreased by 70%.	Voriconazole 400 mg PO q12h or 5 mg/kg IV q12h.
Pimozide	Risk of QTc prolongation may be increased.	Contraindicated.
Quinidine	Risk of QTc prolongation may be increased.	Contraindicated.
Raltegravir (RAL)	Interaction unlikely.	Use standard dose.
Ranitidine	No significant interaction.	No dose adjustment necessary.
Ranolazine	May significantly increase ranolazine serum concentrations.	Avoid coadministration.
Rifabutin (RFB)	RFB serum concentrations may be increased. Voriconazole serum concentrations may be decreased.	Contraindicated.
Rifampin	Voriconazole serum concentrations may be decreased.	Contraindicated.

VORICONAZOLE *(cont.)*

Drug	Effect of Interaction	Recommendations/Comments
Ritonavir (RTV)	RTV 400 mg twice daily: voriconazole AUC decreased by 82%. RTV 100 mg twice daily: voriconazole AUC decreased by 39%.	Contraindicated with RTV 400 mg twice daily. With RTV 100 mg twice daily: avoid or use with close monitoring of voriconazole Cmin (target Cmin >2 mcg/mL).
Secobarbital	Voriconazole serum concentrations may be decreased.	Contraindicated.
Simvastatin	Simvastatin serum concentrations may be increased.	Consider pravastatin, atorvastatin, or rosuvastatin.
Sirolimus	Sirolimus serum concentrations may be increased.	Contraindicated. Use tacrolimus with close TDM.
Tacrolimus	Tacrolimus AUC increased by 300%.	Reduce tacrolimus dose to 1/3 of original dose with close TDM.
Terfenadine	Risk of QTc prolongation may be increased.	Contraindicated.
Tipranavir (TPV)	Voriconazole serum concentrations may be decreased.	Avoid coadministration. Consider voriconazole TDM (target Cmin >2.05 mcg/mL) with TPV/r coadministration.
Triazolam	Triazolam serum concentrations may be increased.	Consider lorazepam, oxazepam, or temazepam.
Verapamil	Verapamil serum concentrations may be increased.	Monitor.
Vinblastine	Vinblastine serum concentrations may be increased.	Monitor closely for ADR and consider dose adjustment.
Vincristine	Vincristine serum concentrations may be increased.	Monitor closely for ADR and consider dose adjustment.
Warfarin	Anticoagulation may be increased.	Monitor INR closely.

DRUG-DRUG INTERACTION – ZIDOVUDINE (AZT)

Drug	Effect of Interaction	Recommendations/Comments
Acetaminophen	Theoretical concern of competing hepatic metabolism (glucuronidation) that has not been demonstrated *in vivo*.	Not clinically significant. Intermittent use of acetaminophen is considered safe. Adverse effects not consistently reported.
Adriamycin	Possible additive bone marrow suppression.	With coadministration, monitor for bone marrow suppression (especially neutropenia).
Amphotericin B	Possible additive anemia.	With coadministration, monitor for anemia.

Drug	Effect of Interaction	Recommendations/Comments
Atazanavir (ATV)	AZT trough decreased 30%, but no change in AUC.	Clinical significance unknown. Use standard dose.
Atovaquone	AZT: AUC increased by 31%.	Clinical significance unknown. Use standard dose.
Buprenorphine	No change in AZT AUC.	No significant interaction. Use standard dose.
Clarithromycin	AZT: no significant change in AUC.	Not clinically significant. Use standard dose.
Dapsone	Possible additive anemia.	With coadministration, monitor for anemia.
Fluconazole	Slight increase in AZT half-life. No change in fluconazole PK.	Not clinically significant. Use standard dose.
Flucytosine	Possible additive bone marrow suppression.	With coadministration, monitor for bone marrow suppression, especially neutropenia.
Food	AZT AUC decreased by 57% with a liquid fat meal. Intracellular AZT triphosphate was not measured.	Clinical significance of fatty meal unknown. Administration AZT with food improves GI tolerance.
Ganciclovir	Additive bone marrow suppression.	Close monitoring of CBC recommended. Switch to alternative ART or use concomitant filgrastim if neutropenia is severe. *In vitro* antagonism; clinical significance unknown.
Hydroxyurea	Possible additive bone marrow suppression.	With coadministration, monitor for bone marrow suppression.
Interferon	Possible additive bone marrow suppression.	With coadministration, monitor for bone marrow suppression.
Methadone	AZT AUC increased 43%.	Clinical significance unknown, but monitor for AZT-associated ADR.
Probenecid	May increase AZT levels by inhibiting renal tubular secretion of AZT.	High incidence of probenecid rash with coadministration.
Pyrimethamine	Possible additive bone marrow suppression.	With coadministration, monitor for bone marrow suppression.
Ribavirin	*In vitro* antagonism but not *in vivo*.	Antagonism not observed *in vivo*, however, patients should be closely monitored for severe anemia.
Rifampin	AZT AUC decreased.	Clinical significance unknown; consider switching to RFB.
Saquinavir (d4T)	*In vitro* and *in vivo* antagonism.	Do not coadminister. Switch to an alternative NRTI.

Drug	Effect of Interaction	Recommendations/Comments
Sulfadiazine	Possible additive bone marrow suppression.	With coadministration, monitor for bone marrow suppression especially anemia.
Tipranavir (TPV)	AZT AUC decreased by approx. 42% with TPV/r 250/200 mg twice daily administration.	Clinical significance unknown. AZT intracellular triphosphate levels not measured.
Trimethoprim + Sulfamethoxazole (TMP + SMX)	Possible additive bone marrow suppression.	With coadministration, monitor for bone marrow suppression.
Valproic Acid	AZT serum concentrations increased 2-fold.	Clinical significance unknown, but monitor for AZT-associated ADR.
Vinca Alkaloids (vincristine, vinblastine)	Possible additive bone marrow suppression.	With coadministration, monitor for bone marrow suppression.

Index